D1129021

27 Alcohol Emergencies, 450

28 Toxicologic Emergencies, 456

29 Environmental Emergencies, 490

30 Genitourinary Emergencies, 511

31 Infectious Diseases, 527

32 Allergies and Hypersensitivity, 559

33 Facial, Ocular, ENT, and Dental Emergencies, 568

IV   TRAUMA, 597

34 Assessment of the Trauma Patient, 599

35 Head Trauma, 613

36 Spinal Cord and Neck Trauma, 637

37 Chest Trauma, 650

38 Abdominal Trauma, 678

39 Musculoskeletal Emergencies, 690

40 Facial, Ocular, ENT and Dental Trauma, 739

41 Burns, 762

42 Obstetric Trauma, 773

43 Pediatric Trauma, 779

44 Geriatric Trauma, 788

V   SPECIAL POPULATIONS, 797

45 Obstetric and Gynecologic Emergencies, 799

46 Pediatric Emergencies, 824

47 Abuse and Neglect, 857

48 Mental Health Emergencies, 871

49 Substance Abuse, 891

50 Intimate Partner Violence, 901

51 Sexual Assault, 907

SHEEHY'S MANUAL OF
EMERGENCY CARE

SHEEHY'S MANUAL OF
EMERGENCY CARE

SIXTH EDITION

Emergency Nurses Association
Des Plaines, Illinois

Edited by

Lorene Newberry, MS, RN, CEN
Clinical Nurse Specialist
Emergency Services
WellStar Health System
Marietta, Georgia

Laura M. Criddle, MS, RN, CCNS, CEN, CFRN, CNRN
Emergency and Trauma Clinical Nurse Specialist
Doctoral Student, Oregon Health and Science University
Portland, Oregon

With **310** illustrations

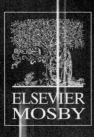

ELSEVIER
MOSBY

ELSEVIER
MOSBY

11830 Westline Industrial Drive
St. Louis, Missouri 63146

SHEEHY'S MANUAL OF EMERGENCY CARE
Copyright © 2005, Mosby Inc.

Notice

Previous editions copyrighted 1999, 1995, 1990, 1984, 1979

ISBN-13: 978-0-323-02799-1
ISBN-10: 0-323-02799-7

Executive Editor: Susan R. Epstein
Senior Developmental Editor: Robyn L. Brinks
Publishing Services Manager: John Rogers
Senior Project Manager: Beth Hayes
Design Manager: Bill Drone

Printed in the United States of America

Last digit is the print number: 9 8 7 6 5 4 3 2

To Robert
who has always championed my dreams.
And who could ask for more than that?

Contributors

Colleen Andreoni, APRN, BC, NP, CCNS, CEN
Nurse Practitioner
Dr. Susan Rife, Family Medicine
Orland Park, Illinois

Nancy M. Ballard, RN, MSN
Cardiovascular Outcomes Coordinator
WellStar Health System
Marietta, Georgia

Gwen Barnett, RN
Emergency Room Supervisor
Wellstar Kennestone Hospital
Atlanta, Georgia

Darcy T. Barrett, RN, MSN, CNRN
Clinical Nurse Specialist, Critical Care
WellStar Health System
Marietta, Georgia

Nancy M. Bonalumi, RN, MS, CEN
Director, Emergency Nursing
Children's Hospital of Philadelphia
Philadelphia, Pennsylvania

Elizabeth Burke, BA
Executive Director
Domestic Violence HELP
Pittsburgh, Pennsylvania

Patricia M. Campbell, RN, MSN, CCRN, ANP-CS
Adult Nurse Practitioner
Banner Good Samaritan Regional Medical Center
Phoenix, Arizona

Patricia L. Clutter, RN, MEd, CEN
Staff Nurse/Educator
Strafford, Missouri

Nancy J. Denke, RN, MSN, FNP-C, CCRN
CNS, Emergency Department
Banner Estrella Medical Center
Phoenix, Arizona

Kathy M. Dolan, RN, MS, CEN
Risk Management and Safety Coordinator
Mercy Medical Center
Cedar Rapids, Iowa

Gretta J. Edwards, RN, BS, CEN
Staff Nurse, Emergency Department
University of Colorado Hospital
Denver, Colorado

Faye P. Everson, RN, CEN, EMT-B
Professional Development
Jordan Hospital
Plymouth, Massachusetts

Clinical Coordinator for Paramedic Training
Emergency Medical Teaching Services, Inc.
Dennis, Massachusetts

John Fazio, MS, RN
Clinical Nurse Specialist
San Francisco General Hospital Medical Center
San Francisco, California

LCDR Andrew A. Galvin, APRN, BC, MSN, CEN
NMC Portsmouth Emergency Department
Portsmouth, Virginia

Tamara Gentry, RN, BSN
Staff Nurse, Emergency Center
WellStar Cobb Hospital
Marietta, Georgia

Nicki Gilboy, RN, MS, CEN
Nurse Educator, Emergency Department
Brigham & Women's Hospital
Boston, Massachusetts

Chris M. Gisness, RN, MSN, CEN, CS, FNP-C
Nurse Practitioner, Associate Provider
Emergency Care Center
Department of Emergency Medicine
Emory University, Grady Campus
Atlanta, Georgia

Donna S. Gloe, BSN, MSN, EdD, RN, BC
Senior Consultant, Genesis Project
Sisters of Mercy Health System
St. Louis, Missouri

Katy Hadduck, RN, BSN, CFRN
Flight Nurse/Business Development Coordinator
Mercy Air Services, Inc.
Simi Valley, California

Jeff Hamilton, RN, BA
Clinical Nurse, Emergency Department
St. John's Mercy Medical Center
St. Louis, Missouri

M. Lynn Herman, RN, MSN
Associate Professor
Floyd College School of Nursing
Rome, Georgia

Robert Herr, MD, MBA, FACEP
Attending Emergency Physician
Northwest Emergency Physicians (A TeamHealth Affiliate)
Mercer Island, Washington

Reneé Semonin Holleran, RN, PhD, CEN, CCRN, CFRN
Nurse Manager of Adult Transport Services
IHC Life Flight
Salt Lake City, Utah

Mary Jagim, RN, BSN, CEN
Emergency Center Nurse Manager
Merit Care Health System
Fargo, North Dakota

Anita Johnson, RN, BSN
Emergency Services
Wellstar Healthcare System
Marietta, Georgia

LCDR Jeffrey S. Johnson, NC, USN, RN, MSN, CEN
Bureau of Naval Personnel
Millington, Tennessee

Kimberly P. Johnson, RN, BSN
Registered Nurse, Emergency Department
University of Colorado Hospital
Denver, Colorado

Mara S. Kerr, RNC, MS
Patient Care Specialist, Women's Services
Legacy Health System
Portland, Oregon

Cheri Kommor, RN, CEN
Resource Nurse
Wellstar Kennestone Hospital Emergency Department
Marietta, Georgia

Louise LeBlanc, RN, BScN, ENC(c)
Patient Care Director Emergency/Urgent Care
The Scarborough Hospital
Scarborough, Ontario

Anne Marie E. Lewis, RN, BSN, BA, MA, CEN
ED Staff Nurse
Sturdy Memorial Hospital
Attleboro, Massachusetts

JEN Associate Editor
Emergency Nurses Association
Des Plaines, Illinois

Diana Lombardo, MSN-FNP, MHA, RN, CCRN
Family Nurse Practitioner
Urgent Care Southwest Medical Associates
Las Vegas, Nevada

Adjunct Faculty, Department of Nursing
Nevada State College
Henderson, Nevada

Dennis B. MacDougall, RN, MS, ACNPBC, CEN
Director, Emergency Department
Johns Hopkins Bayview Medical Center
Baltimore, Maryland

Donna L. Mason, RN, MS, CEN
Nurse Manager, Adult Emergency Services
Vanderbilt University Medical Center
Nashville, Tennessee

Kay McClain, RN, MSN, CEN, CNA
Nurse Director, Emergency and Walk-in
Mount Auburn Hospital
Cambridge, Massachusetts

Jule Blakeley Monnens, RN, MSN
Clinical Nurse RN
University of Colorado Hospital
Denver, Colorado

Jessie M. Moore, APRN-BC, MSN, CEN
Obesity Center Coordinator/Nurse Practitioner, Department of Surgery
Hospital of Saint Raphael
New Haven, Connecticut

Andrea Novak, MS, RN, CEN
Director of Nursing, Continuing Education
Southern Regional Area Health Education Center
Fayetteville, North Carolina

Lisa Murphy Pruner, MS, RN
Clinical Nurse Specialist
Wellstar Kennestone Hospital
Marietta, Georgia

Terri Roberts RN, BSN
Staff Nurse
Atlanta, Georgia

Susan Rolniak, RN, MSN, CRNP
Nurse Practitioner/Clinical Research Coordinator, Emergency Department
Mercy Hospital of Pittsburgh
Emergency Medicine Association of Pittsburgh
Pittsburgh, Pennsylvania

Anita Ruiz-Contreras, RN, MSN, CEN, MICN, SANE-A
Emergency Staff Developer
Santa Clara Valley Medical Center
Sexual Assault Nurse Examiner
Santa Clara County, California

Christopher Schmidt, APRN, BC, MSN, CEN, ENP, CDR, NC, USN
Clinical Nurse Specialist/Emergency Nurse Practitioner
Navy Nurse Corps Specialty Leader, Emergency Nursing
Naval Hospital
Jacksonville, Florida

Janice R. Sisco, RN, BSN
Assist Manager, Adult Emergency Services
Vanderbilt University Medical Center
Nashville, Tennessee

Jeff Solheim, RN, CEN
Manager, Emergency Services
Salem Hospital
Salem, Oregon

Previous Contributors

Joan Elaine Begg-Whitman, RN, CEN

Judith Boehm, RN, MSN

Anne Phelan Bowen, MS, RN

Suzanne L. Brown, RN, BSN, CEN, SANE

Peggy Cass, EMT-Paramedic, MEd

Jorda Chapin, RN, CEN

Donna E. Chase, RN, BS

Debra DeLorenzo, RN, BS

Jane deMoll, RN, CEN

Christine DiGeronimo, RN, BSN, CURN

Mary Dahlgren Gunnels, RN, MS, CHES, CEN

Deborah C. Harcke, RN, BSN, CEN

Lisa Schneck Hegel, RN, BS, CEN

Deborah Parkman Henderson, PhD, RN

Stephen H. Johnson, MD

Linda J. Kobokovich, RNC, MSCN

Diane Panton Lapsley, RN, MS, CS

Genell Lee, RN, MSN, JD

Judith E. Lombardi, RN, MSN, ENP, CEN

Kelly F. Malmquist, RN, BSN

Anne P. Manton, RN, PhD, CEN

Benjamin E. Marett, RN, MSN, CEN, COHN-S

Lisa B. McCabe, MS, CCRN, ARNP

Margaret McCarthy-Mogan, MS, RN, CEN

Brenda M. Moore, RN, CEN

Ingrid B. Mroz, MS, CCRN, ARNP

Delberta Murphy, RN, BS, CEN

Marybeth Murphy, MS, RN

Carla Obar, RN, CSPI

Suzanne O'Connor, MSN, CS

Sandra Thomas Ouellette, RN, CPTC

Tracy Pike-Amato, RN, BSN, CEN

Gail E. Polli, RN, MS, CS

Maureen Quigley, RN, BSN, CEN

Carol Rittenhouse, RN, CCRN

Kathy Sciabica Robinson, RN, CEN, EMT-P

Jaye M. Sengewald, RN, MSN, CDE

Peggy Shedd, MSN, RN, CS

Daun Smith, RN, MS

Patricia M. Speck, MSN, RN, CS, FNP

Susan F. Strauss, RN, CEN, CCRN

Janet L. Sudekum, RN, BSN, CCRN

Geoffrey Tarbox, RN, MS

Barbara A. Tilden, RNC, BSN

Lori Tucker, RN, CEN

Anne Cassels Turner, RN, BA

Deborah Upton, RN, BSN, CEN

Kathleen Waine, RN, CEN

Mary E. Wood, RN, MS, CDE

Andrea B. Wyle, RN, ONC

Mary Young, RN, MSN

Polly Gerber Zimmerman, RN, MS, MBA, CEN

Reviewers

Cynthia J. Abel, RN, MSN, CEN
Value Analysis Program Director
University HealthSystem Consortium
Oak Brook, Illinois

Susan A. Barnason, PhD, RN
Associate Professor
University of Nebraska Medical Center
Lincoln, Nebraska

Karen Delrue, RN, MSN, CEN
*Clinical Nurse Specialist, Emergency and
   Trauma Services*
Spectrum Health
Grand Rapids, Michigan

Mary Martha Hall, RN, MSN, FNP, CEN
Nurse Practitioner
Houston, Texas

Steven A. Weinman, RN, BSN, CEN, EMT
Instructor, Emergency and Trauma Care
New York Presbyterian Hospital,
Cornell Medical Center
New York, New York

Mary Ellen Wilson, RN, MS, FNP, CEN
Nurse Manager, Emergency Department
Cherry Point Naval Hospital
PhyAmerica Government Services
Havelock, North Carolina

Preface

Sheehy's *Manual of Emergency Care* provides complete coverage of the fundamental principles of emergency care, including basic and advanced life support, intravenous therapy, medical emergencies, traumatic injuries, and emergency care of special populations. Each condition described includes a detailed discussion of signs and symptoms, diagnoses and diagnostic testing, treatments and other interventions, age and developmental considerations, as well as information for patient and family education.

Developed in conjunction with the Emergency Nurses Association, this sixth edition features contributions by expert emergency personnel from across the country. Thirteen new chapters address areas of concern for today's emergency nurses. This compact volume contains up-to-date, practical, and portable information for clinical practitioners and nursing students.

Thirteen new chapters cover Communication in the Emergency Department, Cultural Diversity, Intrafacility and Interfacility Patient Transport, Emergency Operations Preparedness, Triage, Patient Assessment, Weapons of Mass Destruction, Pain Management, End of Life Issues for the Emergency Nurse, Complementary and Alternative Therapies, Airway Emergencies, Elder Trauma, and Substance Abuse Emergencies.

Acknowledgments

A work of this magnitude is never born without the contribution of many dedicated individuals. A debt of gratitude is owed to those who patiently endured though the bumps in the road to publication; the deadlines were short and the waits seemed endless. The authors shared their words and experience, the reviewers lent us their expertise, and the editorial and production staff at Elsevier contributed their determination to see this through.

Special thanks to Donna Massey and the Emergency Nurses Association for their support and faith in me and to Elsevier's Robyn Brinks who both held my hand and kicked my butt throughout this project.

And to Lorene Newberry, prolific writer and editor, thank you. Your words and works have enlightened thousands of emergency nurses over the years. Lorene conceptualized and launched this project and then passed on the torch, leaving big shoes to fill and a tough act to follow.

Detailed Contents

I BASICS OF EMERGENCY CARE, 1

1 Communications in the Emergency
Department, 3
Mary Jagim

2 Diversity, 14
Anita Ruiz-Contreras

3 Basic Legal Issues for Emergency Nurses, 21
Kimberly P. Johnson

4 Intrafacility and Interfacility Patient
Transport, 31
Katy Hadduck

5 Emergency Preparedness: Managing Mass
Casualty Incidents, 44
Jeff Hamilton

II CLINICAL BASICS, 59

6 Triage, 61
Nicki Gilboy

7 Patient Assessment, 82
Diana Lombardo

8 Intravenous Therapy, 99
Jessie M. Moore

9 Laboratory Specimens, 123
Nancy M. Bonalumi

10 Rhythm Recognition and Electrocardiogram
Interpretation, 137
Nancy M. Ballard

11 Hemodynamic Monitoring, 174
Darcy T. Barrett

12 Wound Management, 195
Robert Herr

13 Weapons of Mass Destruction, 214
Jeff Hamilton

14 Pain Management, 228
Anita Johnson

15 End-of-Life Issues for Emergency
Nurses, 245
Kay McClain

16 Organ and Tissue Donation, 254
Diana Lombardo

17 Complementary and Alternative
Therapies, 261
Reneé Semonin Holleran

III MEDICAL EMERGENCIES, 275

18 Cardiopulmonary Arrest, 277
Donna S. Gloe

19 Airway Management, 294
Gretta J. Edwards

20 Respiratory Emergencies, 307
Gretta J. Edwards

21 Cardiac Emergencies, 326
Donna S. Gloe

22 Shock, 357
Cheri Kommor

23 Neurologic Emergencies, 374
Kathy M. Dolan

24 Abdominal Pain, 389
Anita Johnson, Terri Roberts

25 Hematologic and Immunologic
Emergencies, 408
Christopher E. Schmidt, Jeffrey S. Johnson

26 Metabolic Emergencies, 424
Lisa M. Pruner

27 Alcohol Emergencies, 450
Gwen Barnett

28 Toxicologic Emergencies, 456
Tammy Gentry

29 Environmental Emergencies, 490
Nancy J. Denke

30 Genitourinary Emergencies, 511
Louise LeBlanc

31 Infectious Diseases, 527
Patricia M. Campbell

32 Allergies and Hypersensitivity, 559
Faye P. Everson

33 Facial, Ocular, ENT, and Dental
Emergencies, 568
Anne Marie E. Lewis

IV TRAUMA, 597

34 Assessment of the Trauma Patient, 599
Andrew A. Galvin

35 Head Trauma, 613
Laura M. Criddle

36 Spinal Cord and Neck Trauma, 637
John Fazio

37 Chest Trauma, 650
Christopher Schmidt

38 Abdominal Trauma, 678
Dennis B. MacDougall

39 Musculoskeletal Emergencies, 690
Chris M. Gisness

40 Facial, Ocular, ENT, and Dental Trauma, 739
Anne Marie E. Lewis

41 Burns, 762
Janice R. Sisco

42 Obstetric Trauma, 773
Mara S. Kerr

43 Pediatric Trauma, 779
Jeff Solheim

44 Geriatric Trauma, 788
Andrea Novak

V SPECIAL POPULATIONS, 797

45 Obstetric and Gynecologic
Emergencies, 799
M. Lynn Herman

46 Pediatric Emergencies, 824
Colleen Andreoni

47 Abuse and Neglect, 857
Patricia L. Clutter

48 Mental Health Emergencies, 871
Jule Blakeley Monnens

49 Substance Abuse, 891
Donna Mason

50 Intimate Partner Violence, 901
Susan Rolniak, Elizabeth Burke

51 Sexual Assault, 907
Anita Johnson

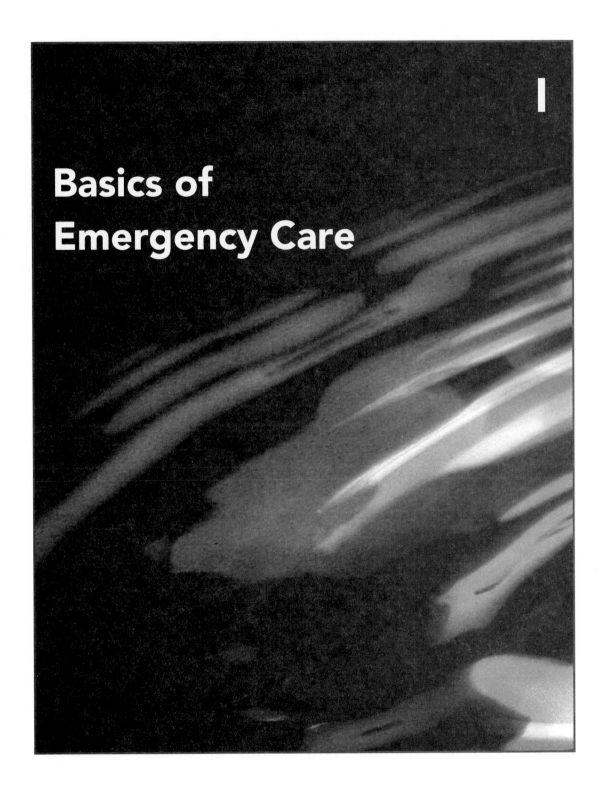

Basics of Emergency Care

1 Communications in the Emergency Department

Mary Jagim, RN, BSN, CEN

Communication is pivotal to successful emergency department (ED) operations. Obtaining information, planning and implementing care, coordinating patient flow, and maximizing teamwork hinge on communication between individuals, disciplines, and departments. The rapid pace, high patient volume, and critical situations that define the ED demand effective communication at all levels.

Poor communication is one of the most common patient complaints in the ED. Specific concerns include lack of information about wait times, diagnostic studies, test results, medications, diagnoses, home care instructions, and admission plans. Frustration increases when patients are asked the same questions repeatedly at triage, by ED nurses and doctors, and again by their admitting physician. Similar frustrations develop among ED staff members when essential patient information is not communicated between shifts and hospital departments. Effective communication requires education, self-awareness, defined yet fluid systems, and commitment from all those involved. Table 1-1 summarizes concepts that can be used to facilitate communication with patients and colleagues to create a positive environment for all. This chapter addresses communication issues specific to the ED, including communication between individuals, between departments, with emergency medical services personnel, and during critical situations.

CRISIS COMMUNICATION

Emergency departments frequently operate in crisis mode. The need to communicate when every room is occupied, the hallways are full, and ambulances are still arriving is a challenge nurses face daily in EDs across the country. During times of tension, it is essential that communication with all those involved be clear, direct, and honest. Patients, families, and staff

Table 1-1   **Key Concepts for Successful Communication With Patients and Colleagues**

Concept	Discussion
Assertiveness	Assertiveness is the ability to express ideas and thoughts in a respectful manner, without undue anxiety about how they will be received by others. Assertiveness is demonstrated by being positive, direct, honest, and genuine and by maintaining eye contact and giving the same message verbally and nonverbally.[1]
Responsibility	Personal and professional responsibility is manifested by a willingness to take action, admit errors, and seek solutions.[1]
Caring	Caring involves a patient approach that takes into account the whole person and responds to individual needs. Caring is situation specific and entails taking time to do "extra" things for someone such as providing a warm blanket, offering a drink, contacting a friend, or taking a moment to listen.[1]
Warmth	Warmth is displayed primarily in nonverbal ways: through facial expressions and eye contact, use of caring, and positive words spoken in soft tones.[2]
Respect	Respect is demonstrated through acceptance of another person's thoughts, feelings, and actions. Respect can be displayed by maintaining eye contact, addressing the person in his or her preferred manner, making physical contact with a handshake or gentle touch. Respect also involves maintaining information confidentiality.[3]
Genuineness	Geniuneness is responding in a way that is real and congruent (verbal and nonverbal behaviors match). This conveys genuineness to others and builds trust.[4]
Empathy	Empathy is insight into how others feel and what makes them feel that way. Empathy is a sense of understanding and acceptance of individuals without judgment or questioning.[5]
Specificity	Specificity in communication prevents frustrations and clarifies misinterpretations by both parties.[6]
Humor	Used in a positive manner, humor promotes relaxation and puts others at ease. Humor can help convey the fact that we all choose our attitudes and approaches to situations.[7]

may respond to stressful incidents with fear, anger, panic, guilt, or denial. Using tools that facilitate transmission of critical information is one way to decrease anxiety and confusion. Table 1-2 offers suggestions on how to minimize panic in the ED.

Communicating Through Patient Representatives

During peak hours in the ED, patient representatives (also called patient advocates or customer service representatives) can serve as liaisons between patients, families, and staff by answering questions, providing information about estimated wait times, supplying resource materials, and greeting patients. Their support can prove invaluable in assisting patients and families who are anxious, angry, or in need of additional aid.[8,9] The presence of patient representatives demonstrates the commitment of an organization to a caring, person-focused environment.

Written Communication

The standards of emergency nursing care, as outlined in the Emergency Nurses Association's *Standards of Emergency Nursing Practice,* include assessment, diagnosis, outcome identification, planning, implementation, evaluation, and triage.[10] Each step in this process involves communication and collaboration with patients, families, and colleagues. Documentation of the nursing process is required to provide a factual record of the patient's condition,

Table 1-2   **Crisis Communications in the Emergency Department**

Principle	*Benefit*	*Potential Emergency Department Application*
Legitimize the fear or guilt.	Acknowledge and accept fear or guilt expressed by emergency department staff, patients, or family members.	A novice emergency department nurse who sees a cardiac arrest, major trauma, pediatric death, or child abuse victim for the first time. A child accidentally injured by a parent.
Do not provide excessive reassurance.	Being honest, clear, and direct gives the person a realistic view of the situation.	Speaking to family members of a patient with a lethal brain injury.
Provide action opportunities.	Persons frequently feel useless in crisis situations. Efficacy is a powerful antidote to denial.	Assignment of a novice nurse to a specific task during a cardiac arrest situation. Asking volunteers to provide blankets to victims of a house fire.
Focus on those who most need help and protection.	Maximize resources by prioritizing and directing actions to areas of greatest need.	Instigation of triage principles. Providing verbal and nonverbal support when an individual is feeling victimized.
Be candid.	Gentle candor provides realistic information without increasing anxiety and stress.[9]	Explaining long treatment delays to patients and families in the waiting room.

care rendered, and responses to interventions. Essential documentation elements include the following:

- Subjective information gathered from patients, family members, emergency medical services providers, or bystanders
- Assessment findings, including vital signs
- Interventions and patient responses to interventions
- Patient and family education information, including any verbal instructions, handouts, or demonstrations/return demonstrations[11]

Communication Standards

The Joint Commission on Accreditation of Healthcare Organizations (JCAHO) standards do not identify specific patient care documentation requirements. However, the 2004 prepublication standards regarding patient care describe hospital requirements related to the provision of care, treatment, and services to patients, including a list of four core processes. These core processes are assessing patient needs; planning care, treatment, and services; providing the care, treatment, and services the patient needs; and coordinating care, treatment, and services.[12] Box 1-1 reviews documentation expectations related to these processes.

Communicating Patient Identification

Accurate patient identification is an essential first step in safe patient care. The 2003 JCAHO National Patient Safety Goals[13] focus on the need to improve the process of patient identification. All hospital staff members should use at least two patient identifiers when performing diagnostic tests or administering medications. Suggested identifiers are a patient's first and last names, birth date, and medical record number. Ideally this information will be

Box **1-1** Documentation Expectations Related to JCAHO Core Processes

General Activities Related to Core Elements

Providing access to appropriate levels of care and disciplines for patients
Providing interventions based on the plan for care, treatment, and services
Teaching patients what they need to know about their care, treatment, and services
Coordinating care, treatment, and services, if needed, when the patient is referred, transferred, or discharged[3]

Documentation Components Related to Core Elements

Initial assessments as defined by the organization; reassessment as needed; physical assessment as appropriate; psychological and social assessment as appropriate
Symptoms associated with a disease, condition, and treatment
Nutritional status, when warranted by patient condition
Functional assessment, when warranted by condition
Pain assessment and treatment provided
Diagnostic testing, including laboratory and radiologic studies
Physical, developmental, visual, communication, behavioral, and emotional disorders
Alcohol and substance abuse assessments, as needed
Medication administration
Education and training specific to patient needs
Screening for victims of abuse; focused screening of those identified as potential victims
Conscious sedation: preassessment and monitoring during the procedure to include heart rate, respiratory status, and oxygen saturation
Interdisciplinary and collaborative care rendered
Restraint/seclusion (See Box 1-2 for specific requirements for restraint/seclusion.)[12]

From the Joint Commission on Accreditation of Hospitals: *2004 patient care standards pre-publication edition.* Retrieved September 5, 2003, from www.jcaho.org/accredited+organizations/hospitals/index.htm.

Box **1-2** JCAHO Requirements for Documentation of Restraint and/or Seclusion

Decision to restrain/seclude patients must be based on the patient's condition at the time.
Alternative therapies attempted before restraint must be documented.
Explanations to patient and family must be documented.
Less restrictive approaches must be attempted first.
The least restrictive device should be used first.
A physician's order must have the date and time and must indicate the type of restraint and purpose for the restraint and must specify a time limit within established guidelines. As-needed orders or restraint/seclude for the duration of the emergency department visit are not acceptable.
The first hour of restraint requires continuous face-to-face observation.
Assessment of the patient must occur at specified intervals; for example, every 15 minutes while in seclusion or nondisposable restraints.
The patient must be offered food, toileting, and hydration every 2 hours while awake.
The patient's condition and response to treatment must be documented.
Condition of the patient's limb before restraint must be documented.
Condition of the patient's skin in the area of the restraints must be documented.
Restraint must be loosened at regular intervals.
The patient's position should be documented.

From the Joint Commission on Accreditation of Healthcare Organizations: *2003 national patient safety goals.* Retrieved September 5, 2003, from www.jcaho.org/accredited+organizations/patient+safety/npsg/npsg_03.htm.

located on the patient identification band. If possible, the staff member should ask the patient (or family member) to state the patient's first name, last name, and birth date before any intervention.

When an unresponsive patient arrives without identification, most EDs use some type of generic name such as "John/Jane Doe" or Greek alphabet names such as "Alpha/Beta," place a temporary name band, and assign a patient number that can be merged later with the correct name once the patient is identified. This allows emergent tests to proceed before formal registration.

Communicating Confidentially

Protection of health-related patient information is an important aspect of emergency care. Rules issued by the U.S. Department of Health and Human Services to implement the Health Insurance Portability and Accountability Act (HIPPA) of 1996 govern communications regarding health information. Emergency department staff must be familiar with these rules and adhere to hospital policies regarding communication of patient information. Protected health information may be used by the hospital for treatment, payment, and health care operations activities without consent of the patient. Treatment is defined as the provision, coordination, or management of health care and related services including consultation between providers regarding a patient and referral of a patient by one provider to another.[14]

In daily ED operations protection of a patient's personal information is important. Protection includes minimizing the release of any patient information in public or uncontrolled settings such as the ED lobby, triage area, nurses' station, or in less-than-private treatment areas. Physical safeguards should be used to provide visual and sound barriers, and conversations with patients must be conducted in a voice that is no louder than necessary for the patient to hear. Communicate only with patients or their authorized representatives. After obtaining patient consent, information may be shared with family members or close friends. Systems should be in place to alert staff if the patient does not wish any information to be shared. See Chapter 3 for additional discussion of Health Insurance Portability and Accountability Act regulations.

Communicating With Mass Media Representatives

Whether the case is a high profile homicide, an outbreak of West Nile virus, or a routine motor vehicle crash, ED staff may encounter members of the media. Reporters can be an important avenue for conveying information to the public regarding health risks and health promotion facts. Most hospitals have policies related to media relations; check with your specific facility for details. When a media representative contacts your ED to inquire about a patient, it is important to be aware of rules that regulate the use and release of patient data. If a direct inquiry is made using the patient's name, facilities can release information only about the patient's general condition unless they have specific authorization from the patient or the patient's representative. The American Hospital Association[15] recommends using a standardized list of brief patient condition descriptions (Table 1-3). States and hospitals may impose stricter guidelines.

Communicating Critical Patient Reports

Critical laboratory values or radiology results fall into two categories: those reported while the patient is still in the ED and those received after the patient has been discharged or transferred. How these reports are communicated varies with the mechanisms and technologies available within a specific ED. Regardless of the process, all critical reports must be tracked to

Table 1-3   American Hospital Association Guidelines for Reporting the Patient's Condition

Condition	Description
Undetermined	Patient is awaiting physician assessment and/or assessment.
Good	Vital signs are stable and within normal limits. Patient is conscious and comfortable. Indicators are excellent.
Fair	Vital signs are stable and within normal limits. Patient is conscious but may be uncomfortable. Indicators are favorable.
Serious	Vital signs may be unstable and not within normal limits. Patient is acutely ill. Indicators are questionable.
Critical	Vital signs are unstable and not within normal limits. Patient may be unconscious. Indicators are unfavorable.

From American Hospital Association: *HIPAA privacy regulations: overview.* Retrieved September 13, 2003, from www.whprms.org/HIPAA%20info/HIPAA%20Overview.PDF.

ensure that none are missed. Policies and procedures should clearly outline accountability for follow-up and documentation.

Critical results reported while the patient is still in the ED may be called to the patient's nurse or physician or to the shift charge nurse. Each institution will have guidelines concerning which laboratory values are consider critical and warrant a call to the ED. These values should include serious or life-threatening abnormalities of electrolytes, blood gases, and cardiac markers. Figure 1-1 gives an example of one process used to manage critical values called to the ED.

Cultures and final radiology reports (those that differ from preliminary readings) received after the patient is discharged may be reported electronically or verbally. Culture reports should be reviewed along with the medical record to determine whether the discharge plan requires revision. If no change in treatment is necessary, the patient may or may not need to be informed. If additional treatment is indicated, processes should be in place to ensure that the patient is notified. In a busy ED, this important communication can be overlooked easily.

Patients generally are contacted by telephone to communicate laboratory or radiology report information. When calling a patient, the emergency care provider first should ensure correct patient identification by asking the patient to state his or her first name, last name, and date of birth. Documentation of patient contact, and the information provided, should be placed in the medical record. Unsuccessful attempts to notify the patient also should be documented. If the patient cannot be reached by phone, a registered letter should be sent to the patient, along with a copy of the laboratory or radiology report.[16] Figure 1-2 illustrates a sample form used to track laboratory culture reports.

COMMUNICATING WITH EMERGENCY MEDICAL SERVICES PERSONNEL

Emergency medical services reports regarding incoming patient information may occur via radio, telephone, or through computer transmission. Local practice protocols and state regulations dictate what information is provided in a prehospital report. Priority patient information should be given first, and if time allows, further details may be added. Table 1-4 identifies the typical priority of information for these communications. The use of signals and

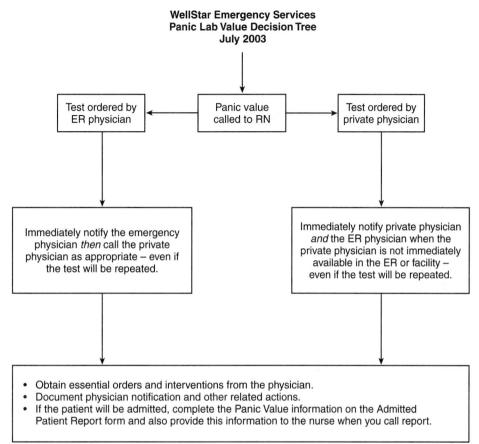

Figure 1-1. Process for managing critical laboratory values called to the emergency department. (Used with permission of WellStar Health System.)

abbreviations is guided by provider protocols and regulatory agencies. Emergency medical services reports may be audiotaped for later review and discussion. A written summary sheet, containing report information, usually is completed as well. This document may be reviewed and discarded after a specific period of time or may be placed in the medical record.

COMMUNICATION WITH INPATIENT UNITS

When ED patients are admitted to an inpatient unit, a report must be provided to the nurse who will be assuming patient care. This traditionally is done by telephone, but many EDs now rely on faxed or written reports.

Faxed Report

Once the decision has been made to admit a patient, the ED nurse completes a report form. When a bed number is assigned, this document is transmitted to the floor, and a phone call

Patient Label	Preliminary Results:	Source:
		Diagnosis:
		Medication treatment
		Admit: Wt:
Provider:	Date/Time Patient Contacted: RN	

Figure 1-2. Sample form used to track laboratory culture reports.

Table 1-4   **Guidelines for Emergency Medical Services Communications**

Priority	Specifics
Priority information	Unit's name or call sign
	Emergency medical services provider identification
	Patient age and gender
	Level of consciousness using the AVPU mnemonic (see Chapter 34, Box 34-3.)
	Chief complaint
	Mechanism of injury
	Destination
	Estimated time of arrival
Important information	Respiratory status
	Level of distress
	Skin color and condition
	Vital signs
Significant information	Scene description, if pertinent
	History of present illness
	Medications taken by patient
	Pertinent technical findings: pulse oximetry, glucometer, electrocardiogram
	Head and neck assessment
	Glasgow Coma Scale score or trauma score
Additional information as time allows	Further neurologic assessment, as appropriate
	Abdominal assessment, pelvic stability
	Extremity assessment
	Allergies
	Field treatment provided and response to treatment

From ASTM F2076-01 "Standard Practice for Communicating an EMS Patient Report to Receiving Medical Facilities." ASTM International. For referenced ASTM Standards, visit the ASTM website, ww.astm.org, or contact ASTM Customer Service at service@astm.org. For Annual Book of ASTM Standards volume information, refer to the standard's Document Summary page on the ASTM website.

is made to ensure its receipt. About 30 minutes later, the patient is transferred. Most facilities still require a verbal report before intensive care unit admission.[18] This system reduces delays and provides consistent and complete reporting. The faxed form may or may not become a permanent part of the patient's medical record.

Written Report

After receiving notification that an inpatient bed is ready, the emergency nurse completes a written report (Figure 1-3) and transports the patient to the floor. The patient and written report form are left with the receiving nurse. A contact name and phone number are included on the report in case there are questions. Written report forms also can serve as a guide for novice emergency nurses learning to give an effective verbal report.

USING TECHNOLOGY TO AID COMMUNICATION

Technologic advances are rapidly changing the face of emergency care communications. From computerized patient tracking and documentation programs to radiographic image retrieval systems, information technology is revolutionizing the way the ED functions. These advances are not yet universal but are increasingly present in EDs across the country. Future technology is expected to integrate patient information further, enhance productivity, eliminate waste, provide rapid references, support patient safety efforts, improve quality of care, and enhance overall job satisfaction.[19]

An ideal automated system would include point-of-care devices such as handheld computers or mobile terminals with voice recognition capability and easy interface with patient care equipment such as monitors, ventilators, and intravenous pumps. Other possible features include the following[19]:

- Online consolidated patient summaries that display current patient status information; for example, diagnostic reports, vital signs, cardiac rhythms, and assessment information
- Computerized provider order entry with imbedded real-time clinical decision support and automated order communication to all departments
- Online work lists and medication administration records that allow the nurse to indicate patient care activities completed and then automatically display the appropriate tool for data entry
- Automatic reminders for scheduled tasks that are overdue
- Real-time alerts that prompt providers—through online flags or paging—to review newly entered orders and patient data and that communicate the level of urgency associated with that data
- Online current reference material related to drug information and clinical practice guidelines
- Automatic referrals to other disciplines based on the data entered
- Intelligent, rule-driven admission assessments and other charting tools that copy/forward pertinent and appropriate patient information (such as medications, allergies, and vital signs) while allowing for validation and modification
- Easy documentation of abnormal and "within normal limits" assessment findings.

Communication is the key to quality, safe, efficient patient care. The time, effort, financial, and educational resources spent enhancing communication systems not only will improve patient care and patients' emergency care experience but also will enhance the job satisfaction of emergency care providers.

WellStar Health System
Emergency Services REPORT Form

Patient Sticker

From: ☐ ER ☐ CA ☐CER   To: _____
(Transferring Unit)   (Receiving Unit)
☐ Verbal Report Summary   ☐ **Written Report**

Date	Time	Attempts @ Verbal: First call _____ Second call _____
Diagnosis		
Pertinent Historical Information	☐Non-English Speaking ☐Blind ☐Hearing Impaired ☐Isolation ☐DNR	
	☐Diabetic ☐Seizures ☐Prisoner	
Mental Status	☐Alert ☐Confused ☐Unresponsive ☐Other	☐Ambulatory w/o assistance ☐Ambulatory with assistance
Respiratory Status	☐Normal ☐Shallow ☐Labored ☐Irregular **Other:**	
Oxygen	LPM _____ ☐NC ☐NRM ☐Venturi Mask Other:	

Pain Scale @ report	0	1	2	3	4	5	6	7	8	9	10

Vital Signs ≤ 1 hr before report	BP		T	P	R	SaO$_2$

Abnormal Lab and Diagnostic Data	
Pending Lab and Diagnostic Tests	Next BBG due @ Other:
IV Access	☐INT ☐IVF Amount in bag @ report
IV Infusions	☐Heparin drip ☐Nitroglycerin ☐Dopamine Other
Time Hung/Rate➔	

Medications	☐Hospital Medications/IVF with patient ☐Home Medications with patient
	Medications due in next two (2) hours:
	PRN Medications in last 4 hours
Bowel/Bladder/Drains	☐Foley ☐NGT ☐Suction Other
Diet	☐NPO ☐Regular Other:
I & O (if applicable)	Intake Output ☐Since arrival ☐Past 4 hours ☐Past 8 hours Other:
Dressings/Wounds	
Other Treatment	
Belongings	☐Given family ☐Taken Floor with patient ☐Given to Security
ER Nurse Signature	Extension
Print Name ➔	

Figure 1-3. Written report form. (Used with permission of WellStar Health System.)

References

1. Balzer-Riley JB: Responsible, assertive, caring communication in nursing. In *Communication in nursing,* ed 4, St Louis, 2000, Mosby.
2. Riley JB: Warmth. In *Communication in nursing,* ed 4, St Louis, 2000, Mosby.
3. Riley JB: Respect. In *Communication in nursing,* ed 4, St Louis, 2000, Mosby.
4. Riley JB: Genuineness. In *Communication in nursing,* ed 4, St Louis, 2000, Mosby.
5. Riley JB: Empathy. In *Communication in nursing,* ed 4, St Louis, 2000, Mosby.
6. Riley JB: Specificity. In *Communication in nursing,* ed 4, St Louis, 2000, Mosby.
7. Riley JB: Humor. In *Communication in nursing,* ed 4, St Louis, 2000, Mosby.
8. Sandman P: Beyond panic prevention: addressing emotion in emergency communication. Retrieved September 2, 2003, from www.psandman.com/articles/beyond.pdf.
9. Stephens N: One emergency department's responses to the increasingly complex challenges of patient care at century's change, *J Emerg Nurs* 26(4):319, 2000.
10. Emergency Nurses Association: *Standards of emergency nursing practice,* ed 4, Des Plaines, Ill, 1999, The Association.
11. Loeb S: Caring for patients. In *Surefire documentation,* St Louis, 1999, Mosby.
12. Joint Commission on Accreditation of Hospitals: 2004 patient care standards pre-publication edition. Retrieved September 5, 2003, from www.jcaho.org/accredited+organizations/hospitals/index.htm.
13. Joint Commission on Accreditation of Healthcare Organizations: 2003 national patient safety goals. Retrieved September 5, 2003, from www.jcaho.org/addredited+organizations/patient+safety/npsg/npsg_03.htm.
14. Office for Civil Rights: Summary of HIPAA privacy rule. Retrieved April 2003 from www.hhs.gov/ocr/hipaa.
15. American Hospital Association: HIPAA privacy regulations: overview. Retrieved September 13, 2003, from www.whprms.org/HIPAA%20info/HIPAA%20Overview.PDF.
16. Sheehy S: A duty to follow up on laboratory reports, *J Emerg Nurs* 26(1):56-57, 2000.
17. American Society of Testing Materials: F 2076-01 standard practice for communicating an EMS patient report to receiving medical facilities. Retrieved September 8, 2003, from www.astm.org.
18. Perlman K: Faxed report to the floors for admitted ED patients: a pilot project, *J Emerg Nurs* 28(3): 231-234, 2002.
19. Sensmeier J et al: Improving operational efficiency through elimination of waste and redundancy work group report, Healthcare Information and Management Systems Society, 2002. Retrieved September 13, 2003, from http://www.himss.org/asp/issuesbytopic.asp?TopicID=14.

2

Diversity

Anita Ruiz-Contreras, RN, MSN, CEN, MICN, SANE-A

Much has been written in recent years about diversity becoming a new way of life, but diversity is hardly a novel concept. Since the beginning of time, human beings have recognized that they are not all the same. Diversity has always existed and has colored world history in positive and negative ways. War, immigration, and struggles for freedom demonstrate the extent to which people are willing to go to maintain the individuality or diversity of their group.

Diversity has been defined variously as the fact or quality of being diverse, differing one from another, made up of differences, or composed of distinct characteristics, qualities, and elements. In 1988 the National Emergency Nurses Association Diversity Task Force defined diversity simply as the ways in which persons differ. These differences (Table 2-1) occur in age, class, culture, ethnicity, gender, nationality, race, religion, sexual orientation, and extent of marginalization. In the health care arena, diversity among patients and staff members directly affects perceptions of health and health care. Emergency nurses need to develop an understanding of a wide range of human differences.

Historically, Western health professionals have assumed that those in our care must conform to standard treatment modalities, regardless of the patient's own cultural, religious, or lifestyle beliefs. Alternative health rituals and customs usually are not promoted in modern health care facilities. Patients find hospitals a difficult place to sustain even simple cultural traditions such as maintaining religious dietary practices.

Today, more providers are realizing that the delivery of competent health care is enhanced by an appreciation and understanding of patient diversity. This trend is reflected in the growing number of patient educational materials and other resources published in multiple languages. Beyond merely complying with the law, health care systems have learned that to survive in today's world they must address issues of diversity directly. Appealing to new patients and learning what strategies make a health care program more attractive to particular groups are emphasized.

Table 2-1   **Areas of Diversity**

Areas	Definitions
Age	A period of existence
Class	A group of persons who share the same attributes, such as social rank or socioeconomic status, and adhere to traditional roles and principles
Culture	Patterns of behavior and thinking that persons living in social groups learn, create, and share
Ethnicity	A conscious choice regarding identity based on beliefs, values, practices, and loyalty to a certain group or groups
Gender	Self-described identity as male or female
Nationality	Belonging to a particular nation by birth, family origin, or naturalization
Race	The biological variation in humankind, scientifically defined in three categories: Mongoloid, Negroid, and Caucasoid
Religion	Organized or unorganized belief systems
Sexual orientation	One's lifestyle identity based on sexual expression
Marginalized status	Individuals seen as possessing relatively little social power

Modified from Emergency Nurses Association Diversity Task Force, 1988.

STAFF MEMBERS

Much of the emphasis on sensitivity to diversity has been directed toward patients and their families. However, openness to diversity must extend to colleagues and other staff members as well. By accepting diversity among patients and co-workers, nurses are able to look at the whole person and understand alternative ways that an individual might perceive an experience. A staff composed of health care professionals from a variety of backgrounds is a staff better suited to meet the needs of the patients they serve.

Obtaining a measure of diversity competence does not require knowledge of each nuance of every group. Caring for diverse populations in a sensitive manner implies a recognition of differences and that individual differences are not seen as wrong or unworthy of respect. Such caring also implies thoughtful consideration of how to work best with these differences to promote patient health. Emergency nurses should be prompted to ask questions, to learn, and not to rely on stereotypes or assumptions.

VISIBILITY VERSUS INVISIBILITY

Although a person may appear to identify with a certain group, such an assumption is not universally correct. Likewise, significant diversity is not always visible. Communication is the most effective means of determining invisible differences, but because of common biases and prejudice, individuals may not feel comfortable discussing these issues. Nonetheless, if it will potentially impact patient care, nurses have the responsibility to "ask the questions that need to be asked." Phrasing queries in a neutral manner generally will yield the desired information.

DIVERSITY PRACTICE MODEL

The Diversity Practice Model (Table 2-2) was developed to assist health care professionals in approaching diversity issues. The model is meant to stimulate discussion and uses an A-B-C-D-E mnemonic to guide relevant ideas and questions. The Diversity Practice Model can generate discussion, even at times when discussion might be difficult, such as when a staff member senses discrimination as a result of subtle comments or jokes.

Assumptions

The Diversity Practice Model begins with the health care professional asking, *"What are my assumptions and what are they based on?"* Assumptions are ideas or thoughts, often rooted in limited experience, bias, or generalizations. Assumptions may or may not be true. Frequently, assumptions are based on contact with a limited number of individuals, wrongly supposed to characterize an entire group. Nurses may have experience with a small sample or subgroup and believe that all members of the larger group will respond in a similar manner. Such stereotyping can involve positive or negative images of a group. Interacting openly with diverse patients allows nurses to assess the validity of their own assumptions. An important step is to gauge to what extent these assumptions influence your relationship with a patient or another individual (visitor, family member, colleague).

Beliefs

The fundamental question when examining beliefs is, *"How do my beliefs affect the care that I give patients who are different from me?"* Beliefs are learned behaviors. Children are raised to accept the beliefs of their families. Families in turn have viewpoints that are congruent with those of their greater community. Not uncommonly, these values involve bias toward other groups. Health care based on negative beliefs only serves as a barrier to good patient–caregiver relationships. A bottom line must exist where respect for others—regardless of assumptions, beliefs, or attitudes—becomes an inalienable feature of care. All patients must be treated with respect and dignity despite their diversity or a health care provider's opinion of it.

Communication

Communication is the process by which meanings are exchanged between individuals. Effective communication is a vital component of professional nursing care. The nurse must

Table 2-2   Diversity Practice Model

	Mnemonic	*Meaning*
A	Assumptions	The act of taking for granted or supposing that a thought or idea about a group is true
B	Beliefs	Beliefs are shared ideas about how a group operates
C	Communication	The two-way sharing of information that results in an understanding between the receiver and the sender
D	Diversity	The way in which persons differ and the effect that these differences have on health perception and health care
E	Education	The act of attaining knowledge about diversity

From Emergency Nurses Association: *Emergency nursing pediatric course provider manual*, Des Plaines, Ill, 2004, The Association.

make an early assessment regarding the patient's ability to comprehend what is being said. If a potential language barrier exists, the nurse should address the patient in English and attempt to determine what language is preferred for communication. Many non–English-speaking patients are able to identify their language in a way that can be understood by speakers of English. In times of stress or crisis, some patients are more comfortable using their first language, even if they are fluent in English.

When communicating with a non–English-speaking patient, talk in a normal tone. One often has a tendency to speak louder than usual because of an assumption that the patient simply may not have heard what was said. When using a translator, speak directly to the patient and not to the translator. Avoid complicated medical terminology with all lay patients, whether they are English speaking or not. Present information in a manner consistent with the patient's language, background, and educational level. Ensure comprehension by asking patients to repeat instructions.

Communication involves far more than words; *it is not just what you say, but how you say it.* Negative nonverbal communication can be damaging to the patient–provider relationship. As communication begins, the nurse's body language should indicate acceptance and respect. Simple gestures may be used to garner basic information until a translator is available. Keep in mind, however, that some groups attribute different meanings to gestures, body contact, and facial expressions and that your intent may be misinterpreted.

Non–English-speaking patients commonly bring someone along to serve as a translator. This person may be a spouse, sibling, friend, or child. Reliance on such individuals is discouraged because one cannot assess the translator's ability to comprehend medical information. Additionally, some of the information requested may be of a sensitive or personal nature and difficult for a family member or friend to discuss. When possible, use only translators approved and certified by the governing agency of the institution. In most health care facilities, regulatory requirements mandate that professional translation services be readily available.

Diversity

The question here is, "How does diversity affect the patient's responses to health and illness and the nurse's response to the patient?" Diverse groups exhibit a wide variety of health behaviors, including the following:
- Some cultures loudly verbalize their discomfort, whereas others consider it cowardly to express pain.
- Individuals from certain groups are reluctant to say "No" to a health care professional because it is considered disrespectful.
- Folk remedies may be used as a primary source of health care.
- Because of fear, lack of information, or limited access, medical attention may be sought only as a last resort, when disease has progressed to a critical stage.
- Preventative health care may be infrequent or absent and may be limited by education, resources, or access.
- Patients may "doctor shop" for a "better" treatment because of a lack of understanding of disease processes and effective options.

To provide optimal care, it is imperative that emergency nurses address patient diversity. A host of diversity issues can affect a patient's ability or desire to follow a treatment plan. For example, the homeless patient prescribed a regimen of antibiotics that require refrigeration necessarily will be noncompliant. Even the definition of normal activities of daily living is highly diverse and cannot be taken for granted. In some areas of the world, bathing is a luxury and body odors are considered natural. Nurses need to ask questions, in a nonjudgmental tone, to gain a better understanding of the patient's situation, beliefs, and customs.

Diverse family practices may influence interventions when a caregiver brings young children or an elder into the emergency department. In many cultures, child care centers and nursing homes are virtually nonexistent because family members assume responsibility for these activities. Individuals acknowledge rites of passage, such as birth and death, in diverse manners. Several cultures greet the birth of a boy differently than that of a girl. Mourning practices vary dramatically among societies. Death may be viewed variously as a highly emotional, a somber, or a peaceful event. In some groups death means nonexistence, damnation, or going to a place of rest, whereas for others death signifies rebirth.

Education

Emergency nurses should seek to learn about various groups common to their health care setting. Information can be gleaned by reading printed material, viewing audiovisual presentations, attending classes, or speaking with patients and health care professionals from different groups. Learning about human diversity can be fascinating. Many ways to explore and celebrate diversity are available: staff members can teach each other, plan meetings around a cultural theme, or even organize a potluck with food from different countries. The ability to work well with diverse groups makes a health care professional a more valuable employee.

END-OF-LIFE CARE

Attitudes and practices related to the end of life, including tissue and organ donation, may be influenced greatly by a patient's culture. See Table 2-3 for a summary of characteristic responses listed according to culture. However, it is essential to remember that these are generalizations that may have no bearing on a particular patient and family. As is true in mainstream American culture, persons from other backgrounds will have highly diverse religious, social, and family practices and must be treated as individuals. Degree of acculturation, socioeconomic status, and educational level account for variations as well.

DIVERSITY DILEMMAS

Occasionally, health care professionals are presented with difficult ethical problems that result from a deeply felt clash of values. Issues regarding customs promoted or condemned by a particular group can cause real personal dilemmas. For example, practices such as abortion, female circumcision, child discipline, autopsy, and blood transfusion may divide care providers and patients. In such cases, one must recognize that everyone is entitled to beliefs and opinions. The mutual goal is communication and understanding.

Table 2-3   Cultural Practices Related to Death and Tissue and Organ Donation

Group	Death Practices	Donation
American Indians	Great intertribal variety exists. A positive attitude may be maintained around the patient. Sadness and mourning are done in private. Traditional practices include turning or flexing the body, sweetgrass smoke, or other purification rituals. Family may want to prepare and dress the body. Some families will take the body home; others prefer to have the body rest at the place of death for up to 36 hours. Several Native American cultures avoid contact with the dead.	Organ donation generally is not desired.
Arabs	Arabs do not openly anticipate or grieve for the dying before death. Nurse should privately inform the head of the family of a death or impending death. Some families bar young women from the dead or dying. "Do not resuscitate" orders may cause the family to lose trust in the health care system.	Arabs may refuse donation so that the whole body can meet the creator.
Blacks/Africans	Nurse should report deaths to the eldest family member, spouse, or parents. Nurse should expect open and public emoting, but this practice varies. Families generally prefer that professionals prepare the body. The dead are highly respected. Cremation commonly is avoided.	Donation is largely considered taboo unless the organ is destined for a relative.
Cambodians	Nurse should inform older family members of the death/ imminent death. The family or a religious representative may want to wash the body, shroud it in white cloth, and burn incense. A monk performs prayers on the night of the death.	Unlikely to permit organ donation because of a belief in rebirth and a desire to be intact.
Central Americans	Nurse should inform eldest male of death/imminent death. Catholic patients often want to see a priest. Death at home generally is considered preferable. Family members consider death a spiritual event and may want to prepare the body and say good-bye.	Organ donation is acceptable if the body is treated with respect.
Chinese	Patients and families may be fatalistic about death and unwilling to discuss it. Families often prefer that the patient remain uninformed of terminal conditions or may choose to break the news. Dying at home can be considered bad luck. Special amulets and cloths may be placed on the body.	Organ donation is not likely.
Cubans	Less acculturated Cubans generally expect the male head of the family to be the person informed; nurse should not inform the patient first. The entire family then will be notified and is expected to visit the patient. Receiving in-hospital care is considered more important than dying at home. Families commonly insist on around-the-clock presence.	Obtaining consent for donation is uncommon.
Ethiopians and Eritreans	News of serious illness is given first to male friends/family members so that they will be available for support. Nurse should never tell a female first. Family members may arrange for a Coptic priest to visit. Great outbursts of emotion are expected at the death of a loved one, including chest beating and tearing of clothing. Standard mortuary body preparation is generally acceptable.	The concept of organ donation is unfamiliar to many in this group.
Filipinos	Nurse should inform the head of the family away from the patient's room. Family may ask a Catholic priest to perform the sacrament of the sick. "Do not resuscitate" decisions are difficult and usually involve the entire family. Patients with chronic diseases often prefer to die at home. Religious medallions, rosary beads, figurines, other objects, and bedside praying are common.	Great respect is afforded the body, which may preclude donation and cremation.

Lipson J, Dibble S, Minarik P, editors: Culture & nursing care: a pocket guide, *San Francisco, 1996, UCSF Nursing Press.*

Continued

Table 2-3   Cultural Practices Related to Death and Tissue and Organ Donation—cont'd

Group	Death Practices	Donation
Gypsies (Roma)	Nurse should inform the head male and ask for help breaking the news to other family members. Family members may call for a priest for purification of the body. An open window allows the spirit to leave. The subject of death usually is avoided. Religious and personal objects are placed in the room. The moment of death and "last words" are highly significant. Relatives may want to sit with the body for a night and day. Immediate embalming is done to remove blood, which is a spiritual danger to family members.	Gypsies rarely agree to donation.
Hmong	Clan elders meet to make decisions regarding care. Immediate family members and females are not considered capable of exclusive decision making. Traditional beliefs hold that the dead appear in the next life as they left this one. Therefore it is considered shameful to die poorly dressed. Nurse should not remove amulets from the patient. A shaman may perform healing rituals. All "hard objects" (buttons, bullets, zippers, metal plates) must be removed before burial.	Traditional Hmong believe one of the body's three spirits must stay with the (whole) body. Christian Hmong may consent to donation.
Koreans	A spokesperson will relay information to the family members, who then unite to prepare for the death. Mourning may be loud and visible. Chanting, incense burning, and praying are common. Cremation is uncommon.	Donation may be viewed as tampering with the body/spirit.
Mexicans	Extended families are obliged to visit the sick and dying to extend their respects. Pregnant women may be exempted from such visits. Religious amulets, rosary beads, or medallions are common. Roman Catholics may request a priest. Wailing is frequent and socially acceptable. Families may want to spend time with the body before its transfer to a morgue.	A desire to keep the body intact for burial usually preempts organ donation.
Puerto Ricans	Customary practice is to have a priest/clergy present when bad news is disclosed. Family usually will arrange for around-the-clock presence. Candles, rosary beads, and figurines are frequently at the bedside. Visitors often want to touch or kiss the body after death. Dramatic emotional and psychosomatic reactions are common.	Donation is not unusual and is viewed as an act of goodwill.
Russians	Nurse should inform the head of the family first. "Do not resuscitate" decisions are seen as a way to allow the patient to die in comfort. A priest, minister, or rabbi may be called. Postmortem practices vary greatly by religion.	Most Russians will refuse donation.
Samoans	Patients and family members prefer to be told the prognosis early. Home care generally is considered preferable to hospital care. Family members often wish to prepare the body. Autopsy and cremation are rare.	Donation is unusual.
South Asians (e.g., Indians)	Death beliefs and practices vary widely among Hindus, Muslims, and Sikhs. Hindus and Sikhs believe in reincarnation. It is unusual for families to inform a patient of impending death. Death at home is preferred, and religious rituals are common. Dramatic grieving is typical. Special postmortem body care rituals may be required. Muslims bury bodies as soon as possible; Hindus and Sikhs favor cremation.	Hindu, Muslim, and Sikh religious practices prohibit donation.
West Indians	Close family and friends want to gather at the dying patient's bedside to pray and witness the loved one's passing. Most prefer home (versus hospital) care. No typical postmortem rituals.	Donation is unlikely.

3

Basic Legal Issues for Emergency Nurses

Kimberly P. Johnson, RN, BSN

Legal issues have a profound effect on the practice of nursing in today's increasingly technologic and evolving health care arena. Emergency care can be a highly litigious area of practice. This chapter provides a basic overview of some of the legal issues that affect emergency nurses and their delivery of care. However, this chapter is not a substitute for professional advice. Nurses should discuss specific legal problems related to emergency nursing with an attorney.

NURSE PRACTICE ACTS

Licensed professional nurses are accountable to the public for their nursing judgment and the consequences of that judgment. Licensure creates standards for entry into practice and is one of the ways the government protects the public. Nurse practice acts are statutory laws created by legislative bodies that oversee the practice of nursing. State Boards of Nursing (known as Boards of Nurse Examiners in some jurisdictions) are the administrative bodies tasked with enforcing the nurse practice act of a state through rules, regulations, hearings, and investigations. Nurse practice acts were originated to do the following:
- Protect the public
- Define and limit the practice of nursing
- Provide scope of practice guidelines
- Set standards for nursing
- Allow for disciplinary action

Every state has its own nurse practice act that determines qualifications for entry into professional nursing, defines educational responsibilities, and regulates advanced practice nurses. Nurse practice acts affect all aspects of nursing. Each licensed practitioner should be aware of the scope of practice delineated in the practice act of the state in which he or she practices.

Copies can be obtained from the State Board of Nursing or from the office of the state nursing association.[1] Nurse practice acts are also available online at state board websites.

Supervision of unlicensed personnel is a growing responsibility of the licensed practitioner. Many hospitals have replaced registered nurses with unlicensed assistive personnel such as emergency medical technicians, paramedics, and certified nursing assistants. Delegation of nursing functions to these individuals can create legal problems for the licensed practitioner. The American Nurses Association defines unlicensed individuals as those who are "trained to function in an assistive role to the licensed nurse in the provision of patient/client activities as delegated by a nurse. The activities generally can be categorized as direct or indirect care." A licensed practitioner cannot delegate activities to unlicensed personnel that rightfully should be performed only by a licensed practitioner. These activities include any task that involves professional judgment related to the diagnosis and treatment of patients.[2]

Violations of the nurse practice act can result in denial of authorization to practice, license suspension or revocation, probation, refusal to renew licensure, mandated submission to treatment or therapy as a prerequisite to continued practice, private/public reprimand, or even criminal prosecution. Categories for which disciplinary action may be taken include the following:

- Fraud and deceit
- Incompetence
- Unethical conduct
- Negligence or risk to clients
- Physical or mental incapacity
- Criminal activity
- Drug or alcohol use (impairment)
- Any other infringement of the rules and regulations of the nurse practice act

All nurses have a duty to report violations of the nurse practice act. State nurse practice acts require such reporting, and most will hold nonreporting nurses accountable. This requirement protects nurses from defamation lawsuits if they report violations in good faith. When faced with a situation that appears to be a violation of the practice act, first notify the nurse's immediate supervisor. Administrative personnel then have a duty to take action regarding the violation and to report it to the State Board of Nursing.[1,2]

CONFIDENTIALITY AND HIPAA REGULATIONS

Confidentiality is essential to the relationship between emergency nurses and their patients, and patients have an expectation of privacy regarding personal health information. In this world of computer technology, opportunities for violation of patient privacy related to easy access to medical data are increased. Federal and state laws exist to protect medical information. Emergency nurses have a legal and ethical duty to ensure patient privacy. Health care organizations (e.g., health maintenance organizations and preferred provider organizations) and institutions are also accountable and liable for breaches in health record confidentiality.

The Health Insurance Portability and Accountability Act of 1996 (HIPAA), enacted in part to simplify administration of health insurance, provides for protection of personal health information by directing ways it may be stored, shared, or released.[3] Under the regulations of the act, individuals are entitled to do the following:

- Receive information regarding how their health data will be used and disclosed
- Access their personal medical records (with an option to amend the record)
- Access a list of nonroutine disclosures of their information
- Authorize the use of their medical records

- Object to or restrict the use of their medical records
- Seek recourse through the U.S. Department of Health and Human Services if privacy protections are violated

Patient confidentiality is everyone's concern. Hospitals are required to devise policies and procedures that address privacy issues, and all health care providers must be diligent in their efforts to protect personal medical data. Vigilance and sensitivity to patient privacy concerns are required whenever discussing or disclosing personal health information. Practitioners should limit conversations about patients to those persons who need to know and should discuss patient issues only in suitable areas. Severe civil and criminal penalties exist for wrongful disclosure of individually identifiable health information including the following:

- $50,000 fine, imprisonment for 1 year, or both
- Up to $100,000 fine, up to 5 years imprisonment, or both if the offense is committed under false pretenses
- $250,000 fine, up to 10 years in prison, or both for offenses committed with the intent to sell, transfer, or use health information for commercial advantage, personal gain, or malicious harm.[4]

Privacy statutes do not limit authorized public health or required state regulatory reporting. In fact, federal and state laws exist that mandate reporting of certain illnesses, injuries, and suspicions, including the duty to warn third parties if a psychiatric patient has made threats toward a specific individual. See Box 3-1 for a list of situations in which reporting is required.

EMTALA AND INTERFACILITY TRANSFERS

Federal and state laws mandate that emergency departments (EDs) have a duty to provide services to those seeking emergency care, regardless of a patient's ability to pay. The Emergency Medical Treatment and Active Labor Act (EMTALA) was enacted to prevent "dumping" (interfacility transfer) of patients unable to pay for treatment. The law applies to all institutions with Medicare provider agreements in effect. The act defines an emergency medical condition as "any condition manifesting itself by acute symptoms of sufficient severity

Box **3-1 Situations That Mandate Reporting in Most States***

Any death in the emergency department and deaths within 48 hours of hospital admission
Child abuse
Communicable diseases such as human immunodeficiency virus, hepatitis, and tuberculosis
Disabled adult abuse
Elder abuse
Elopement of psychiatric patients
Extensive burns
Gunshot and stab wounds
Homicide
Infectious outbreaks
Internal disasters
Rape/sexual assault
Serious injury, illness, or death reasonably suggested to be related to the use of a medical device
Sexually transmitted diseases
Suicide (including attempted suicide)

*From the Joint Commission on Accreditation of Hospitals, 2004. *Patient care standards, pre-publication edition.* Retrieved Sept 5, 2003, from www.jcaho.org/accredited+organizations/hospitals/index.htm. Refer to local regulations for specific state requirements.

(including pain) that if medical treatment is not rendered, the individual or the unborn child would be subject to serious injury or death."[5] The act provides that a hospital with an ED must do the following[5]:

- Provide appropriate medical screening—to determine the nature and severity of the emergency condition—to any individual presenting to the ED and requesting treatment.
- Provide appropriate stabilizing treatment (within the capability of the hospital ED) for emergency medical conditions and active labor.
- Obtain written informed consent from the patient or the patient's representative before transfer to another facility.
- Verify that the receiving facility has available space and qualified personnel to treat the patient.
- Ensure that the receiving facility and an attending physician have accepted the patient.
- Forward all medical records with the patient at the time of transfer.

Under the stipulations of EMTALA, stabilizing treatment must be provided for medical conditions (including active labor) that within reasonable medical certainty likely would deteriorate if not treated. Unstable patients transferred to other hospitals must have physician certification that the benefits of transfer outweigh the risk associated with the move.

Although triage is an important tool for establishing treatment priorities, it is not equivalent to a medical screening examination as defined by EMTALA. Hospital bylaws must delineate clearly which providers can perform the medical screening examination. This person can be a physician, nurse, nurse practitioner, or physician's assistant. Emergency nurses charged with completion of the medical screening examination should be trained and guided appropriately by written protocols for assessment, identification, and evaluation of acute conditions. Penalties for EMTALA violations are as follows[5]:

- $50,000 fine against the hospital and/or the physician
- $25,000 fine against a qualified rural hospital
- Potential loss of Medicare provider status
- Potential civil litigation by the injured patient or the hospital that received the inappropriate transfer
- Potential revocation of Medicare licensing

CONSENT

Consent is the patient's acknowledgment and acceptance of medical treatment. Unconsented treatment of a patient can constitute battery, which is defined as intentional, unwanted touching. Consent may be implied or express. In health care, express consent often goes way beyond a simple "yes" or "no," through a process known as informed consent. Table 3-1 summarizes types of consent.

Express consent, written or oral, is the patient's agreement to treatment. By law, consent is implied when a patient is unable or incapable of giving or denying permission for treatment, as in cases of unconsciousness, where immediate decisions must be made to prevent loss of life or limb. Additionally, emergent procedures may be performed on minors, without parental consent, to protect life or limb when a legal guardian is unavailable. In these cases the law assumes that a reasonable person, in the same or similar circumstances, would provide consent. Therefore the law implies consent on the patient's behalf.

Most laws concerning consent related to health care involve informed consent. Informed consent requires the capacity to consent. The age at which an individual may provide informed consent (or refusal) varies among states and according to the patient's condition.

Table 3-1   **Types of Consent**

Type	*Description*
Implied consent	Allows any appropriate treatment in an emergency situation when the patient is unable to give consent. Based on the assumption that a patient, if able, would provide consent for life-saving treatment.
Express consent	Written or oral agreement to treatment. Includes assessment, evaluation, medications, x-ray films, and laboratory studies.
Informed consent	The patient has a full understanding of risks and benefits of the proposed treatment, is not under the influence of mind-altering substances, and has the legal capacity to consent. Examples of situations requiring informed consent include surgery, invasive procedures, and participation in research protocols.
Involuntary consent	When an individual refuses to consent to needed medical treatment a physician or police officer can ensure that the individual receives treatment. Examples include suicidal, delusional, or demented patients.

Importantly, the age of consent differs from the age of majority. Emancipated minors (e.g., active duty military, married or pregnant minors) are recognized legally as adults.

Informed consent occurs after full disclosure to the patient of the medical procedure and includes the following:

- An explanation of the procedure
- Discussion of potential risks and benefits of the procedure, including the risk of death and the risk of doing nothing
- The names and qualifications of persons who will perform the procedure and those who are assisting
- An explanation that the patient has the right to refuse a suggested treatment and continue with alternative or supportive therapy
- An explanation that the patient is free to refuse to continue any procedure or therapy that has been initiated already

Involuntary consent may be necessary when the capacity to consent is considered impaired (e.g., suicidal patients and intoxicated patients) and the individual refuses indicated medical treatment. By signing papers (along with a psychiatrist), emergency physicians or police officers can ensure that the patient will be held for treatment for a specified period of time. However, prisoners, criminal suspects, and detainees retain the right to consent to or refuse treatment except in cases of emergency or in matters of routine care.

Obtaining consent from patients with language or cultural barriers is challenging. Authorized translation services must be provided to ensure that these individuals are able to ask questions and receive full disclosure related to proposed medical interventions.

Lack of consent does not remove EMTALA requirements to provide a medical screening examination and necessary treatment should never be delayed while seeking consent to treat a minor.

REPORTABLE CONDITIONS

State laws govern situations that require a breach of patient confidentiality for the reporting of certain patient conditions. Mandatory reporting laws vary from state to state, and each ED should have policies and procedures related to these laws, indicating which agencies require notification. Reporting is generally the responsibility of the physician. However, if a situation falls within the realm of mandatory reporting, the emergency nurse has a duty to ensure that a report is made. Box 3-1 lists common reportable situations mandated by law. Some states require that patients who experienced an epileptic seizure while driving be reported to the Department of Motor Vehicles.

DOCUMENTATION

Thorough and accurate documentation, without excess, is an important defense against liability exposure. Nurses' notes are intended to do the following:
- Reflect the care administered to the patient
- Provide a chronology of patient progress
- Communicate clinically significant information to other members of the health care team

Hospitals accredited by the Joint Commission on Accreditation of Healthcare Organizations are required to provide certain information on the medical record (Box 3-2).

Optimally, nurses' notes will be written in a timely manner. However, events, observations, and interventions should always be documented, even after the event. Late entries should be identified as such; indicate the date and time of the entry to signify that it is out of order.

Ensure that the medical record is as follows:
- Clear and objective
- Realistic and factual
- Composed of your own observations
- Free of opinions, generalizations, and ambiguities
- Grammatically written, without spelling errors
- Devoid of unapproved abbreviations

The nurse's signature or initials should appear after each entry, and the medical record should *never* be altered or destroyed. Change mistakes in an obvious manner; draw a single line through the erroneous entry and then initial, time, and date the correction. Chart on each line sequentially or line-through any blank spaces.

Document unusual or variant situations in an institutional incident, variance, or occurrence report, *not* in the health care record. Incident reports function to evaluate patient care. In most states these reports are confidential. Nonetheless, use caution and complete incident reports as though they could be discoverable. The incident report should contain no

Box 3-2 Joint Commission on Accreditation of Healthcare Organizations Required Documentation

Initial assessment data
Time when rapid interventions occurred
Evidence that critically ill patients are receiving intensive care, such as frequent taking of vital signs
Problems and procedures
Interventions
Patient responses to interventions (resolutions)
Nursing observations
Communications with other members of the health care team
Communications with family members
Patient teaching, including discharge instructions
Any patient refusal of care
Use of translators

*From the Joint Commission on Accreditation of Hospitals, 2004. *Patient care standards, pre-publication edition*. Retrieved Sept 5, 2003, from www.jcaho.org/accredited+organizations/hospitals/index.htm. Refer to local regulations for specific state requirements.

language admitting liability or blaming others. State only the facts of the incident. Do not infer, assume, draw conclusions, or indicate what could have been done to prevent the incident. These questions are better answered in a peer review or risk management forum. In the patient's chart, never refer to the existence of an incident report.

SAFETY

To avoid potential liability regarding patient safety, emergency nurses must be cognizant of risks common to the ED population. Box 3-3 identifies areas with the greatest occurrence of associated liability.

Emergency nurses must know and comply with workplace policies to prevent unsafe conditions that can lead to patient injuries. Policies should address reporting, evaluating, and reducing patient injuries, near misses, and sentinel events. An educative approach to patient safety is more effective than a punitive one.

RESTRAINTS

The use of restraints can have severe legal and physical consequences. Restraining a person against his or her wishes constitutes false imprisonment when a nurse does not have a duty to restrain the patient. *False imprisonment* is defined as restraining a person or preventing a person from leaving an area and as confinement or prevention of a patient's freedom of movement, no matter how long the confinement occurs. Physical restraints have been associated with skin breakdown, impaired respiratory status, neurologic damage, and strangulation. Medical (chemical) restraints can cause respiratory distress, hemodynamic instability, decreased competency or judgment, severe neurologic damage, and death. Because of increasing concerns, concerted efforts have been made to limit or even eliminate the use of restraints in the United States. The overall standard dictates that patients have the right to be free from restraint or seclusion and that staff coercion, convenience, retaliation, or disciplinary efforts are inappropriate reasons for the use of restraints or seclusion.[6]

Outside of state statutes, two governing bodies have established guidelines concerning use of restraints in health care. The Centers for Medicare and Medicaid Services rules apply to all facilities participating in Medicare and Medicaid. Joint Commission on Accreditation of Healthcare Organizations guidelines apply to all hospitals accredited by that organization. These bodies define physical restraint as "any manual method or physical or mechanical

---

Box **3-3 Patient Care Areas of Significant Risk and Liability**

Errors in assessment, planning, implementation or evaluation of patient conditions (particularly in the area of triage)
Failure to act as a patient advocate or follow up abnormal conditions
Failure to educate patients on their condition and the adverse consequences if the patient is not following the medical regimen
Failure to monitor, adequately assess, and communicate patient conditions and changes in condition
Falls
Medication errors
Patients likely to injure themselves or others
Use of unsafe or malfunctioning equipment

device, material, or equipment attached or adjacent to the patient's body that he or she cannot easily remove that restricts freedom of movement or normal access to one's body." Medical restraint is defined as a drug "used to control behavior or to restrict the patient's freedom of movement and is not a standard treatment for the patient's medical or psychiatric condition."[2] See Chapter 1, Box 1-1, for Joint Commission on Accreditation of Healthcare Organizations' requirements for documentation of restraint and seclusion.

Time limits have been established for behavioral restraint and/or seclusion. Adult patients can be secluded for no more than 4 hours, adolescent patients (9 to 17 years) can be secluded for no more than 2 hours, and children under 9 years can be secluded for a maximum of 1 hour. A new order must be written at the end of these time limits. The order cannot be renewed on an as-needed basis. The patient must be reassessed, a new physician's order obtained, and reasons for continued restraint/seclusion documented. Hospitals are required to have policies in place regarding the appropriate indications for restraints and seclusions. Types of restraints and the required nursing documentation must be specified. An ED-specific restraint/seclusion sheet may be helpful for guiding required assessment and documentation.

ADVANCE DIRECTIVES

The Patient Self-Determination Act of 1991 is a federal law ratified to provide hospitalized patients with information about advance directives. Advance directives are written statements to health care providers regarding a patient's treatment choices in the face of terminal or irreversible illness. These documents go into effect whenever a patient is no longer able to communicate his or her wishes. Table 3-2 describes three types of advance directives.

The Patient Self-Determination Act requires institutions receiving Medicaid and Medicare to ask all patients about the existence of advance directives and to offer information about advance directives to patients. The Joint Commission on Accreditation of Healthcare Organizations has established guidelines that must be instituted in all accreditation-seeking hospitals. Nurses should review the hospital policies or procedures on this topic. Advance directives may not be transferable from one state to the next.

FORENSICS: EVIDENCE COLLECTION AND PRESERVATION

Forensics is the study of evidence used in legal cases. Medical forensics relates to the collection, analysis, and interpretation of medical evidence presented in legal cases.[6] In the ED,

Table 3-2 **Types of Advance Directives**

Type	Description
Living will	Specifies wishes regarding life-sustaining treatment to include withdrawing, forgoing, or restricting life-sustaining treatment. State statute determines the form the living will may take and how it can be revoked or changed after it has been executed. In most states, nurses and other medical professionals employed at the facility where the individual is receiving care are not allowed to be witnesses.
Durable power of attorney for health care	Appoints an agent to make decisions for the patient concerning medical treatment to include end-of-life treatment decisions.
Do not resuscitate (allow natural death [AND])order or medical directive	Instructs the physician regarding initiation of cardiopulmonary resuscitation or ventilatory support in the event of cardiac or respiratory arrest.

forensic issues related to nursing practice include evidence collection, evidence preservation, and chain of custody. Procedures for evidence collection, the role of the nurse in evidence collection, and situations in which nurses collect evidence for potential use in legal cases should be spelled out clearly in hospital policies or procedure instructions. Box 3-4 lists situations that may require the collection of forensic evidence.

The chain of custody involves protecting the viability of evidence (for court purposes) by establishing that no tampering has occurred. Chain of custody is a documented record of how the evidence was collected, labeled, and transferred to law enforcement representatives. Record information regarding forensic evidence collection in the medical record and clearly label each specimen. Destruction of evidence can lead to charges of obstruction of justice. Box 3-5 lists specific guidelines for preservation of evidence.

All individuals, including criminal suspects and prisoners, have rights. Medical personnel must recognize these rights, and medical professionals cannot compel individuals routinely to submit to specimen collection.[1] If principles of consent are not used in the collection of evidence, the nurse could be subject to civil liability for battery. Law enforcement officials

---

Box **3-4** **Evidence Collection in the Emergency Department**

Blood or urine specimens for alcohol and other drug testing
Child abuse/neglect
Deaths by fire
Deaths related to airplane, train, and other federal transportation events
Deaths related to military action
Disabled adult abuse/neglect
Domestic violence
Elder abuse/neglect
Employment-related requests for blood and urine specimens
Medical examiner/coroner cases
Persons who died without being treated by a physician
Specimens from sexual assault victims
Traumatic deaths
Unexpected or unexplained deaths

Box **3-5** **Guidelines for Preservation of Evidence**

Never discard clothing that potentially may be used as evidence. Place wet or bloody clothing in a paper bag. Place garments in a plastic bag only when directed by local protocol.
Do not wash the hands of a patient with a gunshot wound. Cover the hands with paper bags until police examine the patient. Gunpowder residue tests may be indicated.
Cut around bullet holes, powder marks, and knife cuts in clothing; do not cut through them.
Precisely document what the patient says about the event.
Describe the appearance of surface wounds and the presence of blood. Photographs are useful.
Document the patient's behavior in objective terms.
Unless the procedure is essential, delay cleaning the patient or wounds until after a police examination.
Do not handle bullets or other solid evidence removed from the patient. Place objects in a sealed container. Label containers with location found, date, time, and the initials of the person who collected the specimen.

may seek a search warrant or court order to obtain evidence from patients. However, emergency professionals should be careful not to be placed in the position of becoming agents of the law.[6]

References

1. O'Keefe ME: *Nursing practice and the law,* Philadelphia, 2001, FA Davis.
2. Brent NJ: *Nurses and the law,* ed 2, Philadelphia, 2001, WB Saunders.
3. Lorenzo J: HIPPA and healthcare: healthcare marketing. Retrieved July 11, 2003, from http://www.healthleaders.com/news/feature1.
4. Health Insurance Portability and Accountability Act of 1996, Public Law 104-191, Aug 21, 1996.
5. Emergency Medical Treatment and Active Labor Act, Statute 42 USC Sec. 1395dd, January 16, 1996.
6. Lee G: *Legal concepts and issues in emergency care,* Philadelphia, 2001, WB Saunders.

4

Intrafacility and Interfacility Patient Transport

Katy Hadduck, RN, BSN, CFRN

INTRAFACILITY PATIENT TRANSPORT

Patient transport from one area to another within the hospital is a frequent occurrence. With the variety of diagnostic and therapeutic procedures available, patients admitted to the emergency department (ED) may experience one or more intrafacility "road trips," concluding their ED stay with a final trip to the operating room, the intensive care unit, or another inpatient unit. Patient transport within the hospital potentially is fraught with unexpected events such as a cardiac arrest in an elevator, an infant delivery in the hallway, or a seizure while in the computed tomography scanner. However, with proactive thinking and resourceful preparation, patients can continue to have their care needs met outside the confines of the ED. Nursing care throughout intrafacility transport involves anticipatory planning, adherence to institutional policies, and appropriate patient and family education.

General Considerations

Any patient who is to be moved from the ED to another destination within the hospital must be evaluated carefully to ensure safe intrafacility transport. Quality care for patients is essential throughout the journey. Patients who require the presence of a registered nurse (RN) in the ED also must be accompanied by an RN throughout transport. This includes individuals who are hemodynamically unstable, those with airway or respiratory compromise, and anyone at risk for sudden neurologic decompensation. Also in this category is any patient requiring ongoing cardiac monitoring, continuous infusion of intravenous (IV) vasoactive medications, artificial airway support, or mechanical ventilation.

Stable ED patients who do not require continuous monitoring may be transported safely to destinations within the hospital by ancillary support staff such as emergency medical technicians or nursing assistants. Examples of stable patients include the following:

- Those with isolated traumatic injuries with stable vital signs
- Those with closed head injuries without neurologic impairment, altered level of consciousness, or severe agitation
- Those with abdominal pain with stable vital signs
- Those who are pregnant without abdominal trauma, persistent contractions, or signs of imminent delivery
- Those with mild illnesses or injuries with minimal risk of deterioration

Some facilities employ personnel dedicated to transporting patients to and from various departments within the hospital. Because they provide care to patients without reducing ED nursing staff, these employees can be a valuable resource for emergency nurses. However, it is essential that transporting nurses be trained adequately in advanced life support procedures and be prepared to administer whatever care may be required throughout the journey.

Planning

Safe, successful, intrafacility transport requires planning. Anticipating needs and preparing for the unexpected can ensure a consistent level of care for critically ill patients anywhere within the hospital.

Equipment and supplies

Each ED should have equipment and supplies readily available for intrafacility transport. Items that need to accompany critically ill or injured patients may be stored in a tackle-style box, a carryall tray, a soft-sided transport bag, or even in a small cart. Because drugs and certain other supplies have expiration dates, establish a protocol to check for and replace soon-to-expire items regularly. Intrafacility transports that require RN attendance should include the following equipment and supplies:

- A full oxygen cylinder with a regulator attached
- Airway equipment as appropriate (e.g., manual resuscitation bag, oral/nasal airways, end-tidal carbon dioxide detector, and suction supplies)
- A pulse oximeter for continuous oxygen saturation monitoring
- A cardiac monitor (consider a defibrillator)
- A sphygmomanometer and stethoscope or an automatic (invasive or noninvasive) blood pressure monitor
- Advanced cardiac life support first-line drugs (epinephrine, vasopressin, amiodarone, lidocaine, atropine)

Additionally, if the transport RN is expected to stay and provide care for the patient throughout a diagnostic or interventional procedure, ensure that the site has the following:

- Wall or portable suction
- Wall oxygen outlets
- A stocked crash cart with a defibrillator
- Sufficient electrical outlets
- A mechanism for rapid communication with the hospital operator or the ED in case of emergencies

Documentation

The care a patient receives during intrafacility transport should be charted as thoroughly as any other nursing care. Routine transport from the ED to an inpatient unit, in which care is transferred to another provider, may be noted briefly in the medical record. Document the patient's condition, to whom report was relayed, and any other information required by institutional policy.

If the patient will be returning to the ED for further observation and care after a diagnostic or interventional procedure, more extensive documentation is required. The accompanying nurse should ensure that vital signs, medications, and patient condition are recorded in the patient's medical record on an ongoing basis.

Safety considerations

Throughout transport, patient safety must remain a nursing priority. Nonambulatory patients and those with a potential for lightheadedness must be transported in a wheelchair or on a stretcher. Keep gurney side rails in the upright position. Pediatric patients should be transported in an age-appropriate bed or crib.

Safe transport of patients who require an artificial airway, mechanical ventilation, or multiple IV infusions generally requires more than one provider. This person may be a respiratory therapist, an emergency medical technician, a physician, or a second RN. Extreme care must be taken to avoid accidental extubation or inadvertent removal of invasive lines, particularly when lifting and moving patients from one surface to another.

Transport to the Operating Room

Many patients admitted to the ED eventually are taken to the operating room for surgical intervention. Ordinarily, this process is methodical and controlled. A typical example is the patient who has abdominal pain, requires multiple diagnostic tests and procedures, receives a surgical consult, and then is transferred to the operating room for an appendectomy. Conversely, the critically injured trauma patient may have a short initial ED assessment and resuscitation before being rushed to surgery for lifesaving interventions (Table 4-1).

Emergency nurses can influence greatly the speed with which patients move between the ED and the operating room. Patients requiring emergent surgery must have their care expedited, but safety considerations remain crucial. In such cases, ED interventions should be limited to emergency procedures (such as management of airway, breathing, or circulatory problems), initial assessment, and basic diagnostic studies (e.g., chest and cervical spine radiographs and laboratory tests). Patients with less critical conditions may undergo multiple interventions and diagnostic procedures safely before operating room admission.

Transport to an Inpatient Unit

Emergency departments frequently serve as the point of entry for many other destinations within the hospital. Patients may be admitted to the intensive care unit, a medical or surgical floor, or the labor and delivery suite. An emergency medical technician or nursing assistant can transfer a stable patient safely to a noncritical inpatient bed. The critically ill or injured patient destined for the intensive care unit requires accompaniment by an RN capable of managing sudden deterioration.

As in all patient admissions the accepting unit must be notified adequately (preferably not during shift change) and given sufficient time to prepare for the patient's arrival. Preparation

Table 4-1   Examples of Clinical Severity When Transporting Patients From the Emergency Department to the Operating Room

Patient Condition	Characteristics	Examples
Life-threatening	Critically ill or injured Deteriorating vital signs Uncontrolled hemorrhage	Nontraumatic aortic dissection Traumatic aortic rupture Massive hemothorax with ongoing blood loss Myocardial rupture Pelvic fractures with uncontrolled hemorrhage
Emergent	Critically ill or injured Hemodynamically stable	Ruptured tubal pregnancy Contaminated open fractures Traumatic amputation with potential reattachment Vascular injury with circulatory compromise Gastrointestinal bleeding uncontrolled by other measures
Urgent	Illness or injury less critical Hemodynamically stable	Acute appendicitis Closed hip fracture Cleansing, debridement, and repair of wounds

may be as simple as turning down the patient's bed or as complex as setting up a ventilator and obtaining multiple IV pumps for various drip medications. Admission orders, a copy of the ED chart, a list of personal belongings, and any other documentation required by institutional policy should accompany the patient.

Pregnant patients in labor frequently present to the ED. Hospital policy should address what level of caregiver (RN, technician, assistant) can accompany these patients to the labor and delivery unit. Selection of appropriate personnel depends on patient condition, transport time, and distance to the delivery area. Many facilities insist that a RN transport laboring patients because precipitous deliveries have been known to occur in elevators, hallways, and lobbies.

Transport for Procedures

Emergency department patients commonly require diagnostic procedures, such as imaging studies, that are performed outside the ED. Stable patients may be delivered to the receiving department and left in the care of its personnel with the understanding that the ED will be notified immediately of deterioration in the patient's status. Provide the receiving department with a brief patient report, any physician orders necessary for the procedure, and the name of a contact person in the ED to call if the patient requires additional care. Before diagnostic tests or interventions outside the ED, administer analgesics to patients who are in pain and to those who will undergo painful procedures or positioning. If the study is prolonged, the ED nurse may need to return while the procedure is in progress to administer additional pain medication.

Critically ill or injured patients must be accompanied by an RN throughout any procedure that requires the patient to leave the ED. This can have a significant impact on ED staffing. Nevertheless, a patient who requires cardiac monitoring, has an artificial airway, or is hemodynamically unstable must remain in the care of an adequately trained and equipped RN. Use of a designated intrahospital transport nurse can greatly attenuate staffing difficulties presented by these circumstances.

INTERFACILITY PATIENT TRANSPORT

Patients are moved from one medical care facility to another for a variety of reasons. Access to a higher level of care or specialty services, transport to the center where a patient's physician practices, and even patient or family convenience are valid reasons for interfacility transport. In recent years, transport of critically ill patients has become a nursing specialty area, with its own subspecialties such as pediatric, neonatal, and obstetric transport. Patient care equipment and transport vehicles constantly are being improved to make interfacility travel smooth and safe. As with intrafacility transport, safe transit from one facility to another requires planning and preparation.

Types of Interfacility Transport

Three types of vehicles are available for patient transport. Ground ambulances (also referred to as surface transport) may be staffed with paramedics or critical care nurses. Airplanes and helicopters (fixed and rotary wing aircraft) are available to transfer patients to and from almost any point in the world. Vehicle selection and level of care are determined based on a variety of factors. Patient condition, travel distance, and the availability of transport resources must be taken into account when planning an interfacility move. Issues such as weather and traffic conditions can influence decisions as well (Table 4-2).

Ground

Paramedic ambulance

Standard ambulances, staffed with paramedics and advanced life support equipment, are used frequently for interhospital transport. This resource generally is supplied by a community-based, private provider who bills the patient and/or the insurance carrier. Paramedic ambulances may transport safely patients who do not require the care of an RN. State and local regulations address specific patient conditions and patient care equipment that may be transported by paramedic ambulance. Requests for interfacility transport must not compromise the paramedic scope of practice or the level of care the patient receives.

Ground ambulances may transport patients short distances (e.g., the nursing home across the street) or to destinations far from the point of origin. If conditions are appropriate, it is not uncommon for a paramedic ambulance to drive a stable patient hundreds of miles.

Critical care transport

A growing trend in patient transport is the critical care transport (CCT) concept. Critical care transport uses RNs and specially trained paramedics to provide a higher level of care than a standard ground ambulance. Any ambulance, properly equipped and staffed with a qualified RN, can be a CCT vehicle. Hospitals occasionally supply a staff nurse to travel with the patient in a paramedic ambulance to provide this level of care. Although sometimes necessary, this arrangement is not ideal. Not only does the absence of a nurse affect hospital staffing, but also the RN may be unfamiliar with the ambulance environment and equipment, may lack appropriate emergency protocols, and may be prepared inadequately to handle emergencies in transit. Often additional insurance complexities and licensure issues arise if the ambulance crosses state lines.

The optimal choice for CCT is a ground ambulance with a dedicated crew, staffed with an RN, and specifically equipped for transport. Critical care transport teams deal with the full spectrum of patients, treating critically ill adult, obstetric, pediatric, and neonatal

Table 4-2   Choosing a Transport Mode

	Paramedic Ambulance	Critical Care Transport	Airplane	Helicopter
Route	Road/freeway speeds	Road/freeway speeds	Air	Air
Speed	Slower in high traffic conditions	Slower in high traffic conditions	Very fast	Fast
Cost	Least expensive	More expensive	Expensive Most efficient at distances >150 miles	Expensive Most efficient at distances <150 miles
Staffing	Paramedic level caregivers	RN; may have a respiratory therapist or additional paramedic	Typically RN/RN, physician, respiratory therapist, or paramedic staffing	RN/RN, RN/paramedic staffing
Available equipment	Standard advanced life support equipment	Advanced equipment (isolettes, balloon pumps, invasive pressure monitoring) ICU-type capabilities	ICU-type capabilities	ICU-type capabilities but space is limited
Other considerations/ limitations	—	—	Pressurized cabin (generally) Weight is usually not a factor Commonly capable of instrument navigation in poor weather conditions Must land at an airport; requires ground ambulances for airport-to-hospital transfer	Unpressurized cabin Significant weight and cabin space limitations May or may not have instrument navigation Can land at helipads and a variety of other landing zones; may eliminate the need for any ground ambulance

Registered nurse; *ICU*, intensive care unit.

conditions. Intraaortic balloon pumps, end-tidal carbon dioxide, invasive pressure monitoring, and multiple vasoactive drips commonly are managed on CCTs. Similar to many air medical programs, CCT systems are often hospital based; the patient care facility owns or leases the vehicle, employs the staff, and manages the program. In other locales, the CCT company may be a private, community-based provider.

Air

Airplane (fixed wing)

Airplanes have been used to move the ill and wounded since World War I. The speed and comfort of modern aircraft allow great flexibility in interfacility travel. Short distance transports may involve a small, single-engine, propeller aircraft. Long distance or international flights generally use private jets capable of tremendous speeds. Although most planes used for patient transport are pressurized, this does not eliminate the need to consider the effects of altitude on physiology. For example, a Lear jet cruising at 38,000 ft exposes the patient and crew to a cabin altitude of 8000 ft. This is a significant pressure change if the flight originated at a sea-level location.

Advantages of fixed-wing transport include speed, relative comfort for the patient and crew, and increased cabin room in which to stow equipment or carry a passenger. Most fixed-wing aircraft used for interfacility transport are capable of instrument navigation, which allows flights in less-than-perfect weather conditions. Disadvantages of this mode of travel include its high cost and an inability to land except at approved airports. This method also requires transport by ground ambulance to and from the aircraft. The patient must undergo multiple loading and unloading procedures before reaching the ultimate destination. This process may be highly stressful for an already stressed individual. Fixed-wing transports generally offer the same specialized equipment and staffing found on ground CCT ambulances. Flight personnel must have a thorough grasp of pertinent safety principles involved in air medical transport, including training in altitude physiology and dealing with in-flight emergencies.

Helicopter (rotary wing)

Rotary-wing aircraft are a relatively recent innovation. Early helicopters used for patient evacuation and transport had extremely limited capabilities. Today's helicopters are fast and safe and have earned a position of respect in rapid patient transport.

Moving a patient by helicopter is expensive; the cost can be up to 4 times the cost of ground CCT, depending on a variety of factors. Additionally, these vehicles are not pressurized, an issue that must be taken into account when evaluating patients for transport. The primary advantage of helicopter transport is that the aircraft can land at the scene of illness or injury or at a hospital helipad, eliminating the need for ambulance transport to and from an airport. This allows helicopter flights to make up time on patient transports, even though they cruise at slower speeds than fixed-wing aircraft. However, not all hospitals have access to a helipad, so flights from these facilities involve arranging an alternate landing zone. With hospital and local public safety agency approval and assistance, an alternate landing zone can be established in a nearby field, an empty parking lot, or on a road closed to traffic. If no other options exist, the nearest airport becomes the landing zone, and the patient must be transported by ambulance to the aircraft. Helicopters may or may not have the capacity for instrument navigation, a factor that can limit operation in conditions of limited visibility, particularly fog or low cloud cover. If weather conditions are acceptable, helicopters can fly at night without the need for instrument navigation.

Some flight crews consist of pediatric, neonatal, or obstetric specialty teams. Equipment designed to care for these specialized populations is used to ensure safety and a consistent level of care. Air medical flight crews operating on helicopters must have the same credentials as those on fixed-wing aircraft, including training in safety, emergency procedures, and altitude physiology.

Planning

Transporting patients between medical care facilities can be accomplished safely and rapidly, but advance preparation and knowledge of applicable policies will streamline the process. Emergency Medical Treatment and Active Labor Act legislation significantly affected patient transport decisions by requiring referring hospitals to verify the appropriateness of transport vehicles and personnel, obtain patient consent, and ensure the availability of a bed and an accepting physician before transfer. The ED nurse can facilitate hospital compliance with these regulations by preparing the patient for safe transport and by acting as a patient and family advocate.

Destination Selection

A hospital may have preestablished, formal referral agreements that determine patient destination. Other referrals depend on the specialized services offered by an institution, the patient's insurance carrier's preference, and the availability of an accepting physician and bed. Patients with specialized needs must be referred to centers that offer those services. Examples of specialized care centers with limited availability include the following:

- Burn
- Cardiac surgery
- High-risk obstetrics
- Limb replantation
- Neonatal intensive care
- Organ transplant
- Pediatric intensive care
- Spinal cord injury
- Trauma

The referring physician is ultimately responsible for determining the transport destination and making contact with the receiving physician. The ED nurse, however, may be expected to assist with the process and must be familiar with the referral patterns or contractual agreements of the hospital.

Some medical transport teams will respond to the referring hospital before all arrangements are finalized so as to expedite transfer of critically ill patients. Other teams will not depart to a referring ED until an available bed and accepting physician are confirmed because referrals occasionally are refused.

Patient Preparation

Although the transport team will "package" the patient with their own equipment according to their procedures, the emergency nurse can do much to facilitate patient preparation. Not only will facilitation minimize delays, but also it allows for smoother transition of care between the ED and the transport team.

Equipment

The emergency nurse should do the following:

- Securely tape all IV access sites. Record catheter size on the IV dressing.

- If the patient is receiving IV medications, label each line (close to the patient) to indicate what medication is infusing into which port.
- If the patient is intubated, ensure that the endotracheal tube is placed correctly and secured. Mark the tube size and insertion depth on the tape or securing device.
- Empty the urinary drainage bag, note output, and label the bag with tape to indicate the time it was emptied. Allow uncatheterized patients an opportunity to void before departure.
- Mark the fluid level in closed chest drainage systems, indicating date and time.
- Ensure adequate volume resuscitation and pain management.
- If possible, give patient belongings to family members for safekeeping. If belongings must accompany the patient, store them in a closed and well-labeled bag.

Documentation and record of care

Copies of all relevant ED documentation should be prepared and ready to hand off to the transport team. This documentation includes the following:
- ED medical record
- Patient personal information (the "face sheet")
- Formal documentation of the patient's consent to transport
- Orders from the referring physician regarding care en route
- Copies of imaging studies (on film or compact disc)
- Laboratory results

Communication With the Transport Team

The arrival of a transport team can be a daunting experience. Preparing the patient for transport may include changing out a multitude of monitoring and therapeutic equipment, performing last-minute procedures, and collecting piles of paperwork. This preparation can inflict stress on the patient, the ED nurse, and the transporting team. Cooperative efforts are needed to make the handoff between caregivers as smooth as possible.

Patient report

A variety of patient reporting practices exist. Some transport teams routinely call for detailed information before arriving at the referring hospital; other teams take the report at the patient's bedside. This process can be expedited if the ED nurse has relevant patient information readily available. Facts to include in a patient report are the following:
- Patient's name, age, weight, allergies, medical history, daily medications
- Time of onset of the current complaint and the time of ED admission
- Diagnostic and interventional procedures provided throughout the ED stay
- IV sites and sizes of IV catheters
- Medications given and the patient's response
- Critical laboratory values
- Current vital signs
- Presence of family members
- If the patient is intubated, provide information regarding endotracheal tube size, depth, and ventilator settings.
- If continuous IV drips are infusing, communicate the concentration, dose, and infusion rate. This can expedite changing out IV pumps to the transport team's equipment.

The ED nurse is also responsible for calling the destination hospital and providing a patient report to the receiving RN. The transport team will update information upon patient arrival.

Before Transport
Packaging

"Packaging" the patient for transport is a process that may be simple or complex. Typically, the transport team is introduced to the patient and family. The team then performs a brief but thorough assessment, removes any ED monitors or IV pumps, and replaces these with their own equipment. The emergency nurse can expect that paramedics transporting an advanced life support patient will bring a cardiac monitor. Critical care transport and flight teams generally use monitors capable of tracking noninvasive parameters such as heart rate and rhythm, blood pressure, oxygen saturation, and end-tidal carbon dioxide, as well as invasive arterial, pulmonary artery, or intracranial pressures. Intravenous pumps specifically designed for transport are small, may be capable of managing several simultaneous infusions, and generally require the use of special tubing.

The transport team may request that certain procedures be performed before departure for the patient's safety or comfort while traveling. The insertion of an indwelling urinary catheter facilitates output monitoring and eliminates the need to void during transport. Because even a small pneumothorax will expand at altitude, the flight nurse may request chest tube placement. The preflight insertion of a gastric tube will vent gastrointestinal air and empty material from the stomach, thus reducing the likelihood of vomiting.

Documentation

The transport team will require certain documentation from the referring hospital. Physician certification regarding the necessity of transport and en route patient care orders commonly are requested before departure. Written consent for transport must be included. Transporting personnel should maintain their own record of care provided during the journey and will leave a copy of this record at the receiving hospital. Figure 4-1 provides an example of a transport care record.

Safety Considerations

Maintaining patient and caregiver safety during transport is paramount. Preparing a critically ill patient for transport can be an intense and rapid process, and extreme caution must be taken to protect any IV lines, airways, tubing, and equipment attached to the patient. Transport stretchers and backboards must have multiple securing straps, and these should be used.

Emergency department nurses assisting with loading or off-loading of helicopter patients must be aware of the special precautions required around rotary wing aircraft. If a hospital regularly uses the services of an air medical provider, training can be arranged to orient ED personnel to helicopter safety practices.

Patient and Family Education and Support

Moving a patient from one institution to another can be highly stressful for patients, their family members, and friends. This process can distance a patient from his or her support system at a time when it is most needed. Families who do not have the resources to travel to the new facility can be overwhelmed with concern for the patient's well-being. Basic information, kindness, and patient advocacy go a long way toward helping persons through this frightening experience.

MERCY AIR
...a heartbeat away

MERCY AIR SERVICE, INC.
P.O. BOX 2532
FONTANA, CA 92334-2532

FLIGHT RECORD

BUSINESS (800) 499-9495
DISPATCH (800) 222-3456
FAX (909) 357-1009

FLIGHT INFORMATION

FLIGHT #   DATE: NURSE: EMT-P: PILOT:

SENDING HOSPITAL INFORMATION			LOCATION/TIMES		
SENDING FACILITY	UNIT	MD	LOCATION	ARRIVE	DEPART

SCENE CALL INFORMATION		
REQ AGENCY	UNIT ON SCENE	SCENE LOCATION

RECEIVING HOSPITAL INFORMATION		
RECEIVING FACILITY	UNIT	MD

PATIENT INFORMATION

NAME: _____
LAST, FIRST, MI

ADDRESS: _____
NUMBER & STREET

_____
CITY, STATE, ZIP

D.O.B. ___/___/___ AGE: _____ SEX: (M/F) WT: _____

MAXIMUM ALTITUDE   AMBULANCE COMPANY

REASON FOR TRANSPORT

CHIEF COMPLAINT

MEDICAL HISTORY

MEDICATIONS

MECHANISM OF INJURY / ONSET OF PRESENT ILLNESS   ALLERGIES

ASSESSMENT   TIME:

PRIMARY		SECONDARY			

PRIMARY

AIRWAY
☐ OPEN
☐ PART OBST
☐ TOT OBST

BREATHING
☐ NORMAL
☐ SHALLOW
☐ LABORED
☐ ABSENT

PULSE
☐ NORMAL
☐ WEAK
☐ BOUNDING
☐ IRREGULAR
☐ ABSENT

SKIN SIGNS
TEMP
☐ NORMAL
☐ WARM
☐ COOL
☐ HOT
☐ COLD

COLOR
☐ NORMAL
☐ PALE
☐ FLUSHED
☐ CYANOTIC

MOISTURE
☐ NORMAL
☐ DRY
☐ MOIST
☐ DIAPHORETIC

SECONDARY

NEURO   ☐ A & O X 4

HEAD   ☐ NO DRAINAGE FROM EARS / NOSE

NECK   ☐ NO JVD   ☐ TRACHEA MIDLINE   ☐ C-COLLAR IN PLACE

CHEST   ☐ EQUAL EXCURSION

LUNGS   ☐ CLEAR BILAT   ☐ GTV

ABDOMEN   ☐ SOFT   ☐ NON TENDER

BACK / SPINE   ☐ NO REPORTED INJURY   ☐ ON BACKBOARD

PELVIS

EXTREMITIES   ☐ MAEW   ☐ SMV INTACT X _____

REVISED
TRAUMA SCORE
RR(0-4)_____
SBP(0-4)_____
GCS(0-4)_____
TOTAL:_____
TIME:_____

GLASGOW
EM(1-4)_____
BVR(1-5)_____
BMR(1-6)_____
TOTAL:_____
TIME:_____

VITAL SIGNS (PTA)   PUPILS

TREATMENT PTA
☐ SAGER
☐ IV#1 _____
☐ IV#2 _____

☐ INTUBATED   ☐ EOA   ☐ MAST
☐ O2@ _____ 1/M ☐ FULL C-SPINE ☐ FOLEY

☐ NG TUBE   ☐ CHEST TUBE
☐ OTHER _____
☐ OTHER _____
☐ OTHER _____

PAGE 1 OF 2

Figure 4-1. Example of an air medical patient care record. (Courtesy Mercy Air Services, Inc., Fontana, Calif.)

Continued

FLIGHT RECORD (CONT'D)   FLT # _____   PATIENT NAME _____

TREATMENTS:

TREATMENTS PTA MAINTAINED IN FLIGHT
☐ WITHOUT CHANGE
☐ WITH CHANGE

VITAL SIGNS						INITIATED			
TIME	B/P	P	R	EKG	PULSE OX	PTA	TIME	ORDERS	DOSE/R

NOTES / COMMENTS

☐ ONLOAD – WITHOUT DIFFICULTY
☐ SAFETY STRAPS SECURED

_____

_____

_____

_____

_____

_____

_____

_____

_____

_____

_____

DISCHARGE SUMMARY

INTAKE	PTA	INFLIGHT	OUTPUT	PTA	INFLIGHT
IV			NG		
BLOOD			URINE		
COLLOIDS			EBL		
TOTAL			TOTAL		

R.T.S.	GLASGOW
RR(0-4) _____	EM(1-4) _____
SBP(0-4) _____	BVR(1-5) _____
GCS(0-4) _____	BMR(1-6) _____
TOTAL: _____	TOTAL: _____
	TIME: _____

☐ OFFLOAD – WITHOUT DIFFICULTY
☐ HOT   ☐ COLD

DISCHARGE STATEMENT _____

_____

DOCUMENTATION BY:_____ PT RELEASED TO:_____ TIME: _____
           SIGNATURE   SIGNATURE

Figure 4-1. Cont'd

Ensure that thorough, effective communication has taken place between the patient (or patient representative) and the physician regarding where, why, how, and when the patient is to be moved. Additionally, transport personnel should describe briefly the environment of the transport vehicle, what to expect en route, and safety procedures that will be in place ("You'll be wearing earplugs because the helicopter is loud, and you will have seat belt straps securing you to the stretcher"). Patients who are prone to motion sickness or who are terrified of flying may be offered medications to help make travel more comfortable.

Not uncommonly, a family member or friend may wish to accompany the patient during transport. The decision to bring passengers is based on a variety of factors. Some transport services have policies that preclude anyone from accompanying the patient. If the patient is to be flown in a helicopter, issues of additional weight and lack of cabin space may impose severe limitations. Finally, the health and emotional state of potential passengers must be considered. Requests made to ED nurses to accompany a patient during travel should be passed along to the transporting team. Reinforce with the family that this is not the decision of the referring ED.

Family members and friends who are present at the bedside or in a waiting area should be included in brief pretransport teaching. Driving directions to the receiving hospital can be provided. Information regarding to what unit the patient will be admitted, the telephone number of the unit, and the expected time of arrival are helpful for family and friends. A brief explanation of Health Insurance Portability and Accountability Act regulations may prevent frustration and worry when family members later place calls to the receiving hospital and are refused information regarding the patient's condition.

5 Emergency Preparedness: Managing Mass Casualty Incidents

Jeff Hamilton, RN, BA

Mitigation, preparation, effective response, and recovery are the keys to successful management of mass casualty incidents (MCIs) management. Delivery of medical care in response to an MCI or disaster differs radically from routine emergency care practices.

In disaster or MCI, health care providers must focus on the following:

- Implementing a comprehensive response plan
- Carefully allotting medical resources, personnel, supplies, and facilities
- Providing interventions that will benefit the greatest number of potential survivors

This chapter presents an overview of community, facility, and departmental activities related to emergency preparedness and MCI management.

MASS CASUALTY INCIDENT MANAGEMENT

The Joint Commission on Accreditation of Healthcare Organizations Environment of Care Standard 1.4 requires that hospitals develop a management plan to ensure an effective response to potential emergencies that could affect the environment of care.

The four essential phases of emergency management are mitigation, preparedness, response, and recovery (Table 5-1). Individual departments, facilities, and the community experience each of these phases to various extents.

An MCI may be caused by natural or human-related events (Box 5-1). Geography, population characteristics, weather patterns, and numerous other variables determine the potential for a specific incident in a given locale. For example, health care facilities near the Atlantic Ocean are susceptible to hurricanes; institutions in the Midwest are at increased risk from tornadoes. Strategic assessment of location-specific threats facilitates the development of a targeted response plan.

Table 5-1   **Phases of Emergency Management**

Phase	*Description/Action*
Mitigation	Identify potential mass casualty incident/disaster emergencies that could affect your hospital and its ability to provide care and treatment. Assess vulnerability to specific hazards.
Preparedness	Develop policies and procedures to manage the effects of emergencies once they occur.
Response	Implement policies and procedures identified in the preparedness planning phase.
Recovery	Design recovery activities that will return the facility to normal operations as quickly as possible.

Box **5-1**   **Examples of Natural and Human-Related Mass Casualty Incidents**

Natural	Human-Related
Avalanches	Building collapses
Blizzards	Chemical spills
Earthquakes	Explosions
Floods	Hostage situations
Heat waves	Mine collapses
Hurricanes	Radiation incidents
Ice storms	Structure fires
Mudslides	Transportation events (train, plane, multiple
Severe thunderstorms	vehicle crashes)
Snowstorms	
Tidal waves	
Tornadoes	
Volcanic eruptions	
Wildland fires	

From the *Joint Commission Perspective* newsletter, 21(12):8, 2001.

MITIGATION

Mitigation, the first step in disaster preparedness, involves evaluation of the practice locale to determine vulnerability to various threats. A hazard vulnerability analysis (Table 5-2) can be conducted to identify risks in three broad categories: probability of occurrence, risk to life and health, and current state of readiness. This analysis then can be used as a guide for the development of specific response plans. Table 5-3 illustrates this process for natural events, Table 5-4 provides an example of the same analysis for technologic events, and Table 5-5 addresses human events.

Each of the hazard vulnerability analysis categories is assigned a numeric rating, and specific risks are scored. Scores for each category then are multiplied to calculate vulnerability to a particular event. In Table 5-2, tornadoes receive a total score of 10, based on a moderate probability of occurrence (score = 2), high threat to life (score = 5), and adequate preparedness (score = 1) ($2 \times 5 \times 1 = 10$). Items with the highest total score represent the most probable threats and require the greatest effort, organizational focus, and emergency preparation resources. Likewise, planning groups should determine a value below which no action is necessary.

Table 5-2   **Hazard Vulnerability Analysis**

Category	Discussion
Probability	Is there a recognized risk for this event based on historical data or geographic or other factors?
Risk	What risk does this event pose to life or health? Will it disrupt, damage, or cause the failure of essential services? Can it lead to loss of community trust? What is the estimated financial impact? Are there potential legal issues?
Preparedness	What is the current state of emergency response plans? What is the training status of essential personnel? Are backup systems or community resources available? Is insurance coverage a factor?

From the *Joint Commission Perspective newsletter*, 21(12):8, 2001.

Hazard vulnerability analysis also is used to quantify the level of threat from known hazards in a specific area. Local emergency planning committees or state emergency management agencies can provide this information. Table 5-6 addresses specific hazards that emergency planners should consider. Once hazards inside the hospital and within the community have been identified, the degree of vulnerability to each threat can be assessed. Determining specific levels of vulnerability provides a roadmap for preparation and serves as a response guide in the event of an actual incident.

PREPAREDNESS

Preparation for an MCI involves: creating a plan; training personnel to respond to the plan; and testing the plan.

The Plan

Designing a single disaster plan, adaptable to all hazards, is more effective than writing specific plans for each potential threat. Tools are available to guide disaster plan development. An excellent general planning template, *Mass Casualty Disaster Plan Checklist: A Template for Health Care Facilities,* is available from the Association for Professionals in Infection Control. See the Association website *(www.apic.org)* for various educational resources.

Ongoing evaluation is crucial for successful plan implementation in the event of an actual disaster. Predicting contingencies that will cause the plan to fail is as important as identifying alternative ways to make the plan work. For example, knowing that a major highway overpass could collapse during an earthquake can prompt discussion with local emergency management agencies to identify alternate routes to the hospital. Likewise, a projected lack of morgue capacity during an MCI can stimulate the development of working agreements with managers of indoor ice-skating rinks or refrigerated truck companies.

Disaster Drills

Training exercises are hands-on drills carried out with staff members in their clinical area along with live actors portraying victims. Scenarios must be realistic, and drills should be conducted in real time whenever possible. Include specific parameters for evaluation. Box 5-2 provides guidelines for training drills.

Table 5-3 Example of a Hazard Vulnerability Analysis for Natural Events

	Probability				Risk — Health and Safety			Risk — Disruption Potential		Preparedness			
Event	High	Med	Low	None	Life Threat		High	Mod	Low	Poor	Fair	Good	Total
Score	3	2	1	0	5	4	3	2	1	3	2	1	
Natural events													
Hurricane				X									0
Tornado		X			X							X	10
Severe thunderstorm	X							X				X	6
Snowfall		X						X				X	4
Blizzard			X					X			X		4
Ice storm		X						X			X		8
Earthquake			X		X						X		10
Tidal wave				X									0
Temperature extremes	X								X			X	3
Drought			X						X			X	1
Flood (external)		X						X				X	4
Wildfire				X									0
Landslide				X									0
Volcano				X									0
Epidemic		X					X					X	6

Data from St. John's Mercy Medical Center, St. Louis, Mo. Template copyright American Society for Healthcare Engineering (ASHE) of the American Hospital Association (AHA), 2001. For more information on ASHE, visit www.ashe.org.

Table 5-4   Example of a Hazard Vulnerability Analysis for Technologic Events

Event	Probability — High	Med	Low	None	Risk — Life Threat	Health and Safety	Disruption Potential — High	Mod	Low	Preparedness — Poor	Fair	Good	Total
Score	3	2	1	0	5	4	3	2	1	3	2	1	
Technologic events													
Electric failure		X						X				X	4
Generator failure			X		X							X	5
Transportation failure			X						X			X	1
Fuel shortage			X				X					X	3
Natural gas failure			X				X					X	3
Water failure			X			X						X	4
Sewer failure			X			X						X	4
Steam failure			X			X					X		4
Fire alarm failure			X		X							X	5
Communications failure			X				X					X	3
Medical gas failure			X					X				X	2
Medical vacuum failure			X					X			X		2
Heat, ventilation, air conditioner failure			X			X					X		4
Information systems failure			X					X				X	2
Fire (internal)			X		X							X	5
Flood (internal)		X						X				X	4
Hazardous material exposure (internal)		X				X						X	8
Unavailability of supplies			X						X			X	1
Structural damage		X			X							X	10

Data from St. John's Mercy Medical Center, St. Louis, Mo. Template copyright American Society for Healthcare Engineering (ASHE) of the American Hospital Association (AHA), 2001. For more information on ASHE, visit www.ashe.org.

Table 5-5   Example of a Hazard Vulnerability Analysis for Human Events

Event	Probability				Risk					Preparedness			Total
					Life Threat	Health and Safety	Disruption Potential						
	High	Med	Low	None			High	Mod	Low	Poor	Fair	Good	
Score	3	2	1	0	5	4	3	2	1	3	2	1	
Human events													
Mass casualty incident (trauma)	X				X							X	15
Mass casualty incident (medical)		X			X							X	10
Mass casualty incident (hazardous material)			X		X							X	5
Hazardous material exposure (external)			X		X							X	5
Weapons of mass destruction (chemical)			X		X							X	5
Weapons of mass destruction (biological)			X		X							X	5
Weapons of mass destruction (radiologic)			X		X							X	5
Very important person situation		X						X				X	4
Infant abduction			X					X				X	2
Hostage situation			X					X				X	2
Civil disturbance			X					X				X	2
Labor action			X				X					X	3
Bomb threat			X		X							X	5
Patient elopement		X			X							X	10

Data from St. John's Mercy Medical Center, St. Louis, Mo. Template copyright American Society for Healthcare Engineering (ASHE) of the American Hospital Association (AHA), 2001. For more information on ASHE, visit www.ashe.org.

Table 5-6   **Specific Hazard Considerations**

Category	Considerations
Chemical manufacturing plants	What hazardous chemicals are being manufactured or stored? Material safety data sheets for each chemical at the plant should be accessible.
Bulk chemical storage sites	Identify the location of petroleum tank farms, agricultural chemical depots, and barge or ship storage sites.
Underground pipelines or bulk storage	Determine the location of active and inactive underground storage facilities.
Hazardous materials transportation	Are hazardous materials routinely transported through the local area via truck, train, or ship? What are the most common routes?
Radiation manufacturing facilities	Which radioactive isotopes are manufactured or stored on site? What is the half-life of each isotope?
Nuclear-powered electric generating plants	Is there a nuclear plant located within 100 miles of the hospital?
Explosives, fireworks, or ordinance	Are there explosives, fireworks, or ordinance manufacturing plants or warehouses within the service area?
Natural disaster history information	Review available local information regarding the frequency of earthquakes, floods, hurricanes, tornadoes, volcanic eruptions, landslides, and wildfires.
Potential terrorist targets	Identify potential targets: <ul><li>Areas with high concentrations of persons such as sports arenas, concert halls, convention centers, amusement parks, and airports</li><li>Politically significant venues such as abortion clinics, campaign headquarters, embassies, and government buildings</li><li>Sites with high economic impact such as banking centers and offices of major corporations</li><li>Religiously significant sites including worship centers, mosques, temples, and shrines</li></ul>

Box **5-2   Guidelines for Disaster/Mass Casualty Incident Training Drills**

Define the scope of the drill. Identify who will participate in the event. Will the drill include the entire facility or just the emergency department? Determine when the drill will begin and end.

Create a detailed master schedule of events. This is the most effective method of guiding the exercise. Write down every event, action, or decision to be tested.

Define all contingencies that will be introduced. Be sure each one is realistic.

List vital areas to evaluate, and select individuals to serve as reviewers. Provide clear, written guidelines for the evaluation. Focus on the plan and the process.

Develop goals for the exercise and corresponding objectives that must be assessed. Test no more than five goals for each exercise; more than this number causes confusion and dilutes the energy for revision.

Identify required resources for the exercise including equipment, supplies, and personnel.

Specify injuries for each victim in the exercise; preprint this information on cards that the victims can wear. Brief victims on how to act with specific injuries.

Complete an after-action report. Schedule a meeting with all participants after the exercise is completed. Review objectives to determine what worked and why, what did not work and why, and what needs to be done to make the plan more effective.

Submit an after-action report summary to all participants. Summarize recommendations with timelines for completion. Identify what resources are needed and who will be responsible for meeting each objective.

Tabletop Exercises

Tabletop drills are an effective way to pretest a plan. A tabletop exercise consists of a simulated MCI situation rehearsed while participants gather around a table. This type of interactive learning allows key players to work through operational issues together, develop team skills, and enhance problem-solving abilities. Tabletop exercises are an excellent means of identifying strengths and weaknesses and are an essential early step in the development or revision of an emergency response plan.

RESPONSE

A successful response to an MCI or disaster requires a coordinated approach that involves planning and efficient organization once the event occurs. Components that have proved effective include the use of an incident command system, clear delineation of lines of authority, written guidelines for each job, and skillful triage at the scene and in the emergency department. Fire and police departments have used a formal incident command system for many years. Such systems provide structure to an inherently chaotic situation. This concept has been adapted for use in health care organizations and is known as the hospital emergency incident command system. Figure 5-1 illustrates key components of the command system, including a well-defined organizational structure and clearly delineated lines of authority. An important advantage of this structure is that it can be applied to any size of health care organization. Table 5-7 summarizes essential features of the incident command system. An incident command system template is available through the Federal Emergency Management Agency at *www.fema.gov.* Table 5-8 provides an example of a job action sheet.

Patterns of Hospital Use

Typically, within 90 minutes of an event, 60% to 80% of acute casualties will arrive at the closest medical facility, whereas institutions outside the immediate area may receive few or no victims. Because patients generally are treated in the emergency department for 3 to 6 hours before admission or release, hospitals quickly can become overwhelmed. Careful community coordination will reduce this phenomenon. The most severe injuries in an MCI are major head, thoracic, and abdominal wounds, fractures, burns, and crush injuries. However, the most common injuries are sprains, strains, minor wounds, and damage to the ears or eyes.[1]

Triage Systems

The quality of care in an MCI is related inversely to the number of cases; the larger the number of arriving casualties, the more limited the care available because of finite material resources and trained personnel.[2] Generally, only 10% to 15% of mass casualty victims are severely injured. Therefore use of a system that rapidly triages out patients who require only minimal care and those likely to die despite maximal efforts is crucial. This allows resources to be focused on victims who will benefit most from optimal care.

Two approaches that have proved effective for triage during an MCI are the Simple Triage and Rapid Treatment (START) system (Figure 5-2) for adults and the JumpSTART pediatric MCI triage system (Figure 5-3). JumpSTART modifies the adult START method by substituting a pulse check for assessment of capillary refill time and inserts the step of giving five rescue breaths when a palpable pulse is present in an apneic patient. Figure 5-4 illustrates how both

Hospital Emergency Incident Command System

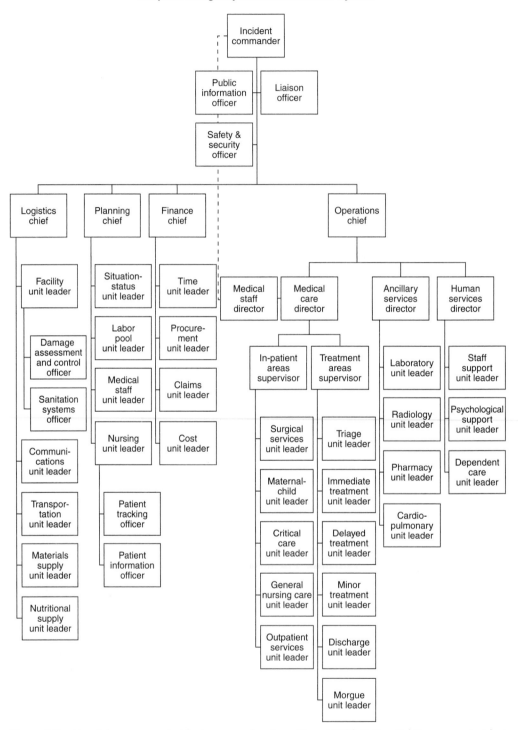

Figure 5-1. Hospital emergency incident command system. (From HEICS III–Hospital Emergency Incident Command System Update Project. Available at www.emsa.cahwnet.gov/Dms2/ORG2.htm. Accessed March 30, 2005.

Table 5-7   **Key Features of the Incident Command System**

Feature	Discussion
Common language	Adhering to established position nomenclature, such as "operations," "logistics," or "liaison" allows easy identification of the position/person responsible for an assigned task. Avoid the temptation of inventing titles to suit your specific needs.
Management by goals and objectives	Using goals, objectives, standardized methods, and established resources provides a roadmap for coordinating the response in all the confusion.
Goals and objectives common to all incidents	Certain common goals are essential for all events: • *Life safety.* This is the primary goal in all incidents. The safety of staff members is as important as that of victims. • *Scene stabilization.* Appropriate attention to triage, media coordination, traffic control, and accommodation of victims' relatives decreases chaos at the scene and in the emergency department. • *Recovery (normalization).* This is the cleanup and damage assessment phase. Examples include coordinating staff members to care for inpatients and inventory control to replace depleted supplies quickly.
Clearly identified lines of authority (who reports to whom)	One person's span of control should involve no more than five direct reports. Chaos is diminished considerably when each person interacts only with a well-defined and limited number of persons. Knowing that it is the job of operations to implement the incident commander's plans, that logistics will obtain needed equipment and personnel, and that finance will be tracking all expenditures allows effective allocation of tasks. In a mass casualty incident, be wary of accepting tasks outside your assigned responsibility; in this situation it is acceptable to say "that's not my job."
Job action sheets	Incident command in a hospital is difficult because key decision makers do not regularly use this system and are uncomfortable interacting with outside agencies. Job action sheets are an excellent guide through an incident. These sheets can be individualized as necessary.

Data from the Federal Emergency Management Agency, www.fema.gov.

algorithms can be combined into a single triage system. This methodology has been used extensively in the prehospital setting and also has been applied successfully to hospital diaster situations.

The triage methodology is as follows:

- Identify all minimally injured victims at triage. This category will constitute the largest number of victims, including those with neuropsychiatric and anxiety disorders. Consider placing minor care patients in a location separate from the emergency department. Treat and discharge patients from this area.
- Identify all critically injured victims with only a minimal chance of survival. Place the mortally wounded in a supportive care area and provide sedation and analgesia. Do not attempt resuscitation. Nurses assigned to this area should have established standing orders or protocols.
- Identify all seriously injured—but potentially salvageable—victims who require surgical intervention. Statistically, this will be about 10% to 15% of the total number injured. Place these individuals near your surgical team. Staff this resuscitation area with a trauma surgeon. Other surgeons should be assigned to operating rooms.
- Ideally, the number of victims received from the scene will be based on the number of available trauma surgeons. Identify all seriously injured victims who do not need immediate surgical intervention. Send these to the emergency department, where your

Table 5-8   A Typical Incident Commander's Job Action Sheet

Job	Action

Mission
Immediate action
	Organize and direct the emergency operations center. Give overall direction for hospital operations.
	• Activate the hospital emergency incident command system.
	• Read the entire job action sheet. Review the organizational chart on the back page.
	• Appoint a section chief each for operations (to implement the plans), logistics (to supply resources to operations), finance (to track expenses), and planning (to anticipate contingencies).
	• Receive situation briefings from the liaison officer.
	• Announce a status/action plan meeting in 30 minutes. Ascertain the following:
	    Readiness of each section
	    Status of the community response plan
	    Inpatient bed availability
	    Issues and contingencies that require immediate attention
	• Establish the following:
	    Goals to meet identified needs
	    Objectives for each goal
	    Methods to implement the objectives
	    Resources needed to accomplish each objective

Intermediate action	• Ensure that all plans are implemented. • Hold frequent update briefings with section chiefs at designated times. • Communicate with the hospital board of directors and chairpersons. • Routinely update current action plans. • Identify successors for yourself and all section chiefs. Effectiveness diminishes with shifts longer than 12 hours. • Remind section chiefs to monitor workers for signs of stress or ineffective action. Use your critical incident stress management team. • Ensure that the action plan minimizes disruption of ongoing hospital functions. • Establish a system of communication with all emergency workers to reduce stress and control rumors.
Extended activities	• Direct all action plans toward ultimately returning the hospital to normal business functions. • As the incident matures, decrease the frequency of staff briefings and allow section chiefs to supervise their direct reports more thoroughly. • Remember that this emergency probably is affecting the entire community and your colleagues and their family members. Anticipate team stress.

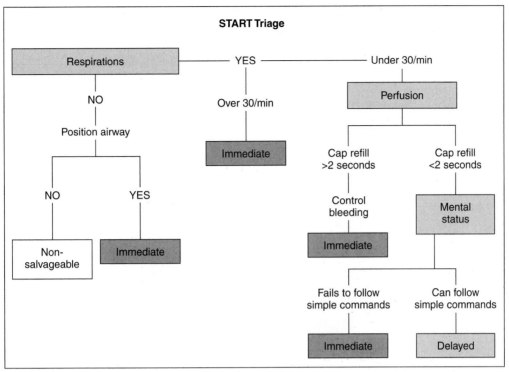

Figure 5-2. START (Simple Triage and Rapid Treatment) system. (Courtesy Newport Beach Fire Department and Hoag Memorial Hospital Presbyterian, Newport Beach, Calif.)

emergency department staff can stabilize and treat. As a rule of thumb, 10% of MCI patients will require immediate surgical intervention. Accept 10 casualties if you have only one trauma surgeon, take 20 victims if you have two surgical teams available, and so on following the 10:1 ratio.

RECOVERY

Hospital planning for disaster recovery begins well before the event occurs. Elements for consideration include the following[1]:
- A process for inventory and rapid resupply
- Incorporation of disaster records into the regular medical record
- Disposal of garbage and other waste
- Restoration of the physical plant (emergency department and other affected areas)
- Critical incident stress management
- Employee assistance programs
- Family support services

JumpSTART Pediatric Mass Casualty Incident Triage©

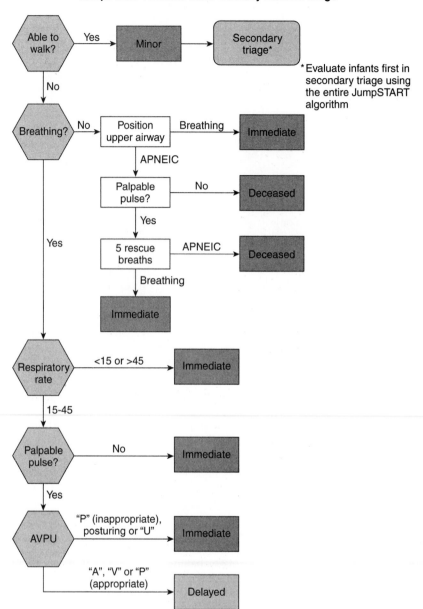

Figure 5-3. JumpSTART pediatric mass casualty incident triage. *AVPU,* Alert, responds to verbal stimuli, responds to painful stimuli, unresponsive. (Courtesy Lou Romig, MD, 2002.)

Combined START/JumpSTART Triage Algorithm

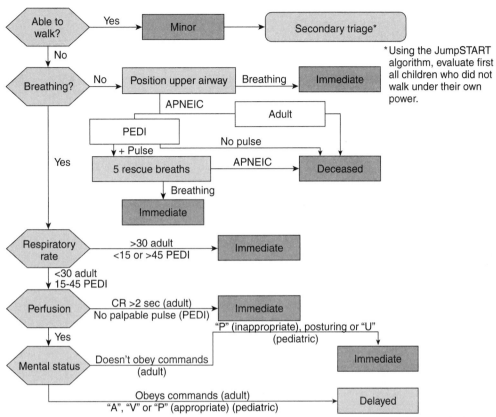

Figure 5-4. Combined START/JumpSTART triage algorithm. *AVPU,* Alert, responds to verbal stimuli, responds to painful stimuli, unresponsive. (Courtesy Lou Romig, MD, 2002.)

References

1. Centers for Disease Control and Prevention: Mass trauma. Retrieved September 1, 2004, from www.bt.cdc.gov.
2. Hirshberg A, Holcomb JB, Mattox KL: Hospital trauma care in multiple-casualty incidents: a critical view, *Ann Emerg Med* 37(6):647-652, 2001.

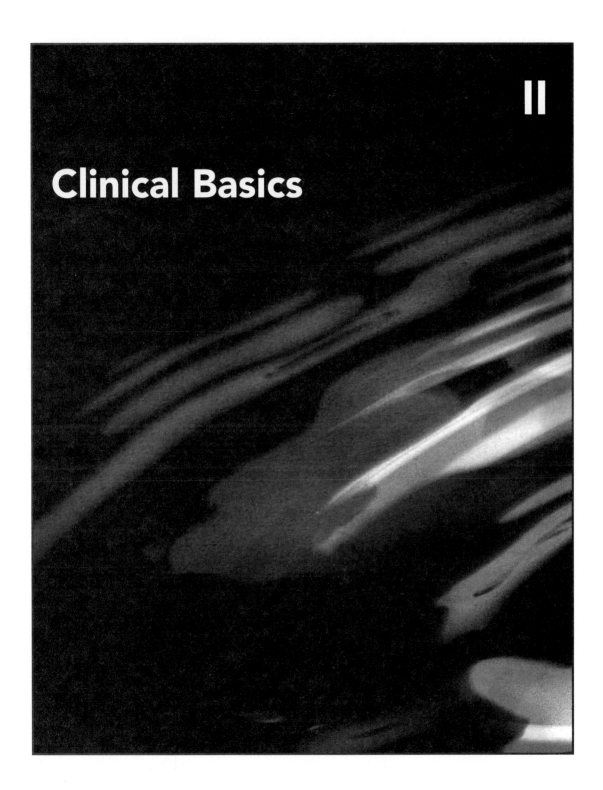

II

Clinical Basics

6

Triage

Nicki Gilboy, RN, MS, CEN

The triage process is an essential component of safe emergency care. Triage involves the rapid sorting of patients who present to the emergency department (ED) to distinguish those who need immediate medical attention from patients who can wait safely to be seen. This process requires the skills of an experienced emergency nurse. The triage concept sounds simple in theory but in practice is actually quite complex.

In today's busy ED, the triage function has become even more critical. The number of persons seeking medical care in EDs grew by 14% between 1997 and 2000.[1] The National Hospital Ambulatory Care Medical Survey, Emergency Department Summary, estimated that 110.2 million visits were made to U.S. emergency departments in 2002.[2] This number is expected to continue to rise in light of the aging population, the number of uninsured patients, and issues surrounding access to primary care. According to the American Hospital Association,[3] 62% of all EDs surveyed indicated they consistently functioned at or above capacity. In 2002 the Joint Commission on Accreditation of Healthcare Organizations[4] (JCAHO) released a sentinel event alert. The JCAHO identified EDs as the location for more than half of all reported sentinel events involving patient death or permanent disability because of delays in treatment. In nearly one third of these occurrences, overcrowding was deemed to be a contributing factor. Given this environment, triage is crucial to the smooth running of an ED. An effective triage process facilitates patient flow through the emergency care system while ensuring that those with the greatest need receive immediate attention.

The word triage comes from the French word *trier*, which means to sort or choose. Today, hospital triage refers to the quick sorting of patients who present to the ED for care. The purpose of triage is to put the right person in the right place at the right time for the right reason. The triage concept has been used since Napoleonic times when soldiers wounded in battle were sorted according to injury severity. Those with mortal wounds were separated from combatants who potentially could be saved. The goal of rapid treatment was to maximize survival and return as many soldiers as possible to the battlefield. The triage concept is still in use in the military and has since become a standard part of civilian ED operations.

In the late 1950s and early 1960s, health care delivery models in the United States changed dramatically. Physicians moved away from independent practices and formed office-based practice groups with regular clinic hours. Instead of house calls, patients now were seen by appointment. At the same time a nationwide move toward medical specialization had begun, leaving fewer doctors available for primary care. Hospitals too were evolving. As a result of advances in diagnostic technology and the introduction of intensive care units, hospitals assumed a new role, becoming 24-hour-a-day medical resources rather than just a place to stay when seriously ill. With the growth of hospital-based services, EDs began to deal with an onslaught of patients, many with nonurgent complaints. The practice of seeing patients on a first-come, first-served basis rapidly became outmoded and severity-based triage systems were developed.

TRIAGE SYSTEMS

Currently, most U.S. EDs use some type of triage system. Thompson and Dains[5] identified three basic types. These systems differ along a number of key dimensions, including the following:
- Triage severity rating systems
- Staffing
- The degree of assessment, reassessment, and documentation
- The extent to which triage staff initiate diagnostic and therapeutic interventions

As part of the 2001 Emergency Nurses Association (ENA) Benchmarking Survey,[6] EDs were asked to identify the type of triage system in place in their facility (Table 6-1).

Type I

Type I, nonnurse, or "traffic director" triage is the most basic system. A receptionist or allied health provider greets the patient, establishes the presenting complaint, and based on this face-to-face contact, makes a decision as to whether the patient is "sick" or "not sick." Those classified as sick are taken to the treatment area and are seen promptly. In type I triage systems, documentation is minimal and may include only patient name and chief complaint. The principal drawback of this approach to triage is that it places a nonprofessional in the position of gatekeeper, making it possible for low-volume, high-risk patient presentations to go unrecognized. This type of system does not conform to ENA Standards of Emergency Nursing Practice.

Table 6-1   **Survey of Triage Types in Use**

Triage System Used	Percent of Respondents
No triage system	5.1%
Type 1, nonnurse, traffic director	3.7%
Type II, spot check	23.5%
Type III, comprehensive	63.1%
Other systems	1.1%
Did not respond	3.6%

Response received from 1380 emergency departments. Data from the Emergency Nurses Association *National Benchmark Guide (2001)* survey of emergency departments.[6]

Type II

In a type II triage system a registered nurse (RN) or physician performs a spot check. The patient presents to triage, and a professional simply takes a quick look. Limited subjective and objective information related to the chief complaint is obtained. Based on this brief encounter, the patient is assigned to one of three levels: emergent, urgent, or nonurgent. Hospitals using this type of system need to have triage protocols and documentation standards in place to guide the process. This approach is appropriate in low-volume EDs where it is not cost-effective to staff a triage area 24 hours a day.

Type III

Comprehensive triage (type III) is the most advanced system and offers many advantages over other triage methodologies (see Box 6-1). Type III is the process recommended by the ENA Standards of Emergency Nursing Practice. "The emergency department RN triages each patient and determines the priority of care based on physical, developmental, and psychosocial needs as well as factors influencing access to health care and patient flow through the emergency care system."[7] The backbone of this approach is the experienced emergency nurse who has completed a competency-based triage orientation process. Comprehensive triage systems have policies, procedures, and protocols (or standards) in place to serve as guidelines. The assessment process involves collecting the chief complaint and any other relevant subjective or objective information. The goal of the comprehensive triage assessment is to gather sufficient information to support a triage severity rating decision. Ratings will vary depending on whether the institution is using a three-, four-, or five-level system. The triage nurse documents initial findings in the medical record and reassesses patients according to individual needs and departmental policy. The ENA recommends that the triage encounter take no more than 2 to 5 minutes.

Two-Tiered Triage Systems

In an ideal world, every patient would receive a comprehensive triage assessment within minutes of arrival at the ED. However, because of high patient volumes, many facilities have recognized that this goal cannot be achieved and instead have adopted a two-tiered system. With this approach the triage process is broken down into steps. First, an experienced triage

---

Box **6-1** **Advantages of Comprehensive Triage**

An experienced emergency registered nurse greets the patient.
Patients in need of immediate care are identified quickly.
A knowledgeable professional performs an assessment.
Immediate reassurance is provided to the patient and the family.
First aid and comfort measures are initiated as needed.
The patient, family, and visitors can be informed about emergency department processes.
During the assessment, the registered nurse has an opportunity for patient teaching.
The registered nurse decides which area of the emergency department is most suitable for the
 patient.
If protocols are in place, medications for fever, pain relief, and tetanus prophylaxis may be
 administered.
Registered nurses may initiate laboratory work and order radiographs based on triage guidelines.
Waiting patients are reassessed regularly according to departmental policy.
A strong communication link is maintained between the triage area and the treatment area.

Modified from Buschiazzo L: *The handbook of emergency nursing management,* New York, 1987, Aspen.

nurse greets the patient and determines the chief complaint while simultaneously conducting a brief assessment of airway, breathing, and circulatory status. This nurse decides whether the patient needs to be seen immediately or can wait safely for further assessment and registration. Patients who require immediate care are taken to the treatment area and are registered at the bedside. Stable patients have a patient chart initiated by the first nurse, who documents chief complaint and then directs these patients to the assessment nurse. This second nurse completes a more detailed (but focused) evaluation and may initiate laboratory work and radiographic studies according to protocols.

A two-tiered system has several advantages. In overcrowded EDs there is legitimate concern that patients who present to the ED with a serious or life-threatening complaint will have to wait to be seen by the triage nurse. The two-tier system virtually eliminates that possibility by immediately identifying patients who require emergent care. Additionally, the first triage nurse will know every patient in the waiting room and can keep an eye on them. This nurse also can answer any questions, address changes in patient status, and perform reassessments as appropriate. The detailed assessment performed by the second triage nurse builds on the rapid initial assessment. If the patient omitted vital information, the triage decision can always be changed.

TRIAGE SEVERITY RATING SYSTEMS

Several different triage severity rating systems are described in the literature and are used in various parts of the world. Each system has unique features that are described briefly later. The type of rating system selected by an ED has significant implications for how the department operates and the quality and quantity of information obtained. The rating system chosen needs to be simple to use and easily understood by all members of the health care team.

Triage severity rating systems are evaluated along several dimensions; two important considerations are validity and reliability. Validity refers to the accuracy of the triage rating system. How well does it measure what it is intended to measure? Do the different triage levels truly reflect differences in severity?

Reliability is another important characteristic of a triage severity system. This refers to the degree of consistency (or agreement) among those using the method. Will different triage nurses assign the same patient the same severity level? Over time, will each triage nurse consistently assign similar patients the same severity level? Importantly, criteria for each triage level need to remain constant. A patient's assigned severity rating cannot vary simply because the department is busy or a particular nurse is performing triage.

A triage rating system serves as more than just a means of scoring an individual's severity of condition; it becomes a language, a precise shorthand, for communicating patient severity to the ED as a whole. If triage data is collected accurately and consistently, an ED can use this information to analyze and trend various patient outcomes such as ED length of stay and hospitalization rates. Reliable data also makes it possible to compare different EDs.

Two-Level Triage

Hospitals in the United States use two-, three-, four-, or five-level triage severity rating systems.[6] In a two-level system the patient is merely designated "sick" or "not sick." The sick patient is in need of urgent care with a condition that is potentially a threat to life, limb, or organ. "Not sick" patients are those with no evidence of immediate jeopardy, who will not be compromised if care is delayed.

Three-Level Triage

Three-level triage systems are the most common in the United States. Sometimes categories are identified by colors (e.g., red, yellow, and green) or they are numbered (Category I to III), but they basically refer to the following levels:

- *Emergent:* The patient requires immediate care. The presenting problem is a threat to life, limb, or organ. Examples are cardiac arrest, major trauma, and respiratory failure. A team response is needed, and reassessment is continuous.
- *Urgent:* The patient requires prompt care, but the patient may wait safely several hours if necessary. Examples are abdominal pain, fractured hip, and renal calculi. Recommended reassessment time is every 30 minutes.
- *Nonurgent:* The patient needs to be seen, but time is not critical and the patient can wait safely. Examples are sore throat, rash, and conjunctivitis. Recommended reassessment time is every 1 to 2 hours.

Unfortunately, several studies have demonstrated poor interrater (between different raters) and intrarater (the same rater on another occasion) reliability with three-level triage severity rating systems.[8-10] This is largely because no universal definition of each level exist. Various institutions and individual nurses use different criteria to assign patients to the three categories.

Four-Level Triage

In an attempt to break down further the large number of patients who fall into the emergent category, some hospitals have moved to a four-level triage system by adding life-threatening to the emergent, urgent, and nonurgent list.

Five-Level Triage

A current movement in the United States is to adopt a uniform, nationwide, five-level triage system. In 2003 a joint Triage Task Force composed of representatives from the American College of Emergency Physicians and the ENA, developed a policy that was approved by the boards of both organizations. "ACEP and ENA believe that quality patient care would benefit from implementing a standardized emergency department triage scale and acuity categorization process. Based on expert consensus of currently available evidence, ACEP and ENA support the adoption of a reliable, valid, 5-level triage scale."[11] This is the first step toward implementation of a uniform patient severity measure in U.S. emergency departments.

Currently, four research-based, five-level triage severity rating scales are in use. In each, level 1 represents the highest severity (most acute), whereas level 5 is used to designate the patients with the least acute conditions.

The Australasian Triage Scale

The Australian emergency medical community adopted the Australasian Triage Scale in 1993 (Table 6-2). Based on research and expert consensus, each category lists clinical descriptors or conditions that correspond to a specific severity level. Objective time frames for physician evaluation are set for each classification. This "time to treatment" is the maximum interval a patient should expect to wait for further assessment and medical intervention. The clock starts when a patient first presents to the ED. The triage nurse selects an Australasian Triage Scale category in response to the statement "This patient should wait for medical assessment and treatment no longer than ..."[12] Vital signs are obtained only if they will assist with making the triage severity decision. Performance thresholds are set for each level and

Table 6-2   **Australasian Triage and Acuity Scale**

	Level	Time to Treatment	Performance Threshold Percent
1	Immediately life threatening	Immediate	100
2	Imminently life threatening	10 min	80
3	Potentially life threatening	30 min	75
4	Potentially serious	60 min	70
5	Less urgent	120 min	70

From Australasian College for Emergency Medicine: *The Australasian Triage Scale (ATS)*. Retrieved July 17, 2002, from http://www.acem.org.au/open/documents/triage.htm.

Table 6-3   **Canadian Triage and Acuity Scale**

	Name	Time to RN	Time to MD	Fractile Response
1	Resuscitation	Immediate	Immediate	98%
2	Emergent	Immediate	<15 min	95%
3	Urgent	<30 min	<30 min	90%
4	Less urgent	<60 min	<60 min	85%
5	Nonurgent	<120 min	<120 min	80%

From Beveridge R et al: Canadian emergency department triage and acuity scale: implementation guidelines, *Can J Emerg Med* 1 (suppl 3):2-24, 1999.
RN, Registered nurse; *MD*, medical doctor.

indicate what percent of the time the ED must comply with time-to-treatment goals. Research has shown the Australasian Triage Scale to be valid and reliable.[13,14] In addition to assigning individual patient severity of condition, this scale has been used to examine case mix and to relate triage levels directly to common outcome measures such as ED length of stay, intensive care unit admission, and resource consumption.

The Canadian Triage and Acuity Scale

A group of Canadian emergency physicians developed the five-level Canadian Triage and Acuity Scale based on the Australasian system (Table 6-3).[15] Working with the National Emergency Nurses Association, the tool was adopted as the countrywide standard and has become part of the ED data regularly reported to the Canadian government. Each triage level is associated with a representative list of presenting complaints. Examples of conditions triaged as level 1 include cardiac arrest, major trauma, and severe respiratory distress. On the other end of the scale, a level 5 is assigned to patients in no acute distress with conditions such as simple sprains or strains. Triage nurses are encouraged to use their experience and instinct to up-triage a patient if any doubt exists regarding severity.

Several studies have indicated that the Canadian Triage and Acuity Scale is valid and reliable.[16,17] Triage categories have been shown to correlate well with resource consumption, admission rates, and other markers of illness severity. As part of the triage process the nurse decides (1) how long this individual safely can wait before an RN performs a comprehensive primary assessment and (2) how long the patient can wait to see a physician and begin treatment.[18] Answers to these questions determine severity level. Fractile response rates are defined for each level. These rates represent the frequency with which the department must meet the criteria for nurse and physician response times.

Table 6-4   The Manchester Triage Scale

Number	Name	Color	Target Time
1	Immediate	Red	0
2	Very urgent	Orange	10 min
3	Urgent	Yellow	60 min
4	Standard	Green	120 min
5	Nonurgent	Blue	240 min

From Manchester Triage Group: *Emergency triage*, Plymouth, 1997, BMJ Publishing Group.

The Manchester Triage Scale

The Manchester triage scale was developed in England by a group of emergency nurses and physicians who created a detailed, flowchart-based system. Each triage level is given a name, number, and color code that identifies the target time frame for a patient to see a treating clinician (Table 6-4).[19] Based on the presenting complaint, the triage nurse chooses from 52 different flowcharts. To arrive at a triage level decision, the nurse follows the flowchart, asking about signs and symptoms (or discriminators). A positive answer to a discriminator determines the severity rating. Documentation consists of simply identifying the presentational flowchart used, which discriminator defined the triage score, and the associated triage level.

The Emergency Severity Index

Two U.S. emergency physicians working with a team of emergency physicians and nurses created the emergency severity index.[20] This research-based, five-level scale categorizes patients by severity and expected resource consumption (Figure 6-1). *Severity* is defined as the stability of vital functions and the potential for life, limb, or organ threat. *Resource consumption,* a component unique to the emergency severity index, is defined as the number of different resources a patient is expected to consume before ED disposition. The experienced emergency nurse is capable of estimating resource consumption based on previous, similar patient encounters.

Like other five-level systems, research has demonstrated that the emergency severity index is valid and reliable.[21,22] The system itself consists of an easy-to-use algorithm designed to sort patients rapidly into one of five mutually exclusive categories. Emergency severity index triage requires the nurse to start at the top of the algorithm and assess whether the patient is intubated, apneic, pulseless, or unresponsive. If the answer is "yes," the patient is assigned an emergency severity index level 1. If "no," the triage nurse moves to the next level of the algorithm and determines whether the patient is high risk, lethargic, confused, disoriented, in severe pain, or in distress. Answering "yes" to any of these questions places the patient in level 2. A "no" directs the triage nurse to address the patient's chief complaint. Based on emergency nursing experience, the triage nurse estimates the number of resources the patient is likely to consume in order for a disposition to be reached. A patient who requires an examination or a prescription, but no other resources, meets the criteria for emergency severity index level 5. Needing one resource places the patient in level 4. If two or more resources are required, the triage nurse considers the patient's vital signs and decides whether they are acceptable. Vital signs that fall outside age-appropriate parameters suggest that the nurse consider up-triaging the patient to emergency severity index level 2. If the nurse is satisfied with current vital signs, the patient may remain at level 3.

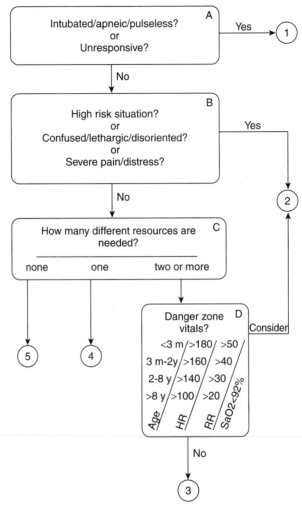

Figure 6-1. Emergency severity index.[19] *HR,* Heart rate; *RR,* respiratory rate; SaO₂, oxygen saturation in arterial blood. (ESI version 3. Copyright 1999-2001. David R Eitel, MD, MBA, and Richard C Wuerz, MD.)

THE TRIAGE PROCESS

The triage assessment should be timely and brief. The purpose of this process is to gather sufficient information about the patient to make a triage severity rating decision. The goal should be for all patients to receive an initial triage assessment within 5 minutes of arrival to the ED. Ideally, triage begins with an across-the-room assessment and then continues in the privacy of the triage booth or room. If at any time the triage nurse identifies a life-threatening airway, breathing, or circulatory problem, the nurse initiates appropriate interventions are initiated immediately, and the patient is transferred to a care area.

Across-the-Room Assessment

Initial assessment begins when the triage nurse first sees the patient; the nurse should observe closely, listen for abnormal sounds, and be aware of any odors. The experienced triage nurse

Table 6-5   **The Pediatric Assessment Triangle**

Appearance	Muscle Tone
	Intractability/consolability
	Look or gaze
	Speech or crying
Work of breathing	Nasal flaring
	Retractions
	Abnormal airway sounds
	Position of comfort
	Altered respiratory rate
Circulation or skin	Pallor
	Mottling
	Cyanosis

From Emergency Nurses Association: *ENPC provider manual,* Des Plaines, Ill, 2004, The Association.

Table 6-6   **Across-the-Room Assessment**

Sense	*Findings*
Observe	Airway patency
	Respiratory rate, obvious distress, use of O_2 devices
	Signs of external bleeding
	Level of consciousness: interacting, unconscious, crying, moaning
	Signs of pain: grimacing, holding, guarding
	Skin color and condition
	Chronic illness: cancer, chronic obstructive pulmonary disease, neuromuscular disorders
	Deformities
	Body habitus: cachectic, morbidly obese
	Activity: ability to ambulate, balance, bear weight
	General behavior: agitated, angry, flat affect
	Presence of splints, dressings, casts, medical equipment
	Clothing: clean, appropriate
Listen	Abnormal airway sounds
	Speech pattern, tone of voice, language
	Interactions with others
Smell	Stool, urine, vomit, ketones, alcohol
	Poor hygiene, cigarettes, infection, chemicals

From Emergency Nurses Association: *ENPC provider manual,* Des Plaines, Ill, 2004, The Association.

can take one look at a patient and, based on general appearance, decide whether immediate care is required. In such cases, triage is considered complete, and the patient is taken directly to a treatment room. If the patient is stable, the triage process continues. The Emergency Nursing Pediatric Course refers to this quick once-over glance as the pediatric assessment triangle (Table 6-5).[23] Table 6-6 lists information that can be obtained from an across-the-room assessment.

The Triage Interview

The triage interview begins with the nurse introducing himself or herself and briefly describing the triage role. During this short interview, the nurse determines the chief complaint and history of the present injury or illness. Based on findings, the nurse conducts a focused assessment of the problem and measures vital signs per protocol. The nurse derives a triage severity level from this information. Next, the patient either goes immediately to a room for treatment and bedside registration or is directed first to the registration area and then to the waiting room.

The initial greeting by a triage nurse can set the tone for the whole ED visit. Although the experienced nurse may view an illness or injury as minor, patients can be stressed and may consider the situation a crisis. Nurses need to be nonjudgmental and empathetic. A few kind words such as "I bet that really hurts" or "You don't look like you feel very well today" can have a positive impact. Patients and their families may feel greatly relieved merely because a professional is now involved in their care. Triage nurses must possess strong interpersonal skills, respond tactfully to questions, and be able to allay anxiety with information and reassurance.

A crucial triage skill is the ability to multitask. Obtaining all necessary triage information, within the 2- to 5-minute time frame recommended by the ENA, requires skill, and every second must be used efficiently. Nonetheless, a 1999 study by Travers[24] (at one tertiary care center) demonstrated that this 5-minute goal was achieved only 22% of the time. Triaging geriatric and pediatric patients tends to take even longer.

Gathering vital information is critical for making appropriate triage decisions. However, to communicate accurately, the nurse and patient need to speak a common language. In some hospitals, medical interpreters are available for non–English-speaking patients. If no interpreter is immediately accessible, family members or others may be used for initial triage; however, this practice is discouraged. AT&T offers interpreter services via telephone. However, this service and those of paid translators tend to be costly. Triage documentation should make reference to the use of an interpreter.

The objective of the triage interview is to establish the chief complaint, obtain a description of relevant signs and symptoms, perform a targeted history and examination, and assign a patient severity rating. The first question asked of patients usually relates to the reason the patient came to the ED. Open-ended questions such as "How can we help you?" or "What seems to be the problem today?" can elicit this information. The chief complaint should be documented in the patient's own words. If the patient identifies several issues, the triage nurse needs to focus the patient to determine the proximate reason for the ED visit. Patients who recite a whole list of medical ailments can be asked, "What is different now?" or "What was it that made you decide to come in today?" When a patient is transported by ambulance, much of the triage information can be obtained from prehospital providers, but it is important to acknowledge the patient and to verify information.

Pediatric triage can be especially challenging. The nurse needs to keep in mind the developmental level of the patient and should tailor the assessment accordingly. For the younger child, the chief complaint and subjective data must be obtained from a caregiver. Older children and adolescents may be able to supply information personally. The Emergency Nursing Pediatric Course uses the mnemonic CIAMPEDS to describe the components of the pediatric assessment (Table 6-7).[23] Family members and caregivers also can be invaluable when triaging elderly individuals.

Multiple tools are available to assist nurses with gathering data relative to the patient's chief complaint. The W questions[25] (Table 6-8) and the PQRST pain mnemonic (see Table 7-5 in Chapter 7) are two systematic approaches frequently used by emergency nurses. If the patient arrives with a traumatic injury, obtain and document data regarding the mechanism and pattern of injury (Table 6-9).

Once the nurse has obtained sufficient information about the chief complaint, the focus shifts to a brief medical history. The mnemonic AMPLE (see Box 7-1 in Chapter 7) can be used to guide questioning.

Triage Vital Signs

The role of obtaining vital signs at triage is controversial and is clearly an area that warrants further research. The triage policy of each ED should address when and whether vital

Table 6-7   **CIAMPEDS**

	Mnemonic	*Assessment Component*
C	Chief complaint	Determine reason for the child's visit to emergency department and duration of complaint (e.g., fever for past 2 days).
I	Immunizations	Evaluate the child's current immunization status. • The completion of all scheduled immunizations for the child's age should be evaluated. • If the child has not received immunizations because of religious or cultural beliefs, document this information.
	Isolation	Evaluation of the child's exposure to communicable diseases (e.g., meningitis, chickenpox, shingles, whooping cough, and tuberculosis). • A child with active disease or who is potentially infectious must be placed in respiratory isolation on arrival to the emergency department. • Other exposures that may be evaluated include exposure to meningitis and scabies.
A	Allergies	Evaluate the child's previous allergic or hypersensitivity reactions. Document reactions to medications, foods, products (e.g., latex) and environmental allergens. The type of reaction also must be documented.
M	Medications	Evaluate the child's current medication regimen, including prescription and over-the-counter medications and herbal and dietary supplements: • Dose administered • Time of last dose • Duration of use
P	Past medical history	Review the child's health status, including prior illnesses, injuries, hospitalizations, surgeries, and chronic physical and psychiatric illnesses. Evaluate use of alcohol, tobacco, drugs, or other substances of abuse, as appropriate. The medical history of the neonate should include the prenatal and birth history: • Maternal complications during pregnancy or delivery • Infant's gestational age and birth weight • Number of days infant remained in hospital after birth The medical history of the menarche female should include the date and description of her last menstrual period. The medical history for sexually active patients should include the following: • Type of birth control used • Barrier protection • Prior treatment for sexually transmitted diseases • Gravida (pregnancies) and para (births, miscarriages, abortions, living children)
	Parent's/caregivers' impression of the child's condition	Identify the child's primary caregiver. • Consider cultural differences that may affect the caregiver's impressions. • Evaluate the caregiver's concerns and observations of the child's condition (especially significant in evaluating the special needs child).
E	Events surrounding the illness or injury	Evaluate the onset of the illness or circumstances and mechanism of injury. Illness • Length of illness, including date and day of onset and sequence of symptoms • Treatment provided before visit to emergency department Injury • Time and date injury occurred

Continued

Table 6-7   CIAMPEDS—cont'd

Mnemonic		Assessment Component
		• *M:* Mechanism of injury, including the use of protective devices (seat belts, helmets)
		• *I:* Injuries suspected
		• *V:* Vital signs in prehospital environment
		• *T:* Treatment by prehospital providers
		• Description of circumstances leading to injury
		• Witnessed or unwitnessed
D	Diet	Assess the child's recent oral intake and changes in eating patterns related to the illness or injury:
		• Changes in eating patterns or fluid intake
		• Time of last meal and last fluid intake
		• Usual diet: breast milk, type of formula, solid foods, diet for age and developmental level, cultural differences
		• Special diet or diet restrictions
	Diapers	Assess the child's urine and stool output:
		• Frequency of urination over last 24 hours; changes in frequency
		• Time of last void
		• Changes in color or color of urine
		• Last bowel movement; color and consistency of stool
		• Change in frequency of bowel movements
S	Symptoms associated with the illness or injury	Identify symptoms and progression of symptoms since the time of onset of the illness or injury event

From Emergency Nurses Association: *ENPC Provider Manual,* ed 3, Des Plaines, Ill, 2004, The Association.

Table 6-8   The Who, What, Where, When, Why, and How Questions

Question	Information Sought
Who	Patient demographics
What	Chief complaint
Where	Location of the problem and any associated symptoms
When	Time of symptom onset
Why	Precipitating events or factors
How	How symptoms affect normal function and how much

From National Nurses in Business: *Emergency nursing bible,* ed 2, Rocklege, Fla, The Association.

Table 6-9   Guidelines for Triaging an Injury

Mechanism of Injury	Triage Questions
Motor vehicle collision	Speed of the vehicle; direction of impact; patient position within the vehicle; use of restraints; airbag deployment; ejection; rollover; fatalities; ambulatory at the scene; entrapment/prolonged extrication
Penetrating injury	Type of object (knife, bullet, impaled object); left in place, removed, broken off
Fall	From how high; landed on which body part(s); what kind of landing surface; why the patient fell
Motorcycle crash	Impact speed; helmet use; other protective clothing; thrown, skidded, pinned, or run over; position of patient relative to the motorcycle
Bicycle crash	Helmet use; collided with a vehicle or object; thrown or run over; impact speed; landed on which body part(s)

From Emergency Nurses Association: *ENPC Provider Manual,* Des Plaines, Ill, 2004, The Association.

signs need to be measured. Care of the emergent patient should never be delayed to obtain vital signs at triage. Many departments have chosen to assess vital signs on all lower-severity patients to collect data to support the assigned severity rating. Cooper et al.[26] studied more than 14,000 patients and concluded that vital signs were an important part of the triage decision process in certain vulnerable populations: individuals with communication problems, those less than 2 years of age, and the elderly. Regardless of the severity rating system used, vital signs outside of age-appropriate parameters can be used to justify up-triaging a patient.

Objective Data

The triage nurse performs a focused physical assessment related to the patient's chief complaint. This physical examination is limited not only in purpose but also by time, space, and privacy constraints. Inspection, palpation, and (occasionally) auscultation can be used to gather information related to the chief complaint. The triage nurse must remove dressings from wounds to assess and document the actual extent of injury. Table 6-10 addresses the focused physical assessment at triage. Assess only parameters pertinent to the chief complaint or patient presentation; this is not a system-by-system or head-to-toe examination.

Triage Severity Rating

Based on the chief complaint and on subjective and objective data, triage nurses use their knowledge, experience, and triage guidelines to assign a severity rating. This decision will be derived logically from the information obtained. The triage decision has a major impact on patient outcomes and patient safety. Undertriaged patients receive delayed care and risk deterioration. The patient who is overtriaged diverts valuable resources away from those who need them the most. (See the preceding section on triage severity rating systems for a detailed discussion of various types.)

Limited first aid may be rendered at some point during the triage process to decrease pain and promote comfort. This treatment may include dressing a wound, splinting potential or obvious fractures, applying ice, elevating affected extremities, and controlling bleeding. Once a severity rating is determined, radiographic and laboratory studies also can be initiated (per protocol). Some triage protocols include the administration of medications for fever control, pain management, and tetanus prophylaxis. Be sure to reassess patients if analgesics or antipyretics are administered.

Safety and Security

The incidence of physical assault on ED nursing staff is increasing.[27] Factors that contribute to ED violence are overcrowding, long wait times, large numbers of psychiatric patients, and violent gangs.[28] Knowledge of what safety measures are in place in the department is essential for the triage staff. These measures may include panic buttons, restricted access doors, security cameras, and visible security guards or police officers. The triage nurse should keep one eye on the waiting room constantly, checking for situations in which the behavior of patients, families, or visitors is escalating. While conducting a triage patient interview, the nurse also must be alert for signs of agitation and potential for violence. Objective indicators of increasing agitation include a piercing stare, pacing, fist clenching, talking rapidly, and using language that is loud or abusive. In such situations it is important to trust your instincts. If a patient makes you uncomfortable, stop the interview, exit the triage booth, and seek assistance. Triage nurses should not place themselves or others at risk, nor should they allow themselves to become the target of aggressive verbal or physical behavior. Often the presence of one or more security guards will deescalate the situation. Triage nurses need to be

Table 6-10   **Focused Physical Assessment at Triage**

System	Assessment Parameter
Respiratory/cardiac	Respiratory rate, rhythm, depth
	Work of breathing; accessory muscle use
	Skin color, temperature, moisture, turgor, mucous membrane status
	Oxygen saturation; peak expiratory flow rate
	Peripheral edema
	Breath sounds
	Position of comfort
	Chest excursion
	Level of consciousness
Gastrointestinal/genitourinary	Abdominal distention, tenderness, rigidity, scars, bruising
Musculoskeletal	Circulation, sensation
(Compare side to side)	Motor function, strength
	Deformity, wounds
	Edema, discoloration
Endocrine	Skin color, turgor; mucous membrane status
	Fingerstick blood glucose
	Level of consciousness
Neurologic	Facial symmetry, droop, ptosis, drooling
	Grip strength, pronator drift
	Speech clarity and articulation
	Level of consciousness
	Behavior
	Pupils size, shape, equality, response to light
	Motor function/sensation in all extremities
	Glasgow Coma Scale score; mental status
	Fingerstick blood glucose
	Oxygen saturation
Psychiatric	Appearance; grooming
	Speech
	Affect
	Behavior: bizarre, appropriate
	Thought content and process
	Memory; orientation
	Potential for danger to self or others
Skin	Description of wounds: size, location, depth, cause, age, bleeding
	Contamination; foreign body
	Signs of infection: general or local
	Rashes, bites, stings, other lesions
Eye	Inflammation, drainage, trauma, foreign body, tearing, photophobia
	Visual acuity: Snellen eye chart, light/dark, shapes

able to identify psychiatric patients who cannot remain safely in the waiting room and need to be escorted directly to a secure room in the treatment area.

Triage Documentation

Triage assessment documentation should be clear, concise, and support the assigned severity rating. Each hospital needs to have a triage policy that includes documentation requirements. Usually a specific area on the patient chart exists for the nurse to record triage findings. This section of the medical record often consists of pick lists or check boxes, or it simply may be a space for narrative notes. Several computerized software programs are available for ED triage; however, further description is beyond the scope of this text. Whether computerized or on paper, the same basic elements usually are required. Information to include in triage documentation can be found in Box 6-2.

In departments that rely on narrative notes, the SOAPIE documentation format may be helpful:

S or *subjective assessment,* is brief and should include pertinent negatives (e.g., denies chest pain, no vomiting).

O is for *objective assessment,* a quick, focused physical examination.

A is for *analysis of data,* which includes the assigned severity rating and the nursing diagnosis.

P is the *plan of care.*

I is for *implementation;* the care provided at triage includes diagnostic tests, first aid, or initiation of infection control procedures.

E is for *evaluation* or reassessment. Any response to interventions or changes in the patient's status would be noted under E.

Each ED needs to decide whether mandated screening assessments (e.g., barriers to learning, nutritional needs, or domestic violence) will be completed at triage or as part of the patient's bedside assessment.

Emergency Medical Treatment and Active Labor Act

The Emergency Medical Treatment and Active Labor Act (EMTALA) has had a profound impact on EDs. The act is a federal law, originally passed in 1985 in an effort to stop hospitals from "dumping" nonpaying patients on another facility. The act came about in response to reports of patients being refused care at an ED or being transferred to another facility before

---

Box **6-2** **Elements of Triage Documentation**

Date and time of arrival at the emergency department
Patient age
Triage interview time
Allergies (medications, food, latex)
Current medications (prescription, over-the-counter, supplements)
Triage severity rating
Vital signs
First aid measures
Reassessment(s)
Assessment of pain
Chief complaint
History of current complaint
Subjective and objective assessment
Significant medical history
Last menstrual period
Last tetanus immunization
Diagnostic testing initiated
Medications administered at triage
Signature of registered nurse
Consider including the following:
  Mode of arrival
  Use of an interpreter

receiving appropriate emergency treatment. Laws now mandate that all persons presenting to an ED that receives federal funding must be given a medical screening examination to determine whether an emergency exists. If an emergency does exist, stabilizing care must be provided. The act has clear implications for the triage process. The U.S. Health Care Financing Administration has made it clear that the triage process is not the same thing as a medical screening examination. The purpose of triage is to identify severity and to determine the order in which patients will be seen. The medical screening examination is an individual patient assessment process (which may include diagnostic tests) designed to establish whether a medical emergency actually exists. Legally, RNs may perform medical screening examinations, but by protocol most facilities delegate this task to physicians, nurse practitioners, or physician's assistants. The triage nurse never accept a medical screening examination role without specific protocols and training.

Left Without Being Seen

In 2000 more than 1.8 million persons walked out of U.S. emergency departments without being seen by a licensed independent practitioner.[1] Emergency department overcrowding has contributed to this growing number. Patients who have been triaged and registered may have to wait for hours before they receive medical care; some prefer to leave. Hospitals must have policies and procedures in place to guide triage staff in such situations because EDs are responsible for documenting patient disposition. Patients, of course, have the right to leave, but the physician on duty should be notified in situations where the nurse feels a significant illness or injury exists that requires emergency care. Patients may or may not let the triage staff know that they are leaving. If they do, the triage nurse has an opportunity to discuss the situation. Incompetent patients can be stopped from leaving. Many EDs request that patients sign a form before departure. These forms document that the patient was offered a medical screening examination but preferred to leave before being seen. If a patient walks out of the department without notifying staff, the triage nurse should document the time it was first noted that the patient was no longer in the ED. Also, the nurse should document any efforts to locate the patient (e.g., "overhead paged × 3 with no response").

Joint Commission on Accreditation of Healthcare Organizations

The JCAHO has several standards applicable to the triage process. The JCAHO considers assessment a nursing function. Therefore triage should be performed by an RN and not by ancillary personnel. Each ED needs to have triage policies and procedures in place that include a system for assigning patient priority. Commission standards also address the issue of staff competency. How does the hospital know that a particular nurse is competent to triage patients? Does the hospital maintain records of orientation and competency validation?

The JCAHO acknowledges that the ED has become the safety net of the health care system, the only place that an individual is guaranteed access to health care. The commission also recognizes that the problem of ED overcrowding is not going away. To address these issues, the JCAHO Emergency Department Overcrowding Standard was adopted in 2004. This standard addresses ED overcrowding as part of a greater, hospital-wide problem and mandates a hospital-wide response.

Infection Control

The triage nurse must use standard infection control precautions in any situation where contact with blood or body fluids could occur. Hand cleansing between patients with soap and water or with a waterless alcohol-based hand sanitizer is essential to reduce the spread of infection. The ED is often the portal of entry for patients with contagious diseases. Therefore all patients should be screened with infection in mind. Any patient identified as potentially having a communicable condition must have the appropriate precautions initiated in order to prevent transmission to staff, patients, and visitors. The nurse should document initiation of infection control precautions in the medical record and provide the patient with an explanation as to why precautions are necessary.

If a patient shows signs of a potential contagion, it is important to inquire about recent foreign travel and to determine whether anyone else in the household has similar signs or symptoms. Once a patient with a suspected communicable condition is triaged, the triage area needs to be cleaned before the next patient enters. Table 6-11 lists suggested infectious disease precautions.

When a patient arrives in the triage area complaining of a cough, rash, or diarrhea, the nurse must always explore the possibility of an infectious cause. If a patient presents to triage with signs and symptoms consistent with exposure to a biologic (bioterrorism) agent, it is essential that the nurse recognize this immediately and initiate appropriate precautions to prevent further spread of the disease. Patients with a rash, fever, symptoms consistent with pneumonia, or neurologic symptoms should trigger further questioning. Table 13-1 (see Chapter 13) includes infection control procedures to be implemented in the event of possible exposure to a biological agent.[29]

The triage nurse also needs to identify patients who are severely immunocompromised. These individuals must be protected carefully from exposure to anyone with even a minor infectious process. Place an N-95 mask, or a surgical mask, on the patient and escort the patient to a positive-pressure room as quickly as possible.

TELEPHONE TRIAGE

Telephone triage is "the practice of performing a verbal interview and making an assessment of the health status of the caller."[30] Some organizations have well-established telephone triage programs with detailed protocols and trained telephone triage nurses. In such circumstances, telephone triage is appropriate. However, all EDs frequently receive calls from the public asking for general medical information, inquiring about what health care actions they should take, and seeking advice as to whether they should come to the ED. The ENA position statement on telephone advice clearly addresses this issue: nurses working in facilities with no established telephone triage program should not offer medical advice over the telephone. In extreme situations the triage nurse may instruct the caller in lifesaving techniques such as cardiopulmonary resuscitation and how to access the emergency medical system. In all other situations, the ENA recommends that callers be informed that the ED is open 24 hours a day and that services are available to anyone who wishes to be seen. Hospitals should have a written telephone advice policy.

TRIAGE QUALIFICATIONS

Rapid, accurate triage requires an emergency nurse with the right qualifications, education, and experience. The ENA recommends the following qualifications for any nurse who functions in a triage capacity[30-32]:
- RN, with a minimum of 6 months of emergency nursing experience
- Formal triage education with a supervised preceptorship

Table 6-11　Infectious Disease Precautions

Patient Symptoms	Initial Precautions During Triage	Possible Diagnoses	Final Precautions Following Assessment
Rash and fever	*AIRBORNE/CONTACT* Put surgical mask on patient. Place patient in a controlled airflow pressure room. If chickenpox is suspected, nonimmune staff should not enter the room. Gowns and gloves are required for anyone entering the room. If smallpox (variola) is possible, use an N-95 mask or powered air purifying respirator (PAPR) for all staff entering the room. Contact the infection control department immediately.	1. Chickenpox (varicella) 2. Measles (rubeola) 3. German measles (rubella) 4. Smallpox (variola)	1. Vesicular rash and lesions commonly occur in successive crops, with several stages of maturity evident at the same time; itching is possible; rash is more abundant on covered parts of the body (trunk); slight fever is common before rash. Only immune staff should not have patient contact. *Airborne/Contact Precautions* 2. Red, maculopapular rash; rhinorrhea; Koplik's spots on buccal mucosa. *Airborne Precautions* 3. Maculopapular rash, sometimes resembles measles or scarlet fever; low-grade fever, malaise, lymphadenopathy; upper respiratory symptoms and conjunctivitis usually precede rash. *Droplet Precautions* 4. Generalized rash with vesicles or pustules; high fever (≥104° F) 1-4 days before onset of rash; vesicles/pustules all in the same stage of development; rash starts on face, forearms, oral mucosa, or palate and spreads to trunk. *Airborne/Contact Precautions*
Headache, stiff neck, and fever	*DROPLET* Put surgical mask on patient. Place patient in a private room.	Meningitis	Viral vs. bacterial? Lumbar puncture can aid in the differential. 1. Viral *No Special Precautions Required* 2. Bacterial; consider meningococcal meningitis. *Droplet Precautions*

Cough and fever	*AIRBORNE* Put surgical mask on patient. Place patient in a negative air pressure room. If tuberculosis is possible, use N-95 respirator mask or PAPR for all staff entering the room.	1. Tuberculosis 2. Petussis (whooping cough) 3. Influenza (flu)	1. Night sweats, cough >2 weeks, weight loss (≥10 lb), history of exposure to tuberculosis *Airborne Precautions* 2. Starts with rhinorrhea, sneezing, and low-grade fever for 1-2 weeks, and then cough becomes more severe and persistent or paroxysmal. *Droplet Precautions* 3. High fever, headache, dry cough, nasal congestion, sore throat, muscle aches. (Usually during November-April "flu season") *Droplet Precautions*
Cough, fever, and history of possible exposure to severe acute respiratory syndrome (SARS)	*STRICT* Place surgical mask on patient. Put patient in a negative air pressure room. Use N-95 mask or PAPR, gown, gloves, and eye protection for anyone entering the room. Contact infection control immediately.	SARS	Consider this diagnosis if World Health Organization or Centers for Disease Control and Prevention report the occurrence of SARS and patient has had possible exposure to SARS. Upper respiratory symptoms with fever >100.4° F; may also have cough, shortness of breath, or difficulty breathing. *Strict Precautions (Airborne, Contact, and Eye)*
Diarrhea	*CONTACT* Put patient in a private room. Use gown and gloves for staff entering the room.	*Clostridium difficile*–associated diarrhea	Associated with recent history of antibiotic usage. *Contact Precautions*

From *Infection control manual*, Boston, Mass, Brigham & Women's Hospital.

- Advanced Cardiac Life Support verification
- Emergency Nursing Pediatric Course verification
- Trauma Nursing Core Course verification
- Certified Emergency Nurse certification (preferred)
- Effective communication skills and ability to work collaboratively
- Ability to use the nursing process effectively
- Flexible personality and adaptable to change
- Role model and suitable hospital representative
- Excellent decision-making skills

THE TRIAGE ROLE

Working as a triage nurse can be mentally challenging and sometimes exhausting. The triage area frequently is noisy and overcrowded; telephones ring constantly; children cry; and patients, families, and visitors are stressed and demanding. Determining which patients need to be seen immediately and which patients can wait safely requires knowledge and experience. The triage process can be accomplished in a variety of ways, but the ultimate goal remains ensuring that the right person is put in the right place at the right time for the right reason.

References

1. McCaig LF, Ly N: *National Hospital Ambulatory Medical Care Survey: 2000 emergency department summary—advance data from vital and health statistics,* no 326, Hyattsville, Md, 2002, National Center for Health Statistics.
2. McCaig LF, Burt C: *National Hospital Ambulatory Medical Care Survey: 2002 emergency department summary—advance data from vital and health statistics,* no 340, Hyattsville, Md, 2004, National Center for Health Statistics.
3. American Hospital Association: Emergency department overload: a growing crisis, *Med Benefits* 19(10):8, 2002.
4. Joint Commission on Accreditation of Healthcare Organizations: Delays in treatment, *Sentinel Event Alert* 26:1, 2002.
5. Thompson J, Dains J: *Comprehensive triage,* Reston, Va, 1982, Reston.
6. MacLean S: *2001 Emergency Nurses Association national benchmark guide: emergency departments,* Des Plaines, Ill, 2002, Emergency Nurses' Association.
7. Emergency Nurses' Association: *Standards of emergency nursing practice,* ed 4, Des Plaines, Ill, 1999, The Association.
8. Gill JM, Reese CL, Diamond JJ: Disagreement among health care professionals about the urgent care needs of emergency department patients, *Ann Emerg Med* 28(5):474-479, 1996.
9. Travers DA et al: Five-level triage system more effective than three-level in tertiary emergency department, *J Emerg Nurs* 28(5):395-400, 2002.
10. Wuerz RC, Fernandes CMB, Alarcon J: Inconsistency of emergency department triage, *Ann Emerg Med* 32:431-435, 1998.
11. Emergency Nurses Association: Position statements. Retrieved March 25, 2005, from http://www.ena.org/about/position/default.asp.
12. Australasian College for Emergency Medicine: The Australasian Triage Scale (ATS). Retrieved July 17, 2002, from http://www.acem.org.au/open/documents/triage.htm.
13. Australasian College for Emergency Medicine: National triage scale, *Emerg Med (Australia)* 6:145-146, 1994.
14. Jelinek GA, Little M: Inter-rater reliability of the National Triage Scale over 11,500 simulated occasions of triage, *Emerg Med* 8:226-230, 1996.

15. Acuity Scale (CTAS) for Emergency Departments. Retrieved April 5, 2002, from http://www.caep.ca/002.policies/002-02.ctas.htm.
16. Beveridge R et al: Reliability of the Canadian emergency department triage and acuity scale: interrater agreement, *Ann Emerg Med* 34:155-159, 1999.
17. Manos D et al: Inter-observer agreement using the Canadian Emergency Department Triage and Acuity Scale, *Can J Emerg Med* 4(1) January, 2002.
18. CTAS: Canadian ED Triage and Acuity Scale, *Can J Emerg Med* 1(suppl 3), 1999.
19. Manchester Triage Group: *Emergency triage,* Plymouth, UK, 1997, BMJ Publishing Group.
20. Tanabe P et al: Reliability and validity of scores on the emergency severity index version 3, *Acad Emerg Med* 11(1):59-64, 2004.
21. Wuerz RC et al: Reliability and validity of a new five-level triage instrument, *Acad Emerg Med* 7(3):236-242, 2000.
22. Wuerz RC et al: Implementation and refinement of the emergency severity index, *Acad Emerg Med* 8(2):183-184, 2001.
23. Emergency Nurses Association: *ENPC provider manual,* Des Plaines, Ill, 2004, The Association.
24. Travers D: How long does it take? How long should it take? *J Emerg Nurs* 25(3):238-240, 1999.
25. Bemis P: *Clinical practice guide of emergency care,* Rockledge, Fla, 2000, Cocoa Beach learning Systems.
26. Cooper RJ et al: Effect of vital signs on triage decisions, *Ann Emerg Med* 39(3):223-232, 2002.
27. American College of Emergency Physicians: Violence in the health care setting: what you should know. Retrieved August 1, 2003, from http://www.acep.org/1,328,o.html.
28. Emergency Nurses Association: Position Statement: violence in the emergency care setting. Retrieved March 25, 2005, from http://www.ena.org/aout/position/violence.asp.
29. *Infection control manual,* Boston, Mass, Brigham & Women's Hospital.
30. Emergency Nurses Association: Position statement: telephone advice. Retrieved March 25, 2005, from http://www.ena.org.
31. Emergency Nurses Association: *Making the right decision: a triage curriculum,* ed 2, Des Plaines, Ill, 2001, The Association.
32. Emergency Nurses Association: *Triage: meeting the challenge,* Des Plaines, Ill, 1997, The Association.
33. Newberry L, editor: *Sheehy's emergency nursing principles and practice,* ed 4, St Louis, 2003, Mosby.

7

Patient Assessment

Diana Lombardo, MSN-FNP, MHA, RN, CCRN

Physical assessment is a vital skill, and rapid, accurate patient evaluation is key to effective care. Not only do emergency nurses treat patients with every possible complaint, but their patients span the age spectrum. Emergency nurses must be comfortable assessing all age-groups, from pediatric to geriatric.

Initial assessment is targeted at addressing immediate needs. The goal of secondary assessment is to identify all relevant injuries or problems. Focused and ongoing assessments supply the data required to customize care to each patient's changing needs. Assessment requires cognitive, problem solving, psychomotor, ethical, and interpersonal skills.[1] Nurses have a responsibility to ensure that their assessment data are documented, accessible, and communicated to other health care providers. The purpose of this chapter is to emphasize general assessment guidelines that can be applied to a variety of patients in the emergency department (ED); specific interventions are not addressed. The reader is directed to pertinent chapters for more detailed discussion.

GENERAL ASSESSMENT

Assessment information is derived from subjective and objective data. Subjective information is data imparted verbally by the patient or significant others such as family members, friends, or caregivers. Although this information can be valuable, patients may or may not be good historians, and their recollection of events sometimes can be misleading. Objective data are those that can be observed or measured. This information is garnered from the physical examination process and from laboratory tests and other diagnostic studies.

Every patient must be viewed with an eye to identifying immediate threats. The focus of the primary assessment process is the ABCs—airway, breathing, and circulation. Determine

Table 7-1 **Components of the Primary Assessment**

Component	Evaluation Points	Action
Airway	Determine whether the airway is patent. Vocalizations? Air movement?	Position the airway to ensure patency. Identify and remove partial or complete airway obstructions such as secretions, foreign objects, and blood. Insert an oropharyngeal or nasopharyngeal airway to maintain airway patency. Protect the cervical spine.
Breathing	Determine the presence or absence of effective breathing. Skin color? Distress? Identify abnormal respiratory patterns or sounds. Stridor? Wheezing? Crackles? Identify any loss of chest wall integrity, the presence of tracheal deviation, chest asymmetry, or jugular vein distention. Evaluate the work of breathing. Labored? Tachypneic? Bradypneic? Accessory muscle use?	Auscultate breath sounds. Position the patient to maximize ventilation. Provide supplemental oxygen. Assist breathing with mouth-to-mask resuscitation, bag-valve-mask ventilation, or endotracheal intubation, as indicated. Occlude open chest wounds. Relieve tension pneumothoraces. Institute therapy for bronchospasm or pulmonary edema.
Circulation	Evaluate pulse presence, quality, character, and equality. Identify the cardiac rhythm and any electrocardiogram abnormalities. Assess capillary refill, skin color and temperature, and the presence of diaphoresis.	Initiate chest compressions, defibrillation, synchronized cardioversion, and medications as indicated. Treat dysrhythmias. Control bleeding. Establish intravenous access. Replace lost volume with isotonic crystalloids or blood products.

whether a life-threatening situation exists and institute appropriate actions (Table 7-1). Once urgent threats are addressed, a secondary assessment can be completed. Variations on the secondary examination are used for pediatric, medical, and trauma patients. Table 7-2 provides an overview of secondary assessment. (See Chapter 34 for further discussion of trauma patient assessment. Chapters 43 and 46 address pediatric trauma and general pediatric emergencies, respectively).

Rarely will any one patient require assessment of every potential examination parameter. Modify your evaluation based on the patient's presenting complaint, history, level of distress, and examination findings. Do not forget to include assessments specific to age-related physiologic changes. Table 7-3 reviews age-specific considerations for pediatric and geriatric patients.

HISTORY

Obtaining a relevant history is an important part of patient assessment. Historical data includes the patient's chief complaint, history of the present illness or problem, medical history, current medications, family history, social history, and a review of systems. However, the process of eliciting a medical history commonly is abbreviated for emergency patients. Factors to consider when deciding on the extent of medical history include the following: the nature and severity of the complaint, the intensity of the situation, how frequently the

Table 7-2   Components of the Secondary Assessment

Component	Considerations
General observations	What is the patient's overall appearance? Note positioning and posture. Is there any guarding or self-protective activity?
	Are there obvious problems?
	What is the general level of distress?
	What is the patient's level of consciousness?
	How is the patient behaving? Calm? Agitated? Lethargic? Cooperative? Restless?
	Can the patient ambulate? Steady or unsteady gate?
	Can the patient communicate verbally? Is speech clear and concise? Confused? Slurred? Aphasic?
	Any odors noted? Urine? Ketones? Ethanol? Chemicals?
	Is there evidence of old injuries, new injuries, or both?
Head and face	Inspect for gross deformity, asymmetry, depressions, or bleeding.
	Are pupils equal and round? Do they react to light?
	Determine gross visual acuity.
	Palpate the scalp for wounds, tenderness, and deformity.
	Palpate facial bones for deformity, asymmetry, and tenderness.
	Inspect the nose for deformity, bleeding, and obstruction.
	Evaluate ears for deformity, lacerations, bleeding, and drainage.
	Examine the oral cavity for color, hydration status, malocclusion, bleeding, obstruction, absent or fractured teeth, edema of the tongue or pharynx, and bruising below the tongue.
	Evaluate for asymmetrical facial expression and slurred speech.
Neck	Inspect the neck for deformity, bleeding, and wounds.
	Observe for tracheal deviation, subcutaneous emphysema, and jugular vein distention.
	Auscultate for carotid bruits.
	Palpate the cervical spine for tenderness, deformity, or wounds.
Chest	Inspect for deformity, wounds, bleeding, impaled objects, and symmetrical rise and fall with ventilation.
	Evaluate rate, depth, and effort of breathing.
	Palpate chest bony structures for deformity, pain, and subcutaneous air.
	Auscultate breath sounds for equality and the presence of adventitious sounds.
	Auscultate the heart for muffling, murmurs, rubs, or other abnormal sounds.
Abdomen	Inspect for injuries, impaled objects, distention, bruising, and surgical scars.
	Auscultate for bowel sounds.
	Auscultate for an abdominal aortic bruit.
	Palpate and compare bilateral femoral pulses.
	Palpate the abdomen for masses, tenderness, guarding, rebound pain, pulsations, and rigidity.
	Percuss to identify air or fluid.
	Palpate the liver to determine its size and the presence of tenderness.
	Compress the symphysis pubis and pelvic ilial wings, checking for instability and pain.
Extremities	Inspect and palpate for deformities, wounds, bleeding, edema, and bruising.
	Note the presence of track marks, pain, or bony crepitus.
	Palpate and compare pulses bilaterally.
	Note distal color, temperature, capillary refill time, movement, and sensation.
Back	If injury is a possibility, logroll the patient while maintaining spinal precautions.
	Inspect and palpate for deformities, wounds, tenderness, bruising, and pain.
	Perform a rectal examination to identify blood, a high-riding prostate, foreign bodies, and loss of sphincter tone.

Table **7-3**   **Age-Specific Assessment Considerations**

Assessment Parameter	Pediatric	Geriatric
History	Consider mother's health during pregnancy; parent-child interactions; developmental level; childhood diseases; and child's ability to give pertinent data.	History may be influenced by patient's attitudes about aging; patient may respond slowly to questions; history may be influenced by deterioration of the senses.
Vital signs	Child may have faster heart and respiratory rates; blood pressure about [70 + (2 × age in years)] mm Hg; and be prone to hypothermia.	Cardiac irregularities may be a normal variable; vital signs are influenced by many medications; seniors are prone to hypothermia.
Cardiovascular	Consider potential congenital heart problems; murmur and third heart sound may be normal variants.	Cardiac output at rest decreases; development of coronary artery disease may occur; heart is less able to adapt to stress.
Respiratory	Infants are obligate nose breathers; abdominal breathing occurs until age 6 or 7; infants more susceptible to respiratory infections; airway is smaller and more easily occluded.	Seniors experience increased anteroposterior chest diameter, decreased pulmonary function, and decreased surface area for gas exchange.
Neurologic	Must consider developmental stage; use pediatric coma scale.	Degenerative changes occur; nerve transmission slows and may be affected by changes in other systems.
Head, ears, eyes, nose, and throat	Visual acuity of 20/20 not obtained until age 7; anatomic differences in eustachian tube predispose to ear infection; hearing develops fully at age 5 years.	Conjunctiva is thinner and yellow; arcus senilis may appear; pupil is smaller; lens loses transparency; seniors are prone to hearing loss.
Gastrointestinal	Abdominal guarding is more common in child with pain; air swallowed with crying causes abdominal distention.	Digestion, gastrointestinal tract motility, and anal sphincter tone decrease with age; seniors are prone to loss of appetite and constipation.
Genitourinary	Ability to control urination is gained between 2 and 3 years old; consider age of puberty.	Renal function decreases after age 40; incomplete bladder emptying occurs.
Musculoskeletal	Bones are flexible—greenstick fractures; subluxation is common.	Seniors have decreased muscle mass and are prone to fractures; degenerative joint disease may occur.
Integumentary	Consider diaper rash, susceptibility to contact dermatitis.	Decreased mobility leads to stasis dermatitis and ulcers.
Endocrine	Growth hormone abnormalities may occur.	Thyroid disorders may occur.
Hematopoietic	Anemias, leukemias, clotting disorders may occur during childhood.	Vitamin B_{12} absorption decreases; levels of hemoglobin and hematocrit decrease.
Immune	Child has passive immunity at birth.	Decreased antibody response occurs with age.

From Newberry L: *Sheehy's emergency nursing: principles and practice,* ed 5, St Louis, 2003, Mosby.

patient experiences this problem, and the extent to which the problem affects quality of life. Box 7-1 presents a simple mnemonic for remembering essential components of history taking.

Certain lifestyle considerations can be important factors in a patient's medical history. Is there evidence of substance abuse? Consider alcohol and other drugs. Box 7-2 illustrates the CAGES questionnaire, a brief tool used to screen quickly for persons with alcohol-related problems. Is the patient's condition potentially related to sexual habits, an alternative lifestyle, or domestic violence? Box 7-3 contains questions that can be posed to discuss sexual orientation in a neutral manner. Use the HITS mnemonic to ask about suspected domestic violence (Box 7-4).

Box **7-1   SAMPLE Mnemonic for History Taking**

Signs and symptoms
Allergies
Medications
Pertinent medical history
Last meal (or medications, or menstrual period)
Events surrounding this incident

Box **7-2   CAGE Questionnaire for Alcohol-Related Concerns***

C	Have you ever felt you should CUT down your drinking?
A	Have people ANNOYED you by criticizing your drinking?
G	Have you ever felt bad or GUILTY about your drinking?
E	Have you ever had a drink first think in the morning to steady your nerves or get rid of a hangover (EYE-opener)?

*A "yes" response in any category is highly associated with problem drinking.[2]

Box **7-3   Questions to Keep the Interview Gender Neutral**

Tell me about your living situation.
Are you sexually active?
In what way?

Box **7-4   HITS Mnemonic for Assessment of Domestic Violence**

In the last year how often has your partner
*H*urt you physically?
*I*nsulted or talked down to you?
*T*hreatened you with physical harm?
*S*creamed or cursed at you?

SUBJECTIVE ASSESSMENT

Interpreting subjective assessment data requires consideration of the patient's culture, cognitive abilities, and developmental level. Pertinent information can be obtained from the patient, family, caretaker, or any person familiar with the patient's history. Start by introducing yourself, clearly stating your name and title. Allow the patient time to respond.

Subjective information includes the chief complaint, the reason for the visit, the patient's present state of health, current medications, allergies, and other information gathered from the medical history. History of medication use should address prescription, over-the-counter, herbal, and recreational drugs. Document the type and severity of reported allergic reactions.

Obtain a thorough description of reported pain, including its severity, nature, location, and duration. Parameters for pain assessment are summarized in the PQRST mnemonic (Table 7-4). If pain is present, use a standardized tool, such as a numeric scale (e.g., 0 to 10)

Table 7-4   PQRST Mnemonic for Pain Assessment

Parameter		Assessment Questions
P	Provokes/ Palliates	What initially provoked the pain? What makes it better? What makes it worse? What were you doing when the pain occurred? Did the pain wake you up?
Q	Quality	Can you describe the pain? Is it sharp, dull, squeezing, pressing, burning, aching, pounding, cholicy, crampy, or stabbing? (Allow the patient to describe pain in his or her own words.)
R	Radiates	Does the pain radiate? To where does the pain radiate? Does the pain move around or is it fixed in one area?
S	Severity	How severe is the pain? Rate pain on a 0-10 scale, with zero as no pain and 10 as the worst pain experienced. (An alternative is to use FACES (Family Adaptability and Cohesion Evaluation Scale) for pediatric patients over 3 years and for anyone with communication difficulties.)
T	Time	When did the pain start? Was the onset slow or sudden? How long has the pain lasted? Is the pain constant or does it come and go? Have you ever had this pain before? Is this the same type of pain or is it different this time?

Box **7-5**   **Pertinent Historical Data**

1. History of present illness or injury:
   a. How and when did the injury or illness first occur?
      - Symptom chronology and duration
      - Travel within days or weeks of symptom onset
      - Others in the household with the same or similar symptoms
   b. Are there influencing factors?
   c. Any related symptoms?
   d. What is the nature and location of any pain or other discomfort (e.g., nausea, vertigo, itching, or shortness of breath)?
   e. What, if anything, has the patient done about the symptoms, including medicines, home remedies, and other treatments?
2. Pertinent medical history:
   a. Has this problem occurred before?
      - If so, was a medical diagnosis made? What was it?
   b. Has the patient ever had surgery? For what reason? What was the result?
   c. Is there any family history that may influence the patient's present complaint?
   d. Are there psychosocial factors that may be influencing the patient's condition?
3. Does the patient have a private physician? (Obtain the full name if possible.)
4. Current medications including prescription, over-the-counter, herbal, and recreational substances:
   a. When were the drugs last taken?
5. Any allergies to medications, latex, or other environmental allergens?
6. What is the patient's age, weight, and height (if appropriate)?
7. When was the last tetanus immunization (if open wounds are involved)?
8. What was the date of the last normal menstrual period (females)?
   a. Is there any chance the patient could be pregnant?
9. Are there any special communication needs related to vision, hearing, or language?

or FACES (Family Adaptability and Cohesion Evaluation Scale), for initial and all subsequent pain assessments. (Refer to Chapter 14 for further discussion of pain.)

In the ED a complete medical history and detailed subjective assessment are rarely practical or desirable. Typically, assessments are focused on the chief complaint but may need to be more global in patients with an indeterminate or complex presentation. Box 7-5 highlights relevant historical data that should be considered for most patients.

OBJECTIVE ASSESSMENT

Objective findings consist of information that can be observed or measured. Like subjective data, this information is essential to the overall assessment process. Examples of objective assessment data routinely collected in the ED include vital signs, patient weight, electrocardiogram tracings, diagnostic tests, and physical examinations.

VITAL SIGNS

Vital signs include temperature, pulse and respiratory rates, oxygen saturation, blood pressure, weight, and evaluation of pain. Pain is unique because although it is evaluated with an objective scale, it is nonetheless a subjective finding and the patient is the one who provides the rating. Table 7-5 lists normal vital signs parameters for specific age groups.

Temperature

Temperature measurement commonly is performed at oral, tympanic, axillary, and rectal sites. A sophisticated, noninvasive option includes a digital wand, which is passed lightly over the temporal artery to determine body temperature. Core body temperature can be measured using a pulmonary artery catheter, a urinary catheter, an esophageal probe, or an intracranial pressure monitor with thermistor capacity. The accepted route of temperature measurement varies among facilities, but for most adult patients an oral temperature is preferred. Institutional preference will dictate whether temperature is measured in centigrade or Fahrenheit. Box 7-6 gives formulas for converting between the two measures. Temperature is affected by activity, certain disease conditions, environmental factors, infection, and injury. An abnormally high or low temperature reading should always be confirmed by an alternate route, thermometer, or observer.

Table 7-5   Normal Vital Signs by Age

Vital Sign	Preemie	Term	6 months	1 year	3 years	6 years	9 years	12 years	15 years	Adult	Elderly
Temperature (°C)	36.8	36.8	37.7	37.7	37.6	37	37	37	37	37	36
Heart rate	140	80-180	80-140	80-140	80-140	75-120	75-120	50-90	50-90	60-100	60-100
Respiratory rate	40-60	30-80	30-60	20-40	20-40	15-25	15-24	15-24	15-20	12-20	15-20
Blood pressure (mm Hg)	73/55	73/55	73/55	90/55	90/55	95/57	95/57	115/70	120/80	120/80	120/80
Oxygen saturation	>95%	>95%	>95%	>95%	>95%	>95%	>95%	>95%	>95%	>95%	>92%

(The "Age" header spans the columns: 6 months, 1 year, 3 years, 6 years, 9 years, 12 years, 15 years, Adult, Elderly)

From Emergency Nurses Association: *ENPC provider manual*, Des Plaines, Ill, 2004, The Association.

Box 7-6 Conversion Formula for Temperature Readings

$(°F - 32) \times {}^5/_9 = °C$
$(°C \times {}^9/_5) + 32 = °F$

Pulse

Pulse assessment involves determination of heart rhythm, rate, quality, and equality. Peripheral pulses are evaluated by palpation, whereas the apical heartbeat is auscultated. Compare pulses on each side of the body to assess for differences. Pulse or heart rate abnormalities can be an indication of physiologic compromise (shock), environmental conditions (cold), local injuries (compromised arterial flow), or general cardiac dysfunction. Continuous cardiac monitoring and a 12-lead electrocardiogram should be considered for patients with significant bradycardia, tachycardia, or irregular pulses. Oxygen saturation monitoring with a pulse oximeter can be used to detect localized decreases in extremity blood flow.[3]

Respirations

Evaluation of respiratory status includes determining rate, auscultating breath sounds, and inspecting for work of breathing. Signs of increased respiratory effort include nasal flaring, retractions, and tracheal tugging; use of intercostal or accessory (abdominal, neck) muscles; an inability to communicate in complete sentences; and the presence of adventitious or diminished breath sounds. Table 7-6 describes normal and abnormal respiratory patterns.

Oxygen Saturation

Monitoring oxygen saturation with a pulse oximeter is essential for patients with respiratory complaints, an altered level of consciousness, serious illness, or any abnormal vital signs. Unfortunately, pulse oximetry has significant technical limitations in persons who are hypothermic, vasoconstricted, anemic, or hypotensive. Artificial nails and brightly colored nail polish also can interfere with readings. Determine a patient's baseline oxygen saturation as part of the initial vital signs; monitor saturation continuously if indicated. Measurements typically are taken on the fingers or toes but readings also can be obtained on the earlobe, the nasal bridge, or even by wrapping the probe around the entire foot of a neonate or small infant. Some sites require specially designed probes.

Table 7-6 **Respiratory Patterns**

Name	Description	Cause
Eupnea	Normal rate and rhythm	
Tachypnea	Increased respirations	Fever, pneumonia, respiratory alkalosis, aspirin poisoning
Bradypnea	Slow but regular respirations	Narcotics, tumor, alcohol
Cheyne-Stokes	Respirations gradually become faster and deeper and then slower, alternating with periods of apnea	Increased intracranial pressure, cardiac and renal failure, drug overdose
Biot's	Faster and deeper respirations with abrupt pauses	Spinal meningitis, other central nervous system conditions
Kussmaul's	Faster and deeper respirations without pauses	Renal failure, metabolic acidosis, diabetic ketoacidosis
Apneustic	Prolonged, gasping inspiration, followed by short expiration	Dysfunction of respiratory center in pons
Central neurogenic hyperventilation	Sustained regular hyperpnea	Midbrain lesions
Ataxic	Completely irregular	Damage to respiratory center in medulla

From Newberry L: *Sheehy's emergency nursing: principles and practice*, ed 5, St Louis, 2003, Mosby.

An important point to remember is that a pulse oximeter only tells you what percent of red blood cells are saturated, regardless of what has saturated the cell. This has important implications in the event of carbon monoxide exposure. A patient with a toxic carboxyhemoglobin level may have a normal pulse oximeter reading. In cases of suspected exposure, send an arterial blood gas sample for direct measurement of arterial oxygen saturation. Compare this result to that of the pulse oximeter reading. If a significant discrepancy exists, check for carbon monoxide and do not use a pulse oximeter until the carbon dioxide level has dropped to near normal levels.

Blood Pressure

Rather than portending the presence of a life-threatening condition, a single abnormal blood pressure (BP) reading simply may indicate the need for further investigation. Conversely, a normal BP does not necessarily denote that all is well; BP changes may not be evident until compensatory mechanisms are exhausted, particularly in young and healthy individuals. Patient position, as well as cuff length and width, can affect blood pressure results significantly. Many "abnormal" BP readings are simply technical errors. If the cuff is too small, BP is falsely elevated; if the cuff is too big, BP is erroneously decreased.

Blood pressure is not a single entity; it is a complex composite of cardiac contractility, heart rate, circulating volume, and peripheral vascular resistance. Think of systolic pressure as a gross reflection of the cardiac output, how much and how well the heart can eject blood. In shock or preshock states, heart rate increases dramatically to maintain cardiac output. Diastolic pressure, however, is a function of peripheral resistance, how constricted the vessels are. In hypovolemic states, systolic BP (cardiac output) drops, whereas diastolic BP remains the same, drops to a lesser extent, or even rises, as long as the blood vessels can vasoconstrict to compensate for volume loss.

Orthostatic Vital Signs

Orthostatic (or postural) vital signs evaluate the BP and pulse in two or three positions: lying, sitting, or standing. Orthostatic vital signs commonly are obtained in patients with a history of syncopal episodes or suspected volume depletion. Unfortunately, although significant positional changes in BP may be noted, they are deemed too variable to be a reliable indicator of blood loss. When evaluating patients for orthostatic hypotension, consider systolic BP, diastolic BP, and heart rate as three interdependent variables, each adjusting as the body attempts to maintain perfusion. Of the three parameters, only a pulse rise of greater than 30 beats/min or severe dizziness has been shown to correlate consistently with blood volume reduction. Importantly, many drugs and several medical conditions can cause orthostatic changes.[4] Box 7-7 summarizes the orthostatic tilt testing procedure.

Pulse Pressure

Another way to evaluate volume status is to calculate pulse pressure. Pulse pressure is the difference between the systolic BP and the diastolic BP (Pulse pressure = Systolic BP – Diastolic BP). This simple formula can be calculated serially to trend changes over time. A narrowing pulse pressure (smaller number) indicates a drop in cardiac output and a compensatory rise in peripheral vascular resistance. Pulse pressure is much more sensitive to hypovolemic changes than is systolic BP, so it can serve as an early warning of impending BP crash. Pulse pressure is a particularly useful parameter in patients who cannot sit or stand for orthostatic measurements.

Box **7-7** **Summary of Orthostatic Tilt Testing***

Test Procedure

1. Blood pressure and pulse are recorded after patient has been supine for 2 to 3 minutes.
2. Blood pressure, pulse, and symptoms are recorded after patient has been standing for 1 minute; the patient should be permitted to resume a supine position immediately should syncope or near syncope develop.

Positive Test

1. Increase in pulse of 30 beats/min or more in adults, *or*
2. Presence of symptoms of cerebral hypoperfusion (e.g., dizziness or syncope)

From Hedges JR, Hedges JR: *Clinical procedures in emergency medicine,* ed 4, Phildelphia, 2004, Saunders.
*The predictive ability of orthostatic vital signs to assess volume status is often overestimated in clinical practice. This suggested guide is based on the ability of the pulse change and patient symptoms to distinguish between no acute blood loss and a 1000-mL acute blood loss in healthy, previously normovolemic volunteers (sensitivity of 98% for detecting 1000-mL acute blood loss) (Knopp R, Claypool R, Leonardi D: Use of the tilt test in measuring acute blood loss, *Am Emerg Med* 9:29, 1980). This guide may not be applicable to elderly patients, sick children, medicated patients, and those with autonomic dysfunction.

Box **7-8** **Weight Conversion Formula**

Pounds to Kilograms

Divide pounds by 2.2 to determine weight in kilograms.

Kilograms to Pounds

Multiply kilograms by 2.2 to determine weight in pounds.

Shock Index

The shock index is yet another way to assess cardiac output and the compensatory responses of the body. To determine the shock index, simply divide the systolic BP by the heart rate (Shock index = Systolic BP/Heart rate); a result greater than 0.9 indicates cardiovascular dysfunction. However, because the number 0.9 is close to 1, an easy way to use this concept without a calculator is simply to ask, "Is the heart rate greater than the systolic blood pressure?" A "yes" answer indicates that the patient is working hard to compensate (elevated heart rate) simply to maintain a systolic BP (cardiac output).

Height, Weight, and Head Circumference

Whether weights are obtained on all adult patients is a matter of ED policy. Reported weights, although subject to error, generally are considered adequate unless there is a specific need for accuracy (e.g., administration of anticoagulants, vasopressors, or other weight-based medications). Pediatric patients, however, should be weighed with each ED visit to obtain an accurate measurement (exceptions may be made for older adolescents). Because most pediatric medications are dosed by the kilogram, weight should always be documented in kilograms. Many patient scales weigh in pounds and kilograms; Box 7-8 provides the conversion formula. Occasionally, measurement of height may be necessary. For example, patient height is needed to calculate expected peak expiratory flow rates.

The Joint Commission on Accreditation of Healthcare Organizations requires evaluation of head circumference on all patients under the age of 2 years *as appropriate.* Indications for measurement of head circumference in the ED include children who have ventriculoperitoneal shunt problems or any obvious cranial abnormality. Refer to institutional policy for specific requirements.[5]

PHYSICAL EXAMINATION

This section provides a cursory review of basic assessment techniques. For a more complete discussion, consult a physical assessment text.

Inspection

Examination of the patient begins with an across-the-room assessment of overall status. Is the patient alert or altered, cachectic or overweight, unkempt or well groomed? Does the patient appear acutely ill, chronically ill, or generally healthy? Are respirations labored? Can the patient speak complete sentences or only a few words? What color are the skin and mucosa? Is there obvious distress, bleeding, deformity, or swelling? Observe body movement and posture noting pain, neurologic or orthopedic abnormalities, mood, and mental status.

Auscultation

Auscultation is used to evaluate lung, heart, and bowel sounds. The ability to distinguish sounds depends on keenness of hearing, stethoscope sensitivity, ambient noise levels, and practitioner experience. Assess sound quality, intensity, and duration. Perform abdominal auscultation before palpation or percussion. Validate ausculatory finding with additional examination techniques.[1]

Palpation

Touch is used to assess surface characteristics such as skin texture, sensitivity, turgor, and temperature. Use light palpation to evaluate pulses, muscle rigidity, deformities, and chest excursion.[6] Deep palpation will identify masses, tenderness, organ size, and rebound pain. Palpate the abdomen lightly before deep palpation.

Percussion

Percussion transmits sound and tactile vibrations. Various tissues or substances respond to percussion in predicable ways. Table 7-7 highlights sounds associated with manual percussion

Table 7-7   **Sounds Associated with Percussion**

Source	Sound	Quality	Pitch	Intensity	Duration
Gastric bubble; intestinal air	Tympany	Drumlike	High	Loud	Moderate
Liver; full bladder; pregnant uterus	Dull	Thudlike	High	Soft to moderate	Moderate
Hyperinflated lungs: emphysema or asthma	Hyperresonance	Booming	Very low	Very loud	Long
Normal lungs	Resonance	Hollow	Low	Moderate to loud	Long
Muscles	Flat	Flat	High	Soft	Short

Modified from Dillon PM: *Nursing health assessment: a critical thinking case studies approach,* Philadelphia, 2003, Davis.

findings. Percussion with the examiner's hands is used to evaluate organ or cavity densities and can distinguish solid, air-filled, and fluid-filled structures. Two factors influence the sounds elicited: examiner technique and thickness of the surface being percussed.[1] Indirect percussion is performed by striking the nondominant hand with the index finger of the dominant hand. Percussion with a reflex hammer is used to evaluate deep tendon reflexes.

SYSTEMS ASSESSMENT

The patient's chief complaint (or presenting problem) is used to guide investigation of pertinent body systems. For example, the patient with cardiac dysfunction requires assessment of the cardiovascular system but also may have respiratory and gastrointestinal complaints that need evaluation. Following initial stabilization, critically ill or injured patients must have a complete head-to-toe evaluation. A brief discussion of systems assessment follows. Refer to related chapters throughout the text for greater detail.

Neurologic

The most important indicator of neurologic function is the patient's level of consciousness. Begin the examination by determining current status. Is the patient alert, oriented, and ambulatory? Can the patient answer a series of basic questions (What is your name? What is this placed called? What day of the week is it?). If level of consciousness is impaired, ascertain from family members or caregivers the patient's baseline status. The Glasgow Coma Scale for adults (Table 7-8) and the Pediatric Glasgow Coma Scale for preverbal pediatric patients are widely accepted tools for communicating neurologic status and for trending changes over time. Avoid vague patient descriptors such as *lethargic, comatose, stuporous, obtunded,* or *drowsy.*

Occasionally, ED patients require a detailed neurologic assessment that includes mental status, physical strength, speech, sensation, and cranial nerve function (Table 7-9). To evaluate strength and sensation, compare the patient's right and left sides. Refer to Chapters 35 and 36 for a discussion of neurologic assessment in the patient with brain or spinal cord trauma.

Table 7-8   **Glasgow Coma Scale**

Category	*Adult/Child*	*Infant (Preverbal)*	*Score*
Eye opening	Spontaneous	Spontaneous	4
	To speech	To speech	3
	To pain	To pain	2
	No eye opening	No eye opening	1
Verbal	Oriented	Coos, babbles	5
	Confused	Irritable	4
	Inappropriate words	Cries to pain	3
	Incomprehensible sounds	Moans to pain	2
	No verbal response	No vocal response	1
Motor	Obeys simple commands	Normal spontaneous movement	6
	Localizes noxious stimuli	Withdraws to touch	5
	Withdraws to pain	Withdraws to pain	4
	Abnormal flexion	Abnormal flexion	3
	Abnormal extension	Abnormal extension	2
	No response	No response	1
Total score ranges from 3 to 15.			

A score of 8 or less indicates coma and requires airway protection.

Table 7-9   **Cranial Nerves**

Number	Nerve	Origin	Function
I	Olfactory	Upper third of nasal septum	*Sensory:* Smell
II	Optic	Lateral geniculate body	*Sensory:* Vision and light reflex
III	Oculomotor	Midbrain	*Motor:* Pupil constriction to light, elevation of upper lid
IV	Trochlear	Midbrain	*Motor:* Downward movement of the eyes
V	Trigeminal	Pons	*Sensory:* Corneal reflexes; sensation to face, cheeks, lips, and mandible *Motor:* Masseter and oral muscles
VI	Abducens	Pons	*Motor:* Abducts the eye
VII	Facial	Pons	*Sensory:* Taste on the anterior two thirds of the tongue *Motor:* Muscles around eyes, forehead, and mouth
VIII	Acoustic	Pons	*Sensory:* Hearing and equilibrium
IX	Glossopharyngeal	Medulla	*Sensory:* Taste on the posterior third of the tongue *Motor:* Control of the pharynx for swallowing
X	Vagus	Medulla	*Sensory:* Pharynx and larynx sensation *Motor:* Pharynx, larynx, soft palate, and uvula movement
XI	Spinal accessory	Medulla and upper spinal cord	*Motor:* Trapezius and sternocleidomastoid muscle function
XII	Hypoglossal	Medulla	*Motor:* Tongue movement

Head, Ears, Eyes, Nose, and Throat

Inspect the head, face, and neck for symmetry and injury, then palpate for deformity or tenderness. Evaluate eye opening. Is ptosis present? Are the pupils equally reactive to light and accommodation? Are the pupil borders circular and symmetrical? Note the presence of exophthalmos. Are extraocular movements intact? If the patient has any eye complaints, determine visual acuity with a Snellen "E" chart or other method. Inspect each naris for deformity, drainage, and obstruction. Evaluate the ears for injuries, discharge, inflammation, or foreign bodies. Examine the oral cavity for color, hydration status, loose or missing teeth, deformities, angioedema, erythema, and obstruction. Is there any tracheal deviation, subcutaneous air, or other neck abnormality present? Does the thyroid gland rise and fall with swallowing?[8]

Cardiovascular

Determine whether the patient requires immediate intervention for a cardiovascular emergency. Is the patient experiencing chest pain? Are vital signs normal? Is the heart rate too fast, too slow, or irregular? Place the patient on a cardiac monitor. What is the heart rate and rhythm? Is there electrocardiogram evidence of an electrolyte abnormality, a bundle branch block, a previous or evolving myocardial infarction, axis deviation, low voltage, or cardiac enlargement? Obtain a 12-lead electrocardiogram if there are abnormalities on the rhythm strip.

Heart sounds

Are normal heart sounds (S_1 and S_2) present? S_3 (Ken-tuc'-ky) and S_4 (Ten'-nes-see) are abnormal heart sounds heard during diastole and indicate left ventricular failure, volume overload, or a noncompliant left ventricle.[9]

Murmurs

Murmurs are produced by turbulent flow across a valve. Heart murmurs are classified by grades 1 to 6. Murmur grade is determined by the loudness of the sound. A grade 1 murmur is faint and may not be heard in all positions. A grade 6 murmur is associated with a palpable precordial thrill and can be heard even when the stethoscope is lifted off the chest.[6]

Pericardial effusion/tamponade

Pericarditis, trauma, uremia, malignancy, myxedema, and coronary artery injury during percutaneous transluminal coronary angioplasty (PTCA) can cause fluid to accumulate in the pericardium. Effusion without tamponade presents as muffled, diminished, or absent heart sounds. Any preexisting friction rub will disappear, and QRS voltage becomes low. On occasion, pericardial effusion can progress to tamponade. Cardiac tamponade most commonly is caused by acute bleeding in the pericardium. Signs of tamponade include distended neck veins (unless the patient is severely hypovolemic), pallor, diaphoresis, mottling, decreased pulse pressure, pulsus paradoxus, tachypnea, dyspnea, anxiety, apprehension, and a drop in the level of consciousness as cardiac output diminishes.

Perfusion

Are there signs of acute or chronic volume loss? What is the skin color? Are pulses strong, regular, and symmetrical? Is capillary refill brisk and equivalent in all digits? Is mottling or edema present? Is there evidence of acute or chronic vascular disease? Is the skin warm and dry? Is there anything (casts, splints, tight clothing, shoes, or jewelry) occluding arterial or venous flow? Is there any evidence of compartment syndrome (pain, pallor, pulselessness, parestheia, or paralysis)

Respiratory

Observe the face, chest, and neck. Can the patient speak in full sentences? Is there evidence of increased work of breathing: nasal flaring, accessory muscle use (abdominal or sternocleidomastoid), or retractions (sternal or intercostals)? Observe the skin color. Is pallor or cyanosis (circumoral or general) present? Are the mucous membranes pink? Is the skin warm and dry or cool and diaphoretic? Does the chest rise and fall symmetrically? Is there good chest excursion? Are adventitious breath sounds audible? Is the breathing pattern abnormal?

Normal breath sounds can be classified as tracheal, bronchial, vesicular, or bronchovesicular. Abnormal (adventitious) breath sounds include stridor, wheezing, rhonchi, rales, crackles and friction rubs. Stridor is a high-pitched, crowing sound heard on inspiration. This condition indicates an upper airway obstruction such as foreign body obstruction, laryngeal spasm, or massive edema (e.g., epiglottitis or anaphylaxis).

Gastrointestinal

Subjective data are important when evaluating the gastrointestinal system. Has the patient had previous abdominal surgery? Is there a history of reflux disease, peptic ulcers, diverticulitis, appendicitis, bowel obstruction, cirrhosis, or pancreatitis? What is the nature of the discomfort/pain? Does the patient have symptoms of nausea, vomiting, diarrhea, hemorrhoids, or fever? What is the character, frequency, quantity, and quality of the stool? Is the stool dark, melanotic, clay colored, or bloody? Are there lifestyle factors that could contribute to gastrointestinal problems such as alcohol abuse, intravenous substance abuse, obesity, or bulimia? Perform a rectal examination (if indicated) to evaluate lower gastrointestinal bleeding and rectal tone. Inspect the abdomen for symmetry, distention, mottling, bruising, masses, and scars. Auscultate all four quadrants. Are bowel sounds normal, hyperactive, diminished, or absent? Palpate for pain, masses, rigidity, and organomegaly. Begin with light palpation and progress to deep palpation, noting guarding, rebound tenderness, and referred pain. Percuss for organ size and to identify areas of intraabdominal air or fluid.

Genitourinary

Inquire about urinary frequency, urgency, incontinence, burning, and foul odor. Assess pain location, severity, migration, and character. Is there a history of urinary tract infections or renal calculi? Is urine color normal? If the patient reports "bloody urine," ask about recent medication use such as anticoagulants or phenazopyridine (Pyridium). Palpate for bladder distention, and tap for tenderness over the costovertebral angles.

Suspect sexually transmitted diseases with complaints of vaginal or urethral discharge or pain. This is particularly relevant in sexually active patients who have had multiple partners, unprotected sex, partners with similar symptoms, or anal intercourse. Question males about scrotal injury and unilateral or bilateral scrotal edema, pain, and erythema. Older men with a history of slow stream, dribbling, urgency, or an inability to urinate should be assessed for urinary retention caused by benign prostatic hypertrophy or urinary tract infection.

Consider the possibility of pregnancy in all females of reproductive age. When was the last normal menstrual period? Is vaginal bleeding present? How many pads or tampons have been used in the past hour? (A saturated pad/tampon holds 20 to 30 mL.) Does the patient have any symptoms of pregnancy-related problems: abdominal, pelvic, or back pain; generalized edema; or elevated blood pressure? Refer to Chapter 45 for discussion of obstetric and gynecologic emergencies.

Musculoskeletal

Musculoskeletal conditions treated in the ED usually are associated with trauma or infection. Assess the patient for deformities, wounds, edema, erythema, pus, and pain. Evaluate the patient for mobility, sensation, and neurovascular status to detect vascular compromise. Initiate basic first aid measures (ice, elevation, immobilization, and rest) to reduce pain and further injury. Remove all jewelry and tight clothing from injured limbs.

Integumentary

Assess the skin to determine color, texture, turgor, and temperature. Is there evidence of pallor, mottling, cyanosis, or jaundice? Evaluate for loss of skin integrity: abrasions, lacerations, avulsions, incisions, or punctures. Are there signs of acute dermal problems such as rashes, burns, bruises, petechiae, wheals, or hives? Does the patient have a chronic skin problem such as eczema, acne, allergic dermatitis, pediculosis, or psoriasis? Are there any unusual or suspicious lesions? Table 7-10 highlights skin color changes and associated conditions.

Hematologic

Examine for signs of bleeding disorders such as bruises, petechiae, pale conjunctiva, and joint pain or swelling. Question patients or family members about prescription, over-the-counter, herbal, and recreational drug use including alcohol. Does the patient have a history of septicemia, anticoagulant use, coagulopathies, or a hematologic disorder (e.g., sickle cell disease, hemophilia, or idiopathic thrombocytopenic purpura)? Is the patient at risk for deep vein thrombosis or pulmonary embolus? Risk factors include polycythemia, recent surgery, pregnancy, obesity, bed rest, and oral contraceptive use.

Table 7-10   **Color Changes in the Skin**

Color	Cause	Location
Brown	Genetic	Generalized
	Sunlight	Exposed areas
	Pregnancy	Localized (exposed areas, palmar creases)
	Addison's disease and some pituitary tumors	
Reddish	Polycythemia	Face, conjunctiva, mouth, hands, feet
	Excessive heat	Generalized
	Sunburn, thermal burn	Exposed areas
	Increased visibility of normal oxyhemoglobin caused by vasodilation from fever, blushing, alcohol, inflammation	Localized
	Decreased oxygen use in skin, as in cold exposure	
	Carbon monoxide poisoning	
Yellow	Increased bilirubinemia caused by liver disease, red cell hemolysis	Sclera in initial stages and then generalized
Blue	Hypoxemia	Central (lips, tongue, nail beds)
	Decreased flow to skin because of anxiety or cold	Localized, peripheral
	Abnormal hemoglobin from combination with methylene or sulfa drugs	Central
Pale or white	Obstructive, hemorrhagic, distributive, or cardiogenic shock	Generalized
	Renal failure	Generalized
	Fear or pain	Generalized and self-limiting

From Newberry L: *Sheehy's emergency nursing: principles and practice,* ed 5, St Louis, 2003, Mosby.

Endocrine

Consider endocrine disorders when the patient has fatigue, weakness, mental status changes, weight changes, hot or cold episodes, low serum sodium levels, polyuria and polydipsia, or sexual abnormalities. Observe for any signs of unusual sexual characteristics such as syndrome of precocious puberty.

Immunologic

A patient's lifestyle, immunization status, and history of diseases are key factors in assessing the immune system. Fever is an important consideration, but not all patients with an elevated temperature are febrile. Noninfectious causes include heat stroke and malignant hyperthermia. Conversely, significant illness and infection can be present without fever in patients who are immunocompromised. In the ED, immediately place persons who are suspected of having or who have a known communicable disease in a protective environment to limit transmission. Additional assessment questions should address travel, particularly within days or weeks of symptom onset. Other considerations include recent immunizations and exposure to persons with similar symptoms.

References

1. Dillon PA: *Nursing health assessment: a critical thinking, case studies approach,* Philadelphia, 2003, Davis.
2. Seidel HM et al: *Mosby's guide to physical examination,* ed 5, St Louis, 2003, Mosby.
3. Docherty B: Cardiorespiratory physical assessment for the acutely ill: 1, *Br J Nurs* 11(11):750-758, 2002.

4. Gorgas DL: Vital sign measurement. In Roberts JR, Hedges JR, editors: *Clinical procedures in emergency medicine,* ed 4, Philadelphia, 2004, Saunders.

5. Behrman RE, Kliegman RA, Jenson HB: *Nelson textbook of pediatrics,* ed 17, Philadelphia, 2004, Saunders.

6. Newberry L: *Sheehy's emergency nursing: principles and practices,* ed 5, St Louis, 2003, Mosby.

7. Engel J: *Pediatric assessment: pocket guide series,* ed 4, St Louis, 2002, Mosby.

8. Estes ME: *Health assessment & physical examination,* ed 2, New York, 2002, Delmar.

9. Docherty B: Cardiorespiratory physical assessment for the acutely ill: 2, *Br J Nurs* 11(12):800-807, 2002.

8

Intravenous Therapy

Jessie M. Moore, APRN-BC, MSN, CEN

INTRAVENOUS THERAPY

Intravenous (IV) therapy is an essential component of emergency care. Intravenous lines are placed for direct infusion of fluids, medications, and blood products into the vascular circulation. Line placement requires a general familiarity with the circulatory anatomy, and one must consider many factors when deciding where to insert a line. Although some sites are clearly preferable to others, consider the situation. Sometimes the need for urgency takes precedence over selection of the optimal long-term location. In emergency situations, when access is critical, the best IV site is the one most accessible.

TYPES OF INTRAVENOUS SOLUTIONS

Fluids used for intravenous therapy are classified broadly as crystalloids or colloids. Crystalloid solutions are composed of water and electrolytes that readily diffuse across capillary membrane. Colloid solutions contain large molecules that do not move easily from the vascular system into the interstitial and intracellular spaces. Hence they serve to increase plasma oncotic pressure.

Dextrose-Containing Solutions

Dextrose-containing solutions are available in various concentrations and in combination with other solutions (such as 5% dextrose in normal saline, dextrose in 0.45% saline, and

5% dextrose in lactated Ringer's solution). These are the only IV solutions routinely used in emergency care that provide patients with any calories. Dextrose 5% in water contains 5 g of glucose (20 calories) per 100 mL. This solution is considered an isotonic solution. Dextrose solutions with higher concentrations (e.g., 10% dextrose in water) are hypertonic. Both 5% and 10% solutions may be given peripherally; concentrations greater than 10% (e.g., total parenteral nutrition) must infused through a central vein. The exception to this rule is the emergency administration of dextrose 50%. This drug may be given in a peripheral vein if it is administered slowly.[1]

Uses

Five percent dextrose in water is used commonly to keep IV lines open, reverse nonelectrolyte dehydration, and provide (minimal) calorie replacement. Hang 10% dextrose in water whenever total parenteral nutrition must be discontinued abruptly. Ten percent dextrose in water also may be indicated for patients with certain conditions such as a hypoglycemic agent overdose.

Precautions

Dextrose-containing solutions should never be infused in the same IV line as blood because they cause red blood cell lysis. Dextrose also may affect the stability of certain drug admixtures (ampicillin, phenytoin). Always check compatibility before administration. Although 5% dextrose in water is isotonic when infused, the dextrose component is metabolized rapidly in the body, leaving only water, a hypotonic solution, which quickly moves from the circulation into the cells. This effect can increase intracranial pressure in patients with head injuries.

Sodium-Containing Intravenous Solutions

Like dextrose solutions, sodium-containing IV solutions are available in a variety of concentrations: hypotonic (e.g., 0.45% NaCl), isotonic (0.9% NaCl or normal saline), and hypertonic (e.g., 3% or 7% NaCl).

Uses

Infusion of a sodium-containing IV solution restores water and salt. These fluids are typically used in patients with dehydration or volume loss of any cause. Because a sodium-containing solution is compatible with blood products, an isotonic sodium-containing solution (normal saline) is used when giving transfusions. Other indications include medication administration and metabolic alkalosis.

Precautions

Use sodium-containing solutions cautiously in patients with conditions involving sodium or water retention, such as congestive heart failure and renal failure. Large infusions can lead to hypokalemia, circulatory overload, hypernatremia, and hyperchloremic acidosis.

Multiple-Electrolyte Solutions

Ringer's injection contains an isotonic mix of sodium, potassium, calcium, and chloride in approximate plasma concentrations. This solution is used rarely today. Lactated Ringer's solution (or lactated Ringer's solution) contains the same ingredients, with the addition of lactate added as a buffer.

Uses

Lactated Ringer's solution expands intravascular volume by replacing extracellular fluid losses. This solution is the standard fluid administered for patients with multiple trauma, severe shock, or cardiac arrest.

Precautions

Excess quantities of lactated Ringer's solution may cause overhydration, electrolyte excess (particularly sodium), and metabolic alkalosis. Use with caution in patients with cardiac or renal disorders. Because lactate is metabolized in the liver, lactated Ringer's is contraindicated in patients with significant hepatic dysfunction.

DELIVERY SYSTEMS

Glass vs. Plastic

With the exception of solutions that are incompatible with plastics (fat emulsions, insulin, nitroglycerin, lorazepam), plastic bags have become the modern standard for IV therapy.[1] When bottles are used, they must be vented so that the solution will flow freely. Venting is accomplished most commonly with the use of a special, vented IV administration set. Plastic bags do not require venting and can be placed in rapid infusion devices such as pressure infusion sleeves. However, bags are susceptible to puncture when they are spiked and when admixtures are instilled. Discard bags if any leakage is detected.

Intravenous Administration Sets

Primary administration sets

The primary administration set is the main tubing that carries fluid to the IV insertion site. Tubing type is selected based on the method of infusion: gravity, infusion pump, or micro-bore syringe pump.

Secondary administration sets

Secondary administration sets are designed to deliver medications or additional fluids. These lines are piggybacked into the primary administration set and may be used intermittently or continuously. Secondary sets should come with a built-in safety device, such as a Luer-Lok connector or blunt plastic cannula, to reduce the risk of accidental stick injuries during connection and disconnection.

Metered volume chamber sets

Metered volume chamber sets (Buretrol, Volutrol, Soluset) are small-volume (e.g., 100-mL) cylinders that are placed between the solution container and the administration set. These devices allow more accurate control of the volume to be infused, preventing accidental overinfusion. Use of metered volume chamber sets is restricted largely to the pediatric population, but such sets are also handy for medication administration in adults. Increased availability of macrodrip IV pumps has decreased use of these devices.

Blood administration sets

Blood administration sets are designed for infusion of blood products. With their Y tubing, two bags can be spiked onto the primary line, making it possible to run normal saline through one arm of the Y and a blood product through the other. This type of tubing has a greater internal diameter and larger drip size (10 drops/mL) than standard tubing. It also contains a filter that screens and removes some of the aggregates found in stored blood. Although designed for blood administration, this type of tubing can be used whenever large volumes of fluid need to be infused rapidly.

Nitroglycerin administration sets

Some studies have indicated that nitroglycerin adheres to standard (polyvinyl chloride) tubing to varying degrees, causing loss of the drug during administration. For this reason, special tubing sets are made from a non–polyvinyl chloride material. They are, however, more expensive. Because nitroglycerin dosing is titrated to effect, many clinicians simply elect to use standard administration sets. If standard tubing is used, it is important to recognize that tubing changes will cause fluctuations in the amount of drug delivered, and dosages may need to be adjusted.

Infusion pump sets

Infusion pump sets are device-specific, and the pump you use may or may not require special tubing to infuse correctly. Always follow the manufacturer's recommendations. To prevent accidental free flow of fluid, be sure that the tubing has a roller clamp in place so that flow rates can be controlled when the pump is not operating.

Patient-Controlled Analgesia

Patient-controlled analgesia pumps can deliver continuous, on-demand, or combination medication doses. These pumps come with several features to prevent tampering. Not only do they have a rate control lockout feature, but their special tubing prevents drug extraction from the line.

Saline or Heparin Locks

A saline or heparin lock is a peripheral IV cannula without tubing attached and with no continuous fluid flow. The distal end of the cannula is plugged. The purpose of this lock is to provide emergency access to a vein, should the need arise. The locks are also appropriate for patients who require only intermittent medication administration or frequent blood sampling. To prevent clotting, the cannula must be filled with a heparinized solution or normal saline. The decision regarding which solution to use is based on institutional policy, but many studies have documented the effectiveness of using a simple saline solution for this purpose.

Drop Factors

The drop factor is the number of drops, delivered by a given tubing, that equal 1 mL. Knowing this number is essential for calculating IV rates any time an infusion is not on a pump.

Box **8-1** Intravenous Flow Rate Calculation

Intravenous flow rates commonly are ordered in milliliters per hour. Calculate the following formula to determine the number of drops per minute.

$$\frac{\text{Drop factor (drops/mL)}}{\text{Minutes/hour (60)}} \times x \text{ mL/hr (ordered)} = \text{Desired drops/min}$$

Example

An intravenous infusion is ordered to infuse at 150 mL/hr using a macrodrip tubing with a drop factor of 15 drops/mL.

$$\frac{15 \text{ drops/mL}}{60 \text{ min/hour}} \times 150 \text{ mL/hr} = \text{Desired drops/min}$$

Answer

38 (37.5) drops/min
When determining drops per minute, always round to a whole number.

Box 8-1 gives information on calculating flow rates based on tubing type. The two general IV tubing classifications are these:

Macrodrip. "Regular" tubing; commonly 10, 12, 15, or 20 drops/mL; must be used whenever rapid fluid administration may be needed

Microdrip. "Pedi" tubing; usually 60 drops/mL; used for pediatric fluid administration, medication drips, and volume-restricted patients

INTRAVENOUS CATHETERS AND CANNULAS

Peripheral Catheters

A wide variety of styles and brands of peripheral IV access devices are on the market, and new versions are introduced regularly. The following section discusses several basic types; each has indications and limitations. Check with your institution for specific equipment availability.

Winged needles

Winged needles, also known as scalp vein needles or "butterflies," consist of a stainless steel needle with two winglike plastic projections mounted where the needle meets the catheter. These wings facilitate catheter placement and anchoring. Because they are easy to secure and easy to place (no plastic catheter to slide off the needle and position in a vein), winged needles are particularly useful for drawing blood. With time, however, steel needles can damage veins, and it is recommended that they be reserved for short-term (1 to 4 hours) use.

Over-the-needle catheters

An over-the-needle catheter is a tapered catheter that is fitted snugly over a needle. The needle is used to puncture the skin and vein, the catheter is advanced over the needle, and the needle then is removed from the patient. Many brands have winged protrusions to improve handling and facilitate securing the catheter. This style of catheter is the one most commonly used in hospitals. Over-the-needle "butterflies" and dual-lumen catheters are also available. Color-coding of IV catheter hubs is not universal in the medical device industry; therefore it is essential that all IV sites be labeled with the size of the catheter placed. Most modern catheters are made of highly specialized plastics designed to reduce thrombogenesis, minimize vein trauma, and lower the incidence of complications. Some materials even expand, increasing in size once they are in the vessel.[1]

Through-the-needle catheters

With this type of device a steel or plastic needle makes the initial puncture, and then a softer plastic catheter is advanced through the needle into the vein. When first introduced, the needle was designed to remain on the device, secured by an outer plastic clip. Newer versions use splittable needles that are removed, leaving only the catheter attached to the patient. Peripherally inserted central catheters commonly are placed using a through-the-needle technique.

Plain plastic catheters

Plain plastic catheters are used when an intravenous cutdown is performed. The catheter (often just a length of IV tubing) is inserted directly into a vein during an open, sterile cutdown procedure. (See the section on venous cutdowns.)

Dual-lumen peripheral catheters

A dual-lumen peripheral catheter has two separate infusion channels. One lumen exits at the tip of the catheter, the second ends more proximal to the hub. This configuration allows simultaneous infusion of incompatible solutions through a single venipuncture site. The combined lumen size of the catheter is fairly large and requires selection of an adequately sized vessel.

Catheter Size

Peripheral intravenous catheters commonly range in length from 5/8 to 2 inches but may be as much as several inches long. Table 8-1 gives information on selecting a catheter gauge.[1]

The rate of fluid administration is limited by the diameter and length of the tubing and catheter. Therefore as a general rule, if rapid volume infusion is required (or potentially required), insert a large-bore ($\geq$16-gauge), short ($\leq$1 1/4-inch) catheter, attached to Y-type (large-diameter) blood tubing, with a single, short extension tubing. This combination maximizes volume infusion. Certain age-appropriate adjustments may need to be made.

Central Venous Access

Several types of catheters and devices are used to access central veins.

Table 8-1 **Catheter Size Recommendations**

Size	Clinical Applications
14-18 gauge	Trauma, surgery, rapid blood product administration
20 gauge	Continuous or intermittent infusion, routine blood product administration
22 gauge	Intermittent or general infusion, particularly in children and the elderly
24 gauge	Infants, small children, and persons with fragile veins

Standard catheters

Standard central lines are inserted by puncturing the subclavian or internal jugular vessel (most commonly). The site then is cannulated with a catheter that extends to the heart. A central venous catheter can have one lumen or multiple lumens. Pulmonary artery catheters are a sophisticated type of central venous catheter.

Peripherally inserted central catheter (PICC) lines are peripherally inserted catheters that are threaded into the superior vena cava position.

Tunneled catheters

Tunneled catheters are silicone-cuffed catheters that have been placed surgically in a central vessel to provide long-term venous access. A tunnel is formed under the skin, from the vein to the catheter exit point. This exit point is located at a site designed to facilitate self-care and maintenance (anterior chest wall, upper abdomen). Brands of tunneled catheters include Hickman, Broviac, Raaf, and Groshong. These may be single lumen or multilumen. See the section on accessing tunneled catheters.

Implanted ports

Implanted ports (e.g., Port-A-Cath [Deltec, Inc. St. Paul, Minn]) come in single- and double-lumen styles. The terminal end of the catheter is situated in the central vena cava. These devices are placed surgically under the skin (usually on the chest) of patients who will require long-term vascular access for fluids, drugs, or blood sampling. Implantable ports have a dense latex or silicone septum overlying a hollow reservoir, and they are easily palpable under the skin (Figure 8-1). This septum is built to withstand 1000 to 2000 needle sticks, but it is essential that only special, noncoring needles (Huber needles) be used to access the device (Figure 8-2). See the section on accessing implanted ports.

Peripherally Inserted Central Catheters and Midline and Midclavicular Catheters

Peripherally inserted central catheters and midline and midclavicular catheters are used for long-term IV access (weeks to months). These long-term access catheters are not inserted in

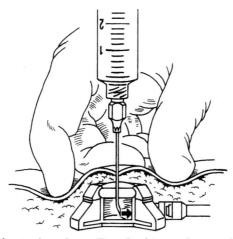

Figure 8-1.   Cross section of an implanted port. (From Bard Access Systems, Salt Lake City, Utah.)

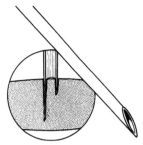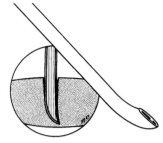

Figure 8-2. Huber tipped needle. **A,** Hypodermic needle. **B,** Noncoring needle. (From Bard Access Systems, Salt Lake City, Utah.)

the emergency department, but many patients with chronic conditions have one of these devices in place. Emergency nurses must be familiar with these lines and know how to access them.

Catheters inserted peripherally that extend all the way to the superior vena cava and are considered central lines. Midline (midarm) and midclavicular catheters are threaded 3 to 10 inches from the insertion site. A midline catheter is defined as a peripherally inserted catheter with a tip that terminates in the proximal portion of the upper extremity (upper arm). A midclavicular catheter is a peripherally inserted catheter with a tip located in the proximal axillary or subclavian vein. Midclavicular lines are associated with significantly higher rates of thrombosis than are peripherally inserted central catheter lines (up to 60% in some reports).[2] These lines are used only when further advancement of the catheter is not possible *and* other IV access options are limited. Because they are not centrally place, midclavicular and midline catheters should *not* be called peripherally inserted central catheter lines. This could result in administration of solutions and medications suitable only for central vein infusion.

Alternative Access Devices

Dialysis access devices

Dialysis access sites traditionally have not been used for routine intravenous therapy or blood collection because of their high potential for infection and thrombosis. However, new silicone dialysis-type catheters now are being used for intermittent therapy in some practice settings. Only trained personnel should access dialysis shunts except in life-or-death situations in which no other access can be established. If a dialysis catheter is accessed, it should always be aspirated first to remove the heparinized saline bolus that was injected to keep the line patent. Higher concentrations of heparin are used in this type of catheter access.

Intraosseous needles

An intraosseous device is a large, steel needle that is inserted directly into the marrow cavity of a bone. Intraosseous devices are an efficient way to get fluids and medications into the vascular system in emergent situations. Any substance that can be infused in a vein (e.g., crystalloids, colloids, blood products, medications, and vasoactive drips) can be infused through an intraosseous line. Use of an intraosseous line has no upper age limit, but these lines are more common in children. Generally, it is easier to find and cannulate a large vein in an

Table 8-2   **Selecting an Intravenous Insertion Site**

Vein	Location	Considerations
Metacarpal	Dorsum of the hand	
Cephalic	Radial aspect of the forearm	
Basilic	Ulnar aspect of the arm	
Median	Ulnar aspect and antecubital fossa	The antecubital fossa veins are at greater risk for mechanical phlebitis and infection and should not be the preferred site except in emergency situations.[1]

Avoid the use of the following*:

Any extremity with an arteriovenous fistula or graft
The affected extremity of a stroke patient
The affected arm in a postmastectomy patient
Lower extremity sites except in children

*Accessing these sites is sometimes necessary in emergency situations. If use is required, follow institutional policy and monitor the site closely for complications.

adult, because as bones calcify with age, it becomes progressively more difficult to drill the intraosseous catheter through to the marrow in adults. An 18-gauge intraosseous line is recommended for infants and small children; use a 15- or 16-gauge intraosseous line in older children and adults.

Special intraosseous needles (Jamshidi Illinois [Baxter Healthcare Corp., Deerfield, Ill]) have been designed and are easiest to use. However, needles used for lumbar puncture can be used in a pinch. See the section on intraosseous catheter insertion.

INSERTION PROCEDURES

Peripheral Intravenous Site Selection

The choice of an IV site depends on a number of factors. Before inserting a line, consider the following:
- The purpose of the IV line and the approximate length of time the catheter will be in place
- The clinical condition of the patient
- The age and size of the patient
- The condition of the vein

Table 8-2 lists other factors to address. Do not forget to inform the patient and family of the rationale for therapy. Explain any special requirements related to positioning, intake and output measurement, and potential adverse reactions.

Ideally, the most distal site on an extremity would be selected first. If repeat venipuncture is necessary, the new site should be proximal to the discontinued site. In the search for an IV site, the external jugular vein often is overlooked. The vein is big, is easy to cannulate, and can accommodate a large-bore catheter. An external jugular vein site should be considered in patients with cardiopulmonary arrest, or any large fluid volume needs. Check the protocol of your institution; in many facilities, only physicians may access this site. Boxes 8-2 and 8-3 address issues related to IV therapy complications.

Box **8-2** **Complications of Intravenous Therapy**

Catheter fragmentation and embolism
Cellulitis
Extravasation
Fluid overload
Hematoma
Infiltration
Phlebitis: bacterial, mechanical, or chemical
Sepsis
Thrombosis

Box **8-3** **Measures to Prevent Intravenous Complications**

When possible, avoid inserting intravenous lines in areas of flexion (e.g., wrist or antecubital fossa).
Use strict aseptic technique for insertion.
Select the smallest gauge catheter that is appropriate for the task.
Large veins provide greater hemodilution when administering irritating medications (e.g., 50% dextrose, phenytoin, vasopressors, and sodium bicarbonate).
Securely tape catheters to prevent excessive movement at the site of entry.
Avoid the use of lower extremity veins (except in nonambulatory children).
Inspect catheters for defects before use.
Never reinsert the stylet into an over-the-needle catheter.
Assess the patient's circulatory and pulmonary status before and during intravenous therapy.

Insertion Site Preparation

To prepare a site for insertion of an IV line, perform the following:

1. Apply a tourniquet to the extremity 4 to 6 inches above the proposed site.
2. Keep the tourniquet in place for no longer than 5 minutes. If the vein does not dilate enough for cannulation, rub the vein or tap it lightly, hold the limb in a dependent position, apply heat with a hot pack or warm towel, or have the patient open and close the fist.
3. Apply 70% isopropyl alcohol for a minimum of 30 seconds. Allow the site to air dry, and then apply a povidone-iodine (Betadine) or chlorhexidine gluconate (Hibiclens) solution. All cleansing solutions should be applied with friction, scrubbing outward from the insertion site.[1]
4. The routine use of 1% lidocaine before catheter insertion is *not* recommended by the Intravenous Nurses Society. Allergic reactions, anaphylaxis, vein constriction, and other untoward responses have been known to occur.[3]
5. Instead of lidocaine, bacteriostatic normal saline can be used intradermally or subcutaneously. The benzyl alcohol preservative acts on nerve endings, producing a short period of local anesthesia. This technique has not been approved for use on neonates or with intrathecal devices.[3]
6. Topical products, such as lidocaine and prilocaine (EMLA) cream, tetracaine 4% cream, and 4% tetracaine and 1% lidocaine (LaserCaine) can be used to reduce pain. Unfortunately, their usefulness in the emergency setting is limited because of the length of time required for the onset of effects (30 to 60 minutes).[3]

Peripheral Venipuncture Techniques

For peripheral venipuncture, perform the following:

1. Always use standard body fluid precautions when initiating IV lines.
2. Use self-sheathing needle protection devices whenever possible to prevent accidental needlesticks and blood exposure.
3. Stabilize the vein by applying traction to the side of the insertion site.
4. The depth of the vein in the subcutaneous tissue determines the angle used to enter the skin (10- to 30-degree angle). The deeper the vein, the greater the angle.
5. Puncture the skin and the vein with the bevel of the needle facing upward (in older children and adults).
6. Advance the needle slowly, check for a blood return ("flashback"), and then thread the catheter into the vein according to the manufacturer's instructions.
7. Remove the tourniquet.
8. Connect the IV tubing or saline/heparin lock.
9. Begin fluid flow (or flush the lock) to ascertain site patency.
10. Tape the device securely according to institutional protocol. Be sure to anchor IV lines with extreme care in an infant or small child; movement can easily dislodge tiny catheters.
11. Label the dressing with the date, time, catheter size, and your initials.

INTRAVENOUS THERAPY IN PEDIATRIC PATIENTS

Site Considerations

The IV sites of choice in an infant or small child are as follows:

- Dorsum of the hand
- Dorsum of the foot
- Scalp (in an infant)
- Umbilical vein (in the newborn). This vein is easy to cannulate, but most facilities limit this procedure to physicians.

Tips for Intravenous Catheter Insertion

To insert an IV catheter into a child, perform the following:

1. Use rubber bands or $3/8$-inch Penrose drains as tourniquets. If these are not available, cut a strip from an adult tourniquet.
2. Have a caregiver hold the child securely or position the young child in a passive restraint device (e.g., Papoose Board) before beginning the procedure.
3. A flashlight placed beneath a small hand or foot helps outline the targeted vein and illuminates the surrounding tissue.
4. Insert the needle with the bevel facing downward to prevent puncture of the back wall of the vein.
5. Spasms can occur in small veins. Stop advancing the catheter and place a warm compress over the vein. Resume advancing the catheter when the spasm has stopped.
6. Use a syringe filled with normal saline, attached to the catheter, to "float" the catheter into the vein once the stylet is removed. This prevents catheter clotting, dilates the vein for easier catheter advancement, and helps confirm correct placement even when a significant blood return is not detected.
7. Padded tongue blades can function as arm boards in little patients; these blades may be placed before venipuncture to help immobilize the extremity.

Scalp Vein Access

The scalp veins of an infant are an important IV sites often overlooked by nurses. These veins are easily accessible in children less than 1 year of age.[5] Scalp sites have less fat than chubby baby hands or feet, they leave the infant's extremities free from armboards and restraints, and they are relatively easy to stabilize. The only major downside to using a scalp site is caregiver perception. Parents may be uncomfortable with the thought of you "sticking a needle in my baby's head." However, when a calm and caring nurse explains the benefits, most parents will find a scalp vein site acceptable. While this site is probably the easiest of all infant sites to cannulate, some special steps and considerations are required:

1. Veins must be differentiated from arteries. Arteries are more tortuous; they pulsate and fill with blood from below while veins fill from above.
2. To prepare the site, shave an area large enough to secure the catheter well. You cannot effectively tape to hair.
3. For a tourniquet, place a rubber band around the head proximal to the venipuncture site. A 1-inch piece of tape, forming a tab around the rubber band, greatly facilitates lifting the band off the patient when the procedure is finished. A pair of scissors nearby also is a good idea. Lifting the tab and snipping the rubber band is much easier than getting an intact rubber band off the head without dislodging the new IV line.
4. Insert the needle in the direction of blood flow (toward the heart) (Figure 8-3).
5. A 23- to 27-gauge butterfly needle generally is used. A 24-gauge over-the-needle catheter also can be placed.
6. Tape the needle or catheter at the point where it enters the skin. A commercial IV protection device or half of a plastic medicine cup can be used to cover and protect the site.
7. The complications of scalp vein use are the same as those at other sites, including the following:
   - Infection
   - Bleeding
   - Extravasation of fluids or medications
   - Inadvertent arterial puncture

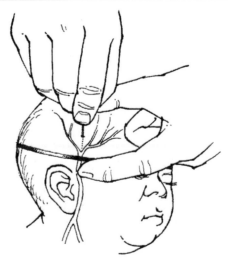

Figure 8-3. Insertion of an intravenous line into the scalp vein of an infant. Using a rubber band as a tourniquet to distend the scalp veins, the needle is introduced approximately 0.5 cm distal to the anticipated site of the vessel puncture. (From Roberts JR, Hedges JR: *Clinical procedures in emergency medicine*, ed 4, St Louis, 2004, WB Saunders.)

INTRAVENOUS THERAPY IN THE ELDERLY

Intravenous therapy in the older adult may require deviation from your standard site selection process. Due to loss of subcutaneous fat and thinning of the skin, dorsal hand sites are less desirable in the elderly. Use can lead to mechanical inflammation and infiltration.

Tips for Intravenous Catheter Insertion

Use the following steps to insert an IV line in an older adult[1,4]:

1. Sidelighting is effective for locating vein shadows below the skin. Bright overhead light may cause a washout effect, making veins hard to visualize.
2. If the vein is visible and already distended, use of a tourniquet can produce excessive distention and may cause vein damage or rupture upon catheter insertion. If veins are not already distended, you may need to allow a few moments longer after placing the tourniquet; venous return is slower in the elderly.
3. Avoid using sclerosed (hard) veins. The walls of these vessels are thickened, leaving only a narrow or occluded lumen.
4. Avoid sites with venous valves or select a smaller catheter size to thread the IV past the valve.
5. Decreased subcutaneous tissue mass causes veins to roll. To immobilize a vein, find the axis of the vessel, place your nondominant thumb directly along the axis 2 to 3 inches below the intended insertion site, and position your index finger above the insertion site.
6. Use of subcutaneously administered lidocaine before IV insertion may cause tissue swelling and other complications in the elderly.
7. Light tapping can enhance vein dilation; slapping may produce vessel rupture.
8. In patients with fragile veins, preflush the catheter with normal saline before attempting access; the preflushed catheter will show blood return more quickly.
9. Maintain stabilization of the skin while using a one-handed technique to advance the catheter.
10. To float a catheter into a tortuous vein, release the tourniquet, remove the stylet, connect the IV tubing, and slowly infuse fluid to distend the vein while gently advancing the catheter.

Central Vein Cannulation

Catheterization of the subclavian or internal jugular veins provides a site for large volume administration and enables measurement of central venous pressures. However, catheterizing these sites carries a risk of pneumothorax, and so these sites should be reserved for urgent situations. Only physicians (or other advanced practitioners) usually perform subclavian and internal jugular vein cannulation.

Assisting With Subclavian Catheter Insertion

For insertion of a subclavian catheter, perform the following:

1. Assemble all necessary supplies and instrument trays: sterile gloves, sterile drapes, catheter of choice, flushing solution (per institution policy), a central line dressing kit, lidocaine, and suture material. Many facilities mandate the use of masks and gowns for central line placement.
2. To increase the size of the vein and decrease the possibility of air embolism, tip the patient into a head down, feet elevated position.

3. Place a rolled towel between the patient's shoulder blades to provide a better insertion angle.
4. Cleanse the neck and upper chest with an antiseptic solution (per institutional policy).
5. Assist with the procedure as directed (e.g., apply sterile drapes, flush all catheter ports, set up IV lines for infusion, and connect equipment for central venous pressure monitoring).
6. Observe the patient's cardiorespiratory status during the procedure.
7. Apply a dry sterile dressing or a transparent occlusive dressing per institution protocol.
8. Label the dressing site with date, time, catheter size, and insertion depth.

Measuring Central Venous Pressure

Central venous pressure is a measurement of the blood pressure on the right side of the heart. From this number, inferences can be made about blood volume and cardiac effectiveness. Pressure can be measured directly (in centimeters of water) with a manual manometer interposed between the catheter and the IV line. Pressure also can measured by a pressurized line, transduced for display on a bedside monitor in millimeters of mercury.

The normal range for central venous pressures is 4 to 10 cm H_2O. A value greater than 10 cm H_2O may indicate cardiac tamponade, failure of the right side of the heart, fluid overload, pulmonary edema, tension pneumothorax, or hemothorax. A value less than 4 cm H_2O can indicate hypovolemia (hemorrhage, dehydration) or vasodilation (septic, anaphylactic, neurogenic, or drug-induced shock).

Measuring Central Venous Pressure With a Manual Manometer

To measure central venous pressure using a manual manometer, perform the following:
1. Place the patient in a supine (flat) position.
2. Determine the location of the phlebostatic axis. This point—the fourth intercostal space, midaxillary line—represents the level of the right atrium. Mark an X at this spot to keep future readings consistent.
3. From the attached IV solution, fill the manometer approximately half way by turning the stopcock of the manometer off to the patient and open to only the manometer and the IV bag. Do not let fluid contact the top of the manometer. The manometer will not function if this filter gets wet.
4. Place the zero marking of the manometer at the phlebostatic axis.
5. Next, turn the stopcock so that it is open to the patient and to the manometer (closed to the IV line).
6. Holding the manometer at the phlebostatic axis, watch the fluid level fall. Eventually the fluid will reach a fairly steady state characterized by minor fluctuations with each breath.
7. When the fluid level appears stable, note where the top of the fluid column reaches.
8. Record this number (in centimeters of water) as the central venous pressure.
9. Adjust the stopcock to close off the manometer and reopen the IV line. Be sure to readjust the IV solution flow rate as needed.

Venous Cutdown

The saphenous vein at the ankle and the basilic vein in the antecubital fossa are the sites most commonly used for cutdown IVs. This surgical procedure is performed when rapid access must be obtained for large volume infusions (usually trauma patients). The steps in the procedure include the following:

1. A skin incision is made perpendicular to the vein.
2. The skin is retracted to expose the vein.
3. The vein is lifted with suture ties that will later be used to control bleeding.
4. The vein is incised and a large bore sterile catheter (or piece of IV tubing) is placed directly in the vessel.
5. The catheter is secured with the sutures.
6. The skin is closed and dressed.
   Complications include the following:
   - Infection
   - Phlebitis
   - Laceration of a nerve or artery

Intraosseous Infusions

An intraosseous infusion involves the IV administration of fluids and drugs directly into the bone marrow. This procedure may be considered for adults and children. However, after 5 years of age, infusion rates are slowed because of the presence of yellow marrow in the bones.[5] Circumstances in which intraosseous placement may be considered include the following:

- Cardiopulmonary arrest
- Hypovolemic shock
- Status epilepticus

Intraosseous infusion also may be considered for any other condition in which the administration of fluid or medication is critical to survival and IV access sites are not rapidly available.

Intraosseous Catheter Insertion Procedure

For infusion by intraosseous catheter, perform the following:

1. In children under the age of 5 the anterior medial surface of the tibia—about 2 cm below the tibial tuberosity—is the preferred site. In adults, the medial malleolus of the tibia is the most common location. Other sites that may be used include the distal anterior femur, the iliac crest, and the sternum.[5]
2. Prepare the area with a povidone-iodine (Betadine) solution.
3. Select a large-bore, metal biopsy needle (an Illinois sternal bone marrow needle or a Jamshidi needle) and advance it through the skin, fascia, and bony cortex using a back-and-forth boring motion. The needle can be inserted perpendicular to the bone but frequently is angled slightly away from the joint space to avoid (hypothetical) injury to the growth plate (Figure 8-4).
4. The needle has entered the bone marrow when you feel a popping sensation, followed by a sudden absence of resistance. The needle should be able to stand upright without manual support.
5. Using a syringe, attempt to aspirate. If bone marrow is returned, the needle has been placed correctly. In shock situations, aspiration may be unsuccessful and does not necessarily indicate misplacement.[5]
6. Once the needle is in the marrow cavity, it should be fairly secure. Minimal padding or taping is required.
7. Begin infusion of solutions and medications. Unlike the venous system, in which blood is constantly flowing, there is no continual flow through the bone marrow. Therefore fluids

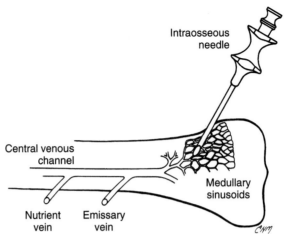

Figure 8-4. Insertion of an intraosseous needle into the tibial tuberosity. (From Roberts JR, Hedges JR: *Clinical procedures in emergency medicine*, ed 4, St Louis, 2004, WB Saunders.

will infuse slowly unless they are under pressure. Provide positive pressure by using a syringe (manual pressure), an infusion pump, or a pressure bag.

Complications of intraosseous infusions include the following[5]:
- Infection (rare; less than 1%)
- Bone fracture
- Fat embolism (adults only)

ACCESSING VENOUS ACCESS DEVICES

Throughout the country, various procedures are used for connecting to long-term venous access devices. Always consult protocols of your institution. However, the fundamental principle of successful venous access device use is strict adherence to aseptic technique. Patients and their families are frequently familiar with the care and use of these devices, and they often have strong preferences regarding venous access device management. Listed below are the basic steps for accessing blood samples from tunneled and nontunneled catheters and from implanted ports.

Tunneled and Nontunneled Catheters

To take blood samples from tunneled and nontunneled catheters, perform the following:
1. Always wear sterile gloves.
2. Gather the necessary equipment:
   - Laboratory tubes/test requisitions
   - Heparinized saline 100 units/mL in a syringe (Institutional protocols for amounts of flush solutions vary with types of catheters. Follow your individual institution policies.)
   - Alcohol wipes and povidone-iodine (Betadine) swabs
   - Two 10-mL syringes, one filled with saline
   - A syringe large enough to draw the required amount of blood. Several smaller syringes should be considered when a large amount of blood is needed, to decrease hemolysis in the collected blood.

- 18-gauge needles for inserting blood into collection tubes
- Sterile Luer-Lok caps (one for each port that will be opened)
3. Prepare a sterile barrier; place sterile supplies on the barrier.
4. Turn off (but do not disconnect) all infusions; clamp each catheter.
5. Disconnect the infusion from the catheter hub (or remove the Luer-Lok cap) of the lumen that will be used for blood sampling. Patients or their family members generally know which lumen is used routinely for blood removal.
6. Attach a 10-mL syringe to the catheter hub; unclamp the catheter and withdraw 6 mL of blood. Reclamp the catheter and discard the blood. One should note that some institutions prefer to use this initial aspirate for blood cultures.
7. Using a syringe (or syringes) large enough to accommodate the blood needed for samples, withdraw the specified amount. Blood for clotting studies should not be drawn from heparinized catheters. Clamp the catheter, remove the collection syringe, and inject the blood into the appropriate laboratory tubes or culture bottles.
8. Flush the catheter with 10 to 20 mL of normal saline, and then reattach and restart the infusion. If the patient has a dual-lumen or triple-lumen catheter, unclamp the other catheters and restart these infusions as well.
9. Following the saline flush, if the catheter is to be capped (no infusion), flush it with heparinized saline (100 units/mL). The protocol of your institution will specify the concentration and amount. Patients and family members are generally aware of the volume of heparinized saline required. Next, clamp the catheter, clean off the hub with an alcohol wipe, seal the catheter with a sterile Luer-Lok cap, and tape the cap on for added security. One should note that Groshong catheters do *not* require a heparin flush.
10. Label blood sample tubes and send to the laboratory.

Accessing Implanted Ports

To access implanted ports, perform the following:
1. Have the patient lie supine or in a semi-Fowler position.
2. Gather the necessary supplies. Place sterile items on a sterile barrier:
   - 10-mL syringe; fill with normal saline
   - Alcohol wipes and povidone-iodine (Betadine) swabs
   - 90-degree Huber needle (ask the patient/family member what gauge and length)
   - Sterile gloves
   - Sterile dressing supplies (e.g., transparent occlusive dressing)
   - Luer-Lok valve if there is no ongoing infusion
   - 5-mL syringe filled with heparinized saline (100 units/mL)
3. Palpate the site to locate the port and the septum; examine the site for signs of infection.
4. Cleanse the site with alcohol and then povidone-iodine (Betadine) swabs, starting at the center and cleaning outward in a circular motion. Allow the site to dry.
5. Prime the Huber needle with normal saline, and leave the syringe attached.
6. With the nondominant hand, stabilize the port, identify the septum, and insert the Huber needle at a 90-degree angle by pushing the needle through the skin and septum until it contacts the rigid back of the port. If the patient has a dual-lumen port, ask the patient or family member which one to use.
7. Check for correct placement by flushing with the saline remaining in the syringe. A correctly accessed port will flush easily without pain or swelling (infiltration).
8. Apply antimicrobial ointment to the site (according to hospital protocol).
9. Stabilize the needle by placing 2 × 2 inch gauze pads under the Huber needle so that the wings lay flat and the needle is stable. Tape and dress according to institutional protocol. If no protocol exists, ask the patient or family member how they care for the site.

10. Clamp the tubing and remove the syringe.
11. Hook up the infusion tubing and ensure that all connections are secure. If no infusion is ordered, flush with heparinized saline (100 units/mL; adults, 5 mL, children, 3 mL) and attach a sterile Luer-Lok cap.

Blood Sampling From Implanted Ports

To take blood samples from implanted ports, perform the following:
1. If access is required, follow the foregoing procedure.
2. If access has been achieved already, gather the necessary supplies:
   - Alcohol wipes
   - Sterile gloves
   - 10-mL syringe filled with saline
   - Syringes of appropriate size and number to draw the required amount of blood
   - Laboratory tubes, culture bottles, test requisitions, and labels
   - 18-gauge needles for inserting blood into collection tubes
   - Luer-Lok valve*
   - 5-mL syringe filled with heparinized saline (100 units/mL)*
   *Needed only if there is no ongoing infusion.
3. Stop any infusions and clamp the Huber needle tubing; disconnect the IV tubing from the needle.
4. If no infusion is running, remove the Luer-Lok cap.
5. Attach a 10-mL syringe, unclamp the tubing, and withdraw 6 mL of blood.
6. Clamp the tubing, disconnect the syringe, and discard the blood.
7. Attach the collection syringe, unclamp the tubing, and slowly withdraw the required amount of blood. Clotting studies cannot be drawn from a heparinized port.
8. Clamp the catheter, remove the collection syringe(s), and inject the blood into the appropriate laboratory tubes or culture bottles.
9. Flush the Huber needle with 10 mL of normal saline; reconnect and restart the infusion.
10. If there is no continuous infusion, flush the Huber needle with heparinized saline (100 units/mL; adults, 5 mL, children, 3 mL), and then attach a sterile Luer-Lok cap.
11. Fill and label blood tubes and culture bottles and send them to the laboratory.

Complications Associated With Venous Access Devices

The following complications may arise with venous access devices:
Infection. Infection may occur at the catheter exit site, along the track of a catheter tunnel, or as septicemia.
Obstruction. Catheter obstruction most commonly is caused by clot formation or drug precipitation.
   - *Withdrawal occlusion* is said to be present when blood cannot be withdrawn but fluid still can be infused.
   - *Intraluminal obstruction* indicates a complete occlusion; blood cannot be withdrawn and fluids cannot be infused. Gentle instillation of a fibrinolytic agent (usually recombinant tissue plasminogen activator) often can declot a catheter. This procedure requires an order from a physician or another advanced-level practitioner.
Extravasation. Extravasation is leakage from the catheter into subcutaneous or deep tissue. Symptoms include pain, swelling, and erythema. Certain drugs can cause tissue necrosis if extravasation occurs. The risk of extravasation is greatest with implantable ports. This usually occurs following Huber needle dislodgment.
Damaged catheters. A tunneled catheter possibly can be repaired if damage is limited to the external portion. Consult your IV therapy department for advice and options.

DISCONTINUATION OF INTRAVENOUS LINES

Remove peripheral catheters immediately if signs of infiltration or phlebitis are observed. Always use standard precautions for body fluid exposure, and remove the catheter with a smooth, steady motion. With dry sterile gauze, apply pressure to the insertion site until bleeding stops. Note catheter integrity, and document any abnormal findings. Only trained personnel should remove long-term, indwelling venous access devices.

To remove a central catheter, perform the following:

1. Place the patient in a supine position with the head of the bed flat.
2. Clip and remove any sutures.
3. Instruct the patient to perform a Valsalva maneuver ("Bear down," or "Take a deep breath and hold it").
4. Remove the catheter with a steady, gentle, pulling motion.
5. With a sterile gauze, hold pressure on the insertion site until the bleeding stops.
6. Apply a sterile, occlusive dressing over the insertion site per institutional policy.
7. Visually inspect the catheter.
8. Document actions and any abnormal findings.

BLOOD TRANSFUSION AND BLOOD COMPONENT THERAPY

Emergency Transfusion

The administration of uncrossmatched type O blood was once the standard approach to emergency transfusion. Now with the advent of modern blood banks, this practice generally is limited to the early resuscitation of patients with massive hemorrhage. Uncrossmatched, type-specific blood usually can be obtained from the blood bank within 10 to 15 minutes. Use of type-specific blood prevents the majority of transfusion reactions. A baseline type and crossmatch sample should always be drawn before administration of any blood products because the administration of uncrossmatched blood products will increase the difficulty of future crossmatching. Table 8-3 gives further information about specific blood products.[6]

Blood Products

Whole blood

Because less than 10% of patients require transfusion of all blood components, whole blood rarely is used today.[6] Each unit of whole blood contains 450 to 500 mL of blood plus a preservative-anticoagulant solution. Clotting factors in banked blood drop within 24 hours of collection, and potassium, hydrogen ions, and ammonia levels start to climb. Potential complications of whole blood transfusion include volume overload and antigen exposure. The plasma portion of whole blood contains antibodies that increase the risk of transfusion reactions.

Packed red blood cells

Packed red blood cells are prepared from whole blood by removing 80% to 90% of the plasma. As a rule of thumb, each unit of packed red blood cells administered should raise an adult's hemoglobin level by approximately 1 g/dL or raise the hematocrit by 3%. Current indications for the transfusion of packed red blood cells are as follows[6]:

- Acute hemorrhage of 25% to 30% of blood volume in an otherwise healthy patient
- Surgical blood loss with a hemoglobin level of less than 7 g/dL or an intraoperative blood loss of 1500 to 2000 mL

Table 8-3   Administration of Blood Products

Blood Component/ Approximate Volume	Composition/Preparation*	Indications	Shelf-Life	Special Considerations
Whole blood 500 mL	RBCs, WBCs, platelets, plasma, clotting factors. Storage of whole blood >24 hours results in destruction of platelets and clotting factors. Contains anticoagulant/preservative.	Restores massive blood volume losses from trauma, hemorrhage, or burn injuries.	42 days	When treating massive blood loss, infuse as fast as the patient can tolerate. Some studies suggest the use of a microaggregate filter. Warm blood by using an approved device (if giving large quantities). Administer with 0.9% saline.
Packed RBCs 250-350 mL	RBCs, minimal plasma, (some nonfunctioning WBCs, platelets, clotting factors). Contains preservative.	Increases the oxygen-carrying capacity of the blood in anemia. One unit raises hematocrit about 3% and hemoglobin about 1 g/dL (in adults).	42 days	Infuse over 2-4 hours. Some studies suggest the use of a microaggregate filter. Administer with 0.9% saline.
Saline-washed RBCs Leukocyte-poor RBCs Frozen-deglycerolized packed RBCs	RBCs, minimal WBCs, minimal plasma, no platelets. Leukocyte-reduced RBCs have negligible WBCs and trace platelets.	Same indications as for packed RBCs in patients with recurrent or severe allergic reactions or in multiparous women. Washed: Use in patients with a history of severe allergic reactions and for neonatal and intrauterine transfusions. Frozen: Prolonged storage of autologous blood and rare types is possible.	Must be infused within 24 hours of saline washing. Frozen: Good for up to 10 years but must be used within 24 hours of thawing/washing.	Washed and frozen RBCs still may contain viable lymphocytes and may induce graft-versus-host disease. Administer with 0.9% saline.
Granulocytes 200-300 mL (rarely used in emergency care)	Granulocytes, lymphocytes, platelets, some RBCs in plasma. From cytomegalovirus-negative donor (preferred). Irradiated (preferred).	To treat infection unresponsive to antibiotics in patients with severe neutropenia (granulocyte count <500 µL). Myeloid hypoplasia	Transfuse within 24 hours of collection.	Infuse over 2-4 hours, observing closely for fever and chills. Consider premedicating with acetaminophen, antihistamines, steroids, and meperidine. Irradiation decreases the risk of graft-versus-host disease. Infuse using a standard filter (not a leukocyte-reduction filter).

Component	Composition	Uses/Indications	Storage	Nursing Considerations
Fresh frozen plasma 100-300 mL	Plasma (with platelets removed) that contains all other clotting factors. Requires 30-40 minutes to thaw.	Used for deficiency of isolated coagulation factors II, V, VII, IX, X, and XI. Corrects bleeding tendencies associated with liver disease. Use for dilutional coagulopathies (e.g., massive transfusion), disseminated intravascular coagulation, and warfarin reversal.	May be stored for up to 1 year at 18° C. Administration must take place within 24 hours of thawing.	Infuse using a standard filter at 5-10 mL/min. No longer indicated as a volume expander, a nutritional source, or to enhance wound healing.
Platelets 30-50 mL per unit or 200-250 mL in 4-6 pooled units	Platelets, plasma, small amounts of RBCs and WBCs.	Thrombocytopenia (usually when platelet count is <50,000) or for platelet dysfunction (thrombocytopathy). Heparin-induced thrombocytopenia.	5 days at 20°-24° C with constant, gentle agitation or 48 hours at 1°-6° C. Administration must take place within 4 hours of pooling units.	Transfused platelets take 4 hours to become fully functional in the circulation. Infuse at 10 mL/min using a standard filter. Check the unit for clumps (aggregates); if present, gently knead the unit. The color of a unit of platelets ranges from clear to straw to light pink. Occasionally platelets have a greenish tinge.
Cryoprecipitate 10-15 mL/bag	Prepared from fresh frozen plasma; a concentrate of plasma proteins containing fibronectin, von Willebrand's factor, factor VIII (80 units), fibrinogen (250 mg), and 20%-30% factor XIII.	Von Willebrand's syndromes. Fibrinogen abnormalities. Factor VIII deficiency. Hemophilia A.	Good for up to 1 year if frozen. Infuse within 6 hours of thawing or 4 hours of pooling units.	Infuse at 5-10 mL/min at room temperature. Must use a standard filter.

RBC, Red blood cell; *WBC,* white blood cell. (From Richards NM, Giullanck KK: Supplement: blood component summary, *AJN,* May, 2002, pp. 18-19.)

- Chronic anemia with a hemoglobin level of less than 7g/dL
- Anemia in patients with symptomatic cardiopulmonary disease

Leukocyte-poor red blood cells

Leukocyte-poor (or leukocyte-reduced) red blood cells are processed to remove 70% to 85% of the white cells. This makes the blood product suitable for transplant recipients and patients with a history of febrile, nonhemolytic transfusion reactions.

Frozen red blood cells

Frozen red blood cells are collected, processed, and stored for use in persons with rare blood types. The military also maintains frozen blood supplies. In their frozen state, red cells can be kept for several years.

Washed red blood cells

Washing red blood cells with isotonic saline makes them suitable for use in neonates and in patients who have had past hypersensitivity reactions to plasma. Once prepared, washed cells must be used within 24 hours because of the risk of bacterial contamination during processing.

Platelets

Platelets usually are ordered in increments of 6 units at a time, for a total of 250 to 350 mL. Each six-pack is expected to raise the platelet count by approximately 50,000 in the average adult. Platelet counts should be checked at 1 hour and 24 hours after the infusion. Use ABO-compatible platelets whenever possible. Rh-negative women of childbearing age should receive Rh-negative platelets.[6]

FRESH FROZEN PLASMA

Once the red blood cells and platelets are removed, the plasma is collected and frozen. Each unit of fresh frozen plasma contains 200 to 250 mL. Transfused fresh frozen plasma should be ABO compatible. The typical starting dose is 8 to 10 mL/kg, or two to four bags of fresh frozen plasma (adults). Transfusion of fresh frozen plasma is indicated only for patients with clotting disorders. Fresh frozen plasma infusion is no longer considered appropriate for volume expansion, nutrition, or wound healing.

CRYOPRECIPITATE

Derived from fresh frozen plasma, cryoprecipitate contains plasma proteins used for the treatment of life-threatening bleeding. Cryoprecipitate is administered in patients requiring massive transfusion or experiencing disseminated intravascular coagulation. One should note that in hemophiliac patients, cryoprecipitate should be used only when recombinant or monoclonal antibody purified factors are not available.

Table 8-4   Adverse Reactions to Blood or Blood Product Transfusion

Adverse Effect or Reaction	Potential Causes	Signs and Symptoms	Prevention
Immunologic			
Intravascular hemolysis or acute hemolytic reaction (rare)	ABO incompatibility Preexisting antibodies against transfused red blood cells Human error	Fever, chills, nausea, dyspnea, low back pain, intravenous site pain, tachycardia, hypotension, cardiovascular collapse, hemoglobinuria, renal failure, disseminated intravascular coagulation	Adhere to blood sample collection and administration procedures. Initiate transfusions slowly with close observation during first 15 minutes. Administer with 0.9% normal saline only.
Anaphylaxis	Severe immune response to foreign substance (usually sensitization to immunoglobulin A from previous transfusion or pregnancy)	Occurs quickly after just a few milliliters of blood: flushing, no fever, respiratory distress, chest pain, hypotention, abdominal cramps, nausea/vomiting, loss of consciousness	Transfuse plasma-free blood products (washed cells).
Febrile nonhemolytic reaction	Recipient antibodies to donor leukocytes Bacterial contamination Inflammatory cytokine release	Temperature >100.4° F (38° C) or >1.8° F (1° C) rise, chills, rigors	Use leukocyte-filtered products for high-risk recipients. Premedicate patient with antipyretics.
Transfusion-related acute lung injury	Presence of anti–human leukocyte antigens or neutrophil antibodies	Respiratory distress, chills, fever, cyanosis, hypotension	None known
Urticaria (plasma allergy)	Allergic reaction to foreign plasma protein	Flushing, hives, itching	Transfuse plasma-free blood products. Premedicate patient with antipyretics/antihistamines.
Transfusion associated graft-versus-host disease	Immunocompetent lymphocytes transfused into an immunocompromised patient	Fever, hepatitis, rash, gastrointestinal distress, bone marrow suppression, infection	Irradiate all blood products containing lymphocytes.
Nonimmunologic			
Nonimmune hemolysis (rare)	Bacterial contamination from infection in donor External introduction of bacteria into (transfused) product	High fever, chills, hypotension, disseminated intravascular coagulation, renal failure, vomiting, sepsis	Properly store and handle blood products. Carefully inspect for abnormalities before administration.
Infectious diseases (rare) (such as hepatitis, cytomegalovirus, human immunodeficiency virus, or malaria)	Incubation of infection in asymptomatic donor	Specific to infectious agent	Screen donor. Use volunteer donors rather than paid donors. Screen and test donated blood supply.

Sources: Weir JA: Blood component therapy. In Hankins J et al, editors: Infusion therapy in clinical practice, ed 2, St Louis, 2001, Saunders; Dreger V, Tremback T: Blood and blood product use in preoperative patient care, *AORN J* 67(1):154-156, 1998; Fitzpatrick L, Fitzpatrick T: Blood transfusion: keeping your patient safe, *Nursing* 27(8):34-42, 1997; Labovich TM: Transfusion therapy: nursing implications, *Clin J Oncol Nurs* 1(3):61-72, 1997.

Blood Administration Process

Absolute identification of the patient and unit to be transfused is essential. Incidents of patients receiving the wrong blood still occur despite the fact that numerous safeguards against this eventuality have long been in place. Blood sampling and administration policies should not be taken lightly.

Transfusion through larger-bore catheters reduces red cell hemolysis and permits rapid infusion if needed. Use normal saline for infusion with packed red blood cells; never use a dextrose-containing solution. Warmed saline (39° to 43° C) can be mixed with cold blood cells before transfusion by holding the blood bag below the saline bag and allowing saline to flow through the Y tubing into the blood. This process warms and thins the blood, reducing patient cooling and red cell hemolysis. Alternatively, an electric blood warmer (e.g., HotLine or Level 1, Smiths Industries, St. Paul, Minn) can be used to limit the cooling effects of banked blood. Blood hemolyzes if warmed to more than 40° C. Never microwave blood products.[6]

Except in emergency situations, blood transfusions are started slowly (for the first 30 minutes). Monitor patients closely for signs of a transfusion reaction. Individuals with normal cardiovascular status easily can tolerate a unit of packed red blood cells infused over 1 to 2 hours. Those with cardiovascular disease will need to be transfused more slowly (over 3 to 4 hours). For rapid blood administration, the use of a pressure infusion device (pressure bags or rapid volume infusers) is acceptable. Modern IV pumps can infuse blood without causing significant hemolysis.

Transfusion Reactions

Up to 20% of all patients receiving transfusions experience some type of adverse reaction. Transfusion-associated complications can occur during the infusion process or can be delayed for hours or years. Table 8-4 details potential adverse reactions from immunologic (allergic response) and nonimmunologic (disease transmission, bacterial contamination) causes.[6]

References

1. Otto S: *Pocket guide to intravenous therapy,* ed 4, St Louis, 2001, Mosby.
2. Carlson K: Correct utilization and management of peripherally inserted central catheters and midline catheters in the alternative care setting, *J Intraven Nurs* 22:(suppl 6):46, 1999.
3. Moureau N, Sonerman A: Does it always have to hurt? Premedications for adults and children for use with intravenous therapy, *J Intraven Nurs* 23(4):213-219, 2000.
4. Weinstein SM: *Plumer's principles and practice of intravenous therapy,* ed 8, Philadelphia, 2005, Lippincott.
5. Tintinalli JE, Kelen GD, Stapczynski JS: *Emergency medicine: a comprehensive study guide,* ed 6, New York, 2004, McGraw-Hill.
6. Richards NM, Giuliano KK: Transfusion practices in critical care: essential care before and after a blood transfusion, *Am J Nurs* 102(suppl):16-22, May 2002.

9

Laboratory Specimens

Nancy M. Bonalumi, RN, MS, CEN

Collection and analysis of laboratory specimens is an important component of emergency nursing practice. Laboratory results may be used to establish a baseline, identify trends, diagnose a particular condition, and monitor the treatment plan. The majority of patients will have some type of blood or body fluid sample collected during their emergency department visit. Because collection techniques affect the reliability of test results, accurate sampling procedures are crucial.

The Joint Commission on Accreditation of Healthcare Organization's National Safety Patient Goals mandate that all patients be identified using two unique identifiers before any invasive procedures are performed or laboratory samples are obtained. Follow the policies of your organization for patient verification. Samples should be labeled clearly at the patient's bedside. Always explain to the patient or family member the reason for the test, the collection process, and the expected time interval for results. This chapter provides nurses with information on how to collect specimens and interpret laboratory data correctly.

BLOOD COLLECTION: VENOUS BLOOD SAMPLES

The median cephalic vein, located in the antecubital fossa, is the site most commonly used for routine blood collection (Figure 9-1). Any other peripheral site that is readily accessible also may be used. If an intravenous line is to be initiated, consider withdrawing blood specimens from the intravenous catheter before connecting the tubing and fluid. This procedure reduces nursing workload and saves the patient an additional venipuncture.[1]

Tips for Finding a Vein

The following procedures can be used to find a vein:
- Lower the extremity so that the site from which the specimen is to be collected is below the level of the heart.

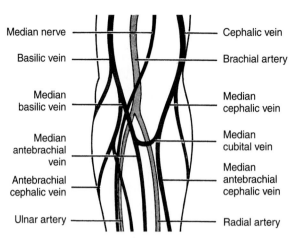

Median nerve — Cephalic vein

Basilic vein — Brachial artery

Median basilic vein — Median cephalic vein

Median antebrachial vein — Median cubital vein

Antebrachial cephalic vein — Median antebrachial cephalic vein

Ulnar artery — Radial artery

Figure 9-1. Veins of the arm. (From Newberry L: *Sheehy's emergency medicine: principles and practice,* ed 5, St Louis, 2003, Mosby.)

- Apply a tourniquet and leave it in place for no longer than 5 minutes.
- Apply a warm compress to the area.
- Have the patient open and close the fist to promote venous filling.
- Use good, direct lighting.
- Feel for a vein with your fingertips. Some large veins are deep and cannot be visualized but can be palpated.
- In emergency situations, when no other site can be located, draw the specimen from the femoral vein. Consult your hospital policy to determine whether this procedure may be performed by registered nurses.

Procedure

Once you have identified a site, cleanse it according to hospital protocol with an antiseptic solution such as alcohol, povidone-iodine (Betadine), or chlorhexidine (Hibiclens). Check to see whether the patient is allergic to any of these preparations. Do not use an alcohol-based solution if you are drawing an ethanol level for a law enforcement agency.

The nurse should follow these procedures:

1. Wear nonsterile examination gloves during the procedure.
2. Palpate the site above the proposed needle entry point; do not touch the actual site.
3. Stabilize the vein with the thumb of your nondominant hand.
4. Draw the skin taut below the site to prevent the vein from moving when punctured.
5. Insert the needle at a 30-degree angle with the bevel facing up (downward in small children).
6. If you are using a needle and syringe, begin to pull back on the syringe plunger.
7. If you are using a Vacutainer system (Becton, Dickinson, Franklin Lakes, New Jersey), pop the blood tube into the Vacutainer holder (Figure 9-2).
8. Once you have collected the correct amount of blood, release the tourniquet.
9. Place a dry, sterile 2 × 2 inch gauze over the venipuncture site and withdraw the needle.
10. Have the patient apply a slight amount of pressure over the puncture site and elevate the arm.
11. Insert blood into the correct laboratory tubes (if the needle-and-syringe technique was used).

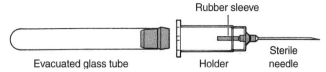

Figure 9-2. Evacuated blood collection system. (From Newberry L: *Sheehy's emergency medicine: principles and practice,* ed 5, St Louis, 2003, Mosby.)

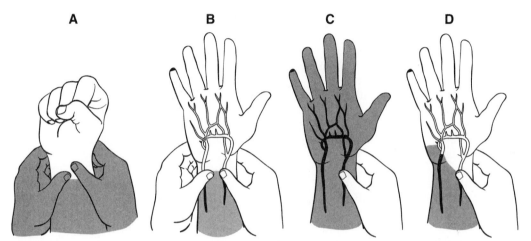

Figure 9-3. Allen's test. **A,** Elevate patient's hand and have patient make a fist. **B,** Compress the radial and ulnar arteries, then have patient open hand. **C,** Release compression from the ulnar artery. The hand should return to normal color within 6 seconds. This is a negative Allen's test. **D,** If normal color does not return to the hand within 6 seconds, the Allen's test is positive. Consider another collection site. (Courtesy Harold May, MD.)

12. Do not exert pressure to force blood through the needle into the tubes. This causes hemolysis.
13. Gently agitate tubes that contain any type of preservative or chemical to allow for mixing.
14. Carefully label all blood tubes with the patient's name and medical record number. Some facilities require the phlebotomist to date, time, and sign or initial the tube (especially for type and crossmatch specimens).[2]

BLOOD COLLECTION: ARTERIAL PUNCTURE FOR BLOOD GAS COLLECTION

General Principles

The nurse should keep in mind the following principles:
- Arterial blood gas samples are drawn from radial, brachial, or femoral artery sites.
- Avoid limbs with poor circulation.
- Avoid sites where hematomas are present.
- If the radial artery is selected, perform an Allen's test (Figure 9-3). Do not use the site if the patient fails the test. (Failure of the test indicates a poor collateral arterial supply to the hand.)

Suggested Equipment

The following equipment is recommended:
- Nonsterile examination gloves
- A container of crushed ice (some facilities run arterial blood gase samples almost immediately, so no ice is required)
- One arterial blood gas kit
- A patient name label for the syringe

Complete a laboratory requisition and include the patient's current supplemental oxygen amount (fraction of inspired oxygen) and route along with the patient's temperature at the time of specimen collection.

Procedure

The procedure for collection of arterial blood samples is as follows:
1. Select the puncture site.
2. Straighten the limb and position it on a firm surface.
3. Apply gloves.
4. Palpate the artery and assess pulse quality.
5. Cleanse the area with a povidone-iodine wipe. Use plenty of friction and allow the site to dry before puncture.
6. Immobilize the artery between two fingers of the nondominant hand (be careful not to contaminate the puncture site).
7. Holding the syringe like a pencil, penetrate the skin and the artery at a 45- to 90-degree angle, depending on the site.
8. If the syringe begins to fill and the plunger moves spontaneously, this usually indicates that the needle is in the artery.
9. If the syringe does not fill spontaneously, reposition the needle.
10. In patients with a systolic blood pressure less than 100 mm Hg (e.g., during cardiopulmonary resuscitation), the syringe may not fill spontaneously. Manually withdraw the plunger.
11. A blood sample that is not bright red indicates that the patient is poorly oxygenated or that the specimen is venous. Determine whether another attempt for an arterial specimen is necessary. Does the patient have other signs of (or risk factors for) hypoxemia?
12. Obtain 1 to 2 mL of arterial blood (some laboratories accept considerably less for analysis).
13. Withdraw the needle quickly.
14. Use a dry gauze to apply direct pressure to the venipuncture site.

Care of the Specimen

Care of an arterial blood gas specimen involves the following:
1. Expel all air bubbles from the sample.
2. Remove the needle and cap the syringe with the rubber cap.
3. Attach a patient name label to the syringe.
4. Place the syringe in a container of ice unless the sample will be analyzed immediately.
5. Send the specimen and the completed request form to the laboratory right away. (In hospitals with limited laboratory facilities, it may be helpful to call before performing arterial puncture so that the blood gas analyzer can be calibrated before the specimen arrives.)

Aftercare

Maintain direct pressure over the puncture site for at least 5 minutes. Patients with blood dyscrasias and those who are receiving anticoagulation therapy may require a longer period of pressure to ensure bleeding has ceased. Observe the puncture site for 1 minute following removal of manual pressure. Check for hematoma formation and reassess the pulse.

INTERPRETATION OF ARTERIAL BLOOD GAS VALUES

Table 9-1 lists normal arterial blood gas values. Table 9-2 gives information on arterial blood gas interpretation. To interpret an arterial blood gas, do the following:
- First, check the pH. Is it acidotic, alkalotic, or normal?
- Next, check the bicarbonate level and the P_{CO_2} to determine the cause of an abnormal pH. Is it metabolic or respiratory? Is there evidence of compensation?
- Finally, examine the Pa_{O_2} to see whether the patient is oxygenating sufficiently.

HEEL-STICK BLOOD COLLECTION

General Principles

In children less than 1 year of age, blood specimens sometimes are best obtained by using the heel-stick method. Figure 9-4 offers a guide to acceptable stick sites on the foot. This technique is not appropriate for blood cultures.

Table 9-1   Normal Arterial Blood Gas Values

Parameter	Normal Values
pH	7.35-7.45
Pa_{CO_2}	35-45 mm Hg
Pa_{O_2}	80-105 mm Hg
HCO_3^-	22-28 mEq/L

Table 9-2   Assessment of Arterial Blood Gas Values

Condition	pH	Pa_{CO_2}	HCO_3^-
Acute metabolic acidosis	<7.3	<30	Depressed
Chronic metabolic acidosis	Normal	Depressed	Depressed
Acute respiratory acidosis	<7.3	>50	Normal
Chronic respiratory acidosis	Normal	>50	Elevated
Acute metabolic alkalosis	>7.5	Elevated	Elevated
Chronic metabolic alkalosis	Normal	>50	Elevated
Acute respiratory alkalosis	>7.5	<30	Normal
Chronic respiratory alkalosis	Normal	<30	Depressed

From Newberry L: *Sheehy's emergency medicine: principles and practice*, ed 5, St Louis, 2003, Mosby.

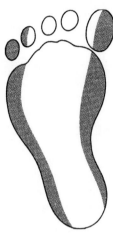

Figure 9-4.   Areas on the infant's foot for obtaining blood specimens. (From Newberry L: *Sheehy's emergency medicine: principles and practice,* ed 5, St Louis, 2003, Mosby.)

Procedure

To collect a capillary blood gas sample by the heel-stick method, do the following:
1. Select a site for blood sampling.
2. Warm the foot for 3 to 5 minutes using a warm, moist cloth. This promotes blood flow to the area.
3. Cleanse the site using an antiseptic agent.
4. Puncture the foot with a commercial lancet.
5. Discard the first drop of blood by wiping with a dry 2 × 2 inch gauze.
6. Collect the required amount of venous blood in capillary tubes or allow it to flow directly into infant-sized blood tubes (microtainers).
7. Apply a small dry dressing at the completion of the procedure.[3]

BLOOD SAMPLING FROM VASCULAR ACCESS DEVICES

For information on obtaining blood specimens from long-term vascular access devices (tunneled catheters, nontunneled catheters, and implanted ports), see Chapter 8.

POINT-OF-CARE TESTING

Point-of-care testing is an approach to specimen analysis that facilitates rapid screening of body fluids at or near the patient's bedside. Screening is done by using various test strips, kits, handheld devices, or semiportable analyzers. Available bedside tests have proliferated rapidly in the last few years, and the number is expected to continue to increase (Table 9-3). Benefits of point-of-care testing include the following:
- Ease of use
- Precise, accurate, laboratory-quality results

Table 9-3   **Available Point-of-Care Tests**

Body Fluid	*Test*
Blood	Glucose
	Sodium
	Potassium
	Chloride
	Ionized calcium
	Total carbon dioxide
	pH
	Pao_2
	HCO_3^-
	SaO_2
	Hemoglobin
	Hematocrit
	Troponin I
	Activated coagulation time
	Human immunodeficiency virus
	Hepatitis C virus
	Prostate-specific antigen
Saliva	Multiple toxicologic tests
Urine	pH
	Specific gravity
	Protein
	Hemoglobin
	Bilirubin
	Leukocytes
	Multiple toxicologic tests
	Human chorionic gonadotropin
Gastric fluid	pH
	Blood
Stool	Blood
Exhaled air	Ethanol
Throat swab	Strep A

- Immediate access to patient results
- Costs that are lower than or equal to those of traditional laboratory methods

Collection and testing procedures vary by specimen and test type. Some processes are as basic as putting a drop of reagent on a test card. Other studies require specialized cartridges and sophisticated machines. Always adhere to the manufacturer's recommendations. Every U.S. institution using point-of-care tests is expected to follow specific quality control and documentation practices. Consult the policy of your facility.

BLOOD FOR BLOOD CULTURES

Unlike other blood samples, specimens collected for culture and sensitivity studies must be obtained under sterile (versus clean) conditions to avoid contamination with skin flora, which leads to false-positive results. Careful skin preparation and sterile specimen handling are essential. Hospitals generally have a written blood culture collection protocol. Although culturing larger amounts of blood is easier, most laboratories can perform this test on much less than the recommended volumes if no more blood is available. Drawing cultures before initiation of antibiotic therapy is important. However, in cases of overwhelming sepsis (e.g., suspected meningococcemia), do not allow difficulty obtaining blood cultures to delay the administration of lifesaving drugs.

Procedure

To obtain a blood sample for culturing, perform the following:
1. Gather equipment:
   A sterile 20-mL syringe (or two 10-mL syringes) and needle for each set of cultures to be drawn; butterfly needles work well
   Alcohol wipes
   Povidone-iodine (Betadine) swabs
   Tourniquet
   Blood culture vials (age-appropriate size); one or two sets as ordered
   2 × 2 inch gauze pad
   Adhesive strip
   Sterile gloves
2. Prepare the venipuncture site using an alcohol wipe. Clean the site by using a circular motion, from the center to the periphery. Repeat this process with a povidone-iodine swab.
3. Allow the site to air dry. Do not touch the site after cleansing. (Some policies suggest a second cleaning with an alcohol wipe to remove the dried povidone-iodine.)
4. Uncap the blood culture vials, and cleanse the rubber stoppers with alcohol wipes (not povidone-iodine).
5. Apply sterile gloves.
6. Perform the venipuncture. Withdraw 18 to 20 mL of blood from adults, and 1 mL of blood for each bottle from pediatric patients.
7. Place a dry, sterile 2 × 2 inch gauze over the venipuncture site and withdraw the needle.
8. Inject 8 to 10 mL of blood into each adult bottle and 1 mL into each pediatric bottle.
9. Label samples, complete the requisition, and transport the specimens to the laboratory.

SPINAL FLUID

General Principles

A lumbar puncture (spinal tap) is performed to remove cerebrospinal fluid (CSF) for analysis. Normal CSF is clear and looks like water. Abnormal CSF may be bloody, cloudy, or yellow. To obtain a specimen, the patient must be positioned adequately. Place the patient in a lateral recumbent position, along the edge of the bed, with the spine exposed and close to the physician. Alternatively, the patient can sit in a chair and lean across an over-the-bed table. Written consent generally is required before performing this procedure. Refer to hospital policy.[1]

Procedure

To obtain a CSF sample, perform the following:
1. Assess and support the patient throughout the process. Monitor respiratory status closely, especially if preprocedural sedatives were given.
2. Usually three to five tubes of CSF are collected. Approximately 1 mL of spinal fluid is drained into each tube.

3. Number the tubes sequentially during collection.
4. Transport specimens to the laboratory immediately; do not allow samples to sit in the department for prolonged periods.
5. If only one tube is collected, send it to the microbiology laboratory. Following aseptic fluid extraction for cultures, the laboratory can divide the remaining CSF for further testing.
6. Upon procedure completion, cover the puncture site with an adhesive strip.

URINE SPECIMENS

General Principles

Urine is collected in the emergency department for a variety of common tests such as urinalysis, culture and sensitivity, toxicologic screening, pregnancy determination, and electrolyte levels. Urine specimens should be collected using a midstream, clean-catch technique, or bladder catheterization. Many practitioners consider stick-on urine collection bags an acceptable means of obtaining urinalysis specimens in young pediatric patients. This technique is not adequate for urine cultures.

Procedure

To collect a urine specimen, perform the following:
1. Collect the urine in a dry, sterile container.
2. Perform urine pregnancy testing only on fresh urine samples. Test results must be read at the designated interval.
3. If you are using the clean-catch technique. Instruct the patient to do the following:
   Cleanse the urethral opening using appropriate materials.
   Start the urine flow and then collect a midstream (not the first, not the last) specimen.
4. If the specimen must be sterile or the patient is unable to perform a clean-catch procedure, a catheterized specimen is required. Use the following:
   • An indwelling urinary catheter (Foley) if the catheter will be left in place for ongoing urine drainage or output monitoring
   • A straight catheter for a simple in-and-out procedure
   • A minicatheter (e.g., FemCath) (This method is the most comfortable and least invasive.)
5. To avoid bacterial overgrowth, send the labeled specimen to the laboratory within 20 minutes of collection.[3]

PERCUTANEOUS ASPIRATION OF FLUID AND WOUNDS

Fluids from body cavities (thoracentesis, paracentesis, joint aspirate) or wounds (abscesses, cellulitis fluid) should be collected in a sterile syringe or an evacuated (vacuum) bottle. Be sure that specimens for anaerobic testing are free of air bubbles. If the patient is taking any antibiotics, indicate the medication on the laboratory requisition.

JOINT ASPIRATION

General Principles

Patients with bleeding disorders and those taking anticoagulants must be monitored carefully during and after the procedure.

Procedure

For joint aspiration, perform the following:
1. Gather supplies:
   - An antiseptic cleanser
   - A local anesthetic solution, needle, and syringe
   - Sterile drapes or towels
   - Needle and syringe for joint aspiration; large (60-mL) syringes may be needed depending on the amount of fluid to be removed
   - Laboratory tubes for specimen transport
2. Cleanse the puncture site.
3. Assist the physician with local anesthesia as needed.
4. Stabilize the joint during the aspiration process.
5. After the needle is removed, apply manual pressure to the aspiration site for 2 to 5 minutes, and then cover the site with a sterile pressure dressing.
6. Place the fluid in an appropriate, well-labeled laboratory tube.[1]

GASTRIC LAVAGE MATERIAL

When collecting gastric lavage fluid for toxicologic testing, be sure to send the sample from the initial aspirate. If the ingested agent is known or suspected (e.g., empty bottle, distinctive smell, or suggestive symptoms), be sure to include your findings on the laboratory slip. This information can aid identification of the toxic substance.

STOOL SPECIMENS

Stool samples should be warm and newly evacuated. Place specimens in a sterile container. If the sample is obtained by rectal swabbing, be sure there is particulate matter on the swab. Do not add saline or any other liquid to the specimen because this can destroy certain parasites.

THROAT SWABS AND SPUTUM SPECIMENS

Throat (oropharyngeal) cultures are obtained using a long, sterile swab. Place the used swab in a sterile culture tube for transportation to the laboratory as soon as possible.

If the patient can expectorate, collect sputum directly in a dry, sterile container. Sputum must come from deep within the tracheobronchial tree. Saliva is not an acceptable sputum substitute. If the patient cannot cough, is unconscious, or is endotracheally intubated, obtain a specimen by suctioning the tracheobronchial tree. To collect the specimen, attach a sputum trap between the suction catheter and the suction tubing. Sputum samples should be sent to the laboratory immediately.

RESPIRATORY SYNCYTIAL VIRUS SPECIMENS

A nasopharyngeal wash or aspirate is the preferred sample source for respiratory syncytial virus, but nasopharyngeal swabs are also acceptable. Place aspirated nasal washings in a sterile container; screw the lid on tightly. Insert nasopharyngeal swabs into a viral transport medium (per hospital policy).

COMMON BLOOD TESTS

A number of common blood tests are performed routinely in the emergency care setting. In some departments, nurses order standard tests when indicated by the patient's condition. In other departments, all laboratory studies require a physician's order. In either case, a working knowledge of common tests, expected results, and their clinical implications are crucial components of emergency nursing practice. Table 9-4 provides a quick overview of frequently ordered laboratory studies and corresponding normal values for each.[3]

Table **9-4   Normal Values for Commonly Ordered Laboratory Tests**

Laboratory Test	Specification	Normal Value
Electrolytes		
Potassium		3.8-5 mEq/L
Chlorides		95-103 mEq/L
Carbon dioxide		24-30 mmol/L
Sodium		136-142 mEq/L
Other Serum Chemistry		
Bilirubin	Total	0.3-1.5 mg/dL
	Direct	0-0.2 mg/dL
Creatinine	Female	0.6-1.1 mg/dL
	Male	0.8-1.3 mg/dL
Urea nitrogen		8-23 mg/dL
Glucose, fasting		65-110 mg/dL
Albumin		3.5-4.8 g/dL
Arterial Blood Gases		
pH		7.35-7.45
Pa_{O_2}		80-105 mm Hg
Pa_{CO_2}		35-45 mm Hg
HCO_3^-		22-28 mEq/L
Complete Blood Count		
Hematocrit	Female	37%-47%
	Male	42%-52%
Hemoglobin	Female	12-16 g/dL
	Male	14-18 g/dL
Red blood cells	Female	$4.2\text{-}5.4 \times 10^6 \text{ mm}^3$
	Male	$4.6\text{-}6.2 \times 10^6 \text{ mm}^3$
Sedimentation rate	Female	Up to 20 mm/hr
	Male	Up to 9 mm/hr
White blood cells		$4.8\text{-}10.8 \times 10^3 \text{ mm}^3$
Platelets		$150\text{-}400 \times 10^3 \text{ mm}^3$
Hematology		
Coagulation	Bleeding time	<8 minutes
	Partial thromboplastin time	24-36 seconds

Continued

Table 9-4   Normal Values for Commonly Ordered Laboratory Tests—Cont'd

Laboratory Test	Specification	Normal Value
	Thrombin time	11.9-18.5 seconds
	Prothrombin time, normal	0.9-1.2 INR*
	Therapeutic range	2-3.5 INR
Troponin I		
	Positive for AMI	>0.14 ng/mL
	Indeterminate for AMI	0.11-0.14 ng/mL
	Negative for AMI	<0.11 ng/mL
Serum Enzymes		
Amylase		15-90 units/L
Creatinine phosphokinase		25-145 milliunits/mL
Lactic dehydrogenase		110-250 milliunits/mL
Alanine transaminase (ALT or SGPT)		5-35 milliunits/L
Aspartate transaminase (AST or SGOT)		10-40 milliunits/mL
Alkaline phosphatase	0-2 months	60-350 units/L
	3-12 years	80-450 units/L
	15 years	30-250 units/L
	≥16 years	30-136 units/L
Urinalysis		
Color/character		Yellow/clear
pH		4.6-8
Specific gravity		1.001-1.035
Glucose		Negative

From Newberry L, editor: *Sheehy's emergency nursing: principles and practice*, ed 5, St. Louis, 2003, Mosby.
*AMI, Acute myocardial infarction; *INR*, International Normalized Ratio.

Complete Blood Count

A complete blood count (CBC) is a routine hematologic screening study. Elements of the CBC include hemoglobin; hematocrit; total red blood cell count; white blood cell count (with or without a differential); platelets; mean corpuscular cell volume; mean cell hemoglobin concentration; and mean cell hemoglobin. Individual components of the CBC can be ordered separately. Three to 5 mL of blood is required.

Blood Glucose

Blood glucose levels can be measured in the laboratory or with a point-of-care glucometer. Fasting glucose levels are considered optimal but are impractical in the emergency department. Collect the specimen before starting oral or intravenous administration of dextrose. If the specimen is to be sent to the laboratory, 2 to 3 mL of blood is required. Finger-stick glucose determinations can be made on a single drop of blood.

Blood Urea Nitrogen

Urea is the end product of protein metabolism and normally is excreted in the urine. The blood urea nitrogen test measures the amount of circulating urea. Blood urea nitrogen elevation indicates renal failure, renal hypoperfusion (dehydration, hypotension, hemorrhage), or obstructive uropathy. One milliliter of blood is required to perform this study.

Serum Electrolytes

Commonly measured serum electrolytes include sodium, potassium, chloride, and carbon dioxide content. Although each element can be tested individually, these electrolytes often change in concert with one another; alterations in one level may have implications for others. Attempt to collect serum electrolyte specimens in an atraumatic manner to avoid hemolysis, which can artificially elevate the potassium level.

Serum Creatinine

The serum creatinine test evaluates renal function by measuring circulating creatinine levels. Creatinine is a skeletal muscle waste product that the renal glomeruli filter easily. In the presence of renal dysfunction, serum creatinine levels rise. Three milliliters of blood is needed for this test.

Cardiac Markers

Elevation of specific cardiac biomarkers supports the diagnosis of acute myocardial infarction. Laboratory studies in this category include creatinine kinase-myocardial band, myoglobin, and troponin I. Five milliliters of blood is required if the blood will be processed in the laboratory.

Toxicologic Studies

A serum drug level may be ordered for a specific agent or to screen for a variety of substances. Serum levels measure the amount of drug per volume of plasma. This is useful for identifying and monitoring drugs with distribution that is largely limited to the circulation. Most substances used therapeutically (phenytoin, digoxin, aspirin, acetaminophen, theophylline, tricyclic antidepressants) stay chiefly in the vascular system and can be tracked and treated by monitoring serum levels serially. Plasma levels are not helpful for substances that leave the circulation and bind to muscle, fat, and organs. With such drugs, serum levels may be low while total body levels are high. Most drugs of abuse fall into this latter category (cannabis, narcotics, cocaine, amphetamines, phencyclidine, benzodiazepines). Qualitative urine screens—which simply indicate a drug is present or absent—are used to identify these substances; tests are not followed serially. The average hospital laboratory can identify and measure common drugs in the serum (phenytoin, digoxin, aspirin, acetaminophen, theophylline, tricyclic antidepressants, phenobarbital). However, a full serum toxicologic screen is expensive, and it takes a long time to get results. Most facilities have to send the specimen to a specialized bioanalysis laboratory. Two to 5 mL of blood is required.

Serum Amylase

Evaluation of serum amylase levels is indicated in patients with upper abdominal pain. This test measures the amount of circulating amylase, an enzyme that digests carbohydrates. Amylase is elevated in cases of acute pancreatitis or pancreatic trauma. This test requires 3 mL of blood.

White Blood Cell Count and Differential

A white blood cell count and a differential are ordered when an infectious process is suspected. These two tests must be ordered and evaluated together because the white blood cell count may not be elevated even in the presence of severe infection, whereas the differential will be. The differential is an evaluation of the different types of leukocytes found in the serum: neutrophils (normally 56% of the total), eosinophils (2.7%), basophils (0.3%), and lymphocytes (34%) (Values for a differential should total 100%). Confusingly, neutrophils also are called "polys," or polymorphonucleocytes, and "segs," or segmented cells. Monocytes are nongranular leukocytes found in small numbers in chronic inflammatory conditions. Bands are "baby" neutrophils, released from the bone marrow in response to an overwhelming bacterial invasion that has taxed the mature neutrophil population. Such a condition (increased bands) is referred to as a *shift to the left* and indicates acute infection. Although a white blood cell and differential study can be collected independent of a CBC (in a clot tube devoid of preservatives or anticoagulants), it more commonly is ordered as a "CBC with diff" and collected in a standard CBC tube. To perform the test, 3 to 5 mL of blood is needed.

Coagulation Studies

A number of studies evaluate various steps in the clotting cascade. The most commonly ordered studies are platelet count, activated partial thromboplastin time, and prothrombin time.

Platelet count

The platelet count identifies the number of platelets in a peripheral smear and confirms defects in stage 1 of coagulation. A platelet count is a standard component of the CBC; it rarely is ordered separately.

Partial thromboplastin time

The partial thromboplastin time study identifies defects in stage 2 of coagulation. The study assesses the function of factors I, II, III, IV, V, VI, VII, and VIII. This test measures the clotting time of plasma when elements of the clotting process are added to calcium-free and platelet-poor plasma in a predetermined sequence.

Prothrombin time

The prothrombin time test identifies defects in stage 3 of coagulation. A calcium-binding anticoagulant is added to the patient's serum; the time between addition of this element and the formation of a fibrin clot is measured and compared to a normalized sample.

References

1. Marx JA et al: *Rosen's emergency medicine,* ed 5, St Louis, 2002, Mosby.
2. Proehl JA: *Emergency nursing procedures,* ed 3, Philadelphia, 2003, Saunders.
3. Miller DT, Lunde JR: Laboratory specimen collection. In Newberry L, editor: *Sheehy's emergency nursing: principles and practice,* ed 5, St Louis, 2003, Mosby.

10 Rhythm Recognition and Electrocardiogram Interpretation

Nancy M. Ballard, RN, MSN

Monitoring the electrical activity of the heart is a cornerstone of emergency nursing practice. Cardiac monitoring consists of two basic types: continuous and periodic 12-, 15-, or 18-lead electrocardiograms. Continuous monitoring is used to identify abnormalities of rate, rhythm, or conduction so as to identify and treat hemodynamic instability. A 12-, 15-, or 18-lead electrocardiogram is required to diagnose many cardiac conditions, including injury, conduction disorders, and complex dysrhythmias. This chapter describes common dysrhythmias, pacemaker rhythms, and basic 12-lead electrocardiogram interpretation.

OVERVIEW OF CARDIAC DYSRHYTHMIAS

Dysrhythmia monitoring requires connecting electrical leads to the patient. A three-lead (Figure 10-1) or a five-lead cable system (Figure 10-2) can be used. Leads are attached according to a standard placement format. By switching negative and positive poles, the cardiac monitor can obtain multiple simultaneous views of cardiac electrical activity. More sophisticated systems provide standardized diagnostic information. Familiarity with the benefits and limitations of the monitoring system used in your facility is important.

Dysrhythmias can originate in the sinus node, the atria, the atrioventricular junction, or the ventricles (Table 10-1). A dysrhythmia occurs in the following situations:
- The sinus node rate falls outside the expected range.
- The sinus node fails.
- Conduction is delayed or blocked at any point in the electrical system.
- Aberrant conduction pathways are activated.
- Ectopic foci initiate impulses.

Refer to a cardiology text for a detailed explanation of cardiac pathophysiology.

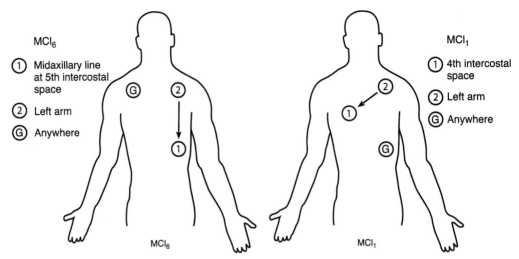

Figure 10-1. Three-lead electrocardiogram monitor. (From Newberry L: *Sheehy's emergency nursing: principles and practice,* ed 5, St Louis, 2003, Mosby.)

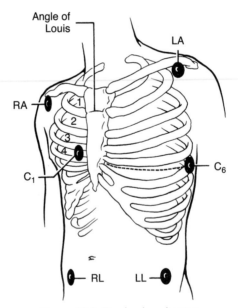

Figure 10-2. Five-lead application.

Table 10-1   Cardiac Rhythms by Point of Origin

Origin	Rhythm
Sinus node	Normal sinus rhythm, sinus tachycardia, sinus bradycardia, sinus arrhythmia
Atria	Premature atrial complexes, atrial flutter, atrial fibrillation, wandering atrial pacemaker, multifocal atrial tachycardia
Atrioventricular junction	Supraventricular tachycardia, premature junctional complexes, junctional escape rhythm, accelerated junctional rhythm, junctional tachycardia
Atrioventricular blocks	First-degree atrioventricular block; second-degree atrioventricular block, type I; second-degree atrioventricular block, type II; third-degree atrioventricular block
Ventricles	Premature ventricular complexes, ventricular tachycardia, ventricular fibrillation, idioventricular rhythm, accelerated idioventricular rhythm
Other	Pulseless electrical activity, asystole

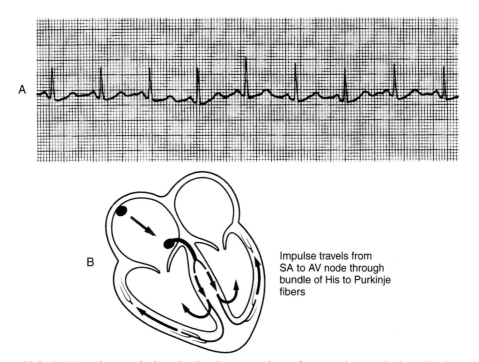

Figure 10-3. A, Normal sinus rhythm. **B,** Conduction pathway for normal sinus rhythm. *SA,* Sinoatrial; *AV,* atrioventricular.

RHYTHMS ORIGINATING IN THE SINUS NODE

Normal sinus rhythm, sinus tachycardia, sinus bradycardia, and sinus arrhythmia are generated by the sinus node. Consult the American Heart Association advanced cardiac life support (ACLS) treatment algorithms for specific interventions.[1]

Normal Sinus Rhythm

The sinoatrial node is the typical pacemaker of the heart, and normal sinus rhythm is the standard rhythm of the heart (Figure 10-3, *A*). Sympathetic and parasympathetic nervous

Table 10-2   **Normal Sinus Rhythm**

Rate	60 to 100 beats/min
Rhythm	Regular
P waves	Present
QRS complex	Present; normal duration (0.04 to 0.11 second)
P/QRS relationship	A P wave precedes each QRS complex.
P-R interval	Normal (0.12 to 0.20 second)

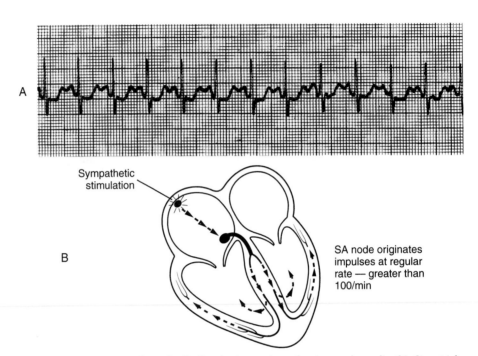

Figure 10-4. A, Sinus tachycardia. **B,** Conduction pathway for sinus tachycardia. *SA,* Sinoatrial.

system stimulation affect cardiac rate by increasing and decreasing sinoatrial node discharge in response to various physiologic signals. A normal sinus rhythm is present when cardiac rate is within the usual parameters, the rhythm is regular, the intervals are normal, a P wave precedes every QRS complex, and impulse formation and conduction follow typical pathways. Table 10-2 lists criteria for normal sinus rhythm. Figure 10-3, *B,* illustrates the normal sinus rhythm electrical pathway.

Therapeutic interventions

No interventions are required.

Sinus Tachycardia

A number of causes can stimulate increased firing of the sinoatrial node (Figure 10-4, *A*). These causes include hypoxemia, anxiety, fever, pain, exercise, nicotine, caffeine, hyperthyroidism,

Table **10-3**   **Sinus Tachycardia**

Rate	100 to 180 beats/min (age dependent)
Rhythm	Regular
P waves	Present, may merge with T waves
QRS complexes	Present; normal duration (width)
P/QRS relationship	A P wave precedes each QRS complex.
P-R interval	Normal

heart failure, hypovolemia, and any disorder that increases tissue oxygen consumption.[2] Conversely, sinus tachycardia also may be caused by any condition that decreases vagal tone (thus reducing parasympathetic input), leaving sympathetic stimulation of the sinus node unopposed. Figure 10-4, *B,* illustrates the path of electrical impulses in sinus tachycardia. Table 10-3 summarizes electrocardiogram characteristics of this rhythm.

Therapeutic interventions

- Sinus tachycardia is a symptom; treat the cause. Because sinus tachycardia is a normal compensatory mechanism, slowing the rate without alleviating the underlying disorder can produce profound hemodynamic instability.
- Hypovolemia is a common cause of sinus tachycardia; replace volume as appropriate.
- No specific drug treatment is available for sinus tachycardia. In cases of myocardial infarction or stimulant overdose (resulting in an outpouring of catecholamines), a beta-blocker may be used to control the rate to reduce myocardial oxygen demands.
- A pulmonary artery (Swan-Ganz) catheter can help determine whether sinus tachycardia is the result of hypovolemia or poor cardiac function.

Sinus Bradycardia

Sinus bradycardia (Figure 10-5, *A*) results when the normal pacemaker of the heart, the sinoatrial node, experiences increased vagal (parasympathetic) stimulation. Causes include sleep, a healthy athletic heart, anoxia, hypothyroidism, elevated intracranial pressure, acute myocardial infarction, and maneuvers that increase vagal stimulation (e.g., vomiting, straining at stool, carotid sinus massage, or ocular pressure). Sinus bradycardia may occur after cardioversion and also can be produced by drugs such as digitalis, verapamil, or beta-blockers. Figure 10-5, *B,* illustrates the path of electrical impulse conduction in sinus bradycardia. Table 10-4 lists electrocardiogram characteristics of sinus bradycardia.

Therapeutic interventions

- Observe for symptoms of decreased cardiac output, such as dropping blood pressure, decreased level of consciousness, syncope, chest pain, shock, or acidosis.
- Do not administer further doses of digitalis, beta-blockers, or calcium channel blockers before consulting with the patient's physician.
- If the patient is symptomatic, keep the patient in a supine position and apply supplemental oxygen.
- Severe symptoms (e.g., hypotension and syncope) can be treated with intravenous atropine or transcutaneous pacing.
- If symptoms remain unresponsive to atropine and transcutaneous pacing, consider an intravenous infusion of dopamine, epinephrine, or isoproterenol.

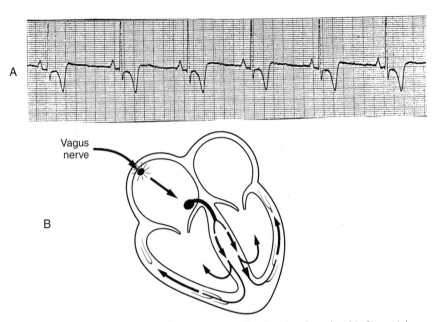

Figure 10-5. A, Sinus bradycardia. **B,** Conduction pathway for sinus bradycardia. *SA,* Sinoatrial.

Table **10-4**   **Sinus Bradycardia**

Rate	Fewer than 60 beats/min (age dependent)
Rhythm	Regular
P waves	Present
QRS complexes	Present; normal duration
P/QRS relationship	A P wave precedes each QRS complex.
P-R interval	Normal

Sinus Arrhythmia

The patient with a sinus arrhythmia has slight to moderate variation in cardiac cycle length (Figure 10-6, *A*). This dysrhythmia is a normal finding in infants, children, and young adults. The rate often varies with the respiratory cycle, slowing with expiration. For cardiac cycle length variance to be considered a sinus arrhythmia, there must be a difference of at least 0.12 second between the longest and shortest cycles. Figure 10-6, *B,* details the electrical pathway for this rhythm. Table 10-5 summarizes specific parameters.

Therapeutic interventions

No interventions are required.

RHYTHMS ORIGINATING IN THE ATRIA

Premature atrial complexes, atrial flutter, atrial fibrillation, and wandering atrial pacemaker, originate in the atria. Symptom severity varies with the rhythm and the patient. Consult the American Heart Association ACLS treatment algorithms for specific interventions.

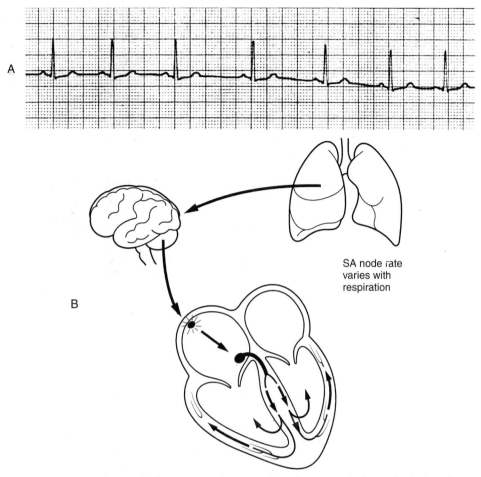

Figure 10-6. A, Sinus arrhythmia. **B,** Conduction pathway for sinus arrhythmia. *SA,* Sinoatrial.

Table 10-5   **Sinus Arrhythmia**

Rate	60 to 100 beats/min; may increase with inspiration and decrease with expiration
Rhythm	Slightly irregular; may be obvious on a rhythm strip but undetectable by palpation
P waves	Present
QRS complexes	Present; normal duration
P/QRS relationship	A P wave precedes each QRS complex.
P-R interval	Normal

Premature Atrial Complexes

Premature atrial complexes (PACs) are initiated by an irritable atrial ectopic focus and are generally a transient phenomenon (Figure 10-7, *A*). Causes of atrial irritation include strong emotions, fatigue, alcohol, caffeine, nicotine, digitalis toxicity, electrolyte imbalance, hypoxia, and ischemia. Any disease state that increases right atrial pressure (congestive heart failure,

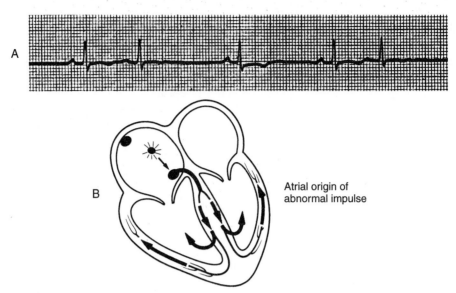

Figure 10-7. **A,** Premature atrial complexes (PAC). **B,** Conduction pathway for PAC.

Table 10-6   **Premature Atrial Complexes**

Rate	60 to 100 beats/min
Rhythm	Irregular because of early beats
P waves	Present, but (because they do not originate in the sinoatrial node) premature P waves have a different configuration
QRS complexes	Present; normal duration; noncompensatory pause
P/QRS relationship	A P wave precedes each QRS complex. If an ectopic P wave appears early in the cardiac cycle, a QRS complex may not follow (nonconducted premature atrial complex)
P-R interval	Normal or prolonged

pulmonary hypertension) can stimulate PACs. These ectopic beats may be a prelude to atrial fibrillation, atrial flutter, atrial tachycardia, or paroxysmal supraventricular tachycardia. Nevertheless, PACs are not unusual in healthy individuals. Figure 10-7, *B,* illustrates the electrical pathway associated with this rhythm. Table 10-6 summarizes PAC characteristics.

Therapeutic interventions

- Intervention is unnecessary unless the patient is symptomatic.
- If PACs are associated with alcohol, caffeine, or nicotine use, discourage future consumption of these substances.
- In symptomatic patients, pharmacologic treatment options include quinidine, procainamide, amiodarone, and digitalis.

Atrial Flutter

A single reentry circuit within the right atrium is thought to be responsible for atrial flutter. In this dysrhythmia, an ectopic atrial focus fires at such a rapid rate that most impulses are

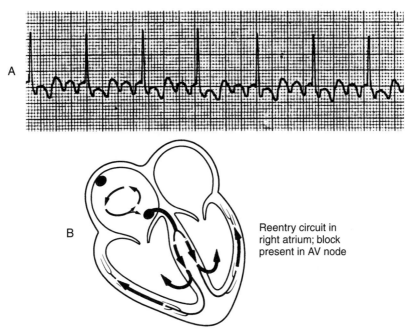

Figure 10-8. A, Atrial flutter. **B,** Conduction pathway for atrial flutter. *AV,* Atrioventricular.

Reentry circuit in right atrium; block present in AV node

Table 10-7   Atrial Flutter

Rate	Atrial rate of 230 to 350 beats/min; ventricular rate varies from normal to rapid
Rhythm	Regular if there is a fixed conduction ratio (a constant number of F waves to QRS complexes); irregular if there is a variable conduction ratio
P waves	A saw-toothed pattern of flutter waves (F waves)
QRS complexes	Present; normal duration
P/QRS relationship	Because of the rapid atrial rate, there will be two or more flutter waves for every QRS; the rhythm may be regular or irregular.
P-R interval	Not applicable

blocked at the atrioventricular node (Figure 10-8, *A*). This allows only every second (2:1), third (3:1), or fourth (4:1) flutter wave (F wave) to reach the ventricles. The ventricular response may be regular or irregular. Atrial flutter generally is initiated by a PAC and may be seen in patients with coronary artery disease, rheumatic heart disease, pulmonary embolism, or chronic obstructive pulmonary disease. This rhythm rarely persists for more than 24 hours; the patient reverts to normal sinus rhythm or progresses to atrial fibrillation. Table 10-6 summarizes atrial flutter parameters. Figure 10-8, *B,* highlights the conduction pathway.

Therapeutic interventions

- Treat the underlying condition.
- Control rapid ventricular rates with calcium channel blockers, beta-blockers, digoxin, diltiazem, or amiodarone.
- If the patient is symptomatic, consider synchronized cardioversion.

Atrial Fibrillation

In atrial fibrillation, multiple atrial pacemakers fire chaotically in rapid succession (Figure 10-9, *A*). The atria quiver but never firmly contract. The ventricles respond to this stimulation in a sporadic fashion (Figure 10-9, *B*). Poor atrial emptying places these patients at risk for mural clot formation and embolization. Without effective atrial contraction, cardiac output drops 15% to 25%. In patients with marginal heart function, this reduction can be significant. Atrial fibrillation is said to be uncontrolled if the ventricular rate is greater than 100 beats/min. This dysrhythmia frequently occurs in the presence of coronary artery disease, pericarditis, congestive heart failure, rheumatic heart disease, hypertension, pulmonary embolus, hyperthyroidism, and digitalis toxicity. Atrial fibrillation may be chronic, and patients can survive for years in this state if the rate is controlled. Table 10-8 lists atrial fibrillation characteristics.

Therapeutic interventions

- Evaluate ventricular response by comparing the electrocardiogram tracing and the apical pulse.
- In hemodynamically stable patients, rate control is achieved with digitalis, beta-blockers, or calcium channel blockers.

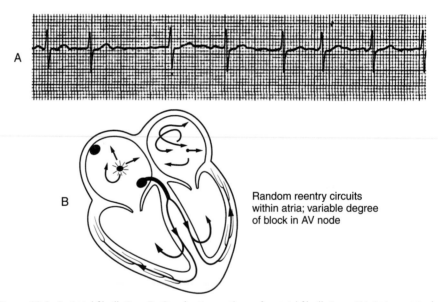

Figure 10-9. A, Atrial fibrillation. **B,** Conduction pathway for atrial fibrillation. *AV,* Atrioventricular.

Table 10-8 **Atrial Fibrillation**

Rate	Atrial rate 400 beats/min or more; ventricular rate varies
Rhythm	The ventricular rhythm is *always* irregularly irregular.
P waves	No identifiable P waves
QRS complexes	Present, normal duration
P/QRS relationship	None identified; irregular ventricular response
P-R interval	Not applicable

- Severely symptomatic patients (syncope, altered level of consciousness, deteriorating vital signs, chest pain) require emergent synchronized cardioversion.
- If the patient has been taking digitalis, draw a serum digoxin sample before cardioversion.
- Unless urgent conversion is indicated, anticoagulation with warfarin is initiated several days before cardioversion to prevent systemic thromboembolism.
- Following successful cardioversion, treat with digitalis or another antidysrhythmic agent.
- Chemical conversion can be accomplished with several agents, including amiodarone, ibutilide, and procainamide.

Wandering Atrial Pacemaker

Wandering atrial pacemaker (or multiformed atrial rhythm) can develop if two or more foci in the sinoatrial node, the atria, or the atrioventricular junction compete for rhythm control (Figure 10-10, *A*). This situation occurs when the sinoatrial node is suppressed or lower

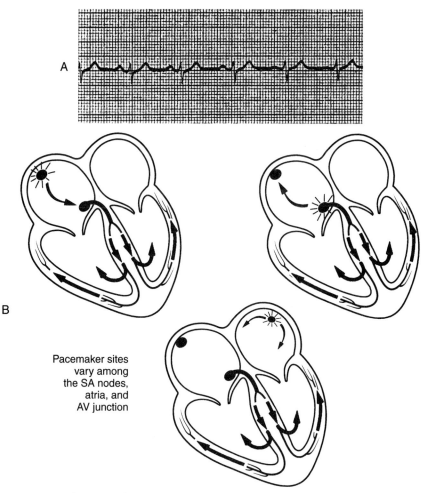

Pacemaker sites
vary among
the SA nodes,
atria, and
AV junction

Figure 10-10. A, Wandering atrial pacemaker. **B,** Conduction pathway for wandering atrial pacemaker. *SA,* Sinoatrial; *AV,* atrioventricular.

Table **10-9   Wandering Atrial Pacemaker**

Rate	50 to 100 beats/min
Rhythm	Regular or slightly irregular
P waves	Present, configuration varies. By definition, at least three different P wave configurations must be present to constitute wandering atrial pacemaker.
QRS complexes	Present; normal duration
P/QRS relationship	A P wave precedes each QRS complex, but the P wave may disappear if it is buried in the QRS complex.
P-R interval	Variable

foci become excited and take over the pacemaker function of the heart (Figure 10-10, *B*). Wandering atrial pacemaker may be observed in normal, healthy individuals (particularly in athletes) and during sleep. Wandering atrial pacemaker also may occur with certain toxicities and some types of heart disease. Table 10-9 provides data on specific parameters for this rhythm.

Therapeutic interventions

- Wandering atrial pacemaker is usually asymptomatic and treatment is unnecessary.
- If the patient becomes symptomatic, treat the underlying condition.

RHYTHMS ORIGINATING IN THE ATRIOVENTRICULAR JUNCTION

Dysrhythmias that originate in the atrioventricular junction are referred to interchangeably as junctional or nodal rhythms. This family of dysrhythmias includes paroxysmal supraventricular tachycardia, premature junctional complexes, junctional escape rhythm, accelerated junctional rhythm, and junctional tachycardia. Consult the American Heart Association ACLS treatment algorithms for specific interventions.

Paroxysmal Supraventricular Tachycardia

Paroxysmal supraventricular tachycardia (PSVT) is a reentrant tachycardia most commonly generated by the atrioventricular node (Figure 10-11, *A*). Under the right conditions, two conduction pathways within the node form an electrical circuit or loop, continuously stimulating the ventricles to depolarize (Figure 10-11, *B*). By definition, PSVT has a paroxysmal onset and cessation. Paroxysmal supraventricular tachycardia can occur in a normal heart or in association with hypoxia, ischemia, electrolyte imbalances, congestive failure, rheumatic heart disease, acute pericarditis, myocardial infarction, and mitral valve prolapse. Some patients are born with accessory conduction systems that predispose them to preexcitation syndromes (e.g., Wolff-Parkinson-White or Lown-Ganong-Levine syndromes). Symptoms include the sudden onset of dyspnea, angina, diaphoresis, fatigue, anxiety, dizziness, and polyuria. Table 10-10 summarizes PSVT characteristics.

Therapeutic interventions

- Record the rhythm in multiple leads before treatment; this helps identify the initiating mechanism.

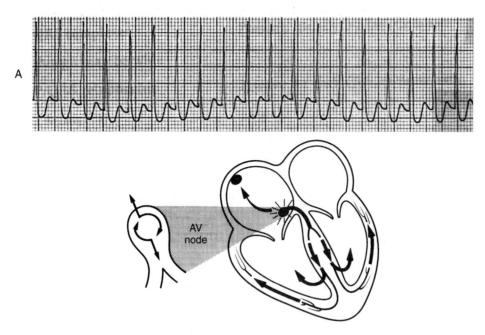

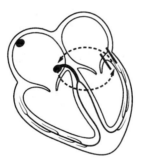

AV junction or atrium originates impulse

Circus movement between
AV node and accessory pathway

Figure 10-11. A, Paroxysmal supraventricular tachycardia. **B,** Conduction pathway for paroxysmal supraventricular tachycardia. *AV,* Atrioventricular.

Table 10-10   Paroxysmal Supraventricular Tachycardia

Rate	100 to 280 beats/min
Rhythm	Regular; sudden start and stop
P wave	May occur before the QRS; often distorted or buried within the QRS complex
QRS complexes	Present; duration is usually normal though the QRS may be wide
P/QRS relationship	A P wave for each QRS or none seen (buried in QRS complex)
P-R interval	Short or none

- Atrioventricular nodal reentry tachycardias are usually benign and self-limiting or are easily terminated with vagal maneuvers such as carotid sinus pressure, gagging, coughing, facial immersion in cold water, or Valsalva maneuver.
- In patients who are symptomatic but fail to respond to vagal maneuvers, adenosine is the drug of choice. Verapamil, digoxin, beta-blockers, diltiazem, and amiodarone also have been used.
- Hemodynamically unstable patients require emergent synchronized cardioversion.
- If the patient has digitalis toxicity, discontinue digitalis therapy and correct any hypokalemia. Preferred antidysrhythmics in this situation are phenytoin, lidocaine, and magnesium sulfate. Administer digitalis-binding antibodies (digoxin immune Fab [Digibind]) to hemodynamically compromised patients.
- Because a PAC usually initiates this dysrhythmia, advise the patient to avoid caffeine, nicotine, alcohol, and stress.
- Permanent prevention of recurrent PSVT episodes can be achieved with radiofrequency catheter ablation or surgical modification of the accessory pathway.

Premature Junctional Complexes

A premature junctional complex occurs when the atrioventricular junction (instead of the usual sinoatrial node) becomes the pacemaker of the heart (Figure 10-12, *A*). This dysrhythmia is seen with digitalis toxicity, ischemia, hypoxia, electrolyte imbalances, and congestive heart failure. Figure 10-12, *B*, illustrates the electrical pathway associated with this event. Table 10-11 summarizes distinguishing characteristics.

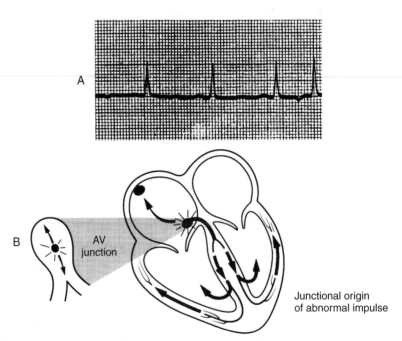

A

B   AV junction

Junctional origin of abnormal impulse

Figure 10-12. A, Premature junctional complex. **B,** Conduction pathway for premature junctional complexes. *AV,* Atrioventricular.

Therapeutic interventions

- If the patient is taking digitalis, withhold further doses and obtain a serum digoxin level. Observe the patient closely for deterioration.
- If the patient is symptomatic, treat with quinidine or procainamide.
- Alcohol, caffeine, and nicotine can stimulate premature junctional complexes, and use should be limited.

Junctional Escape Rhythm

When the sinoatrial node fails, the atrioventricular junction takes over the pacemaker function of the heart. This change is referred to as a junctional escape rhythm (Figure 10-13, *A*). However, the atrioventricular node is an unreliable pacemaker and has an intrinsic rate of only 40 to 60 beats/min. Table 10-12 delineates specific characteristics of the rhythm, and Figure 10-13, *B*, illustrates the associated electrical pathway.

Table **10-11**   **Premature Junctional Complexes**

Rate	Normal or bradycardic, depending on the underlying rhythm
Rhythm	Irregular because of premature complexes
P waves	Absent, or seen just before or just after the QRS; the P wave is commonly inverted
QRS complexes	Present; normal duration
P/QRS relationship	P wave may precede or follow QRS complex or may be nonexistent (buried)
P-R interval	Less than 0.12 second when the P wave is associated with a premature beat

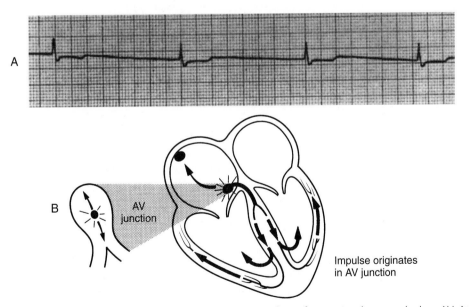

Figure 10-13. A, Junctional escape rhythm. **B,** Conduction pathway for junctional escape rhythm. *AV,* Atrioventricular.

Table 10-12   **Junctional Escape Rhythm**

Rate	40 to 60 beats/min
Rhythm	Regular
P waves	Absent, or seen just before or just after the QRS complex; the P wave is commonly inverted
QRS complexes	Present; normal duration
P/QRS relationship	P wave may precede or follow QRS complex or may be nonexistent.
P-R interval	Less than 0.12 second when the P wave precedes the QRS

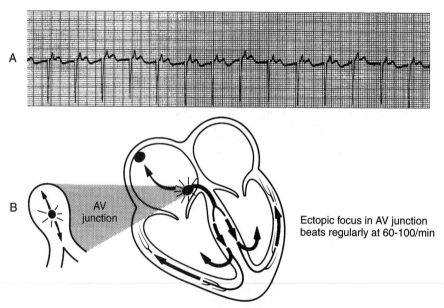

A

B   AV junction   Ectopic focus in AV junction beats regularly at 60-100/min

Figure 10-14. A, Accelerated junctional rhythm/junctional tachycardia. **B,** Conduction pathway for accelerated junctional rhythm. *AV,* Atrioventricular.

Therapeutic interventions

- No specific therapy exists for this dysrhythmia.
- Obtain a serum digoxin level to check for toxicity in patients who are taking digitalis.
- Treat syncope, altered level of consciousness, chest pain, or other signs related to a slow heart rate with atropine sulfate. If atropine is unsuccessful, transcutaneous pacing is indicated.

Accelerated Junctional Rhythm/Junctional Tachycardia

An accelerated junctional rhythm (Figure 10-14, *A*) occurs when a site in the atrioventricular junction begins firing faster than the sinus node, usurping primary pacemaker control (Figure 10-14, *B*). Junctional tachycardia is an ectopic rhythm originating in the pacemaker cells of the bundle of His in which the rate exceeds 100 beats/min These rhythms are usually transient and may be related to digoxin toxicity, congestive heart failure, myocardial ischemia, or cardiogenic shock. Table 10-13 summarizes distinguishing characteristics.

Table 10-13   Accelerated Junctional Rhythm/Junctional Tachycardia

Rate	Accelerated: 60 to 100 beats/min; tachycardia: more than 100 beats/min
Rhythm	Regular
P wave	Absent, or seen just before or just after the QRS complex; the P wave is commonly inverted
QRS complexes	Present; normal duration
P/QRS relationship	P wave may precede or follow QRS complex or may be nonexistent (buried)
P-R interval	Less than 0.12 second when the P wave precedes the QRS complex

Therapeutic interventions

- If the patient currently is receiving digoxin, hold further doses until a serum level is obtained.
- Treat the underlying condition as indicated (e.g., ischemia, acute myocardial infarction, shock, or unstable angina).
- Observe patient closely for the development of hemodynamic instability.

ATRIOVENTRICULAR BLOCKS

Atrioventricular blocks include first-degree atrioventricular block; second-degree atrioventricular block, type I; second-degree atrioventricular block, type II; and third-degree atrioventricular block. Lethality ranges from benign to life threatening. Consult the American Heart Association ACLS treatment algorithms for specific interventions.

First-Degree Atrioventricular Block

A first-degree atrioventricular block exists when an impulse originates in the sinoatrial node but conduction through the atrioventricular node is delayed (prolonged P-R interval) (Figure 10-15*A* and *B*). This condition may be caused by anoxia, myocardial ischemia, atrioventricular node malfunction, edema following open heart surgery, myocarditis, thyrotoxicosis, rheumatic fever, and certain drugs including digitalis, clonidine, and tricyclic antidepressants. Table 10-14 summarizes specific parameters.

Therapeutic interventions

- Treatment for first-degree atrioventricular block is unnecessary unless the patient has other symptoms.
- Discontinue digitalis therapy and obtain a serum digoxin level.
- If the patient becomes symptomatic (syncope, altered level of consciousness, chest pain), treat the underlying cause.
- In the event of symptomatic bradycardia, administer atropine.
- Observe the patient for progression to second- or third-degree block.

Second-Degree Atrioventricular Block, Type I

In second-degree atrioventricular block, type I (also known as Mobitz type I or Wenckebach), successive atrial impulses take progressively longer to travel through the atrioventricular

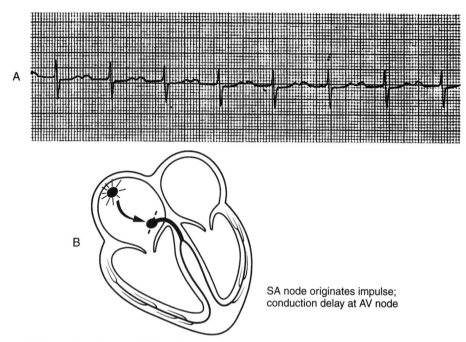

SA node originates impulse;
conduction delay at AV node

Figure 10-15. A, First-degree AV block. **B,** Conduction pathway for first-degree AV block. *SA,* Sinoatrial; *AV,* atrioventricular.

Table 10-14   **First-Degree Atrioventricular Block**

Rate	Usually 60 to 100 beats/min
Rhythm	Regular
P waves	Present
QRS complexes	Present; normal duration
P/QRS relationship	A P wave precedes each QRS complex.
P-R interval	Prolonged (>0.20 second) but consistent

node (lengthening P-R intervals), until a beat (QRS complex) finally is dropped. The cycle then repeats (Figure 10-16). Although the cause is not well understood, this dysrhythmia is transient and commonly occurs following inferior wall myocardial infarction or other disorders that affect conduction through the atrioventricular node or bundle of His. Myocarditis, open heart surgery, and medications such as digoxin, propranolol, or verapamil have been associated with this rhythm. Table 10-15 details distinguishing characteristics.

Therapeutic interventions

- Treatment is usually unnecessary.
- Investigate the cause and withhold digoxin. Observe for atrioventricular block progression.
- If perfusion is impaired, or ventricular escape beats occur, consider administration of atropine or transcutaneous pacing to improve the ventricular rate.

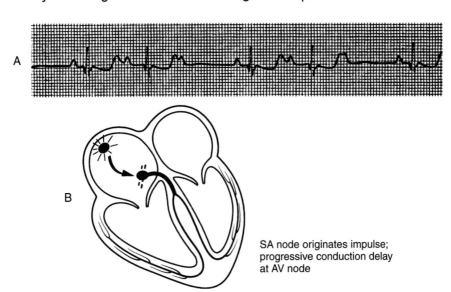

SA node originates impulse;
progressive conduction delay
at AV node

Figure 10-16. A, Second-degree AV block, type I. **B,** Conduction pathway for second-degree AV block type II. *SA,* Sinoatrial; *AV,* atrioventricular.

Table 10-15   Second-Degree Atrioventricular Block, Type I

Rate	Normal
Rhythm	Atrial beats are regular; ventricular beats are irregular.
P waves	One P wave precedes each QRS complex until the QRS is dropped. This pattern recurs at regular intervals.
QRS complexes	Cyclic missed conduction; when the QRS complex is present, it is of normal duration
P/QRS relationship	A QRS complex follows each P wave and then is dropped (absent) at patterned intervals.
P-R interval	Lengthens with each cycle until a QRS complex is dropped, and then the pattern repeats

Second-Degree Atrioventricular Block, Type II

In second-degree atrioventricular block, type II (also known as Mobitz type II), one or more atrial impulses are not conducted through the atrioventricular node to the ventricles (Figure 10-17). This disturbance usually results from infarction of the inferior or anterior myocardial wall. Other causes include anoxia, digitalis toxicity, edema following open heart surgery, or hyperkalemia. This rhythm, in the presence of an anterior myocardial infarction, suggests possible infarction of the major conduction pathway. Progression to complete heart block in not uncommon. Table 10-16 summarizes parameters for second-degree atrioventricular block, type II.

Therapeutic interventions

- Administer supplemental oxygen.
- Monitor the patient closely; this is rhythm considered unstable.

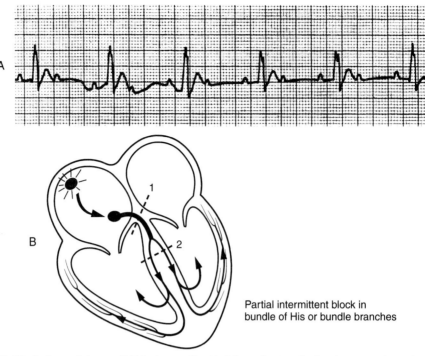

Figure 10-17. A, Second-degree AV block, type II, with 2:1 conduction. **B,** Conduction pathway for second-degree AV block.

Partial intermittent block in bundle of His or bundle branches

Table 10-16   Second-Degree Atrioventricular Block, Type II

Rate	Atrial rate of 60 to 100 beats/min; ventricular rate is often slow
Rhythm	Atrial rhythm is regular; ventricular rhythm is regular with a consistent conduction pattern but is irregular if conduction pattern is variable.
P waves	One or more for every QRS complex
QRS complexes	When present, normal or prolonged duration
P/QRS relationship	One or more P waves for each QRS complex
P-R interval	Normal or delayed for the P wave that conducts the QRS complex

- For patients with a QRS complex of normal duration (width), administer atropine. If atropine is ineffective, transcutaneous pacing is the treatment of choice.
- For patients with a wide QRS complex (>0.11 second), consider transcutaneous pacing or administration of dopamine or epinephrine.
- If hyperkalemia is present, administer sodium polystyrene sulfonate (Kayexalate).

Third-Degree Heart Block

In third-degree heart block (also called complete atrioventricular block), no conduction of sinoatrial node impulses occurs through the atrioventricular node (Figure 10-18, *A*). In response, a junctional or ventricular pacemaker initiates its own impulses. Once this occurs, the atria and ventricles beat independently of each other (Figure 10-18, *B*). Table 10-17

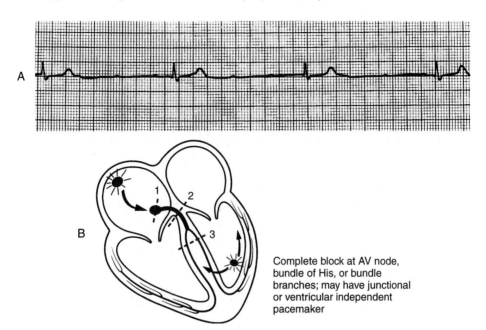

Complete block at AV node, bundle of His, or bundle branches; may have junctional or ventricular independent pacemaker

Figure 10-18. A, Third-degree heart block. **B,** Conduction pathway for third-degree heart block. *AV,* atrio-ventricular.

Table 10-17   Third-Degree Heart Block

Rate	Atrial rate of 60 to 100 beats/min; ventricular rate usually less than 60 beats/min
Rhythm	Regular
P waves	Occurring regularly
QRS complexes	Slow; narrow if the QRS is a junctional escape beat, wide (greater than or equal to 0.12 second) if it is a ventricular escape beat.
P/QRS relationship	The P wave and QRS complex are completely independent of each other.
P-R interval	Inconsistent

summarizes distinguishing characteristics of third-degree block. Patients with this rhythm frequently present to the emergency department complaining of weakness or fatigue. Causes may be temporary or permanent and include digitalis toxicity, diaphragmatic or anterior myocardial infarction, Lyme disease, myocarditis, and accidental injury during open heart surgery.

Therapeutic interventions

- Withhold further doses and obtain a serum level sample if the patient is taking digitalis.
- Observe the ventricular rate closely. If the rate becomes slow enough to cause hemodynamic instability (syncope, altered level of consciousness, chest pain), cardiac failure will soon follow.
- Therapeutic intervention involves cardiac pacing. Transcutaneous pacing may be used as a bridge to transvenous or permanent pacing. Gather pacing equipment, and place pacer pads on the patient for rapid implementation of electrical therapy if needed.

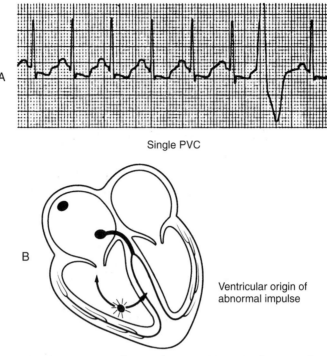

Single PVC

Ventricular origin of
abnormal impulse

Figure 10-19. A, Premature ventricular complexes *(PVCs).* **B,** Conduction pathway for PVC.

- Be prepared to provide basic and advanced life support. (See the ACLS bradycardia algorithm.)
- Do *not* administer antidysrhythmic agents (e.g., lidocaine, procainamide, or amiodarone). These drugs can suppress ventricular response.

RHYTHMS ORIGINATING IN THE VENTRICLES

Dysrhythmias that originate in the ventricles include premature ventricular complexes, ventricular tachycardia, ventricular fibrillation, idioventricular rhythm, and accelerated idioventricular rhythm. Depending on the specific dysrhythmia, pulses may or may not be present. Consult the American Heart Association ACLS treatment algorithms for specific interventions.

Premature Ventricular Complexes

Premature ventricular complexes are referred to by a number of names, including premature ectopic beats and extrasystole (Figure 10-19, *A*). Premature ventricular complexes are indicative of an irritable ventricle. These abnormal impulses are initiated by an ectopic ventricular focus (Figure 10-19, *B*). Causative factors include hypoxia, hypovolemia, ischemia, infarction, hypertrophy, hypokalemia, hypomagnesemia, and acidosis. Many drugs, including alcohol, nicotine, and caffeine, can irritate ventricular cells. Premature ventricular complexes originating from a single focus (unifocal) have the same configuration. Those PVCs arising from various foci (multifocal) present a variety of configurations. Premature ventricular complexes

Table **10-18**   **Premature Ventricular Complexes**

Rate	Varies with underlying rhythm
Rhythm	Irregular because of early beats
P waves	Present with each sinus beat; P waves do not precede premature ventricular complexes (PVCs).
QRS complexes	Sinus-initiated QRS complexes are normal; the QRS complexes of PVCs are wide (>0.12 second) and bizarre and usually have a T wave of opposite polarity. Look for a full compensatory pause.
P/QRS relationship	A P wave precedes each QRS complex in the normal sinus beats; no P wave precedes PVCs.
P-R interval	Normal in sinus beats; none in PVCs

also may occur in repetitious patterns such as bigeminy (every other beat) or trigeminy (every third beat). A pair of PVCs is called a couplet, and three consecutive PVCs form a triplet. A series of three or more PVCs constitutes ventricular tachycardia. Table 10-18 summarizes parameters for this rhythm.

Therapeutic interventions

- Isolated PVCs are not treated unless there is evidence of hemodynamic compromise.
- Administer oxygen if the patient is symptomatic.
- Treat any known underlying cause (e.g., correct acidosis, electrolyte disturbances, or drug toxicities; initiate volume replacement).
- Premature ventricular complexes typically are not treated during the first few hours after myocardial infarction. Little evidence indicates that this dysrhythmia adversely affects mortality or that routine treatment enhances survival.
- If PVCs are related to bradycardia (ventricular escape beats), treat with atropine. Do *not* administer antidysrhythmic agents (lidocaine, procainamide, or amiodarone) until bradycardia has been corrected.
- Other drugs that may be administered include quinidine, phenytoin, or propranolol.

Ventricular Tachycardia

Ventricular tachycardia (VT) is actually a series (three or more) of consecutive PVCs (Figure 10-20, *A*). This rhythm is rare in patients without underlying heart disease. Figure 10-20, *B*, illustrates VT electrical conduction pathways. Loss of atrial function and the rapid ventricular response of VT contribute to hemodynamic deterioration. Individuals with a rate greater than 130 beats/min become dizzy, and loss of consciousness occurs at ventricular rates of about 200 beats/min. Nonsustained VT (lasting less than 30 seconds) may not be treated unless the patient is symptomatic or has underlying heart disease. Sustained VT occurs more commonly in those with prior myocardial infarction, chronic coronary artery disease, or dilated cardiomyopathy. Polymorphic VT (torsades de pointes) may be induced by medications that prolong the Q-T interval (e.g., amiodarone, ibutilide, or quinidine) or by toxic levels of drugs such as tricyclic antidepressants. If rapid VT does not self-terminate, it may deteriorate to ventricular fibrillation. Table 10-19 summarizes defining characteristics.

Therapeutic interventions

- Rapid monomorphic VT (≥150 beats/min) in an unstable patient with a pulse is treated with synchronized cardioversion at 100, 200, 300, then 360 J (monophasic energy dose).

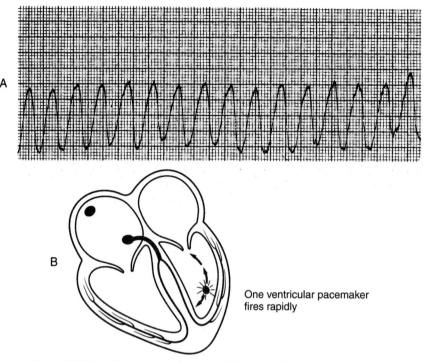

One ventricular pacemaker fires rapidly

Figure 10-20. A, Ventricular tachycardia (VT). **B,** Conduction pathway for VT.

Table **10-19   Ventricular Tachycardia**

Rate	100 to 250 beats/min
Rhythm	Regular
P waves	Not seen
QRS complexes	Wide and bizarre
P/QRS relationship	None

- Treat pulseless VT like ventricular fibrillation with immediate, unsynchronized defibrillation at 200, 300, then 360 J (monophasic energy dose).
- Stable VT is treated with IV antidysrhythmic agents such as amiodarone, lidocaine, or procainamide.
- Pharmacologic interventions for polymorphic VT are magnesium sulfate, lidocaine, isoproterenol, or phenytoin by IV administration or by overdrive pacing (pick one). (See the ACLS tachycardia algorithm for a complete treatment guide.)
- Implantable defibrillators may be placed for recurrent VT unresponsive to pharmacologic intervention. If the site of the irritable ventricular foci can be determined during an electrophysiologic study, ablation or surgical subendocardial resection may be performed.

Ventricular Fibrillation

Ventricular fibrillation (VF) produces no effective cardiac output; death occurs if this rhythm persists more than 4 to 6 minutes (Figure 10-21, *A*). Ventricular fibrillation often follows

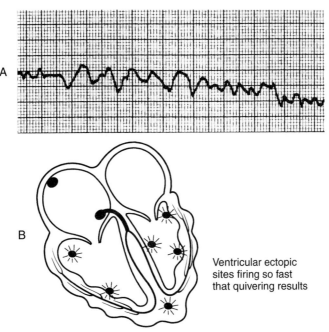

A, Ventricular fibrillation (VF). B, Conduction for VF.

Figure 10-21. A, Ventricular fibrillation (VF). B, Conduction for VF.

Table 10-20   **Ventricular Fibrillation**

Rate	Rapid, disorganized
Rhythm	Irregular
P waves	Not seen
QRS complexes	None
P/QRS relationship	None
P-R interval	None

ventricular tachycardia, but the most frequent underlying cause is coronary artery disease. In this dysrhythmia, ventricular cells fire chaotically; there is no specific pacemaker (Figure 10-21, B). Table 10-20 summarizes patterns associated with ventricular fibrillation.

Therapeutic interventions

- Begin basic and advanced cardiac life support immediately.
- Early defibrillation is the most important factor in successful resuscitation. Defibrillate 3 times in rapid succession (as needed) at 200, 300, and 360 J, respectively (monophasic energy dose). (See the ACLS ventricular fibrillation/pulseless ventricular tachycardia algorithm.)
- Administer 100% oxygen under positive pressure.
- Give epinephrine intravenously and repeat every 3 to 5 minutes. Allow the drug to circulate for 30 to 60 seconds, and then reevaluate the patient's rhythm. (Consult ACLS recommendations for dosing guidelines.)
- For continued ventricular fibrillation, defibrillate again at 360 J. If this is unsuccessful, initiate antidysrhythmic therapy with amiodarone, lidocaine, magnesium sulfate,

procainamide, or (in some cases) sodium bicarbonate. After circulating each dose of medication, defibrillate with 360 J.
- If resuscitation is successful, address the underlying cause of the arrest.
- Patients who survive an episode of cardiac arrest may be candidates for an automatic implantable cardioverter defibrillator.

Idioventricular Rhythm/Accelerated Idioventricular Rhythm

An idioventricular rhythm is associated with a very poor prognosis. The rhythm generally indicates a large area of myocardial damage (Figure 10-22, *A*). Table 10-21 summarizes specific characteristics; Figure 10-22, *B,* illustrates the impulse pathway of this dysrhythmia. Transient accelerated idioventricular rhythms (>40 beats/min) (Figure 10-23) are associated with coronary reperfusion following administration of fibrinolytic therapy (Table 10-22).

Therapeutic interventions

- Begin basic and advanced cardiac life support immediately.
- Intubate the patient, and give 100% oxygen under positive pressure.
- Administer epinephrine and atropine.
- Do *not* administer antidysrhythmic agents (e.g., lidocaine, procainamide, or amiodarone). These drugs can suppress ventricular response.
- Treatment is not indicated if the event is transient (e.g., reperfusion following fibrinolytic therapy for coronary occlusion). Monitor for hemodynamic compromise.

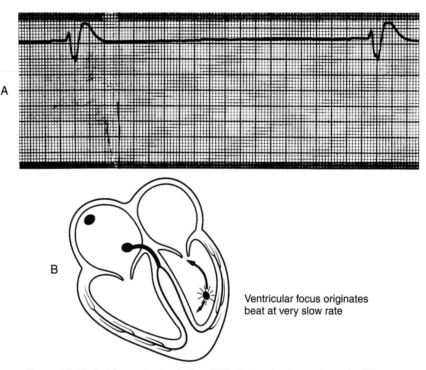

A

B

Ventricular focus originates
beat at very slow rate

Figure 10-22. A, Idioventricular rhythm (IVR). **B,** Conduction pathway for IVR.

Table 10-21   Idioventricular Rhythm

Rate	20 to 40 beats/min
Rhythm	Regular or irregular
P waves	None
QRS complexes	Wide and bizarre
P/QRS relationship	None
P-R interval	None

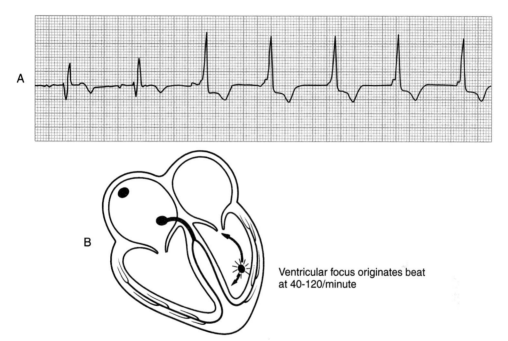

A

B

Ventricular focus originates beat at 40-120/minute

Figure 10-23. A, Accelerated idioventricular rhythm (AIR). **B,** Conduction pathway for AVT. (**A** from Urden L, Stacy K, Lough M: *Thelan's critical care nursing, diagnosis and management,* ed 4, St Louis, 2002, Mosby.)

Table 10-22   Accelerated Idioventricular Rhythm

Rate	40 to 100 beats/min
Rhythm	Regular
P waves	None
QRS complexes	Wide and bizarre
P/QRS relationship	None
P-R interval	None

Box **10-1**   **Causes of Pulseless Electrical Activity**

Acidosis
Cardiac tamponade
Drug overdoses (tricyclic antidepressants, digitalis, beta-blockers, calcium channel blockers)
Hyperkalemia
Hypothermia
Hypovolemia
Hypoxia
Massive acute myocardial infarction
Massive pulmonary embolism
Tension pneumothorax

OTHER DYSRHYTHMIAS

Two more dysrhythmias, pulseless electrical activity and asystole, cannot be categorized by site of origin in the heart. Both dysrhythmias are considered terminal rhythms and indicate severe cardiac dysfunction. Consult the American Heart Association ACLS treatment algorithms for specific interventions.

Pulseless Electrical Activity

Pulseless electrical activity (PEA; formerly called electromechanical dissociation) is a phenomenon in which some type of cardiac electrical activity (other than VT or ventricular fibrillation) is present, but no pulse is palpable. Continue basic and advanced cardiac life support while attempting to identify a treatable cause. In PEA, cardiac output is so low that the patient is functionally in cardiac arrest. Pulseless electrical activity is generally a preterminal rhythm, is followed quickly by death, and is the most common dysrhythmia in patients with traumatic cardiac arrest. However, certain PEA causes are reversible, and survival is possible if the condition is recognized and treated immediately. Box 10-1 lists causes of PEA.

Therapeutic interventions

- Start cardiopulmonary resuscitation, intubate the patient, and administer positive pressure ventilation right away.
- Because hypoventilation and hypoxemia are frequent causes of PEA, ensure optimal airway management and ventilation.
- Administer epinephrine intravenously every 3 to 5 minutes.
- If the underlying pattern is bradycardic, give IV atropine 0.5 to 1 mg (total dose of 0.04 mg/kg).
- Identify any treatable cause, and initiate corrective interventions.
- Reverse hypovolemia with isotonic crystalloids blood products, or both.
- Treat tension pneumothorax with needle decompression.
- Perform pericardiocentesis for pericardial tamponade.
- Treat hyperkalemia, acidosis, and tricyclic antidepressant overdose with sodium bicarbonate.

Asystole

Asystole (ventricular standstill, silent heart) is the complete absence of any ventricular response (Figure 10-24, *A*). Atrial impulses may or may not be present, but no ventricular contractions occur. This rhythm generally implies that the patient has been in cardiopulmonary arrest for

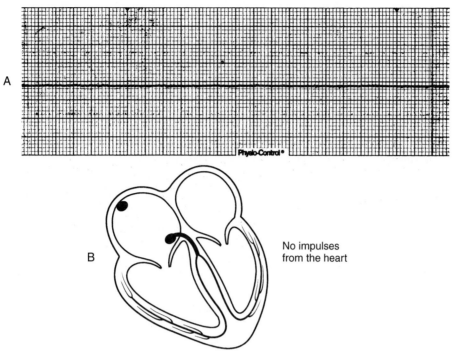

Figure 10-24. A, Asystole. **B,** Conduction pathway for asystole.

No impulses
from the heart

Table **10-23**   **Asystole**

Rate	None
Rhythm	None
P waves	May or may not appear
P/QRS relationship	None
P-R interval	None

a prolonged period; mortality is extremely high (Figure 10-24, *B*). Table 10-23 summarizes the characteristics of asystole.

Therapeutic interventions

- Begin basic and advanced life support immediately.
- Intubate the patient, and provide 100% oxygen under positive pressure.
- Administer epinephrine and atropine intravenously.
- Confirm asystole by switching to another lead; fine ventricular fibrillation can appear as a flat line in some leads.
- Do not defibrillate. Shocking asystole may prevent return of spontaneous heartbeats.
- Transcutaneous pacing may be effective, but only in asystole of short duration.
- Treat the underlying causes if it can be done rapidly, such as needle decompression for tension pneumothorax.
- Consider sodium bicarbonate administration in cases of prolonged arrest or if acidosis is evident.
- Consider termination of resuscitation efforts.

PACEMAKER RHYTHMS

Types of pacemakers include noninvasive (transcutaneous), semiinvasive (esophageal), temporary invasive (transvenous or transthoracic), and implanted (permanent); and each of these categories encompasses a number of devices and options.[3] In the emergency department, transcutaneous pacing is the most commonly initiated type of pacing. Occasionally, esophageal or transvenous pacing wires are inserted emergently.

Permanent pacemakers have become sophisticated over the past decade, and emergency nurses will encounter patients with various combinations of single- and dual-chamber pacers—those pacers that are functioning properly and those that are not. The QRS complexes generated from a ventricular lead have the appearance of an ectopic ventricular (widened) beat because they are conducted through the same pathway that ventricular ectopic beats follow. In dual-chamber pacing, one spike generates a P wave while a second (immediately following) generates the QRS complex. Refer to a current text on pacing modalities for a comprehensive discussion of pacing options. Figure 10-25 provides samples of demand pacemaker rhythms.

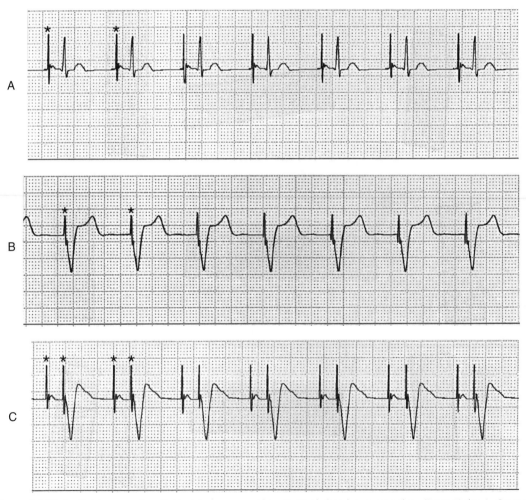

Figure 10-25. A, Atrial pacemaker. **B,** Ventricular pacemaker. **C,** Dual-chamber pacemaker. (From Urden L, Stacy K, Lough M: *Thelan's critical care nursing, diagnosis and management,* ed 4, St Louis, 2002, Mosby.)

An implanted biventricular pacemaker is a new device that resynchronizes the right and left ventricles. The device has been used successfully in patients with heart failure. When working properly, both ventricles are stimulated simultaneously, giving rise to a narrow QRS complex with return of a wide QRS complex only if loss of capture occurs. One must remember that this finding is just the opposite of that seen in the more common demand pacemakers.

PEDIATRIC DYSRHYTHMIAS

Children experience far fewer dysrhythmias than do adults. Instead of ectopic beats, fibrillation, and blocks, children generally have rhythms that are simply too fast, too slow, or absent. The most important treatment distinction between pediatric and adult patients is the heart rate at which therapy is indicated. According to the American Heart Association guidelines,[1] treat children as follows:

- Less than 5 years of age with rates less than 80 or greater than 180 beats/min
- Greater than 5 years of age with rates less than 60 or greater than 160 beats/min

Because young children typically enhance cardiac output by increasing their heart rate, a drop in rate is an ominous sign of cardiac failure. Causes of pediatric bradycardia include hypoxia, acidosis, electrolyte abnormalities, and hypothermia. The most frequently seen pediatric tachydysrhythmia is supraventricular tachycardia; rates can exceed 300 beats per minute. Ventricular tachycardia and ventricular fibrillation are rare but can occur in patients with cardiac disease or certain toxicities. Treatment with countershocks and medications must be adjusted by weight or length. Consult the American Heart Association pediatric advanced life support algorithms for details.

12-LEAD ELECTROCARDIOGRAMS

Rapid interpretation of standard 12-lead electrocardiograms has become an essential component of emergency care, particularly in patients with acute coronary syndromes (myocardial infarction, unstable angina, non-ST elevation myocardial infarction). An electrocardiogram also can be an important tool in diagnosing the cause of wide QRS tachycardias when their origin is not apparent using basic dysrhythmia monitoring.

The 12-lead electrocardiogram takes 12 different, simultaneous views of the cardiac electrical wave as it passes through the heart. Table 10-24 illustrates correct lead placement for a standard 12-lead electrocardiogram, and Box 10-2 summarizes the procedure for obtaining a 12-lead electrocardiogram. Particular areas of the heart are viewed by specific lead groupings. Evaluation of these groupings facilitates identification of the location of injury.

Table **10-24   Location of Electrocardiogram Changes During Myocardial Infarction**

Surface of Left Ventricle	Electrocardiogram Leads	Coronary Artery Usually Involved
Inferior	II, III, aV_F	Right coronary artery
Lateral	V_5, V_6, I, aV_L	Left circumflex
Anterior	V_2-V_4	Left anterior descending
Septal	V_1, V_2	Left anterior descending
Posterior	V_1, V_2	Left circumflex or right coronary
	V_7-V_9 (direct)	artery (reciprocal changes)

From Urden L, Stacy K, Lough M: *Thelan's critical care nursing, diagnosis and management*, ed 4, St Louis, 2002, Mosby.

Box **10-2**   **Procedure for Obtaining a 12-Lead Electrocardiogram**

Attempt to maintain the patient's modesty. Explain what you are doing.
Make sure you enter the patient information, date, and time correctly.
Ensure that all leads are accurately placed:
- "Green and white are on the right, Christmas trees (red and green) below the knees" is a helpful memory aid for limb lead placement.
- Avoid placing electrodes over large muscle masses.
- Remove excess hair (if necessary) to ensure good skin contact. You may need to rub the skin with an alcohol pad to remove dry skin or hair particles.

Ensure that the lead wires are not touching anything metal (this may cause 60-cycle interference).
If 60-cycle interference occurs, check for the following:
- Loose leads
- Leads and wires against metal
- Nearby electrical equipment that could be causing interference; unplug (unless contraindicated)

If the patient will need serial electrocardiograms, leave the electrodes in place to provide consistency between studies.
Evaluate the printout for acute changes, or notify the appropriate practitioner for interpretation.

Left Posterior Leads

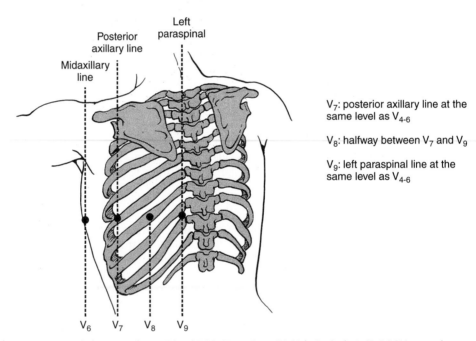

V_7: posterior axillary line at the same level as V_{4-6}

V_8: halfway between V_7 and V_9

V_9: left paraspinal line at the same level as V_{4-6}

Figure 10-26. Lead placement for a 15-lead ECG. (From Lynn-McHale D, Carlson K: *AACN procedure manual for critical care*, ed 4, Philadelphia, 2001, Saunders.)

The electrocardiogram printout is standardized so that the grid pattern on the paper matches the electrical activity of the heart: 1 mV equals 1 mm. Standardization facilitates easy evaluation of ST segment and T wave deviation, and identification of significant Q waves (defined as greater than or equal to 1 mm deep and 1 mm wide). The standard electrocardiogram does not evaluate the right ventricle directly nor the posterior wall of the left ventricle. Special electrocardiogram leads expand the standard 12 leads to 15 (Figure 10-26)

Right Precordial Leads

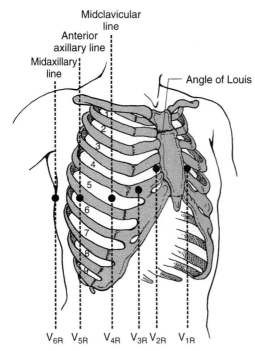

V_{1R}: 4th intercostal space (ICS) at left sternal border (same as V_2)

V_{2R}: 4th ICS at right sternal border (same as V_1)

V_{3R}: halfway between V_{2R} and V_{4R}

V_{4R}: right midclavicular line in the 5th ICS

V_{5R}: right anterior axillary line at the same horizontal level as V_{4R}

V_{6R}: right mid-axillary line at the same horizontal level as V_{4R}

Figure 10-27. Lead placement for assessment of the right ventricle and the posterior left ventricular wall. (From Drew BJ, Ide B: Right ventricular infarction. *Prog Cardiovasc Nurse* 10(2):46, 1995. In Lynn-McHale D, Carlson K: *AACN procedure manual for critical care*, ed 4, Philadelphia, 2001, Saunders.)

or 18 (Figure 10-27). This allows direct assessment of the right ventricle and the posterior left ventricular wall. Current that flows toward a lead (positive electrode) is recorded as an upward deflection on the electrocardiogram tracing. Current that flows away from a positive lead produces a downward deflection. When current travels perpendicular to a lead, biphasic deflections occur.

Interpretation

The process of 12-lead electrocardiogram evaluation involves the same steps used for dysrhythmia interpretation with the addition of ST segment, T wave, Q wave, and axis assessment. Figure 10-28 illustrates typical QRS complex configurations for standard limb leads. Early detection of ischemia, injury, and infarction is of paramount importance. Figure 10-29 details classic T wave and ST segment changes associated with ischemia and injury. Figure 10-30 demonstrates the appearance of significant Q waves. Electrocardiogram changes are considered important when they occur in 2 or more leads that view the same region of the heart.

Accurate assessment of electrocardiogram tracings can be difficult. Figure 10-31 clarifies parameters for measurement based on the location of the J point. Following a standard procedure when reviewing each electrocardiogram reduces interpretation errors. Table 10-25 summarizes recommended steps in electrocardiogram review.

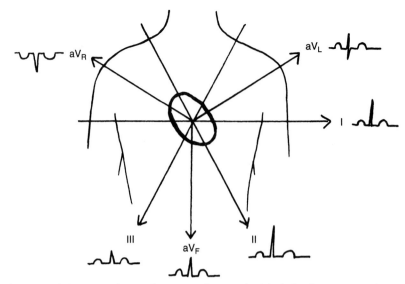

Figure 10-28. Typical QRS complex configurations for standard limb leads (From Newberry L: *Sheehy's emergency nursing: principles and practice*, ed 5, St Louis, 2003, Mosby.)

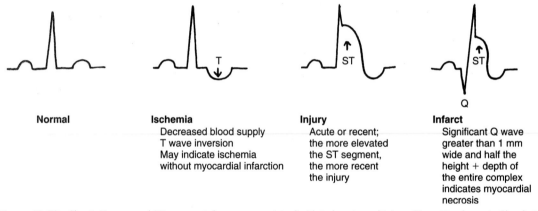

Normal	**Ischemia**	**Injury**	**Infarct**
	Decreased blood supply T wave inversion May indicate ischemia without myocardial infarction	Acute or recent; the more elevated the ST segment, the more recent the injury	Significant Q wave greater than 1 mm wide and half the height + depth of the entire complex indicates myocardial necrosis

Figure 10-29. Classic T wave and ST segment changes associated with ischemia and injury. (From Newberry L: *Sheehy's emergency nursing: principles and practice*, ed 5, St Louis, 2003, Mosby.)

Q Waves

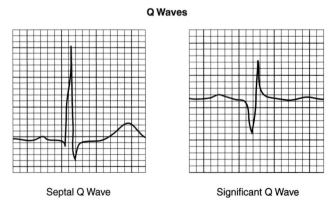

Septal Q Wave   Significant Q Wave

Figure 10-30. Significant Q waves indicate dead myocardium.

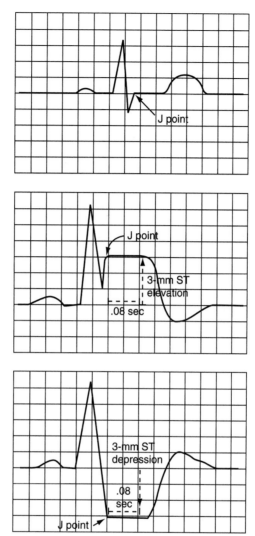

Figure 10-31. The J point is formed by the junction of the QRS complex with the ST segment. To calculate ST elevation or depression, measure the distance from the baseline to the J point. (From Urden L, Stacy K, Lough M: *Thelan's critical care nursing: diagnosis and management,* ed 3, St Louis, 1998, Mosby.)

Table 10-25   **Steps in Reading a 12-Lead Electrocardiogram**

Step	Significance
Measure intervals, identify P wave, and calculate the heart rate.	Determine the origin of the rhythm.
Evaluate ST segment (if no bundle branch block present).	Depression indicates ishemia. Elevation indicates injury.
Evaluate T wave.	Inversion indicates ischemia. Tall, tented configuration indicates ischemia, early injury, or hyperkalemia if generalized.
Evalute QRS complex.	Presence of significant Q wave (≥1 mm deep and ≥1 mm wide) indicates necrosis. *With new left bundle branch block, suspect new myocardial infarction.

*Changes have to present in two or more leads that look at the same wall to be significant.

Box **10-3**   **Causes of Axis Deviation**

> ### Right
>
> Dextrocardia
> Left posterior hemiblock
> Left ventricular ectopic rhythms
> Mechanical shifts, inspiration, emphysema
> Normal variation
> Pulmonary embolus
> Pulmonary hypertension
> Right bundle branch block
> Right ventricular ectopy
> Some right ventricular ectopic rhythms
>
> ### Left
>
> Congenital lesions
> Hyperkalemia
> Left anterior hemiblock
> Left bundle branch block
> Mechanical shifts, high diaphragm (e.g., pregnancy)
> Normal variation
> Right ventricular ectopic beats
> Shift with expiration
> Wolfe-Parkinson-White syndrome

Modified from Driscoll C et al: *Family practice desk reference*, ed 3, St Louis, 1996, Mosby.

Axis

Axis refers to the direction of current flow through the heart. Determining whether the axis is normal, shifted to the left, to the right, or indeterminate can affect the interpretation of certain electrocardiogram tracings. By reviewing leads I and aV_F, one can make a rough determination as to whether the axis is normal or abnormal. If the current flows from the sinoatrial node through standard pathways and there is no physical shifting of the heart, the axis is between 0 degrees and +90 degrees (normal). If current originates in the ventricles and flows in a retrograde manner to the atria, there is often a shift in the axis to abnormal or indeterminate. This shift can be a useful clue when one is trying to determine the origin of a wide QRS tachycardia. Box 10-3 summarizes specific causes of axis deviation (by direction).

References

1. Hazinski M, Cummins R, Field J, editors: *Handbook of emergency cardiovascular care,* Dallas, 2002, American Heart Association.
2. Aehlert B: *ACLS quick review study guide,* St Louis, 2002, Mosby.
3. Overbay D, Criddle L: Mastering temporary invasive cardiac pacing, *Crit Care Nurse* 24(3):25-32, 2004.

11

Hemodynamic Monitoring

Darcy T. Barrett, RN, MSN, CNRN

Diagnosis and management of shock (and other serious cardiopulmonary conditions) require careful hemodynamic monitoring. Hemodynamic status is assessed routinely through noninvasive means such as bedside electrocardiogram monitoring, pulse assessment, noninvasive blood pressure measurement, orthostatic vital signs, pulse oximetry, urine output, and evaluation of mental status. Thanks to a number of technologic innovations, several promising, minimally invasive measures of hemodynamic status have recently become available. Unstable patients and those with complex conditions often require invasive monitoring as well. Such patients may benefit from the use of arterial catheters, central venous catheters, and pulmonary artery catheters.

The role of invasive hemodynamic monitoring in emergency care has been debated for many years; to date there is no consensus on the subject. Although the majority of emergency departments (ED) do not perform any type of invasive monitoring, others use these procedures routinely. Many clinicians argue that the ED is not the appropriate locale for such highly invasive, technical, sterile, expensive, and resource-consuming procedures. Other practitioners counter that patients who could benefit from this technology should not have care delayed while waiting for an operating room, intensive care unit bed, or interfacility transfer. Because the issues raised are not simple and circumstances vary from institution to institution, this discussion undoubtedly will continue.

NONINVASIVE MONITORING

Examples of classic noninvasive monitoring parameters include blood pressure, postural (orthostatic) vital signs, and pulse oximetry. For a more detailed discussion refer to Chapter 7.

Within the last decade, several new technologies have been used to diagnose shock and to trend resuscitation adequacy, including bioimpedance, esophageal Doppler ultrasound, end-expiratory carbon dioxide calculations, sublingual capnometry, near infrared spectrometry, and tissue Po_2 measurement. Each of these monitoring modalities is either noninvasive or minimally invasive. Most of these techniques are easy to use, several are inexpensive, and all show promise of being valid indicators of resuscitation effectiveness. This section discusses few of the newer, noninvasive monitoring techniques.

Bioimpedance

Besides the invasiveness of traditional pulmonary artery catheter monitoring, the issue of validity has long been questioned. Pulmonary artery catheters measure pressure. From this limited information, data regarding volume and resistance are computed through various standardized formulas.[1,2] However, for the trauma patient in particular, volume is of far greater importance than is pressure. In addition, pulmonary artery catheter insertion is a sterile, prolonged, potentially dangerous process. Because impedance cardiography (BioZ, Cardio Dynamic San Diego, CA) overcomes these barriers, it is an attractive monitoring option. Unfortunately, the bioimpedance monitor requires careful placement of a number of electrodes on the chest and neck. Although generally not a problem in the medical patient, placement is difficult in trauma patients, who often are wearing a cervical collar or who require chest exposure for procedures such as chest tube insertion and central line placement.

A large, multicenter trial concluded that bioimpedance monitoring allows for early recognition of low flow and poor tissue perfusion and compared favorably with information derived from pulmonary artery catheters.[3] Nonetheless, impedance cardiography requires a steep initial equipment investment and a clinician mind shift. Because information is reported as volumes and resistance, health care providers long used to working with the pressure readings and calculations associated with pulmonary artery catheters first have to overcome the obstacle of learning an entirely new set of parameters and norms.

Esophageal Ultrasound

Another minimally invasive technique for generating hemodynamic data is esophageal Doppler ultrasound (HemoSonic 100, Arrow International, Cranford, NJ; CardioQ, Deltex Medical London). This device (Figure 11-1), which is almost as simple to insert as an oral gastric tube, has been the subject of many hemodynamic monitoring and fluid management studies, particularly in the United Kingdom.[4-6] The practitioner places the probe in the esophagus via the nasal or oral route to a depth of 35 to 40 cm. The practitioner then manipulates the probe until a characteristic aortic waveform is clearly visible on the monitor.[7] An audible "swoosh" indicates aortic blood flow. Doppler ultrasound waveforms, transmitted from the tip of the probe, are analyzed continuously and are displayed along with numeric readouts. As with bioimpedance, this technique requires users to learn a new vocabulary, a new set of norms, and new waveform interpretation.[8]

End-Expiratory Carbon Dioxide Calculations

Noninvasive cardiac output (NICO), recently touted as an integrated respiratory and hemodynamic monitoring system, measures breath-by-breath volumetric carbon dioxide. Information generated includes cardiac output, cardiac index, stroke volume, and pulmonary capillary blood flow, purportedly measures of cardiac output effectiveness. The partial rebreathing system consists of a disposable sensor that is attached to a conventional endotracheal tube. Because the majority of critically ill persons already are intubated, invasiveness is minimal. Using a modified Fick equation (Box 11-1), cardiac output can be assessed by measuring exhaled carbon dioxide at specific intervals.[9] Data are analyzed and then displayed digitally

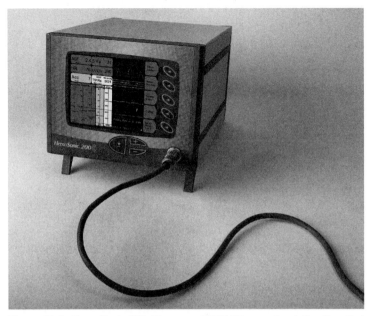

Figure 11-1. HemoSonic 200. (Courtesy ARROW International, Reading, Pa.)

Box **11-1** **Modified Fick Equation**

$$CO = VCO_2/CaO_2 - CVO_2$$

CO, Cardiac output; *VCO₂,* carbon dioxide output; *CaO₂,* arterial oxygen content; *CVO₂,* central venous oxygen content.

and as a waveform on a monitor. This technique has generated numerous studies in operating room settings; however data on critically ill or injured patients is still minimal.[10-12]

Sublingual Capnometry

Recently a thermometer-like, disposable, sublingual probe (CapnoProbe [Nellcor, Pleasanton, CA]) was developed to determine metabolic (versus respiratory) carbon dioxide levels. Clinical trials have supported its validity as a measure of intestinal perfusion.[13-15] Because splanchnic hypoperfusion occurs early in shock—and persists until adequate circulation has been restored to other major organ systems—sublingual carbon dioxide measurement appears to be a reliable marker of resuscitation effectiveness. The CapnoProbe is a portable, handheld device that resembles an electronic thermometer. This monitoring system is particularly attractive because of its ability to measure intestinal perfusion status repeatedly, noninvasively, quickly, and easily at a reasonable cost.

Near Infrared Spectrometry

Other researchers have investigated the use of near infrared spectrometry (also called spectroscopy) as a means of noninvasively monitoring tissue hemoglobin oxygen saturation. Similar in concept to a typical pulse oximeter, these devices involve the use of a single skin probe that emits a deep-penetrating infrared light capable of assessing hemoglobin oxygen content in the underlying muscle. Like the gut, blood is shunted from the skeletal muscles to more essential tissues in hypovolemic states. This modality has shown some success at detecting hemorrhagic shock in trauma patients.[16] A similar version of this instrument can be placed on the scalp for continuous monitoring of cerebral oxygenation during procedures that can affect brain perfusion.[17,18] However, use of spectrometry in the emergent patient population has not been studied.

Tissue Po_2

A slightly more invasive means of monitoring oxygenation status involves insertion of a tiny thermal diffusion microprobe into the tissue of interest. When placed in an undamaged major muscle, continuous, real-time readings purportedly reflect global oxygenation status. This device has been used to assess adequacy of resuscitation and volume administration. Inserted into a specific target muscle or organ, the probe can detect local ischemia and can guide specific interventions aimed at improving tissue perfusion. This device has been studied extensively in the transplant population but remains unproven in critically ill or injured patients.[19-21]

INVASIVE MONITORING

Invasive hemodynamic monitoring provides continuous physiologic data about the cardiovascular system. Many practitioners consider the information provided by this technology a valuable adjunct to other assessment data. Nonetheless, controversy surrounds the use of invasive hemodynamic monitoring, particularly pulmonary artery catheters. Consistent evidence is lacking to show that pulmonary artery catheter monitoring improves patient outcomes. Other legitimate concerns relate to clinician error and practice variations in the interpretation of hemodynamic values.[22] Additionally, these catheters are associated with potentially significant patient risks including pneumothorax, sepsis, air embolism, and pulmonary artery infarction. Despite these challenges, the data can assist practitioners with fluid management and drug administration in patients with significant cardiac, pulmonary, or volume overload or deficits.

Regardless of the modality selected, invasive monitoring requires insertion of a catheter into the vascular system. Specific modalities measure or calculate arterial pressure, central venous pressure (CVP), pulmonary artery systolic and diastolic pressures, pulmonary artery occlusive pressure (PaOP, also called wedge pressure, pulmonary artery wedge pressure, pulmonary artery wedge, or pulmonary capillary wedge pressure), cardiac output and cardiac index, pulmonary vascular resistance, systemic vascular resistance, and left and right ventricular stroke work indexes. Use of invasive monitoring requires knowledge of the basic hemodynamic concepts of preload, afterload, and contractility. These concepts are defined in Box 11-2.

Arterial Pressure Monitoring

Invasive arterial lines provide direct, continuous monitoring of systolic and diastolic blood pressure and easy access for frequent arterial blood gas and other laboratory study sampling. Continuous arterial pressure monitoring facilitates rapid evaluation of the effects of vasoactive agents and other therapeutic interventions.

The radial artery is generally the preferred site. In cases of cardiopulmonary arrest or altered upper extremity perfusion, the femoral artery may become the site of choice.[24] Cannulation of the femoral artery may prove difficult because of its proximity to the femoral vein. The brachial artery also is considered an acceptable site, particularly for short-term arterial

Box **11-2**   **Definitions Related to Hemodynamic Function**

Preload: The degree of myocardial fiber stretch at the end of diastole. Generally, the greater the stretch, the greater the force of contraction. However, Starling's law states that if myocardial stretch is excessive, the force of the contraction will be diminished. Right ventricular preload is reflected in the central venous pressure reading. Left ventricular preload is indicated by pulmonary artery diastolic pressure and pulmonary artery occlusive pressure measurements. Low blood volume and vasodilation reduce preload. Volume overload, poor ventricular function, and high pulmonary vascular resistance increase preload.

   Afterload: The pressure the ventricles must overcome during systole to eject their contents. Afterload is determined by calculating pulmonary vascular resistance for right ventricular and systemic vascular resistance for left ventricular overload. In general terms, the higher the afterload, the harder the myocardium must work to eject volume. Vasoconstriction (pulmonary or systemic) is the most common reason for increased afterload. Aortic or pulmonic stenosis or other restrictors of outflow (aortic coarctation, pulmonary embolus) also increase afterload.

   Contractility: The ability of the myocardium to contract. This ability cannot be measured directly; it must be inferred from other measures (e.g., left and right ventricular stroke work index calculations or ejection fraction measurement) and clinical findings.

From Druding MC: Integrating hemodynamic monitoring and physical assessment, *Dimens Crit Care Nurs* 19(4):25-30, 2000.

Box **11-3**   **Essential Equipment for Arterial Pressure Monitoring**

2-inch, 20-gauge, nontapered Teflon over-the-needle cannula *or* a prepackaged kit with a 6-inch
  Teflon catheter with appropriate introducer and guide wire (available in various sizes)
Pressurized bag of normal saline (heparin is not required) attached to pressure tubing and a
  transducer
Monitoring equipment consisting of a connecting cable, pressure module, monitor display screen,
  and recorder
Nonsterile gloves and goggles
Sterile gloves
Alcohol pads or swabs
Povidone-iodine (Betadine) pads or swabs
Sterile 4 × 4 inch gauze pads
Suture material (sutured arterial lines are much less likely to be removed accidentally)
1% lidocaine without epinephrine, 1 to 2 mL
3-mL syringe with a 25-gauge needle (for lidocaine infiltration)
Absorbent pads (place pads under the proposed puncture site)
Sterile towels or drapes
1- or 2-inch tape
Transparent dressing material
Small wrist board (for radial artery placement)

From Becker DE: Hemodynamic monitoring. In Lynn-McHale D, Carlson K, editors: *AACN procedure manual for critical care*, ed 4, Philadelphia, 2000, Saunders.

monitoring. The artery is cannulated using a sterile, percutaneous technique, and then the cannula is attached to a pressurized system that provides a continuous infusion (about 3 mL/hr) of saline to maintain system patency.

   Before insertion of an arterial catheter, an Allen's test should be performed. The Allen's test assesses the ability of the ulnar artery to maintain collateral perfusion if the radial artery is cannulated or damaged. See Figure 9-3 in Chapter 9 for details on how to perform this test. Box 11-3 identifies essential equipment for arterial pressure monitoring.

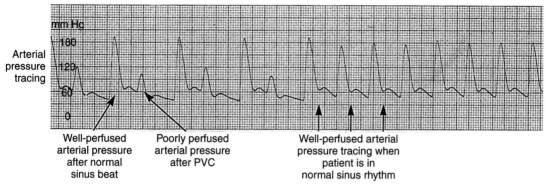

Figure 11-2. Arterial waveform. (From Thelan LA et al: *Critical care nursing*, ed 3, St Louis, 1997, Mosby.)

Box 11-4 Normal Blood Pressure Values

Systolic blood pressure	110 to 120 mm Hg
Diastolic blood pressure	70 to 80 mm Hg
Mean arterial pressure	70 to 105 mm Hg

Arterial pressure waveform analysis

The arterial pressure consists of two phases: systole and diastole. Arterial systole signifies the opening of the aortic valve, with subsequent rapid ejection of blood into the aorta. This event is seen as a large, rapid upstroke on the waveform. Following this ejection is runoff of blood from the proximal aorta to the peripheral arteries (the down slope of the waveform). As the pressure decreases, the aortic valve quickly closes. This closure results in a small elevation in arterial pressure (part way along the down slope of the waveform), known as the dicrotic notch. Diastole (the relatively flat portion of the waveform) occurs following closure of the aortic valve and continues until the next systole (Figure 11-2).[24]

Mean arterial pressure is an important indicator of arterial blood flow. The mean arterial pressure is the average force required to push blood through the systemic circulation and reflects the pressure the organs actually receive. Mean arterial pressure is influenced by the volume of blood in the arterial system (cardiac output) and the elasticity or resistance of the arteries (systemic vascular resistance).[25] Box 11-4 lists normal values for systolic, diastolic, and mean arterial pressure for adults. The formula for calculating mean arterial pressure follows:

$$\frac{\text{Systolic blood pressure} + 2(\text{Diastolic blood pressure})}{3}$$

Potential complications

Every invasive monitoring device involves significant potential complications. Complications associated with invasive arterial monitoring include thrombosis, embolus, local infection, sepsis, neurovascular compromise, distal ischemia, and bleeding.

Therapeutic interventions

Following insertion of an arterial line, check the neurovascular status of the extremity frequently. Assess for bleeding or oozing from the puncture, provide meticulous site care, and immobilize the extremity to reduce vessel trauma and minimize the risk of dislodgment.

Central Venous Pressure Monitoring

Central venous pressure (CVP) monitoring measures pressure in the right atrium or superior vena cava. From this number, information regarding blood volume, general fluid status, preload in the right side of the heart, right ventricular function, and central venous return are inferred.[25] Catheter placement for pressure measurement can be performed percutaneously or via surgical cutdown. Veins commonly used for cannulation include internal and external jugular vein, as well as subclavian veins, and less frequently the antecubital veins. Femoral veins also may be used for central line cannulation, but because of the distance from the femoral vein to the heart, readings may not reflect central pressure accurately. In addition, femoral sites have a much higher rate of nosocomial infection.[26]

Central venous catheters are available with one, two, three, or four lumens. Central venous pressure also can be measured through a pulmonary artery catheter. The decision to place a single-lumen or multilumen central line is determined by the actual or anticipated venous access needs of the patient. Considerations include the need for CVP monitoring, the projected number of blood samples to be drawn; the amount and frequency of medication administration; the potential for blood product administration; requirements for maintenance fluids, fluid boluses, and parenteral nutritional support; and the number of vascular access alternatives. Table 11-1 lists recommendations for the use of ports in multilumen catheters. Any port used intermittently (saline or heparin locked) should be flushed regularly according to institutional protocol.

Central venous pressure can be measured using a pressurized system and transducer (see Arterial Pressure Monitoring) or a water manometer. Central pressures obtained from pressurized systems are measured in millimeters of mercury, whereas values obtained from a water manometer are measured in centimeters of water. Box 11-5 provides the formulas to convert

Table 11-1 Recommendations for Port Use in Multilumen Catheters

Location	Size/Color	Use/Comments
Distal	16-gauge/brown*	Most proximal to the right atrium Use for central venous pressure monitoring, administration of blood products, and general access
Middle	18-gauge/blue*	General access Medication administration
Proximal	18-gauge/white*	Recommended for blood sampling and general access Some facilities reserve this port for administration of total parenteral nutrition.

*Color and lumen size may vary by manufacturer

Box 11-5 Converting Central Venous Pressure Measurements Between Mercury and Water Pressure

Formula	Normal Central Venous Pressure Values
To convert mm Hg to cm H_2O, multiply mm Hg by 1.36	2 to 6 mm Hg
To convert cm H_2O to mm Hg, divide cm H_2O by 1.36	2 to 8 cm H_2O

Data from Urden LD, Stacy K, Lough M, editors: *Thelan's critical care nursing, diagnosis and management,* ed 4, St Louis, 2002, Mosby.

CVP measurements from mercury to water pressure. Chapter 8 contains information on measuring CVP with a manual manometer. All CVP measurements are mean pressures and reflect function of the right side of the heart. The CVP reading does not reflect left ventricular function.

Central venous pressure waveform analysis

The CVP waveform consists of three positive waves: a, c, and v, followed by the x, x_1, and y descents or negative waves. The a wave signifies contraction and is followed immediately by the x descent, or atrial relaxation. The c wave reflects closure of the tricuspid valve during ventricular contraction. This wave may be distinct, appearing as a notch on the a wave, or it may be absent. The v wave signifies right atrial filling, or right ventricular systole. During right ventricular systole, the closed leaflets of the tricuspid valve bulge into the right atrium. The y descent following the v wave represents the opening of the tricuspid valve and right ventricular filling (Figure 11-3).[26] Note the relationship between these events and the electrocardiogram.

Central veins are influenced by intrathoracic pressure changes that occur during the respiratory cycle. During spontaneous inspiration, negative pressure within the intrathoracic space causes the CVP to drop. Conversely, pressures rise during spontaneous expiration. The opposite phenomenon occurs with mechanically delivered breaths. The pressure delivered with mechanically controlled breaths causes positive pressure within the intrathoracic space during the inspiratory and expiratory phases of controlled ventilation. During inspiration (and to a lesser degree during expiration), the CVP will rise.

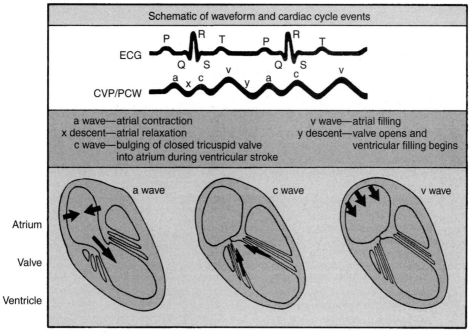

Figure 11-3. Cardiac events and central venous pressure waveform: *a wave*, atrial contraction; *x descent*, atrial relaxation; *c wave*, closed tricuspid valve during ventricular systole; *v wave*, ventricular filling; *y descent*, opening of tricuspid valve and filling of ventricle. *ECG*, Electrocardiogram; *CVP/PCW*, central venous pressure/pulmonary capillary wedge. (From Urden L, Stacy K, Lough M: *Thelan's critical care nursing, diagnosis and management*, ed 4, St Louis, 2002, Mosby.)

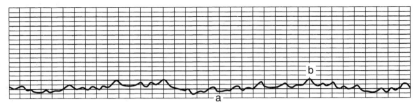

Figure 11-4. Central venous pressure waveform during spontaneous respirations. *a*, Inspiration; *b*, end expiration.

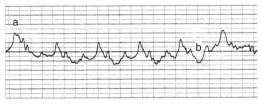

Figure 11-5. Central venous pressure waveform during mechanical ventilation. *a*, Inspiration; *b*, end expiration.

To minimize the influence these changing pressures have on the waveform, CVP should be measured at end expiration, whether the patient is breathing spontaneously or is ventilated mechanically. Intrathoracic pressures at end expiration are closest to zero, and readings will reflect actual CVP more accurately (Figures 11-4 and 11-5).[25]

Potential complications

Pneumothorax, hemothorax, and bleeding are complications of central line insertion. Air embolus can occur during insertion or any time the system is opened. Other complications include site infection, sepsis, thrombosis, catheter occlusion, and neurovascular compromise with use of the antecubital site. Catheters impregnated with antibiotics are available. Studies indicate that these catheters reduce the incidence of bacteremia.[27]

Pulmonary Artery Pressure Monitoring

Pulmonary artery pressure monitoring is achieved through percutaneous cannulation of a central vein. Sites most often used are the internal and external jugular and subclavian veins. Femoral and antecubital veins may be used if necessary but are not ideal. The pulmonary artery catheter allows direct monitoring of pulmonary artery pressures and CVP and indirect measurement of left ventricular function (by measuring pulmonary artery occlusion pressure (PaOP). Other hemodynamic values that can be derived using a pulmonary artery catheter include cardiac output and cardiac index, systemic vascular resistance, pulmonary vascular resistance, stroke volume, left ventricular end-diastolic pressure and volume, left and right ventricular stroke work indexes, core body temperature, and mixed venous oxygen saturation if a fiberoptic catheter is used.

The pulmonary artery catheter is designed with multiple lumens. Several different types of pulmonary artery catheters are available for insertion. Catheter selection is based on patient need and the functions desired. Pacing, venous oxygen saturation monitoring, and continuous cardiac output measurement require specialized pulmonary artery catheters.[28] Once the catheter is inserted, the *proximal* lumen rests in the right atrium and is used for intravenous

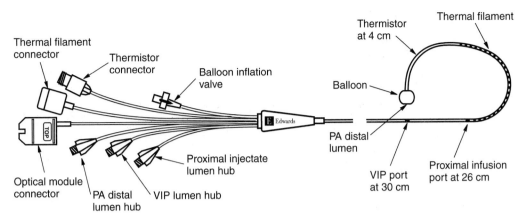

Figure 11-6. Pulmonary artery (PA) catheter. (From Urden L, Stacy K, Lough M: *Thelan's critical care nursing, diagnosis and management,* ed 4, St Louis, 2002, Mosby.)

infusions and CVP measurement. For this reason the proximal lumen also is known as the CVP port. The *distal* lumen is located at the tip of the pulmonary artery catheter and sits in the pulmonary artery. This lumen is used to monitor pulmonary artery pressures continuously and should not be used for infusion. The *balloon* lumen consists of a latex balloon that can be inflated with 0.8 to 1.5 mL of air to obtain PaOP or wedge pressure tracings. The *thermistor* lumen records changes in blood temperature necessary for cardiac output (CO) measurements. Many pulmonary artery catheters have an additional *infusion* lumen called a VIP port.[26] Specialty catheters also may contain a right ventricular pacing port or a fiberoptic venous oxygen saturation connector. Pulmonary artery lines generally are inserted through an introducer, or "straw" or "sheath," that also contains a large-bore side port for infusion. Figure 11-6 shows a standard pulmonary artery catheter with all lumens identified.

Patient preparation

Before pulmonary artery catheter insertion, risks and benefits must always be considered. Relative contraindications to pulmonary artery catheter placement include the presence of a preexisting left bundle branch block, fever, a mechanical tricuspid valve, or a coagulopathy.[29]

The standard pulmonary artery catheter size is 7 to 7.5 French and 110 cm long. The right internal jugular is the preferred point of insertion because this site provides the most direct route to the right artium, minimizing the risk of pneumothorax.[28] Box 11-6 lists essential equipment for this procedure.[29]

Patient preparation is as follows:

1. Set up the pressure bag and tubing, connect the transducer cable to the monitor, level and zero the transducer(s).
2. Place the patient in Trendelenburg position (head down, feet up) to promote venous distention.
3. Prepare the skin with a povidone-iodine solution, and drape the area with sterile towels.
4. Infiltrate the site with 1% lidocaine to provide local anesthesia.
5. Before pulmonary artery catheter insertion, connect pressure tubing to the appropriate ports, and prime all ports with a flush solution (use stopcocks and normal saline–filled syringes). Calibrate fiberoptic catheters before insertion (see manufacturer's instructions).
6. Insert a percutaneous introducer into the patient first; this allows immediate vascular access via the side port.

Box **11-6 Essential Equipment for Pulmonary Artery Monitoring**

Pulmonary artery catheter, check for correct size and type
Introducer (sheath) equipment tray, and sterile catheter sleeve
Pressure cables for interface with the monitor
Cardiac output injectate (normal saline or 5% dextrose in water), tubing, syringe, and monitoring equipment with an injectate sensor
Pressure transducer system, including flush solution (usually normal saline), pressure bag, and pressure tubing with a flush device and transducer. Two systems (or a double system) are required for simultaneous central venous pressure and pulmonary artery pressure monitoring.
Sterile normal saline intravenous fluid, sterile basin/cup, and 10-mL syringes for flushing each catheter lumen and the introducer port
Povidone-iodine (Betadine) solution
Cap, mask, sterile gown, sterile gloves, and sterile drapes
1% lidocaine without epinephrine
Suture material (sutured lines are much less likely to be removed accidentally)
Sterile dressing supplies
Stopcocks (one for each infusion or pressure port)
Dead-end caps (for ports without continuous infusions or pressure lines)

7. Thread the pulmonary artery catheter through a clear plastic sleeve before inserting it through the diaphragm of the introducer. This permits future sterile catheter repositioning.
8. Watch the monitor as the pulmonary artery catheter is advanced into position in the superior vena cava, right atrium, right ventricule, and then the pulmonary artery (Figures 11-7 and 11-8).
9. Continuous cardiac monitoring is required throughout the procedure.
10. During placement, observe for cardiac dysrhythmias (premature ventricular contractions, ventricular tachycardia). These dysrhythmias result from mechanical irritation of the ventricle by the catheter. Treatment is rarely necessary; simply advance or withdraw the catheter.
11. Observe the waveforms and record right atrium, right ventricular, pulmonary artery systolic and diastolic, and PaOP pressures during insertion.
12. Inflate and deflate the catheter balloon as directed. *Always leave the balloon in the deflated position.*
13. Obtain a postprocedure portable chest radiograph to confirm catheter placement and to check for pneumothorax.
14. Do not perform further PaOP measurements until catheter placement is confirmed and the physician has approved the first measurement. Pulmonary infarction may occur if the catheter tip is advanced too far into the pulmonary vasculature.
15. After the line is sutured, dress the site per institutional protocol. Be sure to record the insertion depth. Loop and secure the catheter to prevent pulling.

Pulmonary artery waveform analysis

Pulmonary artery and PaOP pressures are monitored to evaluate left-sided heart function and pulmonary disease.[24] In normal individuals the pulmonary vasculature is a low-pressure, low-resistance system. Pulmonary artery waveform characteristics are similar to those of arterial waveforms; however, the pressures are much lower. Systolic ejection (the peak of the pulmonary artery waveform) reflects right ventricular systolic pressure. The pulmonary artery

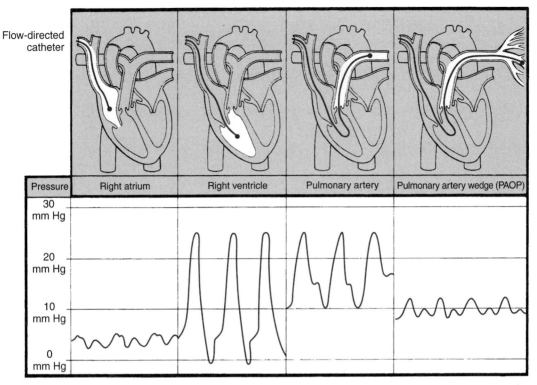

Flow-directed catheter

| Pressure | Right atrium | Right ventricle | Pulmonary artery | Pulmonary artery wedge (PAOP) |

Figure 11-7. Pulmonary artery catheter insertion with corresponding waveforms. (From Urden L, Stacy K, Lough M: *Thelan's critical care nursing, diagnosis and management*, ed 4, St Louis, 2002, Mosby.)

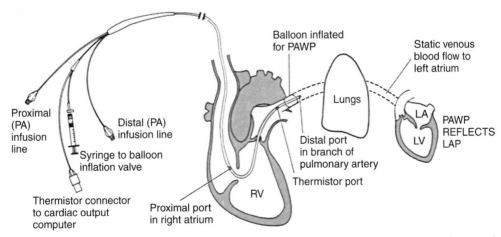

Figure 11-8. Pulmonary artery catheter location within the heart. *PA,* Pulmonary artery; *RV,* right ventricle; *LA,* left atrium; *LV,* left ventricle; *PAWP,* pulmonary artery wedge pressure; *LAP,* left atrial pressure. (From Lynn-McHale D, Carlson K: *AACN procedure manual for critical care*, ed 4, Phildelphia, 2001, Saunders.)

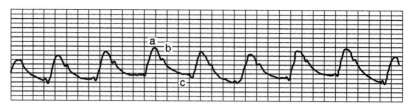

Figure 11-9. Pulmonary artery waveform. *a*, Systole; *b*, dicrotic notch; *c*, diastole.

Box **11-7** **Normal Pulmonary Artery Pressure Values**

Pulmonary artery systolic pressure	20 to 30 mm Hg
Pulmonary artery diastolic pressure	10 to 20 mm Hg
Pulmonary artery mean	10 to 15 mm Hg
Pulmonary artery occlusion pressure	4 to 12 mm Hg

dicrotic notch indicates pulmonic valve closure. This dicrotic notch signals the beginning of the right ventricular diastolic phase (Figure 11-9). The pulmonary artery diastolic pressure correlates with the degree of resistance in the pulmonary vascular bed and the left ventricular end-diastolic pressure.[30] Therefore pulmonary artery diastolic pressure is closely related to PaOP, and this number can be used to trend PaOP continuously. Box 11-7 provides normal adult values for pulmonary artery systolic, diastolic, and mean pressures.

Pulmonary artery occlusive pressure waveform analysis

Pulmonary artery occlusive pressure (also called pulmonary capillary wedge pressure or simply wedge pressure) is obtained by inflating the pulmonary artery catheter balloon. Balloon inflation floats the catheter into position in a small branch of the pulmonary artery where it wedges, occluding blood flow to that segment of the vessel. Inflate the balloon gently and always use the smallest amount of air required to obtain a wedge tracing; never exceed 1.5 mL. The PaOP reflects left atrial pressure, and the tracing has an appearance similar to that of a right atrial (CVP) waveform (presence of a, c, and v waves). The a wave represents left atrial contraction, the c wave (often difficult to observe) signifies closure of the atrioventricular valve, and the v wave reflects filling of the left atrium (Figure 11-10).[29] Like CVP readings, PaOP pressures are recorded as mean values. Pulmonary artery pressures and PaOP readings should be taken at end expiration.

Potential complications

Problems that can occur during pulmonary artery line insertion include hemothorax, pneumothorax, bleeding, air embolus, ventricular perforation, and ventricular dysrhythmias. Complications arising over time include thrombosis, embolus, infection, sepsis, pulmonary infarction, and distal neurovascular compromise if the catheter was inserted in a femoral or peripheral site.

Therapeutic interventions

Ensure that the catheter is inserted under sterile conditions, and provide meticulous site care. Keep the system closed as much as possible. Provide continuous cardiac monitoring,

ECG

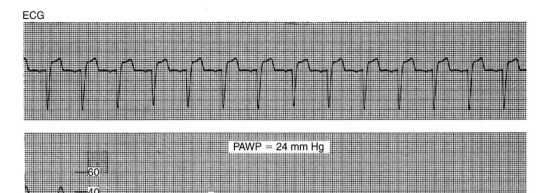

Figure 11-10. Pulmonary artery occlusion waveform. *a*, Atrial contraction; *c*, closure of atrioventricular valve; *v*, left atrial filling. (From Lynn-McHale D, Carlson K: *AACN procedure manual for critical care*, ed 4, Philadelphia, 2001, Saunders.)

Box **11-8**   **Cardiac Output and Cardiac Index**

Formula	**Normal Range**
CO = SV × HR	4 to 8 L/min
CI = CO/BSA	2.5 to 4 L/min

BSA, Body surface area (square meters); *CI*, cardiac index; *CO*, cardiac output; *HR*, heart rate; *SV*, stroke volume.

watching for dysrhythmias. Perform wedge pressure measurements only when indicated; at other times pulmonary artery diastolic pressure can be used for trending PaOP. Routinely assess the pulmonary artery waveform to check for inadvertent wedging. Verify that the balloon is deflated completely after each wedge pressure is obtained. Document catheter insertion depth (in centimeters) and check for dislodgment, especially after transporting or turning the patient.

Cardiac output determination

Cardiac output (CO) is the amount of blood ejected from the left ventricle each minute; it is a product of stroke volume and heart rate (CO = SV × HR). The stroke volume is the amount of blood ejected by the left ventricle with each contraction (Box 11-8).

Using a pulmonary artery catheter, CO is measured with the thermodilution method. This technique is based on the theory that a change in temperature over time is inversely proportional to blood flow.[26] When attached to a CO computer, the thermistor port of the pulmonary artery catheter provides an accurate measurement of blood temperature (core temperature). Each size, brand, and model of catheter has a preset computational constant (a three-digit number) that must be entered into the computer before CO measurement. This number also varies depending on whether iced or room temperature injectate is used.

A predetermined amount (usually 10 mL; 5 mL for some patients with cardiac disease) of 5% dextrose in water or normal saline is injected rapidly through the proximal lumen of the pulmonary artery catheter. This procedure is repeated 3 times, provided each value is

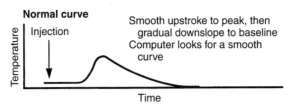

Figure 11-11. Normal cardiac output curve. (From Urden L, Stacy K, Lough M: *Thelan's critical care nursing, diagnosis and management,* ed 4, St Louis, 2002, Mosby.)

within 10% of the others. Totals are averaged. The CO curve displayed on the monitor is a diagrammatic representation of blood flow. The normal CO curve has a smooth upstroke, rounded peak, and gradually tapering down slope (Figure 11-11). If the curve has an uneven pattern, the measurement should be repeated.

The thermistor senses the temperature of the blood in the pulmonary artery, and the injectate sensor measures the temperature of the injectate. Using these known numbers, the CO computer determines the amount of temperature change from the injection site (proximal port) to the measurement site (distal port) and calculates the CO in liters per minute.[26] To ensure accurate readings, injectate temperature and body temperature must differ by at least 10° C, and the injectate must be delivered within a 4-second period. Iced injectate is preferred for patients with low body temperatures and for those who can tolerate only small injectate volumes (e.g., 3 mL for pediatric patients and 5 mL for patients with cardiac disease). Deliver the CO injectate during end expiration. Cardiac index (CI) is the CO corrected for body size, based on body surface area (see Box 11-8). Of the two measures, cardiac index is considered more important because the patient's height and weight are taken into consideration.[30] Any cardiac index less than 2.2 L/min is considered shock.

Physiologic changes that may influence CO and CI include the following:
- Changes in heart rate (affects diastolic filling time)
- Changes in preload
  Increased preload increases CO.
  Decreased preload decreases CO.
- Extreme changes in afterload
  Vasoconstriction increases CO.
  Vasodilation decreases CO.
- Hypothermia (decreases CO)

Systemic vascular resistance

Systemic vascular resistance is the primary determinant of left ventricular afterload. Systemic vascular resistance—the average resistance to blood flow within the systemic circulation—is a calculated value rather than a directly measured number. Factors that influence cardiac workload (e.g., mean arterial pressure, CVP, or CO) also influence systemic vascular resistance. Vasodilatory agents can be used to decrease a patient's systemic vascular resistance; vasoconstrictors are used to raise it.[24] Box 11-9 lists some conditions that alter systemic vascular resistance.

Data accuracy

With any hemodynamic procedure, consistency and technical accuracy are critical. Table 11-2 provides an overview of the hemodynamic parameters and hemodynamic calculations

Box **11-9** **Conditions Associated With Systemic Vascular Resistance Changes**

Decreased Systemic Vascular Resistance

Cardiogenic shock (uncompensated)
Hyperthermia
Hypovolemia (uncompensated)
Neurogenic shock
Overuse of vasodilators

Elevated Systemic Vascular Resistance

Hypothermia
Hypovolemia (compensated)
Low cardiac output (compensated)
Overuse of vasoconstrictors

Table 11-2   **Overview of Hemodynamic Calculations and Normal Values**

Parameter	Normal Value
Cardiac output (CO)	4-8 L/min
Cardiac index (CI)	2.5-4 L/min/m^2
Central venous pressure (CVP)	2-6 mm Hg
Pulmonary artery pressure (PAP)	20-30 mm Hg systolic
	10-20 mm Hg diastolic
	10-15 mm Hg mean
Pulmonary artery occlusion pressure (PaOP)	4-12 mm Hg
Pulse pressure	30-40 mm Hg
Systolic blood pressure – Diastolic blood pressure	
Right atrial pressure	2-6 mm Hg
Right ventricular pressure	20-30 mm Hg systolic
	0-5 mm Hg diastolic
	2-6 mm Hg mean
Stroke volume (SV)	60-80 mL/beat
Systemic vascular resistance	900-1400 dynes/sec/cm^{-5}
$\dfrac{\text{MAP} - \text{CVP}}{\text{CO}} \times 80$	
Pulmonary vascular resistance	20-120 dynes/sec/cm^{-5}
$\dfrac{\text{Mean PAP} - \text{PCWP}}{\text{CO}} \times 80$	

Modified from Druding M: Integrating hemodynamic monitoring and physical assessment, *Dimens Crit Care Nurs* 19(4):25-30, 2000.

discussed in this chapter. To ensure accuracy and reliability from any pressurized hemodynamic monitoring system, the following steps should be taken before data collection:

1. Check all tubing connections for tightness and proper alignment (no leaking, stopcocks in the correct position).
2. Ensure that the pressure bag is inflated sufficiently (usually 300 mm Hg).
3. Check the catheter for correct insertion depth and waveform adequacy.
4. Check the extremity for proper position and alignment.
5. Level the transducer with the phlebostatic axis (Figure 11-12). The phlebostatic axis is approximately the position of the right atrium.
6. Zero the system to atmospheric air.
7. Determine dynamic response by performing a square wave test (see following discussion).

Periodically relevel the transducer to the phlebostatic axis and rezero to atmospheric pressure. If the transducer is not level with the right atrium, hemodynamic values will not be accurate.[31] Once the patient's phlebostatic axis is located, mark the site with an X. A carpenter's level can be used to ensure that the transducer is indeed level. Whether the transducer is pole-mounted or patient-mounted (taped to the lateral chest wall or to the arm), it is paramount that the transducer and phlebostatic axis are in direct alignment. In addition, the head of the patient's stretcher or gurney should be elevated no more than 45 degrees when obtaining hemodynamic measurements.[29]

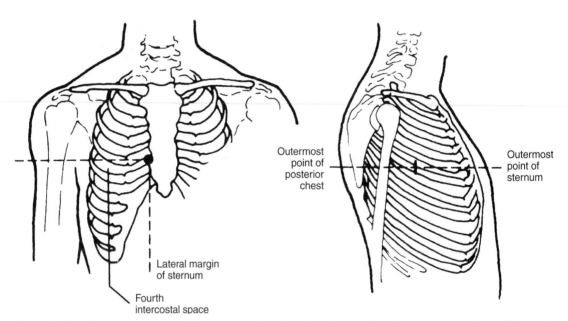

Figure 11-12. The phlebostatic axis. The crossing of two imaginary lines defines the assumed position of the monitoring catheter tip within the body (i.e., right atrial levels). **A,** A line that passes from the fourth intercostal space at the lateral margin of the sternum down the side of the body beneath the axilla. **B,** A line that runs horizontally at a point midway between the outermost position of the anterior and posterior surfaces of the chest. (From Darovic G: *Hemodynamic monitoring: invasive and noninvasive clinical application,* Philadelphia, 1987, Saunders.)

The square wave test reflects the dynamic response of the hemodynamic system and is performed by activating the fast flush mechanism (pull the "pigtail" of the transducer). The portion of the wave that is square is produced by the fast flush. Closure of the fast flush system (letting go) produces the wave or oscillation after the square wave.[32] Figures 11-13 to 11-16 depict how to perform a square wave test.

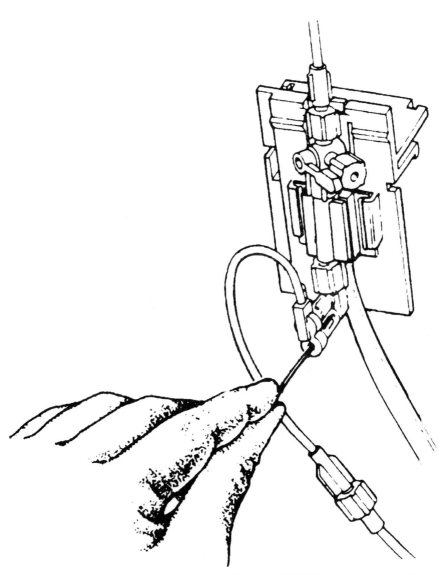

Figure 11-13. Beginning a square wave test. (Courtesy HOSPIRA, Inc., Lake Forest, Ill.)

Square wave test configuration

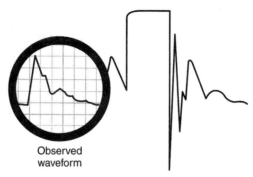

Observed
waveform

Figure 11-14. Optimally damped system. Dynamic response test (square wave test) using the fast flush system normal response. (From Lynn-McHale D, Carlson K: *AACN procedure manual for critical care,* ed 4, Philadelphia, 2001, Saunders.)

Square wave test configuration

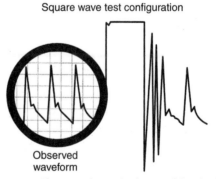

Observed
waveform

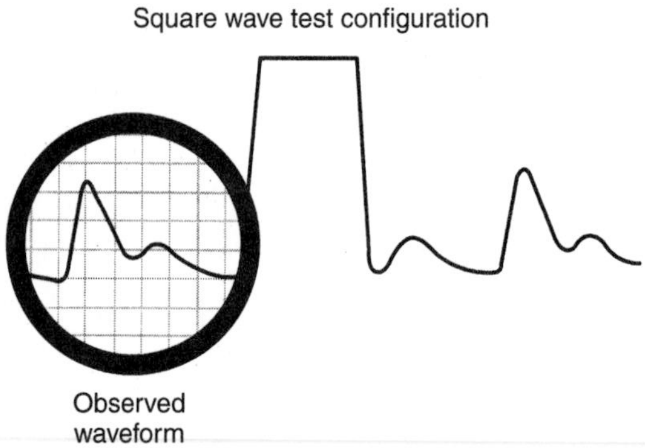

Figure 11-15. Overdamped system. The patient's waveform displays a falsely decreased systolic and falsely high diastolic pressure with an absent dicrotic notch. (From Lynn-McHale D, Carlson *K: AACN procedure manual for critical care,* ed 4, Philadelphia, 2001, Saunders.)

Square wave test configuration

Observed
waveform

Figure 11-16. Underdamped system. The waveform displays a false high systolic and possibly false low diastolic pressure. (From Lynn-McHale D, Carlson K: *AACN procedure manual for critical care,* ed 4, Philadelphia, 2001, Saunders.)

References

1. Haryadii D et al: Evaluation of a new advanced thoracic bioimpedance device for estimation of cardiac output, *J Clin Monit Comput* 15(2):131-138, 1999.
2. Spiess B et al: Comparison of bioimpedance versus thermodilution cardiac output during cardiac surgery: evaluation of a second-generation bioimpedance device, *J Cardiothorac Vasc Anesth* 15(5): 567-573, 2001.
3. Shoemaker W et al: Multicenter study of noninvasive monitoring systems as alternatives to invasive monitoring of acutely ill emergency patients, *Chest* 114(6):1643-1652, 1998.
4. Madan A et al: Esophageal Doppler ultrasound monitor versus pulmonary artery catheter in the hemodynamic management of critically ill surgical patients, *J Trauma* 46(4):607-611, 1999.
5. Penny J et al: A comparison of hemodynamic data derived by pulmonary artery flotation catheter and the esophageal Doppler monitor in preeclampsia, *Am J Obstet Gynecol* 183(3):658-661, 2000.
6. Rodriguez R, Berumen K: Cardiac output measurement with an esophageal Doppler in critically ill emergency department patients, *J Emerg Med* 18(2):159-164, 2000.
7. Turner M: Doppler-based hemodynamic monitoring: a minimally invasive alternative, *AACN Clin Issues* 14(2):220-231, 2003.
8. Lefrant J et al: Training is required to improve the reliability of esophageal Doppler to measure cardiac output in critically ill patients, *Intensive Care Med* 24(4):347-352, 1998.
9. Ott K, Johnson K, Ahrens T: *New technologies in the assessment of hemodynamic parameters, J Cardiovasc Nurs* 15(2):41-55, 2001.
10. de Abreu M et al: Evaluation of a new device for noninvasive measurement of nonshunted pulmonary capillary blood flow in patients with acute lung injury, *Intensive Care Med* 28(3):318-323, 2002.
11. Maxwell R et al: Noninvasive cardiac output by partial CO_2 rebreathing after severe chest trauma, *J Trauma* 51(5):849-853, 2001.
12. Odenstedt H, Stenqvist O, Lundin S: Clinical evaluation of a partial CO_2 rebreathing technique for cardiac output monitoring in critically ill patients, *Acta Anaesthesiol Scand* 46(2):152-159, 2002.
13. Marik P, Bankov A: Sublingual capnometry versus traditional markers of tissue oxygenation in critically ill patients, *Crit Care Med* 31(3):818-822, 2003.
14. Povoas H et al: Comparisons between sublingual and gastric tonometry during hemorrhagic shock, *Chest* 118(4):1127-1132, 2000.
15. Weil M et al: Sublingual capnometry: a new noninvasive measurement for diagnosis and quantitation of severity of circulatory shock, *Crit Care Med* 27(7):1225-1229, 1999.
16. McKinley B et al: Tissue hemoglobin O_2 saturation during resuscitation of traumatic shock monitored using near infrared spectrometry, *J Trauma* 48(4):637-642, 2000.
17. Hirofumi IO et al: The effectiveness of regional cerebral oxygen saturation monitoring using near-infrared spectroscopy in carotid endarterectomy, *J Clin Neurosci* 10(1):79-83, 2003.
18. Nagdyman N et al: Cerebral oxygenation measured by near-infrared spectroscopy during circulatory arrest and cardiopulmonary resuscitation, *Br J Anaesth* 91(3):438-442, 2003.
19. Angelescu M et al: Perioperative monitoring of the cortical microcirculation in clinical renal transplantation by thermodiffusion, *Transplant Proc* 29:2790-2792, 1997.
20. Klar E et al: Thermodiffusion for continuous quantification of hepatic microcirculation: validation and potentials in liver transplantation, *Microvasc Res* 58:156-166, 1999.
21. Mehrabi A et al: Hepatocellular injury early after reperfusion is correlated with liver microcirculation and predicts outcome after transplantation, *Transplant Proc* 30:3716-3717, 1998.
22. Quaal SJ: Improving the accuracy of pulmonary artery catheter measurements, *J Cardiovasc Nurs* 15(2):71-82, 2001.
23. Druding MC: Integrating hemodynamic monitoring and physical assessment, *Dimens Crit Care Nurs* 19(4):25-30, 2000.
24. Williams L: Hemodynamic monitoring. In Swearingen P, Keen JH, editors: *Manual of critical care nursing: nursing interventions and collaborative management,* ed 4, St Louis, 2001, Mosby.
25. Becker DE: Hemodynamic monitoring. In Lynn-McHale D, Carlson K, editors: *AACN procedure manual for critical care,* ed 4, Philadelphia, 2000, Saunders.
26. Urden LD, Stacy K, Lough M, editors: *Thelan's critical care nursing, diagnosis and management,* ed 4, St Louis, 2002, Mosby.

27. Criddle LM et al: Antimicrobial central venous catheters: do they make a difference? *J Emerg Nurs* 27(3):306-307, 2001.

28. Fleck D: Pulmonary artery catheter insertion (perform). In Lynn-McHale DJ, Carlson K, editors: *AACN procedure manual for critical care,* ed 4, Philadelphia, 2000, Saunders.

29. Lynn-McHale DJ, Preuss T: Pulmonary artery catheter insertion (assist) and pressure monitoring. In Lynn-McHale DJ, Carlson K, editors: *AACN procedure manual for critical care,* ed 4, Philadelphia, 2000, Saunders.

30. Hudack C, Gallo B, Morton P, editors: *Critical care nursing: a holistic approach,* ed 7, Philadelphia, 1998, Lippincott.

31. Dietz B, Smith T: Enhancing the accuracy of hemodynamic monitoring, *J Nurs Care Qual* 17(1): 27-34, 2002.

32. Shaffer R: Arterial catheter insertion (assist), care, and removal. In Lynn-McHale DJ, Carlson K, editors: *AACN procedure manual for critical care,* ed 4, Philadelphia, 2000, Saunders.

12

Wound Management

Robert Herr, MD, MBA, FACEP

BASIC CONSIDERATIONS

The goals of wound care are the following:
- Identify underlying injury to bones, nerves, vessels, ligaments, tendons, muscles, and other structures.
- Decrease the incidence of infection.
- Promote optimal healing.
- Minimize scarring.
- Manage pain.

Important considerations in wound management are the following:
- What caused the injury? How did it happen? What were the circumstances surrounding the event?
- When did the injury occur? Where was the patient at the time?
- Where is the wound located? What is the condition of the skin and surrounding tissue?
- What care did the wound receive before the patient arrived at the emergency department (ED)?
- Are motor function, sensation, and perfusion intact distal to the wound?
- Can the wound edges be approximated?
- What is the patient's general physical condition? Current medications? Medical history?
- What is the patient's age and occupation?

WOUND HEALING

Wound healing involves a number of complex physiologic responses that begin immediately after injury. Local vasoconstriction, caused by trauma, is followed quickly by vasodilation.

Vasodilation produces erythema and edema below the epithelial layer. In open wounds, epithelial cells begin to migrate within 24 hours of injury. The process of fibrin formation is followed (within days) by collagen deposition. Epithelialization will close the lesion in 48 to 72 hours if skin margins can be approximated and the wound remains uninfected.[1] Epithelialization occurs more slowly in patients with the following conditions:

- Poor nutritional status
- Compromised vascular supply, such as in diabetes or severe atherosclerosis or smoking
- Medications that slow collagen formation such as corticosteroids or phenytoin
- Wounds of the lower legs, feet, or toes
- Advanced age
- Low tissue oxygen levels, especially in patients with chronic obstructive pulmonary disease and those receiving home oxygen therapy

GENERAL PRINCIPLES OF WOUND MANAGEMENT

Wound care begins with management of the patient, then focuses on the general area of injury, and finally addresses the specific wound. The following principles apply to the management of all wounds, regardless of cause, location, or patient presentation[2]:

Manage the Patient

- Always use standard infection control precautions.
- Address airway, breathing, and circulatory concerns first.
- Complete the primary survey by evaluating the patient's level of consciousness, pupil size, and reactivity.
- Expose the patient (as indicated) to identify any other wounds that may warrant intervention.
- Control bleeding with direct pressure, elevation, and surgery.
- Identify and treat hemorrhagic shock.
- Evaluate the patient's tetanus immunization status.
- Assess for hypothermia, particularly when extensive skin loss is present.

Manage the Injured Area

- Assess distal pulses, capillary refill time, skin color, and temperature.
- Check for motor and sensory function distal to the wound.
- Splint fractures.
- Remove rings and other constrictive clothing or objects.
- Notify the physician immediately if an open fracture is present. An open fracture is defined as any skin disruption near the site of a fracture. Wounds associated with open fractures require irrigation, and the patient should receive intravenous antibiotics as soon as possible. Surgical wound débridement may be required.

Manage the Wound

- Remove current dressings.
- Obtain radiographs if a fracture or foreign body is suspected.
- Immediately notify the physician of any wounds with copious or pulsatile bleeding.

- Remove visible foreign matter.
- According to institutional protocol, perform or assist with the following:
  - Flush abrasions and wounds containing obvious debris.
  - Irrigate puncture wounds and lacerations.
  - Explore the wound for foreign bodies and injury to underlying structures.
  - Debride devitalized tissue.
  - Approximate the wound edges or bandage the wound, if closure is not appropriate.
  - Notify public health authorities of reportable conditions (e.g., dog bites and gunshot wounds). Refer to local guidelines for mandatory reporting requirements.
  - Collect and preserve forensic evidence from gunshot or stab wounds.[1]

WOUND ASSESSMENT

The ultimate size of a scar is determined by the degree of tension on wound margins at the time of approximation. The lower the tension, the smaller the scar. Scar size and wound tension can be predicted by the extent of wound gaping. Wounds that gape more than 5 mm will heal with a wide scar. Ironically, jagged wounds actually cause less scarring than do linear lacerations (as long as the edges can be approximated) because tension is distributed over a wider perimeter. This reduces stress on the margins, causing less scar formation. Therefore jagged edges should not be trimmed unless they are devitalized or contaminated.

Foreign Bodies

Evaluate all wounds for the presence of foreign bodies. Glass and metal objects are identified easily with plain radiographs. Matter with a density similar to that of soft tissue (e.g., wood splinters, thorns, cactus spines, and pieces of plastic) are not found so easily. Ultrasound, computed tomography, and magnetic resonance imaging can be used to locate these objects.[3]

WOUND PREPARATION

Thorough cleansing is crucial for optimal healing and infection prevention. Surface cleaning is the initial step in wound preparation. Issues to be considered include cleanser selection, hair removal, and wound irrigation.

Skin Antisepsis

Bacteria on the outer layer of dead skin quickly migrates into a wound. Fortunately, surface bacteria can be destroyed with chlorhexidine (Hibiclens) or a povidone-iodine (Betadine) solution. Importantly, chlorhexidine and 10% (usual strength) povidone-iodine impair wound defenses, damage delicate tissues, and delay healing. Use these solutions to clean intact skin around wounds, but avoid spilling them into the wound itself. A dilute (1%) povidone-iodine solution is not toxic to tissues and is as effective as a 10% solution at killing *Staphylococcus aureus*. Hydrogen peroxide damages tissues by hemolyzing erythrocytes, occluding local microvasculature, and releasing gas that causes crepitus and tissue distortion. As a rule of thumb, never put any substance in a wound that you would not put in an eye.

Hair Removal

Wounds in hairy areas heal best without hair in the approximated edges. Unfortunately, shaving abrades the skin, increases wound infection rates, and is cosmetically irritating. Snip hair with scissors or trim it with an electric clipper if removal is necessary. Moving hair out of the way and plastering it down with a lubricant (e.g., petroleum jelly), a topical ointment, or tape is generally preferable to removal. One area that should never be shaved is the eyebrow. The eyebrows provide important landmarks for approximating wound margins and, once shaved, may fail to grow back.[4]

Mechanical Irrigation

Irrigation remains the most effective (and sometimes the only) way to decrease the occurrence of wound infection. Infection will occur when (1) wound edges contain more than 10^6 bacteria per gram of tissue, (2) a foreign body is retained, or (3) the wound contains certain types of soil. Clay, commonly found in wounds associated with industrial or farming accidents, contains charged particles that inhibit the action of antibiotics and interfere with leukocyte activity. Mechanical removal of bacteria is also essential in wounds caused by bites and in those with fecal contamination. Fecal matter and the gingival crevices of the teeth harbor concentrations of bacteria up to 10^{11} per gram.

Sand, dirt, and other large particles can be removed by low-pressure irrigation with a bulb syringe. However, small particles such as clay and bacteria require higher-pressure irrigation. Forcing fluid through a narrow catheter or needle (e.g., a 19-gauge needle on a 12- or 35-mL syringe) provides an irrigation pressure of 5 to 8 psi. A disposable irrigation assembly—consisting of a 19-gauge catheter on a 35-mL syringe that attaches to intravenous tubing—is available commercially. Through this, a sterile isotonic solution can be injected easily via a one-way valve on the syringe barrel.[5]

Regardless of the solution or type of irrigation apparatus, place the needle perpendicular to the wound (as close as possible to the surface) and forcefully depress the syringe plunger. Use protective equipment to guard against fluid splatter to the face and eyes and prevent blood-borne pathogen exposure. Splash guards can be attached between the syringe and the catheter to decrease splatter, but they are not a substitute for personal protective equipment.[1]

Mechanical Cleansing

Scrubbing with a saline-soaked gauze has been shown to prolong the effective period of antibiotics, presumably by removing bacteria. Avoid using coarse, bristle-laden brushes that will injure tissue. When combined with a nonionic surfactant (Shur-Clens), a fine-pore sponge is the best way to clean a wound and minimize tissue damage. Chlorhexidine (Hibiclens) and povidone-iodine (Betadine) surgical scrub solutions should never be used. Any solution that causes significant pain when applied to an open wound will also damage tissue defenses, increasing the likelihood of infection.

TETANUS IMMUNIZATION

Tetanus is caused by *Clostridium tetani,* a gram-positive anaerobic bacillus. Because *C. tetani* forms spores, this organism is highly resistant to measures taken against it. *Clostridium tetani* is present in soil and in garden moss, on farms, and anywhere animal and human excreta can be found. The bacteria enter the circulation through an open wound and attach to cells within the central nervous system. The usual incubation period is 2 days to 2 weeks.

However, spores can lie dormant in tissue for years, so scrupulous wound cleansing is crucial. As long as immunizations are current, tetanus is a 100% avoidable condition. Postexposure immunizations should be given only when needed. Individuals can become sensitized by frequent vaccination, and subsequent injections can cause several days of painful swelling. This type of reaction is the usual source of "tetanus allergy" reported by some patients. Recommendations for tetanus immunization are based on current guidelines from the Centers for Disease Control and Prevention. The Centers for Disease Control advise that the tetanus vaccine also should contain diphtheria toxin. This combination, dT(Td), is given as a single 0.5-mL intramuscular dose.[5]

- The tetanus vaccine is given routinely with diphtheria and pertussis vaccines to children aged 2 months, 4 months, 6 months, 18 months, 4 to 6 years, and again as a booster at 16 years.
- A fully immunized individual is one who has had an initial tetanus series and a revaccination within the past 10 years.
- If a patient's immunization status is not clear or not immediately known, the injection can be given up to 72 hours after the wound occurred.
- Patients with a tetanus-prone wound should receive dT(Td) unless a booster has been given within the last 5 years. Tetanus-prone wounds are those that are infected, result from human or animal bites, are greater than 6 hours old, are puncture wounds, or were caused by a crush mechanism.
- Patients without previous vaccinations (or only one of the series) should begin the immunization regimen with 0.5 mL of dT(Td) in the ED. If the wound is tetanus-prone, simultaneous administration of tetanus antitoxin, 250 units intramuscularly, is recommended.
- Patients with partial immunity, from two or more previous tetanus injections, are considered sufficiently immune. The Centers for Disease Control recommend a booster of 0.5 mL dT(Td), even for patients with tetanus-prone wounds.
- Patients over the age of 6 years, who have not completed an initial immunization series, should be referred to their primary care provider or local health department for a second dT(Td) dose (0.05 mL intramuscularly) in 4 to 6 weeks and a third injection in 6 to 12 months.[4,5]

PROPHYLACTIC ANTIBIOTICS

Simple open wounds, less than 8 hours old, rarely become infected with or without antibiotic prophylaxis. Given this low incidence, prophylactic antibiotics generally are not recommended. Antibiotics should always be considered an adjunct to debridement and irrigation rather than a substitute.[4] The selection of a prophylactic antibiotic depends on many factors, including (1) the location of the wound, (2) the type of pathogens usually encountered with a particular injury, and (3) the fact that most contaminated wounds contain a wide variety of organisms. Little evidence exists to support the routine application of topical antibiotics on simple wounds.[1]

ANESTHESIA

Routes of anesthesia administration for wound closure include (1) topical, (2) wound infiltration, (3) regional blocks, and (4) intravenous procedural (conscious, moderate) sedation. The method(s) selected depend on the patient, the wound, and its location.

Anesthetic Agents

The most common anesthetic for local infiltration or regional use is lidocaine, primarily because of its low tissue toxicity. Another advantage of lidocaine is its short duration of action. This short duration is desirable for repairs of areas such as the mouth or lip, where recovery of sensation reduces the incidence of accidental biting of the wound. Likewise, prompt return of sensation to a finger prevents further injury as the patient begins to use the hand. One disadvantage of lidocaine is the pain associated with injection. Warming the solution to 37° C (98.6° F) can minimize this effect. Sodium bicarbonate also reduces the pain associated with lidocaine injection. Buffer lidocaine by adding 1 part 8.4% sodium bicarbonate (1 mEq/mL) to 10 parts 1% lidocaine (i.e., add 1 mL of sodium bicarbonate to 10 mL of lidocaine. (NOTE: This mixture reduces the shelf-life of lidocaine from 3 years to a few days, after which the solution will precipitate in the bottle.[5])

Preparations of lidocaine with epinephrine are also available. Epinephrine increases the duration of anesthesia and decreases bleeding. Use of this combination is contraindicated in heavily contaminated wounds or those with a tentative blood supply such as avulsions. Adverse effects of epinephrine include an increased rate of infection and ischemia when lidocaine with epinephrine is injected into the ear, tip of the nose, digits, or penis.

Another anesthetic agent used for infiltration is bupivacaine (Marcaine, Sensorcaine). The effects of this drug last 4 times longer than lidocaine. This makes bupivacaine ideal for situations in which wound closure will require longer than 2 hours or when prolonged anesthesia is desirable.

Anesthetic Allergy

Patients frequently report an allergy to lidocaine; however, true allergy to injected anesthetics is uncommon.[5] Many reported allergies are actually adverse reactions such as hyperventilation, vasovagal syncope or lightheadedness, cardiovascular stimulation from epinephrine, and various idiosyncratic reactions to the injury and subsequent wound repair. Contact dermatitis, caused by topical local anesthetics, also has been reported. This type of reaction is not immunoglobulin E–mediated and poses little risk. If a true allergy is suspected, an anesthetic from a different chemical class can be used. Sterile saline infiltration, guided imagery, and hypnosis are nonpharmacologic options. If local anesthesia is not possible, needleless wound closure techniques such as tying hair on the scalp or applying adhesive closure strips (e.g., Steri-Strips) should be considered.

Infiltration Anesthesia

Direct injection of an anesthetic agent into the wound is the most common anesthesic technique used in the ED. Infiltration of lidocaine along wound edges anesthetizes subcutaneous nerves. Some authorities recommend injecting through intact, antiseptically cleansed skin at the periphery of the wound to prevent spread of contamination. However, injecting through the edge of the wound is less painful. Several ways are available to reduce discomfort from anesthetic infiltration:

- Use the thinnest possible needle; 30 gauge or smaller works best.
- Minimize the number of skin punctures; a longer needle, inserted to the hub, can cover most of the edge of a wound.
- Perform subsequent needlesticks through already anesthetized skin.
- Inject into the subdermal area rather than into the dermis; raising a wheal is painful.
- Anesthetic agents injected slowly (over 10 seconds) are more comfortable than those injected quickly (less than 2 seconds).

Digital Block

Digital blocks can be used when the nerve supply to the wound is superficial. This technique is particularly superior to infiltration anesthesia in regions where the skin is sensitive, especially the digits, palms, soles, and face. Another advantage of digital or other regional nerve blocks is that they do not distort the wound or interfere with approximation.

Topical Anesthesia

Topical anesthetics eliminate the pain associated with injection, prevent tissue swelling, and cause vasoconstriction, which limits bleeding. TAC (0.5% tetracaine, 0.5% epinephrine [adrenalin], and 11.8% cocaine), the traditional topical anesthetic agent, has been replaced by newer combinations such as LET (4% lidocaine, 0.1% epinephrine, and 0.5% tetracaine). Another name for LET is XAP (xylocaine-adrenalin-pontacaine). The solution is applied topically 20 minutes before wound repair and is left until the skin blanches around the application site. Absence of blanching indicates incomplete anesthesia. TAC has fallen out of favor for several reasons. Toxic reactions, such as methemoglobinemia, have been reported when the solution was applied to mucous membranes. Because TAC produces vasoconstriction, it may cause ischemia when used on the ear, nose, digits, or penis. Most important, use of TAC is associated with a higher incidence of wound infections and necrosis of wound margins. Because of the cocaine in TAC, the solution is relatively expensive; it requires on-site preparation and must be handled as a controlled substance.

Topical anesthesia also can be achieved by applying a mixture of 5% lidocaine and prilocaine (EMLA) for 60 minutes. However, EMLA cream is designed for use on intact skin. Use on lacerations is not recommended because it causes inflammation, which increases infection rates.

Procedural Sedation

Procedural ("conscious" or "moderate") sedation is a medically controlled state in which consciousness is depressed, but the patient still can maintain an airway and respond to commands; protective reflexes remain intact. Procedural sedation can be used to facilitate wound care and anxiety management in pediatric and adult patients who are unable to cooperate because of underlying physical, emotional, or developmental challenges. Procedural sedation commonly is used for reduction of fractures and dislocations but is also a valuable adjunct when extensive cleansing, irrigation, and wound debridement are required. See Chapter 14 for further information on procedural sedation.

SPECIFIC WOUNDS AND ASSOCIATED CARE

Basic wound types include abrasions, abscesses, avulsions, contusions, incisions, lacerations, and punctures. Although each wound is distinct and warrants different treatment, it is important to remember that any number of wound types may occur simultaneously in the same patient. Additional considerations related to specific wounds include their size, location, and cause. Bites from animals and human beings cause a constellation of injuries commonly involving a combination of contusions, crush injuries, puncture wounds, and lacerations. For the purpose of this discussion, bites are addressed as a separate entity.

Abrasions

Rubbing skin against a hard surface removes the epithelium and exposes the dermis or subcutaneous layer. The resulting abrasion, or friction burn, initially may appear yellow, white, pink, or bloody depending on the tissue exposed. Abrasions can be superficial or can involve multiple skin layers. Embedded foreign bodies, such as gravel or asphalt, may cause permanent tattooing if not removed. Abrasions have the same physiologic effect as a second-degree burn. Large abrasions—and their associated disruption of protective outer skin layers—may precipitate significant fluid loss and hypothermia because of evaporation.[2]

Therapeutic interventions

Therapeutic interventions include the following:
- Provide pain control through the use of topical anesthetics or parenteral pain medication before cleaning, particularly when wounds are extensive or contain a large amount of embedded foreign material.
- Cleanse the wound with irrigation and gentle scrubbing.
- Remove all foreign material.
- Apply an antibiotic ointment and a sterile dressing.

Abscesses

An abscess forms when pus does not drain through the skin. The underlying infection may arise from inoculation by an insect bite or sting, a puncture wound, an infected hair follicle, or any injury that has closed without proper drainage. An abscess typically is recognized when it enlarges sufficiently to distend the skin and produce pain. Underlying pus causes the skin to become tense and discolored. When pus makes the skin tent, the abscess is said to "point" and is ready to be drained. Abscesses that point eventually will drain spontaneously. However, these wounds are treated optimally before this time. Therapeutic draining in the ED decreases pain, allows wound packing, and helps prevent the development of cellulitis. Abscesses in the perirectal area are usually much deeper than they initially appear, and drainage may require general anesthesia. Antibiotic therapy is indicated for patients with concurrent cellulitis, immunosuppression, endocarditis, or a facial abscess that is draining into the sinuses.[2]

Therapeutic interventions

Therapeutic interventions include the following:
- Premedicate the patient with analgesics; use procedural sedation for patients experiencing severe discomfort.
- A local anesthetic is injected around the abscess to dull pain.
- A scalpel is used to make an incision in the tense, overlying skin to drain a pointing abscess. Needle drainage will not adequately prevent rapid abscess recurrence. Pus initially is allowed to drain spontaneously; any remaining pus is expressed by pressing on the wound edges.
- The abscess cavity is packed with iodinated (Betadine) gauze to prevent premature closure of the skin and to facilitate further pus drainage. Packing should be inserted snugly against the walls of the abscess cavity. This process is inherently uncomfortable, but adequate drainage and packing are required to prevent recurrence. Packing gauze usually is changed in 1 to 2 days.

Avulsions

An avulsion involves peeling of the skin from underlying tissues. Peeling compromises blood supply to the site and can lead to further tissue devitalization. Avulsions are described as

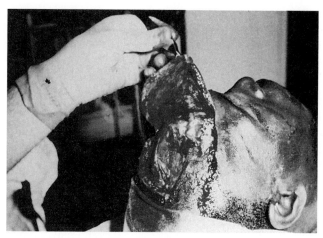

Figure 12-1. Degloving injury of the scalp. (From Newberry L, editor: *Sheehy's emergency nursing: principles and practice,* ed 5, St Louis, 2003, Mosby.)

proximal-based or distal-based. Proximal-based avulsions in general have better circulation. Nonetheless, wound edges may look gray or dusky, indicating the tenuous nature of the blood supply. An avulsion injury is called a degloving injury when skin is separated completely from underlying tissue (Figure 12-1). Degloving injuries typically involve the hand or foot. However, scalp-degloving incidents can occur.[2]

Therapeutic interventions

Therapeutic interventions include the following:
- Clean, irrigate, and debride the wound of devitalized tissue.
- Avoid lidocaine with epinephrine because its vasoconstrictive properties can further compromise blood supply to the avulsed fragment.
- Sometimes, avulsed skin that is crinkled or folded can be extended to cover the entire wound and then can be sutured into place (unless contraindicated by wound age, contamination, or other factors).
- Even skin that appears gray or dusky may heal surprisingly well. Such skin edges should be approximated, not trimmed. If necessary, the edges can be debrided the following day.
- Avulsions are common in patients with thin skin caused by age or long-term corticosteroid therapy. In such cases the skin may be too thin to suture; approximate wound edges with adhesive strips. In patients with extremely thin skin, even these strips can cause tearing. An occlusive dressing such as Tegaderm can be used to hold avulsed tissue in place.

Contusions

Contusions (bruises, hematomas) occur when blunt trauma causes extravasation of blood into subcutaneous tissue. When viewed through the skin, such blood classically looks black and blue. After about 2 days, breakdown of blood pigments changes the color to yellow. Although most contusions are minor and resolve with little or no treatment, large hematomas are painful and can cause tissue swelling in fascial compartments.[2] Continued subfascial swelling will lead to compartment syndrome because fascia does not stretch well enough to accommodate the increase in volume. Rising pressure within a muscle compartment compromises blood supply to nerves and other tissues. See Chapter 39 for discussion of this limb-threatening condition.

Therapeutic interventions

Therapeutic interventions include the following:
- Provide ice, elevation, and systemic analgesia with nonsteroidal, antiinflammatory agents. Stronger analgesia with narcotics may be required for some patients.
- No dressing is necessary.

Subungual Hematoma

In this condition, a direct blow to the fingertip ruptures vessels and blood collects below the nail (Figure 12-2). The resulting hematoma makes the nail appear black or blue. The patient experiences significant pain as pressure builds in the subungual region. A widespread hematoma can lift the entire nail off of its bed. This actually provides significant pain relief because pressure is substantially reduced.[4]

Subungual hematomas are treated as follows:
- Initial treatment involves ice, elevation, and analgesia to minimize the painful throbbing.
- Obtain a radiograph of the digit to rule out a tuft fracture of the distal phalanx.
- If the nail is intact, a hole is drilled through it directly over the hematoma. The nail itself has no nerve endings, so no anesthesia is required. A small battery powered electrocautery can be used to drill through the nail or the nail can be trephined slowly away with a scalpel (Figure 12-3).
- If the nail is loose, it may be removed entirely.

Incisions and Lacerations

Incisions are produced when tissue is sliced with a sharp object, whether it is a scalpel, a kitchen knife, a metal edge, or a piece of glass. In contrast, a laceration results when blunt

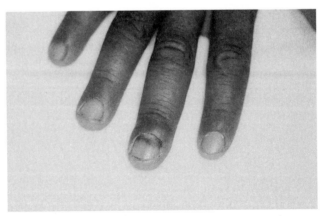

Figure 12-2. This 25% subungual hematoma is enough to cause intense pain and pressure. (Courtesy James R. Roberts, MD.)

trauma causes tissue tearing or crushing. Theses wounds may penetrate only the top layer of skin or can extend well beyond the dermis into deeper structures. Incisions are relatively resistant to infection, and the margins usually can be reapproximated. Lacerations can be linear (Figure 12-4) or stellate, with jagged or smooth edges.

Therapeutic interventions

Therapeutic interventions include the following:
- Determine the age of wound.
- Anesthetize the wound.
- Cleanse the wound using gentle scrubbing and irrigation.
- Explore the wound for bone exposure and damage to underlying structures.
- Remove any foreign bodies.
- Excise necrotic tissue.
- Approximate the wound edges.
- Apply a sterile dressing.

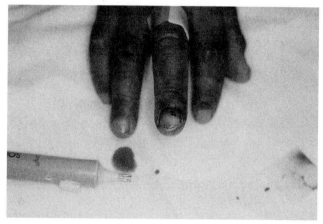

Figure 12-3. Pressure was relieved by repeated application of electrocautery filament to bore a hole down to the trapped blood. (Courtesy James R. Roberts, MD.)

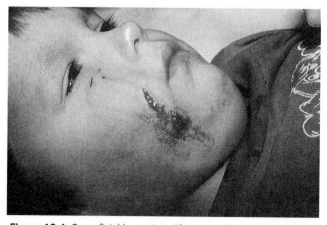

Figure 12-4. Superficial laceration. (Courtesy Thomas Lintner, MD.)

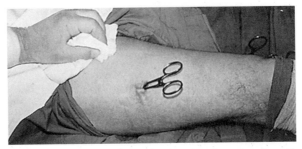

Figure 12-5. An accidental stab wound of the thigh. (From Newberry L, editor: *Sheehy's emergency nursing: principles and practice*, ed 5, St Louis, 2003, Mosby.)

Punctures

A puncture occurs when a sharp object penetrates the skin (Figure 12-5). A depth that is greater than the diameter of the entry hole characterizes these wounds. Because the ability to explore a puncture is limited, a high index of suspicion is needed to predict associated injury. Missiles can cause extensive tissue damage, whereas puncture wounds from nails, glass, pins, and other foreign bodies tend to move vessels and nerves aside, rather than sever the structures. Punctures can introduce bacteria deep into wounds that are inherently difficult to clean and tend to close early.[5]

Evaluate puncture wounds for the presence of foreign bodies. Determine what caused the puncture, and investigate whether a foreign body (or some portion of it) may still remain in the wound. Ask the patient or the person who removed the object whether it appeared to be intact. Inspect the wound for contaminants such as clothing, rust, or dirt.[3]

Punctures into joint spaces can lead to septic arthritis; punctures into cartilage, bone, and periosteum are associated with osteomyelitis. Such wounds warrant exploration in the operating room. Radiographic evaluation is recommended for any puncture wound near a bone or joint. Specific types of punctures that merit separate discussion are bites, gunshot wounds, punctures of the plantar area of the foot, and high-pressure injuries.

Therapeutic interventions

Therapeutic interventions include the following:
- Obtain a plain radiograph of all infected puncture wounds and those with a possible retained foreign body.
- Inspect the entrance site and explore the wound for obvious contaminants.
- Irrigate and clean uncomplicated, uncontaminated puncture wounds that are less than 6 hours old.
- Routine use of prophylactic antibiotics is not recommended for uncomplicated puncture wounds in healthy individuals. Use actually can predispose a patient to a secondary infection with *Pseudomonas*. Prophylactic antibiotics, such as first-generation cephalosporins (e.g., Ancef or Kefzol), are recommended for contaminated puncture wounds, wounds on the plantar area of the foot, or in patients with immunocompromising conditions such as diabetes mellitus, peripheral vascular disease, or systemic immunodeficiency.[5]
- All puncture wounds are considered tetanus-prone and require prophylactic vaccination in inadequately immunized individuals.
- Observe for complications such as cellulitis, abscess formation, joint infection, or osteomyelitis.

Plantar puncture wounds

Wounds over the metatarsal-phalangeal joints require special attention because the injury is usually caused by deep penetration as a result of weight bearing on a sharp object. Penetration to bone is frequent. Such penetration may lead to osteomyelitis in adults or osteochondritis in children. Suspect these conditions when a patient reports pain 4 to 7 days after injury and the wound is red or swollen. *Pseudomonas aeruginosa* has been cultured from the inner soles of tennis shoes and sneakers. Wound inoculation with *Pseudomonas* occurs when a sharp object penetrates the shoe, sole, and skin and contacts bone or cartilage. About half the time, an infected plantar puncture wound contains a foreign body—usually a piece of fabric. For this reason, careful inspection of any puncture wound is essential. Antibiotic prophylaxis is recommended for contaminated puncture wounds.[5]

Gunshot wounds

In contrast to other punctures, gunshot wounds cause extensive damage to underlying tissues and organs. The amount of damage has no relationship to the size of the entrance or exit wounds. Bullets can shatter bone and cause further injury as bone fragments become secondary projectiles. A gunshot wound forms a negative pressure cavity that can pull overlying clothing and debris into the wound in the wake of the bullet. Bullets from rifles have a higher velocity than those from handguns and are associated with greater tissue damage. High-velocity/high-energy missiles cause shock waves to travel through the tissues, shearing and crushing nerves, vessels, muscles, and organs several centimeters (or more) from the actual missile path. At close range, shotgun wounds can embed wadding and other debris (as well as pellets) in the tissues. Notify law enforcement agencies according to local reporting requirements[6]:

- Document the exact location of the wound(s). Photographs and diagrams can be helpful.
- Record the number of wounds. Note that distinguishing entrance from exit wounds is an important forensic task but does not affect how the wounds are managed.
- Place paper bags over the patient's hands to protect evidence such as gunpowder residue.
- Cut around (not through) bullet holes, powder marks, and other possible evidence when removing clothing. (Not all jurisdictions encourage this practice.)
- Place clothing in a paper bag and give it to the police. Some agencies accept clothing in plastic bags, so consult local authorities to determine the procedure in your geographic area.[6]

High-pressure injuries

Paint guns and grease guns are designed to inject these substances into hard to reach places. When forced against the skin, such guns inject paint or grease for several centimeters, typically following tissue planes. In the volar aspect of the hand, paint or grease can travel down tendon sheaths and along the digits. These wounds are serious, and immediate surgical intervention is required to drain the paint or oil and to preserve tissue.[4]

Bites

All bites from human beings or animals introduce bacteria into the wound, which predisposes it to infection. These wounds are considered tetanus prone. Patients may require prophylaxis for viral infections such as hepatitis or rabies, as well. Most clinicians elect to immediately close bites of the face but not those on the hand. Hand wounds are closed after 3 to 5 days or are packed and left open. Bites to the torso, arms, and legs are managed in a variety of ways to minimize infection and scarring. All puncture wounds from bites are closed by secondary intention. Dog and cat bites are addressed specifically in the following sections, but other domestic pets, livestock, birds, and wild animals also bite.

In cases of bites, do the following:

- Document the circumstances surrounding the bite; the source of the bite; signs of infection; number of bites; and the wound type, location, and depth.
- Assess for damage to underlying bone, muscle, tendons, and nerves.
- Irrigate and débride wounds to minimize bacterial contamination.[7]

Dog bites

Dog bites are grouped roughly into two categories: those that are provoked and those that are not. Provoked bites are incurred while petting, teasing, or reaching for the dog or entering the animal's territory. Unprovoked attacks occur without warning or provocation and are more likely to be associated with rabies. Actual tissue damage from a dog bite depends on the size and general state of the animal. The wound may consist of multiple punctures, caused by the animal's teeth, or major tissue loss (avulsion) can result if flesh is torn away from underlying structures. Significant crush injuries occur if the animal bites down on a limb.

The dog bite infection rate for patients not receiving antibiotics is 6% to 16%.[5] The most common pathogens in the animal's saliva include *S. aureus* and *Pasteurella multocida*.[2] Prophylaxis with amoxicillin/clavulanate potassium (Augmentin) is recommended.

If evidence of infection is present, culture the wound and begin antibiotic therapy. Progressive infection and sepsis warrant intravenous antibiotics, hospital admission, and (in some cases) operative debridement.

Cat bites

Cats have long, slender fangs that cause puncture wounds rather than lacerations. The major infecting organism is *P. multocida*. The patient has a rapidly progressive, painful swelling around the bite. The antibiotic of choice for these infections is penicillin. Prophylaxis with amoxicillin/clavulanate potassium (Augmentin) is recommended, especially for bites on the hand. Wounds are left open unless they are located on the face.[5]

Rabies prophylaxis

Rabies is introduced into bites from an infected animal. Theoretically, any mammal can be a carrier of rabies. Common carriers are bats, raccoons, foxes, and wild dogs. Herbivores, such as rodents, also can transmit the disease, although this is unlikely. Your local animal control office can provide information about rabies carriers in your area.

Bites from dogs that have been vaccinated, or from any animal that can be observed for 2 weeks, usually do not require rabies prophylaxis. If the animal dies within the 2-week observation period, the brain is autopsied to look for signs of rabies infection. This allows prompt prophylaxis for the victim if disease is detected.

Rabies has a minimum incubation period of 2 weeks in which the virus migrates along the nerves to the brain. Consequently, extremity bites have a longer incubation than face or head wounds. Rabies prophylaxis must be administered before symptoms begin. The disease is fatal in human beings.

Rabies prophylaxis is initiated routinely if a bat, wild animal, or a domestic animal that cannot be observed adequately caused the wound. Box 12-1 provides current guidelines for rabies prophylaxis.

Many states require that all animal bites be reported. Refer to local guidelines to determine requirements in your practice area.[7]

Box **12-1** Centers for Disease Control and Prevention Recommendations for Rabies Prophylaxis

---

Passive Immunity

Rabies immune globulin (RIG)
- 20 units/kg
- Give half the dose intramuscularly and inject the other half locally into the wound.
- Inject in the deltoid for adults and in the anterolateral thigh in children.

Active Immunity

Human diploid cell vaccine (HDCV)
- Give 1 mL intramuscularly on days 0, 3, 7, 14, 28.
- Give 1 mL intramuscularly only on days 0 and 3 if the patient had been immunized preexposure.

From Herman M, Newberry L: Wound management. In Newberry L, editor: *Sheehy's emergency nursing: principles and practice,* St Louis, 2003, Mosby.

WOUND CLOSURE

The goal of wound repair is rapid healing without infection. As a rule, healing occurs faster in wounds that are primarily closed with sutures, staples, tape, or cyanoacrylate glue. However, bites, other punctures, and contaminated wounds are so prone to infection that irrigation, debridement, and prophylactic antibiotic therapy take priority over closure.[8]

Open skin serves as a fresh culture medium for bacteria. From the moment of injury, wounds play host to increasing numbers of bacteria. Signs of infection can be seen within 8 hours in skin with poor blood supply resulting from crush injury, smoking, or simply a location distal to the heart. Wound closure prevents buildup of bacteria; therefore early closure is preferred. If the wound is more than 8 hours old, closure may not be wise even with adequate debridement or irrigation. After this time bacteria will spread more quickly in wounds that are closed than in those that are left open. The triage implication in these situations is that time matters. Every attempt should be made to close wounds as soon as possible.

The exception to the 8-hour rule is facial wounds. The face has such an effective blood supply that infection is less likely, and clean closure is more cosmetically desirable. Primary closure of wounds on the face may be attempted regardless of wound age.

Contaminated Wounds

Wounds that are contaminated may be obvious. However, contamination with liquids (such as water) is not always apparent. The potential for contamination should be considered in any open wound. Determination of contamination is based on historical evaluation and wound inspection. Establish whether the wounding implement was clean or grossly soiled. Common knife contaminants include meat, poultry, and dirt. A laceration over the knuckle that occurred when the fist struck a human mouth is always considered contaminated. Likewise, a retained foreign body may provide a nidus of infection. Fungal infections may occur in the presence of retained wood fragments. Wound irrigation, debridement, and foreign body removal are critical for healing to occur without infection.[8]

Wound Closure Materials

Options for wound closure include sutures, staples, tape, and adhesive bonding agents. The choice of material and technique depends on the preference of the care provider, the amount

Table 12-1   **Guidelines for Suture Removal**

Location	Time for Removal
Face, eyelid, lip	3 to 5 days
Eyebrow	4 to 5 days
Ear	4 to 6 days
Scalp	5 to 8 days
Back, chest, trunk, arm, hand, and thigh	7 to 10 days
Lower leg and foot	10 to 14 days

From Herman M, Newberry L: Wound management. In Newberry L, editor: *Sheehy's emergency nursing: principles and practice*, St Louis, 2003, Mosby.

of tension at the wound edges, the probability of infection, and the availability of closure materials.

Absorbable suture is degraded in the tissue and loses tensile strength within 60 days. Nonabsorbable suture retains its strength for 60 days but is nonetheless slowly absorbed over a period of months to years. Nonabsorbable sutures should be removed as soon as epithelialization occurs to minimize scaring caused by the suture itself. Epithelialization takes the shortest time in facial lacerations and the longest time in the legs and feet. Table 12-1 lists optimal times for suture removal by various body locations. Leave sutures in place longer in patients with delayed healing caused by debilitation or the use of medications such as corticosteroids. Because the wound does not regain full tensile strength for several weeks, apply tape strips across newly removed suture sites to reduce tension.[8]

Closure Techniques

Tape closure

Closure with a sterile, microporous tape (e.g., Steri-Strips) is appropriate for wounds with well-approximated edges in areas with minimal skin tension. Tape strips commonly are used for transverse lacerations over the brow, under the chin, or across the malar prominence of the cheek (Figure 12-6). This technique is not recommended for wounds that may become edematous. Taping avoids the pain of anesthesia and later suture removal. Tape adheres poorly to wet skin, but adherence can be increased by applying tincture of benzoin to the area around the wound.[8]

Suture

Suture is available in absorbable and nonabsorbable material. A synthetic monofilament, such as nylon, is associated with the fewest wound infections and can be used safely in all types of skin closures. Contrary to popular belief, nylon is absorbed, but usually over a period of a year or more. Therefore nylon is reserved for use on the skin where it can be removed as soon as the wound has healed sufficiently. A variety of stitches are used to close different skin lesions. The type of stitch is based on the wound size, depth, and site. Skin heals at different rates depending on body location and heals more slowly in patients with underlying conditions that retard repair.[5]

Staples

Stapling the skin (Figure 12-7) is faster than suturing and is associated with lower rates of tissue reactivity and wound infection. Unfortunately, stapling cannot align the wound margins

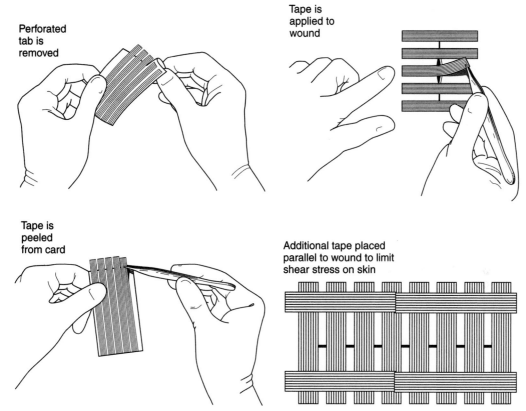

Figure 12-6. Tape closure. (From Newberry L, editor: *Sheehy's emergency nursing: principles and practice*, ed 5, St Louis, 2003, Mosby.)

as neatly as suturing because edges must be prepositioned and held in place while the staple is inserted. Invariably, the margins are slightly malpositioned. Therefore stapling is most appropriate in locations where scarring can be tolerated, such as on the scalp. Stapling does not provide the same degree of hemostasis that is possible with sutures.[2]

Wound glue

The latest approach to wound repair is adhesive bonding. One such wound glue is n-butyl cyanoacrylate monomer (Dermabond). Contact with an alkaline pH causes the glue to polymerize and form a thin, waterproof bandage. This requires 1 second on moist skin and several seconds on dry skin. Adhesive bonding is most effective on wounds that have little tension.[8]

Wound Dressing and Aftercare

Wound dressing and aftercare procedures are as follows:
- Dressings are applied to wounds to absorb drainage, protect the site from contamination, and hold antibiotic ointments in place. The choice of dressing materials depends on the wound type and the purpose of the dressing. Bulky dressings are used to provide

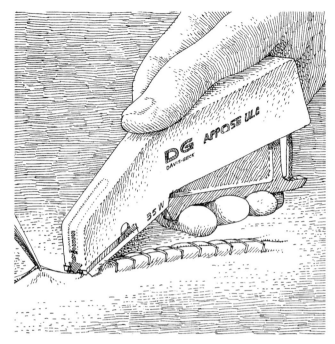

Figure 12-7. Application of skin staples. Staples are centered over incision line, using locating arrow or guideline, and placed approximately ¼ inch apart. (From Newberry L, editor: *Sheehy's emergency nursing: principles and practice*, ed 5, St Louis, 2003, Mosby.)

additional protection and can absorb the significant amount of drainage associated with some wounds in the initial phase of healing. Other wounds, particularly those on the face, may be left uncovered.

- Generally, a dry sterile dressing is applied for 2 days, unless the area is a gingival surface or is too hairy to accommodate a dressing.
- Wounds closed with tape have a lower risk of infection than those closed with suture. Do not put topical antibiotics on taped wounds.
- Patients may shower following wound closure without increasing the incidence of infection.

Provide aftercare instructions to the patient or to the patient's primary caregiver. In addition to the foregoing information, home care advice should incorporate the following:

- Essential wound care follow-up instructions, including the anticipated removal date for sutures or staples
- Any activity restrictions
- Signs of wound infection and indications of circulatory compromise
- Specific reasons to contact a primary care physician or return to the ED
- The need for sunscreen use for 6 months after injury (Abraded skin is sensitized, and hyperpigmentation can occur after sun exposure.)
- Elevation of an injured extremity to limit edema formation[5]

References

1. Lammers R: Principles of wound management. In Roberts J, Hedges J, editors: *Clinical procedures in emergency medicine,* ed 4, Philadelphia, 2004, Saunders.
2. Herman M, Newberry L: Wound management. In Newberry L, editor: *Sheehy's emergency nursing: principles and practice,* St Louis, 2003, Mosby.
3. Stone D, Koutouzis T: Foreign body removal. In Roberts J, Hedges J, editors: *Clinical procedures in emergency medicine,* ed 4, Philadelphia, 2004, Saunders.
4. Tintinalli J, Gabor D, Stapczynski J: *Emergency medicine: a comprehensive study guide,* ed 6, New York, 2004, McGraw-Hill.
5. Simon B, Hern H: Wound management principles. In Marx J, Hockenberger R, Walls R, editors: *Rosen's emergency medicine concepts and clinical practice,* ed 5, St Louis, 2002, Mosby.
6. Smock W: Forensic emergency medicine. In Marx J, Hockenberger R, Walls R, editors: *Rosen's emergency medicine concepts and clinical practice,* ed 5, St Louis, 2002, Mosby.
7. Schaider J et al. In Barkin R et al, editors: *Rosen and Barkin's 5-minute emergency medicine consult,* ed 2, Philadelphia, 2003, Lippincott Williams & Wilkins.
8. Lammers R, Trott A: Methods of wound closure. In Roberts J, Hedges J, editors: *Clinical procedures in emergency medicine,* ed 4, Philadelphia, 2004, Saunders.

13

Weapons of Mass Destruction

Jeff Hamilton, RN, BA

Terrorism and weapons of mass destruction (WMD) are a fact of life in today's world. Countries, states, cities, hospitals, and individuals must be alert to possible threats and must be prepared to deal with them. For emergency nurses to be knowledgeable and ready to handle what was once unthinkable is essential.

MINIMAL SKILLS AND KNOWLEDGE

The information available about WMD is emerging constantly and is changing rapidly. Nonetheless, a framework has been developed to address health care provider learning needs in this dynamic environment. The American College of Emergency Physicians, in collaboration with the Emergency Nurses Association and other organizations, has identified the following minimal level of skills and knowledge required to deal effectively with medical issues in the aftermath of an event caused by WMD.[1]

Recognize and Identify
- Recognize the signs of a terrorist attack; identify the most common types of attacks: nuclear, biological, chemical, radiation, and explosives.
- Identify detection devices that are available to warn of the presence of WMD.
- Understand and use surveillance systems.
- Identify biological attacks, as opposed to an emerging infectious disease.
- List actions to be performed by the hospital in response to notification of a disaster specifically regarding equipment, staffing, and pharmaceuticals.
- Identify how, and to whom a suspected terrorist event should be reported.

- Identify individual staff roles and responsibilities in responding to a terrorist event.
- Know how to use the incident command system to identify roles and responsibilities.
- Understand how the hospital incident command system integrates with the joint command system in the community.
- Be able to assess and communicate the needs of your department for information, supplies, and nourishment.
- Understand security needs related to large numbers of victims and relatives.

Decontaminate and Treat

- Describe the facilities and equipment needed for appropriate, effective decontamination specific to the incident site and type (if the agent is known).
- Track large numbers of persons.
- Use and apply the different triage methods used with WMD incidents, mass casualty incidents, and incidents where resources are limited.
- Perform effective assessment, stabilization, diagnosis, and treatment of victims of specific types of WMD events. This includes required familiarity with the following:
  - Symptoms and disease patterns that indicate exposure to various WMD
  - Appropriate pharmaceuticals and vaccinations
  - Clinical indicators
  - Diagnostic and laboratory testing
- Distinguish between the victims who require decontamination and those who do not.
- Demonstrate appropriate and effective decontamination procedures for all types of victims.
- Select and work effectively with personal protective equipment.
- Minimize contamination risks and preserve evidence.
- Identify the vaccinations and pharmaceuticals required for self-protection and preexposure and postexposure care.
- Identify the psychological and psychosocial effects experienced by WMD victims and health care providers, as well as appropriate interventions.
- Understand the challenges associated with massive numbers of fatalities, including appropriate, safe, and effective means of handling the deceased.
- Implement appropriate techniques for maintaining patient records and belongings.
- Describe the techniques for handling evidence and chain of custody during a WMD event.

WEAPONS OF MASS DESTRUCTION

Experts in the field of WMD have identified four major types of weapons: explosives, chemicals, biologics, and radiation/nuclear weapons.

Explosive Weapons

Most explosions are associated with relatively minor injuries and affect a minimal number of individuals. However, high-energy explosions can cause penetrating, blunt, blast, and thermal injuries to large numbers of victims simultaneously, with devastating consequences. Blast injuries can be divided into three phases: (1) primary, (2) secondary and (3) tertiary. *Primary blast injuries* are produced by sudden changes in atmospheric pressure generated by the blast wave itself. Structures at greatest risk are the air-filled internal organs. There is an increased risk of damage to the lungs during an explosive event, because they are air-filled organs. Pulmonary contusions and lacerations can lead to life-threatening conditions such as tension pneumothorax, bronchial disruption, myocardial infarction, or stroke caused by arterial air emboli. (See Chapters 37, 22, and 23 for further information about specific conditions.) *Secondary blast injuries* are a consequence of flying shrapnel that strikes the victim, causing blunt or penetrating trauma. *Tertiary blast injuries* result when victims are literally blown over or thrown against objects. Two other trauma mechanisms, thermal burns and crush injuries, also result from explosive events.[2]

Signs and symptoms

Signs and symptoms of blast injuries include the following:
- Rapid, shallow respirations
- Dyspnea: Difficulty completing sentences in one breath
- Tachypnea: Respiratory rate may be in excess of 30 breaths per minute
- Dry cough with or without wheezing
- Hemoptysis
- Diminished breath sounds

Therapeutic interventions

Therapeutic interventions for blast injuries include the following:
- Perform immediate needle thoracostomy to decompress a potential tension pneumothorax in victims with asymmetrically decreased breath sounds and evidence of shock.
- Assist with the management of massive hemoptysis, which is accomplished by blocking the mainstem bronchus of the involved lung with an endotracheal tube and unilaterally ventilating the opposite lung.[2]

Chemical Weapons

Toxic substances that can be used as WMD range from chemicals designed for legitimate industrial use to those whose only purpose is weapons. This latter class includes nerve, blister, choking (pulmonary), blood, and riot agents. The effects of exposure to these chemicals can be devastating. Victims will require immediate attention and decontamination. For information about antidotes, see Chapter 28.

Chemical weapons decontamination

Decontaminate every victim believed to have been exposed to any agent with a known secondary contamination risk. To carry out decontamination, staff members must be trained and clad in appropriate personal protective equipment at all times. Personal protective equipment is discussed in depth later in this chapter. To minimize the spread of toxic agents, establish three zones of contamination: (1) hot zone, (2) warm zone, and (3) cold zone.
- *Hot zone.* The hot zone is the area with the highest concentration of the toxic agent. In hospitals, this is usually the decontamination shower area.
- *Warm zone.* This area is adjacent to the hot zone/decontamination shower and is considered minimally contaminated.
- *Cold zone.* The cold zone refers to all hospital areas that are contamination free.

Decontamination procedures for ambulatory victims

Gross decontamination (strip and rinse)

Gross decontamination of ambulatory victims consists of the following steps:
- Brush off any visible dry material.
- Use diapers or paper towels to absorb blister agents. Do not use water; it spreads the agents.
- Remove the patient's clothing; 90% of decontamination can be accomplished simply by disrobing.
- Double-bag all clothing and place in a plastic-lined barrel.
- Place the patient's valuables in a plastic zipper bag, label the bag, and give it to the patient.
- Have the patient step into the decontamination shower area with the arms raised above the head, eyes and mouth closed, while rotating slowly at least twice. The water should be at room temperature and should be sprayed at a pressure of 60 to 90 psi.
- Instruct the victim to step out of the gross decontamination area into the technical (or secondary) decontamination site.

Technical (secondary) decontamination (rinse-wash-rinse)

Secondary decontamination consists of the following steps:
- Rinse the patient's head and face using a handheld sprayer and room-temperature water.
- Rinse all open wounds. Gently wash wounds with a decontamination solution consisting of 1 oz baby shampoo per 1 gallon of water. Rinse wounds again and cover with water-resistant material such as plastic wrap.
- Rinse all other body surfaces, including the axilla and perineal areas, from the neck to the feet.
- Using washcloths or a soft sponge, wash the patient with the decontamination solution and rinse again from head to toes.
- Dry the victim with towels. Have the patient don a clean gown and cover with a blanket. The patient may now enter the cold zone.
- If radiation or nuclear agents are present, radiation safety technicians (nuclear medicine staff) should perform a head-to-toe sweep with radiation detection equipment before the patient exits the decontamination area.
- Rinse-wash-rinse again if the radiation safety technician does not clear the victim. A second elevated reading, after two washes, suggests that the victim has absorbed, inhaled, or swallowed a radioactive substance. These individuals are not contagious and may exit the decontamination area.

Decontamination procedures for nonambulatory victims

Gross decontamination (strip and rinse)

Gross decontamination of nonambulatory victims consists of the following steps:
- Place the patient on a long board or plastic-covered cart. Industrial roller-type conveyor systems are ideal for moving large numbers of victims on backboards.
- Brush off any dry material.
- Use diapers or paper towels to absorb blister agents.
- Cut off clothing and discard into plastic-lined barrels.
- Place valuables in plastic zipper bags. Label the bag and keep it with the victim.

- Shower the patient with a handheld sprayer. Logroll the victim to spray all body surfaces.
- Move the victim to the technical (secondary) decontamination area.

Technical (secondary) decontamination (rinse-wash-rinse)

Secondary decontamination consists of the following steps:
- Using a handheld sprayer and room temperature water, rinse the victim's face starting in the midline and moving laterally.
- Rinse all open wounds; cover with a water resistant material such as plastic wrap.
- Using washcloths or soft sponges, wash all body surfaces (including the perineum and axilla) with the decontamination solution. Logroll the victim to reach all body surfaces and rinse from head to toe, front and back.
- Dry the victim thoroughly with towels, place the patient in a gown, and cover with a blanket.
- Radiation safety technicians will perform a body survey (as indicated). Repeat the technical (secondary) decontamination if the survey reading is greater than background levels.
- Transfer the victim from the original long board onto a clean long board outside the technical decontamination area. Scoop stretchers are ideal for this transfer.[3]

Biological Weapons

Biological weapon attacks are likely to be covert. Dissemination of a biological agent in a public place will not have an immediate impact because of the delay between exposure and onset of illness. Medical offices and hospital emergency departments are the most likely sites where health care providers will initially encounter victims. Public health department surveillance programs, integrated with reports from local emergency departments and clinics, are crucial for early detection of bioterrorism incidences.

The Centers for Disease Control and Prevention (CDC) categorize biological agents according to their potential for dissemination, their degree of lethality, and the public health response required to deal with large-scale events. Box 13-1 gives categorization details. The CDC also has established a list of biological agents that would have the greatest impact on public health and security. These agents, as well as important precautions and patient management information, are presented in Table 13-1.

Mass prophylaxis

Preventive vaccinations and postexposure prophylaxis are key elements in the management of a bioterrorism incident. Not only will the number of victims multiply, health care provider attrition also will be high if clinicians do not feel assured they are safe to practice.

Health care personnel can take the following steps for mass prophylaxis:
- In the event of a communicable disease outbreak, quickly establish a prophylactic program that includes immediate family members of health care workers.
- Coordinate prophylactic programs with the public health department.
- Develop a method that will notify all personnel rapidly when a mass prophylactic program has been initiated.
- Create appropriate signs and literature, as needed, to inform personnel of the risks and benefits of prophylaxis.
- Identify equipment, supplies, staff training, distribution sites, hours of operation, and barriers to prophylactic program implementation.
- Be prepared to reassign any personnel who decline prophylactic medications to nonpatient care areas.

Box **13-1** Biological Weapon Categories

Category A

Agents that can be disseminated or transmitted easily person to person
High mortality, with a potential for major public health disruption
May cause public panic and social disruption
Require special action for public health preparedness

Category B

More difficult to disseminate
Moderate morbidity and low mortality
Require special enhancement of public health surveillance and diagnostic capability

Category C

Emerging pathogens that could be engineered for mass dissemination
Potential for high morbidity and mortality

Modified from www.bt.cdc.gov/agent/agentlist-category.asp#catdef.

RADIATION AND NUCLEAR WEAPONS

Exposure to ionizing radiation can occur in a variety of scenarios—through accidental or intentional events—that range in extent from single-person incidents to large-scale disasters. Despite fears of nuclear holocaust from bombs or a nuclear reactor meltdown, historically most radiation exposures have been unintentional, involving only a modest number of patients. However, the possibility of a terrorist's "dirty bomb" (a conventional explosive device containing radioactive material) has underscored the need for nurses to become familiar with emergency management of radiation exposure. Table 13-2 (p. 222) describes the radionuclides produced from various radiation releases.

Types of Radiation

Ionizing radiation/nonionizing radiation

The term *radiation* encompasses a number of concepts, and it is important to remember that visible light, ultraviolet light, microwaves, ultrasound, and radio waves are forms of radiation. Although these nonionizing types of radiation can certainly do damage over time (e.g., skin cancer), radiation emergencies are related only to ionizing forms of radiation. Ionizing radiation is a high-frequency, low-amplitude form of radiation that interacts significantly with biological systems. Alpha, beta, and neutron particles and gamma and x-rays are forms of ionizing radiation.

Radiation particles versus waves

Additionally, radiation is emitted as particles or waves. This is an important concept for health care providers to understand because of the fact that particles stick to a patient (contaminating them), whereas waves do not. This explains why patients who have had an x-ray (wave radiation) are not radioactive, even following tremendous exposures.

Table 13-1   Bioterrorism Infection Control Practices for Patient Management

BIOTERRORISM
Infection Control Practices for Patient Management

Infection Control Practice	Anthrax	Brucellosis	Cholera	Glanders (rarely seen)	Bubonic Plague	Pneumonic Plague	Tularemia	Q Fever	Smallpox	Venezuelan Equine Encephalitis	Viral Encephalitis	Viral Hemorrhagic Fever	Botulism	Ricin	T-2 Mycotoxins	Staphylococcus Enterotoxin B
(group)	*BACTERIAL AGENTS*								*VIRUSES*				*BIOLOGICAL TOXINS*			
Isolation Precautions																
Standard precautions for all aspects of patient care	X	X	X	X	X	X	X	X	X	X	X	X	X	X	X	X
Contact precautions			X	X	X	X			X			X				
Airborne precautions									X							
Use of N-95 mask by all individuals entering the room						X			X							
Droplet precautions						X				X						
Wash hands with antimicrobial soap		X	X	X					X	X		X				
Patient Placement																
No restrictions	X	X					X	X					X	X	X	X
Group "like" patients when private room unavailable			X	X	X	X			X							
Private room						X			X	X	X	X				
Negative pressure									X							
Door closed at all times									X							
Patient Transport																
No restrictions	X	X					X	X					X	X	X	X
Limit movement to essential medical purposes only			X	X	X	X			X	X	X	X				
Place mask on patient to minimize dispersal of droplets						X			X							
Cleaning, Disinfection of Equipment																
Routine terminal cleaning of room with hospital-approved disinfectant upon discharge	X	X	X	X	X	X	X	X	X	X	X	X	X	X	X	X

	C1	C2	C3	C4	C5	C6	C7	C8
Disinfect surfaces with bleach/water solution 1:10 (10% solution)	X	X		X	X		X	X
Dedicated equipment disinfected before leaving room		X			X		X	X
Linen management as with all other patients	X	X	X	X	X	X	X	X
Routine medical waste handled per internal policy	X	X	X	X	X	X	X	X
Discharge Management								
No special discharge instruction necessary	X	X	X	X	X		X	X
Home care providers should be taught principles of standard precautions	X	X	X	X	X	X	X	X
Patient not discharged from hospital until determined to be no longer infectious			X		X			X
Patient generally not discharged until 72 hours of antibiotic therapy completed			X					X
Postmortem Care								
Follow principles of standard precautions	X	X	X	X	X	X	X	X
Droplet precautions		X						X
Airborne precautions					X			
Use of N-95 mask by all individuals entering the room					X			
Negative pressure					X			
Contact precautions					X			X
Routine terminal cleaning of room with hospital-approved disinfectant upon autopsy	X	X	X	X	X		X	X
Disinfect surfaces with bleach/water solution 1:10 (10% solution)	X		X	X	X		X	

From *Environment of Care Newsletter*, 2003, Joint Commission.
Developed by Suzanne E. Johnson. Template courtesy of Walter Reed Army Medical Center.
Standard precautions prevent direct contact with all body fluids (including blood), secretions, excretions, nonintact skin (including rashes), and mucous membranes. Standard precautions routinely practiced by health care providers include hand washing, use of gloves, use of mask/eye protection/face shield while performing procedures that cause splash/spray, and use of gowns to protect skin and clothing during procedures.

Radiation emergencies

Three forms of radiation are most likely to be involved in an emergency:
1. *Alpha particles.* Alpha particles are heavy, highly charged particles that travel at a low velocity and are readily stopped by matter. Because of their large mass, alpha particles have poor skin penetration, and their energy dissipates quickly. These particles pose little hazard after external exposure but can produce tissue injury when inhaled, ingested, or absorbed in wounds.
2. *Beta particles.* Beta particles have a smaller mass and greater velocity than alpha particles. They will penetrate about 8 mm into exposed skin and can cause serious burns. Like alpha particles, beta particles are also hazardous if internally deposited (through wounds, inhalation, or ingestion), but to a lesser extent.
3. *Gamma rays.* Gamma rays are a form of ionizing radiation that has no mass. Like visible light, gamma rays are waves made of photons. These photons can penetrate deeply while leaving no particles behind (no contamination). Exposure to a high-energy gamma source causes significant whole-body radiation and acute radiation syndrome. Gamma rays are the most devastating external radiation hazard after exposure.[3,4]

Radiation exposure initial interventions

When treating victims exposed to radiologic contaminants, emergency nurses must be aware of appropriate respiratory and skin protection, as well as how to care for patients with concurrent injuries.

Respiratory protection

N-95 masks provide sufficient protection for radiologic contaminates. However, under stressful conditions some wearers may experience breathing difficulties because of reduced airflow that occurs when wearing the mask.

Skin (barrier) protection

Normal barrier clothing and gloves provide excellent personal protection against airborne radioactive particles. If they are available, disposable medical scrub suits or high-density polyethylene coveralls (Tyvek) should be used for splash protection.

Table 13-2   Radionuclides Produced from a Radiation Release

Element	Source	Radiation	Respiratory Absorption	Gastrointestinal Absorption	Primary
Americium	NWD	Alpha	High	Minimal	Skeletal, liver, bone marrow suppression
Cesium	MF	Beta, gamma	Complete	Complete	Whole body
Cobalt	MF, FI	Beta, gamma	High	Minimal	Whole body
Iodine	NWD, NPP	Beta, gamma	High	High	Thyroid
Phosphorus	MF	Beta	High	High	Rapidly dividing cells
Plutonium	NW, NWD	Alpha, gamma	High	Minimal	Lung, bone, liver
Strontium	NWD	Beta, gamma	Limited	Moderate	Bone

FI, Food irradiation facility; *MF*, medical or research facility; *NPP*, nuclear power plant; *NW*, nuclear waste site; *NWD*, nuclear weapon detonation.

Care

Victims exposed to lethal doses of radiation are *not* a serious hazard to health care workers. Health care providers may care for patients with critical injuries safely before decontamination.[3]

Decontamination

Victims of particle (alpha or beta) radiation require decontamination; those subjected to wave radiation (e.g., gamma waves) do not. Ideally, all patients will be surveyed for the presence of contamination upon hospital arrival. However, if radiation meters are not readily available, proceed with decontamination. Use the same procedure described in the discussion of chemical weapons decontamination.

Rapid radiologic triage

Patients exposed to radiation can be triaged on the following basis:
- Time to vomiting less than 4 hours: Refer for immediate evaluation.
- Time to vomiting more than 4 hours: Refer for delayed evaluation if there are no concurrent injuries.
- Victims who experience radiation-induced emesis within 1 hour after a radiation incident require extensive and prolonged medical intervention. An ultimately fatal outcome is expected.
- The Armed Forces Radiobiology Research Institute has developed a Biodosimetry Assessment Tool. This software is designed to be used after a radiation incident.
  Box 13-2 defines various units of measure commonly used to describe radiation doses.

TRIAGING MASS CASUALTY INCIDENTS

Triage during a mass casualty incident must focus on "the greatest good for the greatest number." Switching to this triage philosophy requires a radical mental shift for nurses accustomed to treating the most critical victims first. Each emergency department needs to have clear,

---

Box **13-2** **Radiation Exposure: Units of Measure**

Current Units of Measure	
Becquerel (Bq)	The International System of Units (SI) measurement of radioactivity, defined as decay events per second. 1 Bq = 1 disintegration per second.
Gray (Gy)	The standard SI unit for the energy deposited by any type of radiation, in joules per kilogram. 1 Gy = 100 rad.
Sievert (Sv)	The SI unit for measurement of human exposure to radiation, in joules per kilogram. 1 Sv = 100 rem.
Outdated Units of Measure	
Curie (Ci)	The traditional measure of radioactivity, as measured by radioactive decay. 1 Ci = 3.7×10^{10} disintegrations per second.
Radiation absorbed dose (rad)	The energy deposited by any type of radiation to any type of tissue or material. Replaced by the term *Gray*. 1 rad = 0.01 Gy.
Roentgen equivalent man (rem)	The unit of human exposure to radiation. Replaced by the term *Sievert*. 1 rem = 0.01 Sv.

simple, disaster triage guidelines in place. The decision to switch to a mass casualty triage approach is driven by patient needs and the resources available to meet those needs. Consider the following when deciding whether to change triage modes:

- Total number of victims affected
- Anticipated victim injury severity level
- Expected number of victims who will be transported to your facility by emergency medical services
- Anticipated number of walk-in patients (Historically, 80% of victims self-refer to the closest facility.)
- Availability of specialized equipment such as monitors, ventilators, and operating rooms.
- Availability of decontamination equipment
- Availability of trained personnel who can decontaminate patients
- Availability of resources to transfer victims to other hospitals
- Availability of staffed inpatient beds

Triage Categories in Mass Casualty Incidents

Victims of mass casualty incidents can be triaged into five categories:

1. Victims exposed, but not symptomatic
2. Victims exposed and requiring minimal care
3. Victims exposed and considered salvageable; maximum medical care is required
4. Victims exposed and expected to die (establish minimal qualifications for survival as the event matures)
5. Deceased victims

Supportive Care Area/Expectant Care Area

In mass casualty situations, victims who are not expected to live are placed in a supportive care, or "expectant care" area. Although no life-sustaining measures are implemented, liberal administration of sedatives and analgesics is vital. Standing medication orders or protocols should be available. This area may be staffed by nurse practitioners. Importantly, the supportive care area is not the morgue; those who die should be transferred out.

PERSONAL PROTECTIVE EQUIPMENT

Adequate personal protective equipment (PPE) and training in its use are critical components of any plan for responding to a WMD incident. Staff members must be protected for their own safety, to decontaminate and treat victims, and to prevent further spread of noxious agents. PPE is also essential for dealing with the cleanup and aftermath once all the patients have gone. The following section discusses levels of personal protective equipment; Table 13-3 describes supplemental decontamination supplies.

Levels of Protection

Defining recommended levels of personal protective equipment is difficult and controversial because of minimal regulatory guidance and a lack of research directly applicable to health care facilities. However, general consensus suggests the following levels of protection for suspected WMD incidents involving chemical or radioactive agents:

Table **13-3**   **Supplemental Decontamination Supplies**

Equipment	Quantity
Large barrels for clothing	2
Large barrels for linen	2
Plastic barrel liners	100
Ziplock bags for personal articles	100
Indelible waterproof marking pens	10
Soft brushes (to remove particulate matter)	4
Paper towels	5 rolls
Baby diapers	50
Water resistant covering (e.g., plastic wrap)	50
Towels	100
Washcloths	100
Patient gowns	100
Cotton-tipped applicators	100
Baby shampoo	1 gallon
Bleach (undiluted)	2 gallons
Spray bottles filled with diluted bleach and water (1:10)	4
Old wheeled emergency department carts	4
Plastic covering for carts	4
Long boards	10

Minimum

- Don chemical protective suits with full face mask, air-purifying respirators, gloves, and boots.
- *Gloves:* Wear thin cotton gloves covered by nitrile gloves covered by chemical-resistant gloves (silver shield or 4H) when dealing directly with patients contaminated by chemical agents. Thin cotton gloves covered by nitrile gloves alone allow better dexterity and are usually adequate once patients have been through the initial decontamination process.
- *Suit/glove/boot sealing:* Use a chemical-resistant tape (duct tape is not acceptable) to seal the suit closure and tape all sites where the suit interfaces with gloves or boots.

Better

- A higher level of protection consists of hooded, powered air-purifying respirators, with a chemical protective suit, gloves, and boots.
- Air-filtering canisters (preferably an NTC-1 cartridge) incorporate high-efficiency particulate air filtration to protect against organic vapors, acid gases, and known military nerve agents.

Equipment Selection

Selection of suits (chemical protective clothing) should be based on the principles of permeation, penetration, and degradation.

Permeation refers to how long a suit will keep agents from passing through by means of passive diffusion. The longer the permeation time, the more effective the suit. However, the permeation rate is different for each chemical. A breakthrough time of greater than 480 minutes (8 hours) is considered ideal. Heat-sealed seams offer the highest level of protection and are mandatory for suits. These seams are first sewn and then sealed with heat-activated tape.

Penetration refers to how easy it is to rip the suit. Because hospital personnel are not at the scene digging through rubble, this is generally not a major consideration.

Degradation occurs from contact with chemicals or from aging. Signs of suit degradation include shrinking, swelling, brittleness, cracking, discoloration, and stickiness. To be effective when needed, suits must be inspected and replaced regularly.

MENTAL HEALTH ASPECTS OF TERRORISM

Whether experienced at the personal or community level, no one who witnesses a terrorist event or other major disaster is untouched. Although most persons are able to function during and after a disaster, varying levels of stress and grief are almost always present; these are normal responses to an abnormal situation. Although an incident may be long over, its effects live on, and patients will continue to present to the emergency department as a result of psychological reactions to the horror. Box 13-3 lists common emotional responses that follow exposure to disaster situations.

INTERACTING WITH DISASTER VICTIMS

The CDC's publication *Mental Health Aspects of Terrorism* has the following suggestions for interacting with survivors of terrorist events[5]:

Do say:

- These are normal reactions to a disaster.
- It is understandable that you feel this way.
- You are not going crazy.

Box **13-3** **Typical Emotional Reactions to Disasters**

Alcohol or drug use
Behavior problems
Confusion
Crying, whimpering, screaming
Depression
Disobedience
Excessive clinging
Fear of being left alone
Fear of crowds or strangers
Fear of darkness or animals
Fear and anxiety
Fighting
Irritability
Nightmares
Refusal to go to school or work
Reluctance to leave home
Sensitivity to loud noises
Insomnia or hypersomnolence

- It wasn't your fault; you did the best you could.
- Things may never be the same, but they will get better and you will feel better.

Don't say:

- It could have been worse.
- You can always get another pet/car/house.
- It's best if you just stay busy.
- I know just how you feel.
- You need to get on with your life.

Refer disaster victims for mental health evaluation when the following are present:
- Disorientation
- Mental illness
- Inability to care for self
- Suicidal or homicidal thoughts or plans
- Problematic use of alcohol or drugs
- Domestic violence, child abuse, or elder abuse

BIOTERRORISM RESOURCES ON THE INTERNET

Visit these websites for current information on all aspects of bioterrorism and emerging infectious diseases:
- Association for Professionals in Infection Control: *www.apic.org.*
- Centers for Disease Control and Prevention: *www.bt.cdc.gov.*
- University of Alabama—Birmingham: *www.bioterrorism.uab.edu.*
- Center for Bioterrorism and Emerging Infections at St. Louis University: *www.bioterrorism. slu.edu/.*

References

1. American College of Emergency Physicians–NBC Task Force, final report, April 2001. Retrieved 10/12/03, from www.acep.org.
2. Frykberg ER: Medical management of disasters and mass casualties from terrorist bombings: how can we cope, *J Trauma* 53(2):201-212, 2002.
3. Tintinalli J, Gabor D, Stapczynski J: *Emergency medicine: a comprehensive study guide,* ed 6, New York, 2004, McGraw-Hill.
4. American Academy of Pediatrics Committe on Environmental Health: Radiation disasters and children, *Pediatrics* 111(6 pt 1):1455-1466.
5. Centers for Disease Control and Prevention: Mental health aspects of terrorism. Retrieved 10/12/03, from www.mentalhealth.samhsa.gov/publications/allpubs/KEN-01-0095.

14

Pain Management

Anita Johnson, RN, BSN

Pain management in the emergency department (ED) has undergone progressive change over the past decade. Recognition, assessment, and treatment of pain in the emergency care setting continues to improve. An operational definition of pain that is useful in clinical practice is *"pain is whatever the person experiencing it says it is, and it exists whenever the person says it does."*[1,2] Pain can be classified as acute or chronic. Acute pain is relatively short term and subsides as healing occurs. Pain is considered chronic when it persists for more than 6 months.[3] Table 14-1 compares characteristics of acute and chronic pain, and Table 14-2 describes the physiologic and behavioral responses associated with each pain type. Pain can be differentiated further by its physiologic source (Table 14-3) and intensity. Additionally, an individual's pain experience is affected by many psychosocial factors, including attitudes, beliefs, and personality.[4]

In a 1999 study, Tanabe et al[5] found that 78% of patients presenting to the ED had a chief complaint related to pain. Despite growing awareness of the issue, EDs still commonly undertreat, fail to treat, or delay treatment of pain. Health care providers and their patients are influenced by a number of misconceptions that serve as barriers to effective pain management.[6] Box 14-1 lists common barriers. Interventions for pain are classified broadly as pharmacologic (medications), nonpharmacologic (e.g., mind-body therapies), or a combination of both.

ASSESSMENT

Assessment of a patient's pain should begin at the time of arrival in the ED. Assessment facilitates development of an optimal pain management plan. Each patient should be assessed for the presence and intensity of pain, regardless of the chief complaint. The PQRST mnemonic was designed to guide pain evaluation, and its routine use will ensure thorough and consistent assessment:

P Palliative or precipitating factors
Q Quality of the pain
R Region and radiation of the pain
S Subjective description of the pain
T Temporal nature of the pain (when pain occurs, how long it lasts, has it happened before)[7]

Table 14-1   Comparison of Acute and Chronic Pain

Characteristic	*Acute Pain*	*Chronic Pain*
Experience	An event	A situation, state of existence
Source	External agent or internal disease	Unknown; if known, treatment is prolonged or ineffective
Onset	Usually sudden	May be sudden or develop insidiously
Duration	Transient (up to 6 months)	Prolonged (months to years)
Pain identification	Painful and nonpainful areas generally well identified	Painful and nonpainful areas less easily differentiated; change in sensations becomes more difficult to evaluate
Clinical signs	Typical response pattern with more visible signs	Response patterns vary; fewer overt signs (adaptation)
Significance	Significant (informs person something is wrong)	Person looks for significance
Pattern	Self-limiting or readily corrected	Continuous or intermittent; intensity may vary or remain constant
Course	Suffering usually decreases over time	Suffering usually increases over time
Actions	Leads to actions to relieve pain	Leads to actions to modify pain experience
Prognosis	Likelihood of eventual complete relief	Complete relief usually not possible

From McCance KL, Heuther SE: *Pathophysiology: the biologic basis for disease in adults and children*, ed 3, St Louis, 1998, Mosby. Data from Blach RG: *Surg Clin North Am* 55(4):999,1975.

Table 14-2   Physiologic and Behavioral Responses to Acute and Chronic Pain

Pain Type	*Physiologic Response*	*Behavioral Response*
Acute	Increased blood pressure initially Increased pulse rate Increased respiratory rate Dilated pupils Perspiration	Restlessness Inability to concentrate Apprehension Distress
Chronic	Normal blood pressure Normal pulse rate Normal respiratory rate Normal pupils Dry skin	Immobility or physical inactivity Withdrawal Despair

From Ignatavicius D et al: Biopsychosocial concepts related to health care. In Ignatavicius D, Workman ML, Mischler MA, editors: *Medical-surgical nursing across the health care continuum*, ed 3, Philadelphia, 1999, Saunders.

Table 14-3   **Physiological Sources of Pain**

Type of Pain	Physiologic Structures	Mechanism of Pain	Characteristics of Pain	Sources of Acute Pain	Sources of Chronic Pain Syndromes
Somatic pain	Cutaneous: skin and subcutaneous tissues Deep somatic: bone, muscle, blood vessels, connective tissues	Activation of nociceptors	Well localized Constant and achy	Incisional pain, pain at insertion sites of tubes and drains, wound complications, orthopedic procedures, skeletal muscle spasms	Bony metastases, osteoarthritis and rheumatoid arthritis, low back pain, peripheral vascular disease
Visceral pain	Organs and the linings of the body cavities	Activation of nociceptors	Poorly localized Diffuse, deep, cramping, or splitting	Chest tubes, abdominal tubes and drains, bladder distention or spasms, intestinal distention	Pancreatitis, liver metastasis, colitis
Neuropathic pain	Nerve fibers, spinal cord, and central nervous system	Nonnociceptive Injury to the nervous system structures	Poorly localized Shooting, burning, fiery, shocklike, sharp, and painful numbness	Phantom limb pain, postmastectomy pain, and pain from nerve compression	Diabetes, human immuno-deficiency virus, chemotherapy-induced neuropathies, postherpetic neuralgia, cancer-related nerve injury

From Ignatavicius D et al: Biopsychosocial concepts related to health care. In Ignatavicius D, Workman ML, Mischler MA, editors: *Medical-surgical nursing across the health care continuum,* ed 3, Philadelphia, 1999, Saunders.

The QUESTT mnemonic can be used to assess pain in children[8]:

Q   Question the child.
U   Use a pain rating scale.
E   Evaluate physiologic and behavioral changes.
S   Secure the caregiver's involvement.
T   Take the cause of pain into account.
T   Take action and evaluate results.

A pain assessment should be performed as follows:
- Before and after analgesic administration
- Before and after nonpharmacologic interventions
- Whenever the patient is uncomfortable
- Routinely with vital signs

Documentation

Document a subjective description of the complaint, preferably on a standardized assessment form. A consistent documentation format, easily located in the patient's chart, facilitates pain management. Patients should be asked routinely to rate their pain using a numeric rating scale ranging from 0 (no pain) to 10 (extreme pain) (Figure 14-1). Most children who are 7 years or older can rate their pain on a 0-to-10 scale.

Pediatrics

The Wong-Baker FACES Pain Rating Scale is a pain assessment instrument designed for pediatric patients over 3 years old. The scale also can be used in cognitively impaired or language-limited individuals of any age (Table 14-4).[9] A behavioral observation scale such as FLACC

Box **14-1**   Misconceptions About the Use of Pain Medications

Health Care Providers

Lack of knowledge regarding effective dosages and side effects
Exaggerated fears about addiction or respiratory depression
A belief that clinicians can determine how much pain a patient is experiencing without directly asking the patient

Patients

Fear of addiction
Concern about side effects
A belief that pain is inevitable
A desire to be a "good" patient and not complain

From Gunnarsdottir S et al: Interventions to overcome clinician- and patient-related barriers to pain management, *Nurs Clin North Am* 38(3):419-434, 2003.

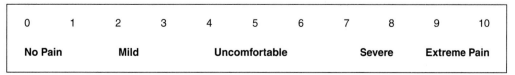

0	1	2	3	4	5	6	7	8	9	10
No Pain		**Mild**			**Uncomfortable**			**Severe**		**Extreme Pain**

Figure 14-1. Numeric pain rating scale.

Table 14-4 Pain Rating Scales for Children

Pain Scale/Description	Instructions	Recommended Age/Comments
FACES Pain Rating Scale* (Wong and Baker, 1988, 2000): Consists of six cartoon faces ranging from smiling face for "no pain" to tearful face for "worst pain"	*Original instructions:* Explain to child that each face is for a person who feels happy because there is no pain (hurt) or sad because there is some or a lot of pain. FACE 0 is very happy because there is no hurt. FACE 1 hurts just a little bit. FACE 2 hurts a little more. FACE 3 hurts even more. FACE 4 hurts a whole lot, but FACT 5 hurts as much as you can imagine, although you don't have to be crying to feel this bad. Ask child to choose face that best describes own pain. Record the number under chosen face on pain assessment record. *Brief word instructions:* Point to each face using the words to describe the pain intensity. Ask child to choose face that best describes own pain and record the appropriate number. 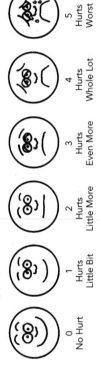	For children as young as 3 years. Using original instructions without affect words, such as *happy or sad*, or brief words resulting in same pain rating, probably reflecting child's rating of pain intensity. For coding purposes, numbers 0, 2, 4, 6, 8, 10 can be substituted for 0-5 system to accommodate 0-10 system. The FACES provides three scales in one: facial expressions, numbers, and words. Use of brief word instructions is recommended.
Oucher (Royer, Denyes, and Villaruel, 1992): Consists of six photographs of child's face representing "no hurt" to "biggest hurt you could ever have"; includes a vertical scale with numbers from 0-100 scales for black and Hispanic children have been developed (Villaruel and Denyes, 1991)	*Numeric Scale* Point to each section of scale to explain variations in pain intensity: "0 means no hurt" "This means little hurts" (pointing to lower part of scale, 1-29). "This means middle hurts" (pointing to middle part of scale, 30-69). "This means big hurts" (pointing to upper part of scale, 70-99). "100 means the biggest hurt you could ever have." Score is actual number stated by child. *Photographic Scale* Point to each photograph on Oucher and explain variations in pain intensity using following language: first picture from the bottom is "no hurt," second is "a little hurt" third is "a little more hurt," fourth is "even more hurt than that," fifth is "pretty much or a lot of hurt," and sixth is the "biggest hurt you could ever have." Score pictures from 0 to 5, with the bottom picture scored as 0.	For children 3 to 13 years. Use numeric scale if child can count to 100 by ones and identify larger of any two numbers, or by tens. Determine whether child has cognitive ability to use photographic scale; child should be able to seriate six geometric shapes from largest to smallest. Determine which ethnic version of Oucher to use. Allow child to select a version of Ouches, or use version that most closely matches physical characteristics of child (Jordan-Marsh et al, 1994).

Below the faces images:

0	1	2	3	4	5
No Hurt	Hurts Little Bit	Hurts Little More	Hurts Even More	Hurts Whole Lot	Hurts Worst

General

Practice using Oucher by recalling and rating previous pain experiences (e.g., falling off a bike). Child points to number or photograph that describes pain intensity associated with experience. Obtain current pain score from child by asking, "How much hurt do you have right now?"

For children as young as 4 years.

Poker Chip Tool[†]

Uses four red poker chips placed horizontally in front of child (Hester et al, 1998)

Say to child, "I want to talk with you about the hurt you may be having right now." Align the chips horizontally in front of child on bedside table, a clipboard, or other firm surface.

Tell child, "These are pieces of hurt." Beginning at the chip nearest child's left side and ending at the one nearest child's right side, point to chips and say, "This [first chip] is a little bit of hurt, and this [fourth chip] is the most hurt you could ever have." For a young child or for any child who may not fully comprehend the instructions, clarify by saying, "That means this [one] is just a little hurt, this [two] is a little more hurt, this [three] is more yet, and this [four] is the most hurt you could ever have."

Do not give children an option for zero hurt. Research with the Poker Chip Tool has verified that children without pain will so indicate by responses such as "I don't have any."

Ask child, "How many pieces of hurt do you have right now?"

After initial use of the Poker Chip Tool, some children internalize the concept "pieces of hurt." If a child gives a response such as "I have one right now," before you ask or before you lay out the poker chips, record the number of chips on the Pain Flow Sheet. Clarify child's answer by words such as "Oh, you have a little hurt? Tell me about the hurt."

Word-Graphic Rating Scale[‡]

(Tesler et al, 1991): Uses descriptive words (may vary in other scales) to denote varying intensities of pain

Explain to child, "This is a line with words to describe how much pain you may have. This side of the line means no pain, and over here the line means worst possible pain." (Point with your finger where "no pain" is, and run your finger along the line to "worst possible pain," as you say it.) "If you have no pain, you would mark like this." (Show example.) "If you have some pain, you would mark somewhere along the line, depending on how much pain you have." (Show example.) "The more pain you have, the closer to worst pain you would mark. The worst pain possible is marked like this." (Show example.) "Show me how much pain you have right now by marking with a straight, up-and-down line anywhere along the line to show how much pain you have right now."

For children 4 to 17 years.

Continued

Table 14-4 Pain Rating Scales for Children—cont'd

Pain Scale/Description	Instructions	Recommended Age/Comments
	With a millimeter ruler, measure from the "no pain" end to the mark and record this measurement as the pain score. No pain Little pain Medium pain Large pain Worst possible pain	
Numeric Scale Uses straight line with end points identified as "no pain" and "worst pain" and sometimes "medium pain" in the middle; divisions along line are marked in units from 0 to 5 or 10 (high number may vary)	Explain to child that at one end of the line is a 0, which means that a person feels no pain (hurt). At the other end is usually a 5 or a 10, which means the person feels the worst pain imaginable. The numbers 1 to 4 or 9 are for a very little pain to a whole lot of pain. Ask child to choose a number that best describes own pain. 0 1 2 3 4 5 6 7 8 9 10 No Pain Mild Uncomfortable Severe Extreme Pain	For children as young as 5 years, as long as they can count and have some concept of numbers and their values in relation to other numbers. Scale may be used horizontally or vertically. Number coding should be same as other scales used in a facility.
Visual Analogue Scale Defined as a vertical or horizontal line that is drawn to a certain length, such as 10 cm, and anchored by items that represent the extremes of the subjective phenomenon, such as pain, that is measured (Cline et al, 1992)	Ask child to place a mark on line that best describes amount of own pain. With a centimeter ruler, measure from the "no pain" end to the mark and record this measurement as the pain score.	For children as young as 4½ years, preferably at least 7 years. Vertical or horizontal scale may be used.

Color Tool

Uses crayons or markers for child to construct own scale that is used with body outline (Eland and Banner, 1999)

Present eight crayons or markers to child in random order. Ask child to "pick a crayon with a color that reminds you of the most hurt (or pain) that you could possibly have"; once that crayon is selected, separate it from the others. Next, ask child to select a crayon with a color that "reminds you of pain that is a little less than the pain we just talked about"; once the second crayon selected, separate it from the group and place it with the first crayon selected. Ask child to select a third crayon with a color "that reminds you of only a little pain"; separate this crayon and move it to the selected group. Finally, ask child to select a crayon with a color that "reminds you of no hurt (or pain)" and separate that fourth color. Show the four crayons selected to the child and arrange them in order of "worst hurt (or pain)" to "no hurt (or pain)" and ask child to show on the body outline "where the hurt is." If child offers any verbal comments, note them.

Children as young as 4 years, provided they know their colors, are not color blind, and are able to construct the scale if in pain.

From Wong DL, Hockenberry-Eaton M: *Wong's essentials of pediatric nursing*, ed 6, St Louis, 2001, Mosby.

*Wong-Baker FACES Pain Rating Scale Reference Manual describing development and research of the scale is available from the Pain/Palliative Resource Center, City of Hope National Medical Center, 1500 East Duarte Road, Duarte CA 91010, (626) 359-8111, ext. 3829; fax: (626) 301-8941; e-mail: mayday_smtplink.coh.org; Web site: www.mosby.com/WOW/. A compilation of many pain scales, including the FACES, is available free from Purdue Frederick Company, 100 Connecticut Ave., Norwalk, CT 06850-3950, (800) 733-1333 or (203) 853-0123, ext. 7378 or 7314; Web site: www.partnersagainstpain.com. The use of FACES with children is demonstrated in *Whaley and Wong's Pediatric Nursing Video Series*, "Pain Assessment and Management," narrated by Donna Wong, PhD, RN. Available from Mosby, 11830 Westline Industrial Drive, St. Louis, MO 63146, (800) 426-4545; fax: (800) 535-9935; Web site: www.mosby.com.

†Developed in 1975 by N.O. Nester, University of Colorado Health Sciences Center, School of Nursing, Denver, CO 80262. Also available in Spanish and French.

‡Instructions for Word-Graphic Pain Rating Scale from *Acute Pain Management Guideline Panel: Acute pain management in infants, children, and adolescents; operative and medical procedures; quick reference guide for clinicians*, ACHPR Pub. No. 92-0020, Rockville, Md, 1992. Agency for Health Care Policy and Research, Public Health Service, U.S. Department of Health and Human Services. Word-Graphic Rating Scale is part of the Adolescent Pediatric Pain Tool and is available from Pediatric Pain Study, University of California, School of Nursing, Department of Family Health Care Nursing, 2 Kirkham St., Box 0606, San Francisco, CA 94143-0606, (415) 476-4040; e-mail: savedra@Linex.com.

Table 14-5   **FLACC Behavioral Scale**

Categories	Scoring*		
	0	1	2
Face	No particular expression or smile	Occasional grimace or frown, withdrawn, disinterested	Frequent to constant frown, quivering chin, clenched jaw
Legs	Normal position or relaxed	Uneasy, restless, tense	Kicking or legs drawn up
Activity	Lying quietly, normal position, moves easily	Squirming, shifting back and forth, tense	Arched, rigid, or jerking
Cry	No cry (awake or asleep)	Moans or whimpers; occasional complaint	Crying steadily, screams or sobs, frequent complaints
Consolability	Content, relaxed	Reassured by occasional touching, hugging, or being talked to; distractible	Difficult to console or comfort

Reprinted from *Pediatric Nursing*, 1997, volume 23, number 3, pp 293-297. Reprinted with permission of the publisher, Jannetti Publications, Inc., East Holly Ave, Box 56, Pitman, NJ 08071-0056; phone 856-256-2300; fax 856-589-7643. For a sample copy of the journal, please contact the publisher.
*Each of the five categories Face (F), Legs (L), Activity (A), Cry (C), and Consolability (C) is scored from 0 to 2, which results in a total score between 0 and 10.

(Face, Legs, Activity, Cry, and Consolability) provides a tool for evaluating pain in the preverbal or noncommunicative child (Table 14-5).[9,10]

Geriatrics

Because patients with advanced dementia cannot describe their pain, this group is consistently undertreated. A 2003 study by Manfredi et al[11] noted that clinicians were able to assess the presence of pain accurately in the dementia population 80% to 90% of the time by closely observing facial expressions.

PHARMACOLOGIC INTERVENTIONS

Each individual is unique and thus experiences various responses to medications. Therefore pharmacologic pain management strategies must be tailored to the individual. Classes of drugs used for the treatment of pain include the following:
1. Local anesthetics: Primarily used for minor surgical procedures such as laceration repair (Table 14-6). This group includes lidocaine, bupivacaine, lidocaine and prilocaine (EMLA cream), and tetracaine/epinephrine (adrenaline)/cocaine (TAC).
2. Analgesics: Nonopioids and opioids
   a. Nonopioid analgesics are used commonly. This category includes nonsteroidal antiinflammatory agents and acetaminophen (Table 14-7).
   b. Opioids are the most effective agents for severe acute pain (Table 14-8).[3] These drugs are commonly underutilized for fear of addiction. Addiction is actually a rare complication, occurring in less than 1% of patients treated.[8]
3. Adjuvants: Medications that have analgesic properties but are used primarily for other functions (Table 14-9).
   a. Sucrose is an effective tool for the management of minor pain in infants. The recommended dose is 2 mL of a 12% to 24% solution for full-term neonates and 0.1 to 0.4 mL for premature infants. Give orally 2 to 5 minutes before a procedure.[12]

Table **14-6**   **Topical Anesthetics**

Name	Ingredients	Indications	Special Considerations
TAC	Tetracaine Adrenaline Cocaine	Topical anesthetic for minor wounds not involving fingers, toes, penis, nose	Wear a glove when preparing TAC; hold TAC in place on wound; observe for blanching of skin; additional lidocaine filtration may be needed.
LET	Lidocaine Epinephrine Tetracaine	Topical anesthetic for minor wounds not involving fingers, toes, penis, nose; may be safer than TAC (does not contain cocaine)	Wear a glove when preparing LET; hold LET in place on wound; observe for blanching of skin; additional lidocaine infiltration may be needed.
EMLA cream	Lidocaine Prilocaine	Topical anesthetic (cream based) that is applied to body area before procedure to decrease pain (venous cannulation site; lumbar puncture site)	Requires at least 30-60 minutes to work; may require reapplication if first procedure attempt is unsuccessful.

From Albrecht S et al: Pain management. In Newberry L, editor: Emergency nursing core curriculum, ed 5, Philadelphia, 2000, Saunders.

Table **14-7**   **Nonopioid Agents for Pain Management**

Generic Name (Trade Name)	Typical Dose (Maximum Dose)	Approximate Equivalent	Onset Effect (min)	Peak Effect (min)	Duration Effect (hr)
Acetaminophen (Tylenol, Tempra, etc.)	650 mg PO; 650 mg PR (4000 mg/day)	Aspirin 650 mg	30	60	3-4
Acetylsalicylic acid (aspirin)	600 mg PO; 600 mg PR (5200 mg/day)	Morphine 2 mg IM	30	60	3-4
Ibuprofen (Motrin, Advil, etc.)	200 mg PO (3200 mg/day)	Aspirin 650 mg	30	60-120	4
Choline magnesium trisalicylate (Trilisate)	2000-3000 mg PO (3000 mg/day)		5-30	60-180	3-6
Diflunisal (Dolobid)	500 mg PO (1500 mg/day)	Aspirin 650 mg	60	120-180	8-12
Ketoprofen (Orudis)	25 mg PO (300 mg PO)	Aspirin 650 mg	30	30-120	6
Naproxen (Naprosyn)	250 mg PO (1250 mg/day)	Aspirin 650 mg	60	120-240	6-8
Ketorolac (Toradol)	30-60 mg IM initially (120 mg IM/day × 5 day, max 30 mg IM × 20 doses over 5 days)	Morphine 6-12 mg IM	10	60	3-6
Piroxicam (Feldene)	20 mg/day		60	180-300	>12
Sulindac (Clinoril)	200 mg/day		1-2 days	60-120	Unknown
Indomethacin (Indocin)	25 mg PO (100 mg/day)	Aspirin 650 mg	60	60-120	4
Nabumetone (Relafen)	1000 mg PO (2000 mg/day)	Aspirin 3600 mg	1-2 days	Days-2 weeks	Unknown
Etodolac (Lodine)	200-400 mg PO (1200 mg/day)	Aspirin 650 mg	30	60-120	4-12

Copyright DJ Wilkie, 1998.
IM, Intramuscular; IV, intravenous; PO, oral; PR, rectal.

Table 14-8   **Opioid Agents for Pain Management**

Generic Name (Trade Name)	Typical Dose (Maximum Dose)	Approximate Equivalent	Onset Effect (min)	Peak Effect (min)	Duration Effect (hr)
Opioid-Agonist Drugs					
Codeine	30-60 mg PO (200 mg PO)	Aspirin 650 mg Morphine 10 mg IM	30-45	20-120	4
	15-60 mg IM	Morphine 10 mg IM	10-30	30-60	4
Immediate release					
Oxycodone (Roxicodone, w/aspirin—Percodan, w/acetaminophen—Percocet)	5 mg PO (30 mg PO)	Codeine 60 mg PO Morphine 10 mg IM	10-15	60	3-4
Hydrocodone (Vicodin, Lortab, Lorcet, and others)	5 mg PO (30 mg PO)	Morphine 10 mg IM	10-30	30-60	4-6
Meperidine (Demerol, Pethidine)	50 mg PO (300 mg PO)	Aspirin 650 mg Morphine 10 mg IM Demerol 75 mg IM	15	60-90	2-4
	75 mg IM	Morphine 10 mg IM	10-15	30-60	2-4
	50 mg IV	Morphine 10 mg IM	1	5-7	2-3
Propoxyphene HCl (Darvon, Dolene);	65 mg PO	Aspirin 600 mg	15-60	120	4-6
Propoxyphene napsylate (w/aspirin—Darvon-N, w/acetaminophen—Darvocet-N)	100 mg PO	Aspirin 600 mg			
Tramadol (Ultram)	50-100 mg	Codeine 60 mg PO	60	2 hr	4-6
Agonist-Antagonist Drug					
Pentazocine HCl (Talwin)	60 mg IM	Morphine 10 mg IM	15-20	30-60	2-3
	30 mg PO (180 mg PO)	Aspirin 600 mg Morphine 10 mg IM or pentazocine 60 mg IM	15-30	60-90	3
Agonist Drugs					
Morphine sulfate *Immediate*-release tablets and liquids	30 mg PO 30 mg PR	Morphine 10 mg IM Morphine 10 mg IM	20-60	120	4-5
Sustained release					
(MS Contin, Oramorph SR)	30 mg PO	Morphine 10 mg IM		210	8-12
Injectable					
(Astramorph/PF; Duramorph, Infumorph)	10 mg IM	Morphine 10 mg IM	10-30	60	4-5
	5 mg IV	Morphine 10 mg IM	5	20	2-4

Table **14-8** **Opioid Agents for Pain Management—cont'd**

Generic Name (Trade Name)	Typical Dose (Maximum Dose)	Approximate Equivalent	Onset Effect (min)	Peak Effect (min)	Duration Effect (hr)
Oxycodone Immediate release					
(Roxicodone)	5 mg PO	Codeine 60 mg PO	0-15	60	3-4
	30 mg PO	Morphine 10 mg IM			
		Morphine 30 mg PO			
Controlled release					
(OxyContin)	30 mg PO	Morphine 30-60 mg PO	30-60	60, 420	12
Methadone (Dolophine)	20 mg PO	Morphine 10 mg IM	30-60	90-120	4-6
		Methadone 10 mg IM			
	10 mg IM	Morphine 10 mg IM	10-20	60-120	4-5
	5 mg IV	Morphine 10 mg IM	5	15-30	3-4
Hydromorphone (Dilaudid)	7.5 mg PO	Morphine 10 mg IM	30	90-120	4
	3 mg PR	Hydromorphone 1.5 mg IM	15-30	30-90	4-5
	1.5 mg IM	Morphine 10 mg IM	15	30-60	4-5
	1 mg IV	Morphine 10 mg IM	10-15	15-30	2-3
Oxymorphone (Numorphan)	1 mg IM	Morphine 10 mg IM	10-15	30-90	3-6
	0.5 mg IV	Morphine 10 mg IM	5-10	15-30	3-4
	10 mg PR	Oxymorphone 1 mg IM	l5-30	60	3-6
Levorphanol (Levo-Dromoran)	4 mg PO	Morphine 10 mg IM	10-60	90-120	4-5
		Levorphanol 2 mg IM		60	4-5
	2 mg IM	Morphine 10 mg IM	10-15	15	3-4
	1 mg IV	Morphine 10 mg IM			
Fentanyl (Sublimaze, Duragesic)	0.1 mg IM	Morphine 10 mg IM	7-15	20-30	1-2
	25-50 mcg/hr transdermal	Morphine 30 mg sustained-release q8h	6 hr	12-24 hr	72
Agonist-Antagonist Drugs					
Butorphanol (Stadol);	2 mg IM	Morphine 10 mg IM	10-30	30-60	3-4
	2 mg IV	Morphine 10 mg IM	2-3	30	2-4
Nalbuphine (Nubain);	10 mg IM	Morphine 10 mg IM	15	60	3-6
	10 mg IV	Pentazocine 60 mg IM	2-3	30	3-4
Dezocine (Dalgan)	10 mg IM	Morphine 10 mg IM	30	60-120	3-6
Partial Agonist Drug					
Buprenorphine (Buprenex)	0.4 mg IM	Morphine 10 mg IM	15	60	6

Copyright DJ Wilkie, 1998.
IM, Intramuscular; *IV,* intravenous; *PO,* oral; *PR,* rectal.

Table 14-9　Adjuvant Analgesic Agents for Pain Management

Generic Drug (Trade Drug)	Approximate Daily Dose	Onset Effect	Peak Effect	Duration Effect (hr)
Carbamazepine (Tegretol, Epitol)	200-1600 mg PO	8-72 hr	2-12	Unknown
Phenytoin (Dilantin)	300-500 mg PO	2-24 hr	1.5-3	6-12
Gabapentin (Neurontin)	900-1800 mg PO	60-120 min	2-4 hr	Up to 24 hr
Sumatriptan (Imitrex)	6-12 mg subcut	30 min	Up to 2 hr	to 24 hr
Amitriptyline (Elavil and others)	10-150 mg PO	3-4 days	1-2 wk	Days-weeks
Doxepin (Sinequan, Adepin)	25-150 mg PO	3-1 days	1-2 wk	Days-weeks
Imipramine (Tofranil and others)	20-100 mg PO	60 min	2-6 wk	Weeks
Trazodone (Desyrel and others)	75-225 mg PO	2 wk	2-4 wk	Weeks
Paroxetine (Paxil)	20-50 mg PO	3-4 days	1-2 wk	Days-weeks
Hydroxyzine (Vistaril, Atarax, and others)	300-450 mg IM	15-30 min	2-4 hr	4-6 hr
Lidocaine	5 mg/kg IV	2 min	2 min	10-20 min
Mexiletine (Mexitil)	200-400 mg PO	30-120 min	2-3 hr	8-12 hr
Dexamethasone (Decadron and others)	16-96 mg PO/IV	2-4 days	1-2 hr	2.75 days
Dextroamphetamine (Dexedrine and others)	10-15 mg PO	1-2 hr	Unknown	2-10 hr
Methylphenidate (Methidate, Ritalin)	10-15 mg PO	Unknown	1-3 hr	4-6 hr
Nefazodone (Serzone)	200-600 mg PO	3-4 days	1-2 wk	Days-weeks

Copyright DJ Wilkie, 1998
IM, Intramuscular; *IV,* intravenous; *PO,* by mouth; *subcut,* subcutaneous.

NONPHARMACOLOGIC INTERVENTIONS

Nonpharmacologic pain management strategies may be used along with pharmacotherapy to enhance a patient's coping abilities. Table 14-10 summarizes nonpharmacologic pain management strategies for pediatric patients that can be implemented readily in the ED. Examples of nonpharmacologic treatment include the following:

- Place the patient in a position of comfort.
- Immobilize an affected area to minimize further pain.
- Have the patient focus on a stimulus other than the pain. Examples of distractions include listening to music, viewing videotapes, telling stories, and engaging in conversation.
- Create a pediatric treasure chest filled with various distraction tools. Magic wands, bubbles, squeezable balls, and stuffed animals distract toddlers and school-age children.
- Magazines, audiotapes and videotapes, games, television, and puzzles are effective distractors for adolescents and adults.
- Consider hypnosis, guided imagery, and relaxation; it is important note that hypnosis is rarely practiced in the ED because of a lack of personnel.
- Guided imagery assists the patient to imagine pleasant images associated with calm, soothing sensations.
- Relaxation refers to any number of techniques aimed at anxiety reduction. Deep breathing is one technique that can be taught quickly in the ED.[1,3,13,14]

Table **14-10**   **Nonpharmacologic Treatment Strategies**

Developmental Age	Strategy
Infant	Relaxation: Rocking, swaddling, sucking
Toddler	Relaxation: Rocking, cuddling
	Distraction: Singing, pictures, toys, favorite stuffed animals, or comfort articles (blanket, pillow)
Preschooler	Distraction: Blowing bubbles, counting, singing, storytelling
	Relaxation: Rocking, cuddling
School age	Relaxation: Rhythmic breathing patterns
	Distraction: Storytelling
	Imagery: Superheroes, favorite places (beach, amusement park, playground)
Adolescent	Imagery: Favorite places
	Distraction: Music, hobbies

From Tanabe P et al: A prospective study of ED pain management practices and the patient perspective, *J Emerg Nurs* 25(3): 174, 1999, with permission from the Emergency Nurses Association.

- Cutaneous therapy involves stimulating the skin to provide pain relief.
- Superficial heat, such as a warm compress, relieves the pain of an infiltrated intravenous line.
- Superficial cold (an ice pack) applied to fractures and sprains reduces pain and swelling.
- Massage can minimize muscular tension.
- Transcutaneous electrical nerve stimulation (TENS) occasionally is used in emergency care settings. This procedure requires initial and ongoing education before implementation.[3,5]

PROCEDURAL (CONSCIOUS) SEDATION

The purpose of procedural sedation (also referred to as conscious sedation or moderate sedation) is to minimize pain awareness and intensity while preserving the patient's ability to maintain an airway and respond to verbal commands.[1,3,13] Procedural sedation often is used for procedures such as deep laceration repair, joint relocation, abscess drainage, and fracture reduction. In infants and children, procedural sedation also is used to facilitate diagnostic testing such as imaging studies. These medications primarily are given intravenously. However, several agents also may be administered orally, rectally, intramuscularly, or nasally. Drugs commonly used for moderate sedation in the adult include the following:
- Midazolam: Sedative, amnesic agent
- Diazepam: Anxiolytic
- Lorazepam: Anxiolytic
- Fentanyl: Narcotic analgesic
- Morphine: Narcotic analgesic
- Chloral hydrate: Sedative

A combination of sedation and analgesia can optimize management of anxiety and pain; titrate doses to the desired response. The appropriate antagonist should be readily available to reverse undesired sedation. Naloxone (Narcan) is a short-acting opioid antagonist; flumazenil (Romazicon) reverses acute benzodiazepine overdose.

Figure 14-2 provides a sample procedural sedation flowsheet. Table 14-11 summarizes pediatric sedation dosage guidelines. Box 14-2 describes guidelines for moderate sedation.

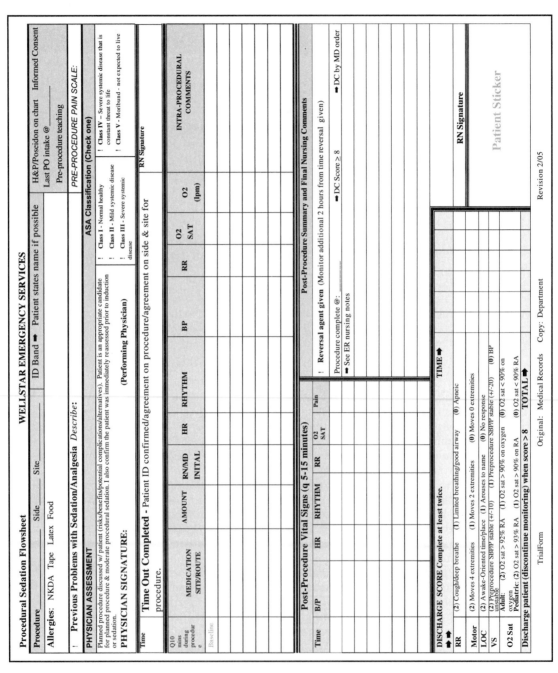

Figure 14-2. Procedures sedation flowsheet. (Courtesy WellStar Health System.)

Table 14-11   Pediatric Procedural Sedation Dosage Guidelines

The dose ranges are provided to guide the clinician. However, clinical judgment must be used to tailor therapy to each patient. Decreased doses may be necessary in patients undergoing multiple procedures on the same day. When used along with central nervous system depressants or when two or more of the listed agents are used together, consider decreasing the dose by 25% to 50%. Patients who have a history of tolerance to medication may exceed the initial dosage guidelines, or in longer procedures where the clinical situation indicates, smaller doses may be repeated as long as vital signs and ventilation are stable.

Drug	Pediatric Dose	Onset (min)	Duration (hr)	Comments
Chloral hydrate	PO/PR: 50-75 mg/kg/dose given 30-60 min before procedure (Max: 1 g/dose for infants, 2 g/dose for children)	30-60	4-8	Renal or hepatic impairment may prolong effects.
Diazepam (Valium)	PO/PR: 0.2-0.3 mg/kg/dose given 45-60 min before procedure (Max: 10 mg/dose) IV: 0.1-0.2 mg/kg/dose (Max: 10 mg/dose)	PO: 30-60	PO: less than 3	Incomplete and erratic absorption occurs via IM route. In children do not exceed 1-2 mg/min IV.
Fentanyl	IM/IV: 1-2 mcg/kg/dose May repeat after 10 min × 5 PRN	IM: 7-15 IV: 1	IM: 1-2 IV: 0.5-1	Rapid IV injection may produce thoracic muscle rigidity. Reduce dose to 1 mcg/kg/dose when given with benzodiazepine.
Ketamine	PO: 6-8 mg/kg/dose (mix in juice) IM: 1-4 mg/kg/dose IV: 0.2-2 mg/kg/dose (Total IV dose not to exceed 3 mg/kg.)	PO: 30 IM: 3-4 IV: 0.5-1	IM: 12-25 IV: 5-10 Average recovery time: 1-2	Infuse over 60 seconds. May repeat IV dose or half dose after 5-10 min. Consider benzodiazepine with ketamine and antisecretory agent glycopyrrolate (Robinul) 0.005 mg/kg.
Lorazepam (Ativan)	IM/IV: 0.05-0.1 mg/kg/dose (Max dose: 4 mg)	IV: 5-15 IM: 15-45	IV: 0.5-12 IM: 4-12	Dilute with equal volume of NS, D5W, or sterile water.
Meperidine (Demerol)	IM: 1-2 mg/kg/dose IV: 0.5-1 mg/kg/dose (Max dose: 100 mg)	IM: 10-15 IV: 5	IM/IV: 2-4	Infuse over at least 5 min. Avoid in patient with history of seizures and renal failure.
Midazolam (Versed)	IM/IV: 0.06-0.1 mg/kg/dose May repeat with 0.1-0.2 mg/kg in 5-10 min (Max per dose: 2 mg) NAS: 0.25-0.5 mg/kg/dose (Max per dose: 5 mg) PO: 0.5 mg/kg PR: 0.25-0.5 mg/kg/dose	IM: 15 IV/NAS: 1-5	IM: 2-6 IV/NAS: 0.5-1 (but may persist for 3-4)	No more than 2.5 mg should be administered over a period of 2 min. Additional doses may be administered after 2 min. If narcotics or other CNS depressants are administered, the midazolam dose should be reduced by 30%.
Morphine	IM/subcut/IV: 0.05-0.2 mg/kg/dose Up to a total of 15 mg	IM/subcut: 10-30 IV: 5	IM/subcut/IV: 4-5	Administer IV over 4-5 min. May affect systemic vascular resistance. Watch for hypotension.

Data from *The Harriet Lane drug handbook*, ed 14, St Louis, 1996, Mosby.
CNS, Central nervous system; *D₅W*, dextrose 5%; *IM*, intramuscular; *IV*, intravenous; *Max*, maximum; *NAS*, intranasal; *NS*, normal saline; *PO*, by mouth; *PR*, rectal; *PRN*, as needed; *subcut*, subcutaneous.

Box **14-2** **Guidelines for Procedural Sedation**

Ensure that the physician has obtained consent for both the procedure *and* sedation.

Perform a brief preprocedural assessment of respiratory, cardiovascular, and neurologic status.

Have resuscitation equipment, suction, oxygen, and drugs readily available.

Place the patient on an oxygen saturation monitor. Some institutions also require a cardiac monitor and an automatic blood pressure cuff.

The patient must be monitored continuously by a licensed staff member (trained in sedation and resuscitation) whose only responsibility is monitoring the patient.

Reassess the patient every 5 to 15 minutes during the recovery period.

Complete a postrecovery assessment.[1,3,13,14]

References

1. Albrecht S et al: Pain management. In Newberry L, editor: *Emergency nursing core curriculum,* ed 5, Philadelphia, 2000, WB Saunders.
2. McCaffery M, Pasero C: *Pain: clinical manual,* ed 2, St Louis, 1999, Mosby.
3. Troutman D: Pain management. In Newberry L, editor: *Sheehy's emergency nursing,* ed 5, St Louis, 2003, Mosby.
4. Cepeda M, Carr D: Overview of pain management. In Joint Commission Resources: Approaches to pain management—an essential guide for clinical leaders, Oakbrook Terrace, Ill, 2003, Joint Commission on Accreditation of Healthcare Organizations.
5. Tanabe P et al: A prospective study of ED pain management practices and the patient's perspective, *J Emerg Nurs* 25(3):171-177, 1999.
6. Gunnarsdottir S et al: Interventions to overcome clinician- and patient-related barriers to pain management, *Nurs Clin North Am* 38(3):419-434, 2003.
7. Krohn B: Using pain assessment tools, *Nurse Pract* 27(10):54-56, 2002.
8. Wong D et al: Family centered care of the child during illness and hospitalization. In *Wong's essentials of pediatric nursing,* ed 6, St Louis, 2001, Mosby.
9. Ellis J et al: Keeping pediatric patients comfortable, *Nursing 2003* 33(7):22, 2003.
10. Willis M et al: FLACC Behavioral Pain Assessment scale: a comparison with the child's self report, *Pediatr Nurs* 29(3):195-198, 2003.
11. Manfredi P et al: Pain assessment in elderly patients with severe dementia, *J Pain Symptom Manage* 25(1):48-52, 2003.
12. Coleman M et al: Assessment and management of pain and distress in the neonate, *Adv Neonat Care* 2(3):123-136, 2002.
13. American Academy of Pediatrics, American Pain Society: The Assessment and management of acute pain in infants, children, and adolescents, *Pediatrics* 108(3):793-797, 2001.
14. Bishop-Kurylo D: Pediatric pain management in the emergency department, *Top Emerg Med* 24(1): 19-30, 2002.

15

End-of-Life Issues for Emergency Nurses

Kay McClain, RN, MSM, CEN, CNA

Emergency clinicians are frequently involved with the 10% of deaths in the United States that occur suddenly and unexpectedly as a result of motor vehicle crashes, penetrating trauma, massive cerebrovascular events, or myocardial infarctions. However, emergency nurses are just as likely to care for a significant number of patients with terminal illnesses for whom death is expected. As the illness progresses visits to the emergency department (ED) often become more frequent. Nurses play an important role in caring for—and advocating on behalf of—these patients, as the focus of intervention shifts from curative to palliative. The end of life is defined as the period in which (1) there is little likelihood of cure, (2) further aggressive therapy is considered futile, and (3) patient comfort becomes the primary goal. The trend toward offering patients in-home palliative care earlier in their dying process is having an impact on how patients die in our society. Nonetheless, emergency providers still have many opportunities to improve care at the end-of-life.

ADVANCE DIRECTIVES

An advance directive is a means of documenting an individual's wishes regarding future health care. An advance directive may include a living will or health care proxy and is based on the supposition that patients have a right to make their own treatment decisions. An advance directive is *not* equivalent to a do not resuscitate order. Rather, the purpose of an advance directive is to encourage patients and their families (or significant others) to understand, reflect on, and discuss treatment options before the need for resuscitation or other emergency interventions. Although state law (usually a natural death act) is the legal basis for advance directives, laws differ in respect to format, forms, witness requirements, and the need for a notary public.

Statements made in an advance directive reflect the values and beliefs of the individual and may change over time as illness progresses or an emergency arises. Discussion and formal documentation before such a crisis is more likely to ensure that a patient's wishes are respected and carried out. Two possible components of an advance directive are the following:

- A *living will* allows individuals to specify whether they would accept or refuse particular life-sustaining interventions such as dialysis, mechanical ventilation, cardiopulmonary resuscitation (CPR), tube feeding, intravenous (IV) hydration, and blood transfusions.[1]
- A *health care proxy* (or durable power of attorney for health care) identifies a specific individual who can make medical decisions on behalf of the patient once the individual is unable to make decisions for himself or herself.[1]

Living wills and health care proxies are flexible documents that can be changed easily or revoked. This can be done in a variety of ways, including simply telling a health care provider. In the emergency setting, one must exercise care to make sure the latest version of these documents is available. In some states, nursing home residents wear colored wristbands to indicate they have an advance directive.

The Patient Self-Determination Act of 1990 is a federal law that requires all health care agencies that receive federal funding to recognize advance directives. Hospitals must do the following:

- Ask patients if they have an advance directive.
- Offer patients and families information about advance directives.
- Inform patients of state laws that pertain to advance directives.
- Notify patients about any hospital policies that affect advance directives.

Standards may differ from state to state and from institution to institution. Patients are never required to have advance directives, and facilities may not discriminate against persons who have or do not have one. Most hospitals try to honor a patient's wishes, but specific exceptions may exist, and institutional policies must identify these situations clearly. If a health care provider is not willing or able to honor an advance directive, the provider should inform the patient and family of this and arrange for orderly transfer of care to a new practitioner. Hospitals need a clear method for identifying patients with advance directives and must have a plan for making these documents readily available.

If a patient does not have an advance directive and is unable to make his or her own medical decisions, then clinicians must seek guidance from a spouse, adult child, parent, or friend, or they must pursue appointment of a legal guardian. At times, consultation with the ethics committee of the hospital is advisable. Unfortunately, this is usually difficult or impossible in emergent situations. Potential problems should be identified proactively and addressed with any patient nearing the end of life who uses the ED frequently. Consult your ethics committee or legal counsel if there appears to be a misunderstanding or disagreement about treatment options and patient preferences. Table 15-1 provides a list of Internet resources related to advance directives.

DO NOT RESUSCITATE

Do Not Resuscitate, No Cardiac Resuscitation, and *Do Not Attempt Resuscitation* are terms that refer to patients for whom life-sustaining efforts are limited at the request of the patient, family, or health care team. Other variations include *Do Not Intubate* and *Do Not Defibrillate.* Some institutions prefer the phrases *Allow for Natural Death* or *Comfort Care Only* because patients and families may misconstrue the use of the word *not* to mean that no care will be given. Positively worded phrases emphasize that care will be continued (e.g., pain control and comfort measures) and that the patient is not being abandoned.

Table 15-1   Internet Resources Related to Advanced Directives

Organization/Group	Internet Address
American Association of Retired Persons	http://www.aarp.org/index.html
Aging With Dignity—Five Wishes	http://www.agingwithdignity.org/5wishes.html
American Bar Association (ABA Network)	http://www.abanet.org/home.cfm
American Medical Association	http://www.ama-assn.org/
Choice in Dying	http://www.choicesindying.com/
Compassion in Dying	http://www.compassionindying.org/

A problem unique to the emergency setting is the patient who presents in a state of crisis, requiring an immediate decision to act or not act. Initial information is frequently limited or confusing. Therefore emergency providers are justified in starting or continuing care that may later be determined to be contrary to patient or family wishes.

OUT-OF-HOSPITAL DO NOT RESUSCITATE ORDERS

About half of the states in the United States have passed legislation allowing out-of-hospital do not resuscitate (DNR) orders.[2] These laws go by a variety of names including portable DNR, community-based DNR, and physician order for life-sustaining treatment (POLST). These laws require the following:
- If an individual with an out-of-hospital DNR order experiences a cardiac or respiratory arrest, emergency medical services personnel should *not* initiate cardiopulmonary resuscitation. However, they can provide the following:
  - Assessment
  - Assistance if the patient is choking (airway clearance, oxygen, and medications for dyspnea)
  - Aggressive pain management
  - Grief counseling
  - Other appropriate services for the patient and family
- Some states limit access to out-of-hospital DNR orders to patients who are terminally ill or elderly, whereas other states make them available to any competent adult.
- To be valid, an out-of-hospital DNR order requires the health care provider's signature *and* the patient's or surrogate's signature.
- To avoid potential confusion, patients should have a copy of the original order and some form of wearable identification such as a MedicAlert bracelet.
- Most states include a provision allowing emergency medical services personnel to perform CPR if the family persistently and strongly requests it, even if the patient has an out-of-hospital DNR order. However, in these difficult situations, emergency medical services personnel are trained to counsel families to forgo CPR.
- Ideally, medical facilities will have a policy that defines the circumstances under which an out-of-hospital DNR order will be honored within the health care facility. In particular, policies should address care of the person with an out-of-hospital DNR in the ED, clinic, or inpatient setting. In addition, discussion regarding out-of-hospital DNR orders should be part of the nursing discharge plan for all appropriate patients.

Table 15-2   Clinical and Legal Distinctions between Advance Directives and Do Not Resuscitate Orders

Component	Advance Directive	Institutional-Based DNR	Out-of-Hospital DNR
How do you obtain one?	From many sources including the Internet, hospitals, physicians, or clinics	The physician writes a DNR order in the medical record.	Forms can be obtained only from a licensed, independent health care provider.
Who signs the document?	Only the person for whom it applies (witness required)	The physician	The physician and the patient or a legal surrogate
When does it apply?	Only when the patient is unable to speak for himself or herself. Some state laws specify certain conditions (e.g., permanent vegetative state or coma).	Immediately	Immediately
What should occur if the person suffers cardiopulmonary arrest?	Start CPR. When patient is stabilized, evaluate the situation and communicate with the patient or legal surrogate.	Do not begin CPR.	Do not begin CPR.
Does the document represent informed consent?	No. The document is a written statement of a person's wishes. It does not require disclosure of specific information by a health care provider, so it does not represent an informed decision.	Yes. The order results from a discussion between the physician (or team) and the patient or legal surrogate. Like any other order for treatment, informed consent should be part of the process.	Yes. The form is signed by the physician and the patient or legal surrogate. The form is written evidence that informed consent has occurred.

From Wilkie DJ: *Toolkit for nursing excellence at end of life transition,* Seattle, 2001, University of Washington (CD-ROM). *DNR,* Do not resuscitate; *CPR,* cardiopulmonary resuscitation.

- Many states are working to make out-of-hospital DNR orders the standard for nursing homes and other community-based care facilities so that emergency medical services personnel responding to these facilities can honor DNR requests.

    Importantly, an out-of-hospital DNR order is *not* an advance directive. The out-of-hospital DNR order is a physician's order to withhold life-sustaining therapy, and it requires a patient's or surrogate's signature as evidence that informed consent occurred, similar to consent for a surgical procedure. Table 15-2 summarizes specific differences between advance directives, institutional-based DNR orders, and out-of-hospital DNR orders.

COMMON MEDICAL EMERGENCIES AT THE END OF LIFE

Patients with a terminal illness may present to the ED with a problem that requires rapid intervention. Examples include uncontrolled pain, delirium, hemorrhage, bowel obstruction, and spinal cord compression. Attempts should be made rapidly to determine the wishes of the patient and family and to explore what alternatives exist.

Table 15-3   **Causes and Treatment of Delirium in End-of-Life Patients**

Cause	Treatment
Opioid toxicity	Switch to another opioid.
Sepsis	Start antibiotic therapy (with the approval of the patient or family).
Drugs	Discontinue drugs that aggravate delirium such as tricyclic antidepressants and benzodiazepines.
Dehydration	Consider intravenous hydration after consultation with the patient and family. This intervention can have undesired side effects such as increased urine output, decreased catecholamine release, increased pressure from tumors, and increased pulmonary congestion.
Metabolic disorders (hypercalcemia, uremia, hepatic failure, hyponatremia)	Correct the underlying problem when possible.
Hypoxia	Provide supplemental oxygen. This may involve simply blowing oxygen across the face.
Brain metastases	Consider corticosteroid therapy, which may provide temporary improvement.

Uncontrolled Pain

Effective pain control is possible for the vast majority of end-of-life patients. (Refer to Chapter 14 for a discussion of pain management.) If the patient is comatose or otherwise unable to verbalize, closely monitor the patient for signs of pain such as grimacing, increased restlessness, and heart rate elevation. Provide pain medication when indicated. Analgesic doses and routes are likely to be different from those used in routine practice. End-of-life patients often receive their drugs through transdermal patches, intrathecal infusions, or continuous IV drips at doses many times greater than those used for standard therapy.

Delirium

Distinguishing between pain, dementia, and delirium can be difficult. Delirious patients may moan, groan, and be restless in the absence of pain. Conversely, delirium can limit a patient's perception of and ability to express pain. Essential criteria for the diagnosis of delirium are (1) disordered attention and cognition and (2) disturbances of psychomotor behavior. Behavioral disturbances include agitation, hallucinations, and paranoia, with an acute or subacute onset and course.

Preexisting cognitive problems, such as dementia and Alzheimer's disease, may become more evident at the end of life. Delirium can be distinguished from dementia in that dementia is more likely to have a gradual onset, exist as a chronic condition, and coexist without alteration in level of consciousness. One must identify and treat the underlying cause of delirium (Table 15-3).

Agitation and hallucinations can be managed with orally or subcutaneously administered haloperidol (Haldol) to prevent patient and family expressions distress. Doses range from 1 mg (orally or subcutaneously) every 8 to 12 hours to 2 mg every 30 minutes in severe cases. The maximum dose of 20 to 30 mg/day may be necessary. If haloperidol is not effective, alternatives include methotrimeprazine (Levoprome, Nozinan) and midazolam (Versed). Discussion with the patient and family should emphasize that confusion and agitation are expression of brain malfunction and that the aim of controlling symptoms is not to prolong life but

to provide comfort. Common pitfalls in delirium management include failure to do the following:
- Recognize depression as a variant of delirium and provide antidepressants.
- Distinguish between delirium and poor pain management, subsequently aggravating the problem by giving more opioids.
- Identify urinary retention or constipation, easily treated problems that can mimic signs of delirium.

Bowel Obstruction

About 95% of patients on high-dose opioid therapy experience constipation if a prophylactic bowel regimen is not started concomitantly. Untreated constipation can progress to incomplete or complete bowel obstruction. Metastases are another common cause of obstruction. Findings associated with bowel obstruction include nausea, vomiting, abdominal pain, distention, high-pitched or absent bowel sounds, tympanic sounds on percussion, a history of infrequent bowel movements, and absence of flatus. For a limited number of patients, surgical intervention (bowel resection, gastrostomy tube insertion) may be an option. Gastric or duodenal (Miller-Abbott) tubes can provide temporary relief. Medical management with prokinetic agents such as metoclopramide (Reglan) or cisapride (Propulsid) and hyoscyamine butylbromide (Anaspaz, Gastrosed) or octreotide (Sandostatin) may be used but these agents are contraindicated in complete malignant bowel obstruction.

Spinal Cord Compression

About 5% of patients with end-stage cancer experience spinal cord compression. Treatment delays can lead to paralysis and loss of bowel and bladder control. Central back pain—worsened by movement, coughing, and straining—is the usual initial symptom and may be present for days to weeks before the onset of neurologic symptoms. Back pain is followed by progressive sensory loss, motor weakness, incontinence, reduced muscle tone, and diminished reflexes.

Plain radiographs have limited diagnostic value; magnetic resonance imaging or computed tomography scans are preferred. The initial treatment of choice is steroid therapy but radiation or surgery may be needed.

Seizures

Seizures are common in patients with cerebral tumors or meningeal involvement but may also be related to metabolic disturbances, infection, toxicity, drug withdrawal, metastases, or intracerebral hemorrhage. First seizures are upsetting to patients and families. If the patient is not going to be admitted to the hospital, provide educational information about seizure management. Active seizures may be controlled with diazepam (Valium) 10 mg IV or per rectum. Alternatively, lorazepam (Ativan) 2 mg subcutaneously or midazolam (Versed) 5 mg subcutaneously or IV can be given. To prevent future seizures, prophylactic treatment with phenytoin (Dilantin), carbamazepine (Tegretol), or valproic acid (Depakene) may be started. Drugs with a greater sedative effect, such as subcutaneously administered phenobarbital and midazolam by IV, may be required for seizures that are difficult to control.

Massive Hemorrhage

Tumors (especially of the head and neck) can infiltrate large vascular structures, producing catastrophic bleeding. Other causes of end-of-life hemorrhage include thrombocytopenia, liver failure, massive gastrointestinal bleeding, and disseminated intravascular coagulation.

Few treatment options may be available once such bleeding has started, and such bleeding is often a preterminal event. Direct pressure can minimize external bleeding. Turning the patient to the side may prevent aspiration in those with hemoptysis or hematemesis. Reducing or stopping vasopressor agents can decrease blood loss. Sedation with midazolam reduces patient anxiety over the event. Great sensitivity and support for the patient and family are needed in the face of such frightening blood loss.

DEATH NOTIFICATION AND POSTMORTEM CARE

About 75% of patients who die in the ED have family members (or other significant persons) present at the time of death or shortly thereafter. In such instances, notification of death is given face to face.[3] Depending on the circumstances, the family may or may not be prepared to receive this information. In cases of chronic progressive illnesses, families have had time to prepare for such news and may be further along in the bereavement process than the family of a patient whose death was unexpected. Witnessing the actual events and observing prehospital care may or may not provide loved ones with insight into what has happened.

Ideally, families are given the opportunity to be with the patient before death pronouncement. This has been shown to be a beneficial part of the bereavement process. With proper support and information before entering the room, family members typically do not become disruptive. Before viewing the patient, provide families with information about what they are likely to see: tubes, activities, medications, and the condition of the patient. The accompanying staff member can be a role model for families by speaking directly to and touching the dying patient.

For those with chronic illnesses, the family may choose to hold a death vigil, waiting continually at the bedside. If all treatments are stopped, a quiet private room is desirable; one without monitors, IV bags, and other medical paraphernalia. The ED is not the optimal location for such an event, and attempts should be made to facilitate transfer to an inpatient area. Unfortunately, this is not always possible. In such cases the emergency nurse should continue to monitor the patient and family regularly and offer assistance to the family such as drinks, telephones, chairs, tissues, and bathrooms. Other interventions include repositioning the patient for comfort; managing pain, seizures, and agitation; and informing the family about what the normal progression is likely to be. If the family does not choose to remain in the room, frequent updates are helpful. Ideally, loved ones can be directed to a quiet, separate location. The triage nurse, security personnel, and registration staff members also should be kept informed of any family members who are expected to arrive so that they can be intercepted and directed to the appropriate location. Many hospitals have social workers, psychiatric counselors, and even trained volunteers to help families at these times. Offering to contact the hospital chaplain or the patient's spiritual advisor also may be helpful and comforting.

When family members must be notified of a death, certain steps should be taken. A physician-and-nurse team approach works well. These individuals should be free of other distractions (e.g., pagers turned off) and then should sit down, introduce themselves, and identify the family members. The team should briefly ascertain what the current understanding of the situation is, then provide a synopsis of what occurred, and describe the result of these actions. Simple words including *died* or *dead* are appropriate. Use of euphemisms and medical jargon ("didn't respond," "coded," "flat lined," and "failed resuscitative efforts") may be confusing to the family. Ideally, the physician will stay in the room for a time to answer questions and provide support, but this is not always possible because of the needs of other patients in the department.

The emergency nurse may be left to review the events and provide essential information again, answer general questions, and present new information (e.g., medical examiner notification, the possibility of an autopsy for legal reasons, and the option of organ/tissue donation). (See Chapter 16 for discussion of organ and tissue donation.) Families may show a variety of reactions based on past experiences and cultural considerations. Often the nurse just being present and acknowledging the grief the family members are experiencing is beneficial. Silence and a gentle touch may be appropriate; however, phrases such as "I know what you are going through" or "I can imagine what you are feeling" are not helpful. Rather, statements such as "I am so sorry for your loss" or "It must be hard to accept what happened" provide openings for the family to express their grief.

If family members were not present at the death, the nurse should offer the family an opportunity to see the deceased. For families that choose cremation, this may be the last time they see their loved one. If the family accepts the offer, the nurse should excuse herself or himself to ensure that the corpse is presentable. The following preparations may be necessary:

- The body may need to be moved to another room for the department to continue to function. This also applies in situations in which family members wish to view the remains but will be delayed in arrival.
- Although certain tubes must remain in place in medical examiner cases, IV catheters, indwelling urinary catheters, and chest tubes can be plugged and made less obvious.
- Except in medical examiner cases, blood should be washed off. In some cultures and religions, the family (or other designated party) may wish to perform this activity. Familiarity with local cultures and customs is helpful. (Refer to Chapter 2 for additional discussion of cultural variations.)
- Large wounds should be covered.
- Place clean sheets and a clean gown on the body and tidy the room as much as possible.
- Dimming the lights, or aiming mobile lights away from the deceased, makes the dead person's skin appear more lifelike.
- Arms should be at the side, the jaw shut, dentures in the mouth, and eyes closed.

The nurse should prepare the family for what they will see. If the nurse touches the deceased, the nurse will model that touching is acceptable. Lower stretcher or gurney side rails and provide chairs. Determine from the family's nonverbal cues whether to stay in the room or to leave. If the family prefers to be alone, check frequently to offer assistance and answer any questions that may have arisen.

Before the family's departure, certain formalities are usually necessary, such as completion of demographic or contact information and transfer of valuables and clothing (in non–medical examiner cases). Provide the family with instruction sheets containing information related to funeral arrangements and whom to contact about the death. Any interaction with the family should be done with great sensitivity and support. A friend, neighbor, taxi driver, or even the police may be needed to help get the family members home.

Pediatric Death

The death of a child is an extremely emotional event, and families may need to spend a lot of time with the deceased child. Wrap small infants and children snugly so that parents can hold their child. Provide a rocking chair if possible. An offer to snip a lock of hair for the parents to keep may be appreciated. (This should be documented clearly in the medical record.) Some families may ask that photographs be taken and imprints made of the hands and feet.

Fetal Loss

The legal differentiation between "products of conception" and a "fetus" typically is based on weight or gestational age. Individual states may have more specific parameters. However, it is important to remember that gestational age does not predict the degree of loss experienced. The woman an emergency nurse thinks of simply as the "the woman with vag bleeding in room 3" may be, in the patient's perception, a mother whose only baby just died. Parents may request a photograph, lock of hair (if available), and imprints of the hands or feet and may desire to hold funeral services.

References

1. Monagler JF, Thomasma DC: *Health care ethics,* Gaithersburg, Md, 1998, Aspen.
2. Wilkie DJ: *Toolkit for nursing excellence at end of life transition,* Seattle, 2001, University of Washington (CD-ROM).
3. Isaacs E: Grief support in the ED. Retrieved July 30, 2003, from www.emedicine.com/emerg/topic694.htm.

16

Organ and Tissue Donation

Diana Lombardo, MSN-FNP, MHA, RN, CCRN

More than 6000 American adults and children die each year while awaiting organ transplantation. Most organ donors are individuals who suffer a traumatic brain injury, anoxic event, or stroke that causes brain death. Emergency nurses are in a key position to identify potential donors. Federal law mandates that health care professionals offer the option of organ and tissue donation to all who qualify.

In 2004 there were 14,154 deceased and living organ donors, which resulted in 27,035 transplants.[1] Nevertheless, more than 88,000 children and adults remained on waiting lists. Unfortunately, no national registry exists for potential organ donors. Even if an individual clearly makes his or her wishes known on a driver's license or donor card, in practice, family members will always be consulted before donation.

Researchers began experimenting with organ transplantation on animals and human beings in the eighteenth century. By the mid–twentieth century, successful organ replacement was a regular occurrence. Transplantation of kidneys, livers, hearts, pancreases, intestines, lungs, and heart-lung combinations now are considered routine medical treatment. Box 16-1 gives a list of transplantable tissues and organs.

In the past 20 years, important medical breakthroughs, such as tissue typing and immunosuppressant drugs, have lengthened survival and increased the number of transplants performed. Most notable was the discovery of the immunosuppressant cyclosporine, which was approved for commercial use in 1983. Box 16-2 highlights milestone events in the history of organ and tissue donation and transplantation.

Membership in the United Network for Organ Sharing is divided into 11 geographic regions (Table 16-1) to facilitate equitable organ allocation and to provide individuals the opportunity to identify concerns regarding organ procurement, allocation, and transplantation that are unique to their particular geographic area.

Box **16-1**   Transplantable Organs and Tissues

Organs	Tissues
Heart	Bone marrow
Intestines	Bones
Kidneys	Cornea
Liver	Heart valves
Lungs	Ligaments
Pancreas	Pancreatic islet cells
Spleen	Skin
	Blood
	Tendons
	Veins, arteries, nerves
	Vertebral bodies
	Lymph nodes

Box **16-2**   Timeline of Key Events in U.S. Organ and Tissue Transplantation

1954	The first successful kidney transplant is performed.
1966	The first simultaneous kidney-pancreas transplant is performed.
1967	The first successful liver transplant is performed.
1968	The first successful isolated pancreas transplant is performed.
	The Southeast Organ Procurement Foundation (SEOPF) is formed as a membership and scientific organization for transplant professionals.
1977	SEOPF implements the first computer-based organ matching system, the United Network for Organ Sharing (UNOS).
1981	The first successful heart-lung transplant is performed.
1982	SEOPF establishes the Kidney Center, the predecessor to the UNOS Organ Center.
1983	The first successful single lung transplant is performed and cyclosporine is introduced.
1984	The National Organ Transplant Act is passed.
	UNOS separates from SEOPF and is incorporated as a nonprofit organization.
1986	The first successful double lung transplant is performed.
	UNOS receives a federal contract to operate the organ procurement and transportation network.
1987	The first successful intestinal transplant is performed.
1988	The first split-liver transplant is performed.
1989	The first successful living donor lung transplant is performed.
1992	UNOS prepares the first comprehensive report on transplant survival rates.
	UNOS helps found the Coalition on Donation to build public support.
1995	UNOS launches its first Web site.
1998	The first successful living adult-adult liver transplant is performed.
1999	UNOS launches UNet, an Internet-based transplant information database for all organ matching.
2000	The U.S. Department of Health and Human Services publishes the final rule, federal regulations for the operation of the organ procurement and transplantation network.
2001	For the first time, the total number of living donors for the year (6528) exceeds the number of deceased organ donors (6081).

Table 16-1   **United Network for Organ Sharing**

Region	States and Territories
1	Connecticut, Maine, Massachusetts, New Hampshire, Rhode Island
2	Delaware, District of Columbia, Maryland, New Jersey, Pennsylvania, West Virginia
3	Alabama, Arkansas, Florida, Georgia, Louisiana, Mississippi, Puerto Rico
4	Oklahoma, Texas
5	Arizona, California, Nevada, New Mexico, Utah
6	Alaska, Hawaii, Idaho, Montana, Oregon, Washington
7	Illinois, Minnesota, North Dakota, South Dakota, Wisconsin
8	Colorado, Iowa, Kansas, Missouri, Nebraska, Wyoming
9	New York, Vermont
10	Indiana, Michigan, Ohio
11	Kentucky, North Carolina, South Carolina, Tennessee, Virginia

Box **16-3**   **Minimum Exclusion Criteria for Organ/Tissue Donation**

Unresolved septicemia
Metastatic cancer (not a barrier to eye donation)
Injectable drug use
Positive for human immunodeficiency virus infection or in a group that is at high-risk for such
  infection

GENERAL TISSUE DONOR CRITERIA

Tissue donations are derived from individuals who are brain dead and from those without a beating heart. Almost anyone who dies can donate tissue. Donor requirements change frequently; consult your local organ and tissue bank for current criteria. Box 16-3 summarizes the minimal exclusion criteria for organ and tissue donation. Procurement specialists are always available to assist with evaluation of potential donors. These individuals also are willing to talk to family members who are considering donating the "gift of life." The procurement specialist can anticipate and answer most questions or concerns related to donation. Table 16-2 highlights the critical pathway for organ donation.

WEST NILE VIRUS

Recently, several cases of West Nile virus transmission have been reported following organ transplantation. The benefits of transplantation still outweigh the minimal risk of West Nile virus transmission. Nonetheless, the Centers for Disease Control and Prevention recommend that clinicians and their patients be aware of the potential risks of this disease.

Cultural Aspects

When caring for a potential donor, health care providers must consider the family's cultural, religious, and emotional situation. Contrary to widely held beliefs, the majority of the major religions approve of organ and tissue donation and consider donation the greatest gift. Families should be offered the option of donating organs. In August 1998 the Centers for Medicare

Table **16-2**   **Critical Pathway for Organ Donation**

Phase	Action
I	Referral of a potential donor
II	Declaration of brain death (Obtain donation consent.)
III	Donor evaluation
IV	Donor management
V	Recovery phase

Box **16-4**   **Criteria for Determination of Brain Death**

1. A person with irreversible cessation of circulatory and respiratory function is dead.
   a. Cessation is recognized by clinical examination and criteria.
   b. Irreversibility is recognized by persistent cessation of all functions during a period of observation, trial of therapy, or both.
2. A person with irreversible cessation of all functions of the entire brain, including the brainstem is dead.
   a. Cessation is recognized when evaluation discloses the following:
      i. Cerebral functions are absent.
      ii. Brainstem reflexes (pupillary, corneal, gag) are absent.
   b. Irreversibility is recognized when evaluation discloses the following:
      i. Reversible conditions such as hypothermia and hyponatremia have been corrected and the vital signs are hemodynamically stable.
      ii. The cause of the coma is established and is sufficient to account for loss of brain function.
      iii. The possibility of brain function recovery is excluded.
      iv. Cessation of all brain functions persists for an appropriate period of observation, trial of therapy, or both.[1]

From Uniform Determination of Death Act, 1978.

and Medicaid Services published their final rule on organ donation. This rule contains two key provisions:
1. Hospitals must contact their organ procurement organization in a timely manner about any individual who dies in the hospital or whose death is imminent.
2. Only organ procurement organization staff or trained hospital staff members may approach the patient's family about organ donation.

DETERMINATION OF DEATH FOR ORGAN DONATION

The Uniform Determination of Death Act (1978) plays an integral role in identifying criteria that must be met to determine brain death (Box 16-4). It is important to note that, emergency nurses can help family members understand that patients who are brain dead *are* dead and not in some separate or potentially recoverable state.

Once brain death is determined, the date and time of death must be documented in the medical record. The physician notifies the family of death, but the organ procurement coordinator is the person who obtains signed consent from the family and reviews the patient's medical and social history. Figure 16-1 provides a sample consent form. Conditions that require medical examiner notification vary from state to state but commonly include (1) homicide, (2) suicide, (3) accidental death, (4) death within 24 hours of admission, (5) patients admitted

---

ANATOMICAL GIFT BY A RELATIVE OR THE GUARDIAN OF THE PERSON OF A DECEDENT

I hereby make this anatomical gift from the body of _____
(Name)

who died on _____ in _____
(Date)   (City and state)

The marks in the appropriate squares and the words filled in the blanks below indicate my relationship to the decedent and my desires respecting the anatomical gift.

1. I survive the decedent as: ☐ Adult brother or sister
   ☐ Spouse   ☐ Grandparent
   ☐ Adult son or daughter   ☐ Guardian of the person
   ☐ Parent   ☐ Person authorized to dispose of the body

2. I hereby give the following body parts:
   ☐ Heart   ☐ Heart valves (heart)   ☐ Eyes
   ☐ Liver   ☐ Skin grafts   ☐ Ribs
   ☐ Kidneys   ☐ Long bone segments   ☐ Tendons
   ☐ Pancreas   ☐ Iliac crest (hip bone segments) ☐ Ligaments
   ☐ Lungs   ☐ Small bones (humerus, etc.) ☐ Veins, arteries, nerves
   ☐ Small bowel   ☐ Soft tissue (fascia, etc.) ☐ Vertebral bodies (bone marrow)
   ☐ Spleen, lymph nodes, and vessels

3. To the following person (or institution): _____

4. For the following purposes:
   ☐ Any purposes authorized by law ☐ Therapy
   ☐ Transplantation   ☐ Medical research and education

5. I give consent for the release of any medical information necessary for these donations.

6. I give consent for infectious disease tests to be performed with blood, spleen, or lymph nodes for the detection of transmissible diseases, including but not limited to: HIV, HTLV, hepatitis, and syphilis. If positive tests are reported, I am aware that I will be notified, as well as appropriate health officials.

7. After the donated organs, tissues, or eyes are removed, the remains of the body shall be disposed in the following manner: _____; at the expense and responsibility of the following persons: _____

_____   _____
Date   City and state

_____   _____
Witness   Signature of survivor

_____   _____
Witness   Address of survivor

Executed in triplicate:
    Original retained on donor's chart
    1 copy accompanies donated organs/tissue
    1 copy available for family at their request

Anatomical Gift by a Relative or the Guardian of the
Person of a Decedent, CL-105-2
H:\clinical policies\noteform\105-2.doc
Revised 9/24/2001

Figure 16-1. Consent form for donation of anatomical gift. (Courtesy Lifeline of Ohio, 2000).

in a comatose state, and (6) death of a minor. These conditions do no necessarily exclude donation, and many medical examiners will act quickly to release the body. Because these patients are dead, their care and management does not have to be directed by a physician. Orders written by authorized transplant coordinators are valid and should be followed. The procurement coordinator will need to do the following:

- Collect blood for serologic testing for HIV, hepatitis, syphilis, and cytomegalovirus.
- Obtain lymph nodes or blood for tissue typing.
- Inform the surgical team of a pending donation.
- Notify the appropriate institution or facility supervisor of a potential donor.
- Determine chest and abdominal circumference.
- Obtain a cardiology consult.
- Ascertain which organs are available for transplant.
- Initiate and direct a postmortem patient management protocol.

DONOR MANAGEMENT

In most settings, donor management occurs in the intensive care unit. However, there will be times and situations when the emergency nurse must initiate the process. In general, initial evaluation of a potential organ donor includes the following:

- Age and social/medical history
- Assessment of family dynamics
- Accurate weight
- Blood type
- Complete blood count with differential
- Full blood chemistry studies including liver function tests
- Arterial blood gases on the current ventilator settings
- Serial vital signs with hourly (or more frequent) calculation of intake and output (Table 16-3 summarizes the target hemodynamic parameters for organ procurement in adults.)
- Monitoring and evaluation for septicemia
- Management of the complications associated with loss of cerebral function:
  - Neurogenic diabetes insipidus
  - Neurogenic pulmonary edema
  - Neurogenic shock
  - Neurogenic hypothermia

Table 16-3   Hemodynamic Parameters for Organ Procurement (Adults)

Parameter	Value
Systolic blood pressure	>100 mm Hg
Pao_2	>100 mm Hg
Sao_2	>95%
Central venous pressure	5-15 mm Hg
Urine output	100 to 500 mL/hr
Hematocrit	>25%
Temperature	35°-39° C (95°-102° F)

From Newberry L, editor: *Sheehy's emergency nusring principles and practice*, ed 5, St Louis, 2003, Mosby.

- Consent for organ donation
  The Uniform Anatomical Gift Act recommends the following order of priority for relatives asked to consent to donation:
- Spouse
- Adult son or daughter
- Either parent
- Adult brother or sister
- Grandparent
- Legal guardian

THE PROCUREMENT PROCESS

Tissue procurement (eyes, corneas, bone, heart valves, and skin) can occur up to 10 hours following asystole, but shorter intervals are preferable. Ideally, the body should be kept in a refrigerated room. If the eyes are to be donated, elevate the patient's head 20 degrees and tape the eyelids shut with paper tape. Ice applied to the eyelids reduces edema and facilitates the recovery process. Enucleation is performed as a clean procedure using sterile technique. This process takes about 30 minutes and does not require an operating room. The entire globe may be recovered, or surface tissue can be recovered with a corneal punch procedure. Corneas are usually transplanted within 24 to 48 hours.[2]

Recovery of solid organs (beating heart patients) occurs in the operating room and can require multiple teams, depending on how many organs will be recovered. The process to prepare the patient for organ recovery is in-depth, time-consuming, and requires the use of valuable resources. One should note that the patient's family will not be billed for any medical costs related to donation or recovery. Once the patient becomes a donor candidate, the recipient, the recipient's insurance, Medicaid, or Medicare pays all costs. To facilitate this shift in billing, most facilities generate a new account number for the patient once the consent to donate has been signed.

Reference

1. The Organ Procurement and Transplantation Network: *Data*. Retrieved May 22, 2005 from www.optn.org.
2. Campbell CE: Organ and tissue donation. In Newberry L, editor: *Sheehy's emergency nursing: principles and practice*, ed 5, St Louis, 2003, Mosby.

17

Complementary and Alternative Therapies

Reneé Semonin Holleran, RN, PhD, CEN, CCRN, CFRN

The use of complementary and alternative therapies (CAT), also referred to as complementary and alternative medicine (CAM) is not new to the management of health and well-being. The traditions of acupuncture, herbal therapy, and ayurvedic medicine are thousands of years old. The majority of persons in this world use what Western (allopathic) medicine would consider "alternative" approaches to the cure of disease and other disorders. (See Chapter 2 for a discussion of human diversity and health care.) Because of this, emergency nurses undoubtedly will encounter patients using alternative methods to manage their health problems.

Only in recent years has contemporary Western medicine been challenged to base practice on evidence. This drive toward evidence-based medicine has made it clear that drawing a clear distinction between contemporary medicine and complementary practices is in fact irrelevant. Rather, there are simply evidence-based practices and there is everything else—whether contemporary or complementary—and practitioners need to be open to all effective therapies.

A panel established by the National Center for Complementary and Alternative Medicine at the National Institutes of Health described CAT as a broad domain of healing resources that encompasses health systems, modalities, and practices and their accompanying theories and beliefs other than those intrinsic to the dominant health system of a particular society or culture at a given historical period.[1] Table 17-1 summarizes some of the CAT that may be used by patients presenting to the emergency department (ED).[2]

Multiple studies have reported that the majority of patients use some sort of complementary or alternative therapy to manage their health.[2,4-8] Snyder and Lindquist[3] cited several factors that have contributed to the use of CAT in the United States. These factors include the following:

- An increase in the number of immigrants from areas of the world where alternative therapies are routine
- A belief (and continued evidence) that biomedical treatments do not always take care of a patient's problems
- A wish to avoid the side effects of medications used to treat some illnesses, such as chemotherapy

Table 17-1   **National Center for Complementary and Alternative Medicine: Classification of Therapies**

Therapies	Examples
Mind-Body Therapies	
Behavioral, psychological, social, and spiritual approaches to health and healing	Yoga, tai chi, meditation, guided imagery, hypnosis, biofeedback, group therapy, music therapy, dance therapy, use of a journal, prayer, prayer circles, humor, sweat lodges, soul retrieval, and faith healing
Alternative Medical Systems	
Systems of theory and practice developed outside of Western medicine	Traditional Chinese medicine including herbal therapy and acupuncture, Native American medicine, ayurvedic medicine, traditional African medicine, traditional aboriginal medicine, homeopathy, Wiccan practices, naturopathy, "local" healers, curanderos
Biological-Based Therapies	
"Natural" and biological-based Practices, interventions, and products	Herbs, animal parts, special diet therapies, nutritional counseling, bee pollen, bee stings, aromatherapy, electrodiagnostics, iridology
Manipulative and Body-Based Systems	
Systems based on manipulation or movement of the body	Chiropractic medicine, massage, Trager body work, Alexander technique, acupressure, hydrotherapy, color therapy, colonics
Energy Therapies	
Systems that use energy to heal	Therapeutic touch, healing touch, natural healing, Reiki, magnets, crystals, pyramids

Data from Hageness S, Kreitzer MJ, Kinney ME: Complementary, integrative and holistic care in emergency nursing, *Nurs Clin North Am* 37(1):123-133, 2002; and Snyder M, Lindquist R: Issues in complementary therapies: how we got where we are, *Online J Issues Nurs* 6(2):1, 2001.

- A desire to work with care providers who listen and pay attention to the individual
- A longing to be treated in a holistic manner
- A need to have input and control over one's own health care
- Evidence-based research that has demonstrated the effectiveness of certain therapies
- A preference for magical thinking versus scientific thought

Historically, emergency nurses have recognized that the patient's body, mind, and spirit cannot be separated. These systems continually interact, and when one is affected, reactions occur in the other systems. For example, for the patient who has suffered physical injury from a sexual assault, sutures and sedatives will not heal all the wounds from this trauma. The limitations and the sometimes serious consequences of Western medicine are becoming more and more evident. In response, patients are turning to CAT.

PATIENT HISTORY RELATED TO COMPLEMENTARY AND ALTERNATIVE THERAPIES

Patients may not realize the importance of providing information regarding CAT use to their health care providers, or they simply may forget to mention nonprescribed therapies.

Therefore the emergency nurse needs to inquire about CAT use. Consider the following questions when asking patients about CAT:
- Are there patient factors present that may contribute to the use of CAT versus contemporary medicine?
  - Ethnicity or country of origin
  - Religious or spiritual beliefs
- What over-the-counter medications, herbs, or remedies is the patient currently taking?
- Has the patient or family sought advice from an alternative healer? What type of healer?
  - What advice or treatment was prescribed?
  - Has the patient tried the treatment or taken prescribed medications? For how long?
- If treatments were stopped, when and why?

Also assess for signs and symptoms known to be related to problems with certain CAT drugs, including the following:
- Abdominal pain (associated with CAT drug toxicity)
- Agitation
- Anxiety
- Confusion
- Fatigue
- Headache
- Hypertension
- Nausea and vomiting
- Palpitations
- Pruritus
- Psychosis
- Skin discoloration
- Tachycardia

When performing a physical assessment, observe for evidence of CAT treatments or beliefs such as the following:
- Presence of creams or poultices
- Significant tattoos or body markings
- Symbolic jewelry, icons, or amulets
- Pattern bruising or trauma to the skin (e.g., marks made by cupping or coining, especially on the back and buttocks)
- Jaundice (associated with drug-induced liver failure)

INTERACTIONS AND TOXICITIES

Herbal (may or may not contain herbs), supplemental, or natural therapies have become common in the United States. An estimated 60% to 70% of the population has taken or routinely takes at least one of these products.[9] More than 30,000 over-the-counter products contain herbs, vitamins, minerals, and a wide variety of other active and inactive ingredients. Some products can cause toxicity or produce potentially serious problems when they interact with prescribed medications (Table 17-2). Unlike the arduous Food and Drug Administration testing processes that prescription medications are required to undergo, supplement manufacturers are under no obligation to prove the efficacy or safety of their products. In addition, there are no quality assurance requirements to guarantee that what the patient has purchased is actually what its maker claims it is. "Natural" products (e.g., homeopathy drugs) purposely can contain or can be contaminated with potentially deadly ingredients such as arsenic or lead. These toxic ingredients may be what brings the patient to the ED for treatment.

Table 17-2   Drug-Herb Interactions: "Do Not Take Together"

Herbal Product	If Drug/Vitamin/Mineral Product Contains	Results In
Internal aloe vera, soaked flax seeds, fenugreek, sarsaparilla, slippery elm, plantain, psyllium seeds (Metamucil), marshmallow	All drugs	Binds with drugs, separate by at least 2 hr.[1,10,25]
Flaxseed	With niacin	Increases flushing.[1,11]
Evening primrose oil	Phenothiazines	Increased likelihood of seizures.[1, 11]
Bilberry fruit, bromelain, chamomile, chondroitin, cinchona bark, dan shen, devils claw[1], dong quai, fenugreek, feverfew, garlic, ginger,[6] gingko,[1] ginseng (Asian, American), goldenseal, guarana,[5] horse chestnut, huang qin, meadowsweet, MSM, pau d'arco, papain, red clover, shiitake (water-soluble extracts), turmeric, vitamin E (above 2000 international units), willow bark, fish oils[7]	Warfarin (Coumadin), low molecular weight heparin, and maybe aspirin	Increases bleeding tendency. May elevate International Normalized Ratio (INR), alters bleeding times.[10] Stop herbs at least 7 days before surgery.[23,25] Platelet aggregation inhibitors. May inhibit thromboxane synthesis.[5]
Coenzyme Q10, ginseng	Coumadin	May increase effects of Coumadin; therefore, more prone to clotting.[1]
Bittermelon, burdock, chromium picolinate, fenugreek, garlic, ginseng (Asian, American), gymnema, psyllium seeds	Antidiabetic drugs	May increase likelihood of hypoglycemia.[11]
Vitex	Estrogen	Do not use together.[1,9,10,11,20]
Black cohosh	Estrogen	Probably safe.[9,11,35]
Dong quai	Estrogen	Unknown effect—do not use together.[9,11]
Licorice	Estrogen	Safe together.[1,9,11]
Flax, soy	Estrogen	Safe together.[9,11]
Ginseng (Asian)	Coffee, tea, cola	Increased stimulation, tachycardia, hypertension.[10]
Ginseng (Asian)	Antipsychotics, MAOI	May increase insomnia, headache, tremulousness.[10]
Ginseng (Asian)	Corticosteroids	May potentiate medications or increases side effects.[10]
Ginseng (Asian), guarana	Phenelzine sulfate (Nardil) and other MAOIs	Increases likelihood of headache, tremulousness, and manic episodes; increases blood pressure.[9,10]
Hawthorn, ginseng, dan shen	Digoxin	Increases likelihood of digitalis toxicity or may interfere with effectiveness.[1,4,11,28]
Ginseng (Korean), licorice	Beta lockers	Reduces effectiveness of beta blockers; do not use together.[4]
Ginseng (Siberian)	Digoxin	May falsely elevate digoxin levels.[1,4]
Cranberry	Ura Ursi	Reduce each others effectiveness.[10,25]

Table 17-2   Drug-Herb Interactions: "Do Not Take Together"—cont'd

Herbal Product	If Drug/Vitamin/Mineral Product Contains	Results In
Licorice, uzara root, ginseng (Siberian) (?), buckhorn (bark/berry)	Digoxin	May interfere with both monitoring and its pharmacodynamic activity.[25]
Aloe (latex), buckthorn, cascara sagrada, castor bean, horsetail, licorice, rhubarb, senna	Cardiac glycosides, antidysrhythmics, diuretics, or laxatives	All increase K^+ loss, and all listed drugs may have increased toxicity and lead to confusion, weakness, and dysrhythmia.[4,10,31]
Licorice	Corticosteroids	Interferes with β-reductase, thus steroid reduces elimination, increasing side effects and toxic effects.[1]
Valerian	Sedatives	May intensify effects.[8]
Valerian	Metronidazole (Flagyl), sleeping pills of any kind	Wake up hung over and groggy.[5]
Blue cohosh	Nitrates and Ca^{++} channel blockers	Theoretically, may antagonize the hypotensive effect. Use cautiously together.[25,28,31]
Guggul as guggulipid	Beta blockers, with Ca^{++} channel blockers	May diminish the effectiveness of drugs.[10,25]
Hawthorn, guarana	Beta blockers	May potentiate.[28,31]
Plantain, psyllium	Lithium, carbamazepine	May reduce absorption; separate by 2 hr.[25,28]
Diuretic herbs: dandelion (often found in products to treat PMS, diet products)	Antihypertensives, diuretics	Avoid concurrent use. May potentiate effects (but not K^+ loss as dandelion contains K^+). Avoid concurrent use.[10,11,25]
Thiazide, diuretics	Guarana, licorice	Increases urinary secretion of K^+. Cautious use together.[5,4] Increases urinary secretion of K^+. Could be a problem after 4–6 wk of continuous use. Do not use licorice in doses of 100 mg/day with thiazides. Monitor K^+ levels.[5]
Yohimbe	Diuretics	May interfere with effectiveness.[5]
St. John's wort 5-Hydroxytryptophan	Cough and cold products containing dextromethoraphan; all SSRIs	Increases likelihood of serotonin syndrome.[14,15,18]
Alfalfa, St. John's wort, motherwort, parsley, celery	Chlorpromazine, tetracycline	Increased photosensitivity.[11,14,15,18]
St. John's wort, saw palmetto	Iron	Tannic acids in both herbs may inhibit the absorption of iron. Separate by at least 2 hr.[18]
St. John's wort ashwagandha, kava kava, California poppy, gotu kola, hops, valerian, black cohosh, German chamomile, motherwort, passion flower, SAMe	Alcohol, barbiturates, benzodiazepines	Synergistic effect and increases sedative effect; may result in coma.[11,12,14,29,30]
Valerian	Barbituates	Enhanced sedation.[1,5,25]

Continued

Table 17-2   Drug-Herb Interactions: "Do Not Take Together"—cont'd

Herbal Product	If Drug/Vitamin/Mineral Product Contains	Results In
Schisandra	Pentobarbitol, barbitol	Use cautiously together; may have increased sedation.[28]
Dan shen	Caffeine, amphetamines	
Ashwagandha		May antagonize CNS-stimulating effect.[1]
Evening primrose oil, ginkgo, kava, St. John's wort	Anticonvulsants	May interfere with seizure control.[5]
Alfalfa, green tea[8,9,10]	Coumadin	Green tea source of vitamin K; be consistent with intake.
Blue cohosh, lobelia	Nicotine patches	May increase side effects or potentiate patches. Cautious use together.[1]
Kava kava	All anti-Parkinson's drugs	Increased tremor; medications less effective. Do not use together.[29,30]
Kava kava	Risperidone, codeine	Potentiates hallucinogen effects of drug.[8,30,29] Potentiates CNS effects. Avoid with higher doses of opiates.[29,30]
Vitamin C, kava kava, St. John's wort, yohimbe	Tricyclics	Decreases effectiveness, Potentiates and increases side effects.[10,18,20]
Hops, kava kava, passion flower	Hydroxyzine HCL, visteral (Atarax), hydroxyzine pamoate, loratadine (Claritin)	May, in combination, have sedative action and exacerbate drowsiness and fatigue side effects.[10,3,30]
Tumeric, willow	NSAIDs	May increase bleeding and increase GI irritation.[1]
Selenium, vitamin C, fiber	Zinc	Decreases zinc absorption.[13]
Ma huang (ephedra)* (½ L 5.2 hr)	Cardiac glycosides and anesthetics	Increased likelihood of dysrhythmias.[8] Hemodynamic instability; increases risks of MI and stroke.[2]
Ma huang (ephedra)*	Quanethidine, stimulants, MAOIs, decongestants, guarana, antianginals	Enhances sympathetic activity; increases blood pressure[8]; increases angina.[1]
Ma huang (ephedra)*	Beta blockers, theophylline, antidepressants, and all antihypertensives	Possible hypertensive crisis; elevation of blood pressure; tachycardia; and increased anxiety.[8,34]
Hawthorn	Anesthetics	Theoretically, enhances hypotension.[22,23,32,34]
Night shade vegetables	Muscle relaxants	Enhances side effects; interferes with two enzymes that break down muscle relaxants and anesthetics.[11,32]
Arnica, golden seal, kava, licorice, yohimbe Asian ginseng, fenugreek	Antihypertensives	Interferes with blood pressure control.[1,4,23,29]
Cat's claw, black cohosh, hawthorn	Antihypertensives	May potentiate activity and increase risk of hypotension.[4,31]
Arnica	Antihypertensives	May reduce effectiveness of drugs.[4,10,30]
Most tinctures	Metronidazole (Flagyl)	Anabuse reaction.[1,11]

*Banned in the United States in 2004.

Table **17-2**   **Drug-Herb Interactions: "Do Not Take Together"—cont'd**

Herbal Product	If Drug/Vitamin/Mineral Product Contains	Results In
Flax seeds, aloe, senna, yellow dock	Laxatives	Potentiates laxative effect.[13]
Red yeast rice, echinacea, astragalus, licorice, alfalfa	Cholesterol-lowering drugs	Potentiates side effects of drugs[11]; may interfere with drugs effectiveness.[1,2]
St. John's wort	Cyclosporine (Sandimmune)	May decrease activity and increase risk of rejection; may increase activity of hepatitic enzyme CYP3A4, thus lowering levels of drug.[3,8,12,17,18,21,24,27]
St. John's wort	Indinavir (Crixivan) and other non-nucleoside inhibitors	Irinotecan (Camptosar) (chemotherapy drug). One study has found reduced levels of drug thereby increases drug resistance and treatment failure. More study is necessary.[12,14,18,19,21,26,27]
St. John's wort	Digoxin	Decreases digoxin serum level by as much as 25%. May reduce efficacy; do not use concurrently.[5,12,13,14,27]
St. John's wort	Theophylline, amitriptyline (Elavil)	Worsening of asthma symptoms; same possible mechanism as noted above. Worsening of depression; same mechanism as above.[8,14,21,24,27]
St. John's wort	Estrogen (BCP), selective serotonin reuptake inhibitors (SSRIs)	Breakthrough bleeding.[12,24] Increased incidence of serotonin syndrome. Lethargy, confusion, muscle stiffness.[12,14,21,24,27]
St. John's wort	Irinotecan (Camptosar) (chemotherapy drug)	Blood levels of the drug dropped significantly in participants when the herb was in their system compared to when it was not.[8,14,21,24,27,28,33]
Guarana [8,9,10]	Respiratory drugs Digoxin Lithium Adenosine (Adenocard) Benzodiazepines	Increased likelihood of side effects as guarana contains theophylline; do not use concurrently. May increase sensitivity to digoxin with prolonged use due to increased K^+ excretion.[4,5,31] May inhibit clearance of lithium; do not use concurrently. May lower response; do not use concurrently.[31] Drugs may be less effective; do not use concurrently.[25]
Devil's claw	Antidysrhythmics	Possibly interfere with drug activity.[2,32]
Lemon balm, bugleweed	Thyroid drugs	Interferes with thyroid hormone.[11]
Nettles	Diuretics Calcium carbonate and other antacids Chromium carbonate and other antacids	Reduces absorption.[10]

Continued

Table 17-2   Drug-Herb Interactions: "Do Not Take Together"—cont'd

Herbal Product	If Drug/Vitamin/Mineral Product Contains	Results In
5-Hydroxytrypotan	All antidepressants; anti-Parkinson's drugs, barbiturates; all tranquilizers, weight loss products, antihistamines, cold medications, alcohol, chemotherapy, antibiotics	All may be potentiated—particularly their side effects; do not take concurrently.[14,25]
Bromelain[8,15]	Antibiotics	Improves effectiveness and efficacy of drugs.[1]
Echinacea	Immunosuppressive drugs	No concrete evidence of interaction, but caution is advised.[25]
Garlic, ginger	Antacids	May decrease effectiveness of drug; increases gastric secretory activity.[4,25]
Gingko biloba	SSRIs	May reduce sexual dysfunction associated with drug; safe together.[5]

Contraindicated Herbs

Moderate or occasional consumption of herbs is safe even if they are "contraindicated." However, when products (aloe, senna, cascara, comfrey) are used daily for many years, severe complications such as cancer may result.

Contraindicated In	Rationale	Herbs
Women with estrogen-positive tumors	Tumor growth may increase.	Ginseng? Dong quai?
Persons who are hypothyroid	Thyroid hormones are antagonized.[2]	Lemon balm, bugle weed, horseradish
Asthmatics who are taking methylxanthines	Toxicity increases.	Ma hang[†]
Patients with schizophrenia	Symptoms may worsen.	Yohimbe, ginseng
Persons with diabetes	Blood glucose control may be more difficult; more likely to cause hypoglycemia	Ginseng (Asian), aloe, marshmellow, flax seed, psyllium, fenugreek, bilberry leaves, stinging nettle
Allergic sensitivity	Exacerbations may occur	Blessed thistle, burdock, chamomile, dandelion, feverfew, chicory, mug wort, papaya, yarrow leaves
Persons with liver disease	As these herbs are hepatotoxic.*	Sassafras, borage (not the oil), chaparral, coltsfeet, comfrey, eucalyptus

*Pittler MH, Ernst E: Systematic review: hepatotoxic events associated with herbal medicinal products, *Aliment Pharmacol Ther* 18(5):451-71, 2003.
†Banned in the United States in 2004.

Table 17-2   Drug-Herb Interactions: "Do Not Take Together"—cont'd

| Persons with hypertension | Blood pressure may be elevated. | Asian ginseng, lobelia (due to a adrenergic activity), night blooming cereus |
| Persons with Parkinson's disease | Tremor may be increased. | Kava kava[29,30] |

Herbs Contraindicated During Pregnancy

Abortifacients (may cause abortion)	Uterine stimulants (may cause uterine contractions)	Teratogenic (may cause birth defects)
Aloe exudates (*Aloe*)	Arnica flowers (*Arnica montana*)	Betelnut seeds (*Areca catechu*)
Black pepper fruit (*Piper nigrum*)	Barberry root bark (*Berberis vulgaris*)	Cinchona bark (*Cinchona* spp.)
Blue cohosh (*Caulophyllum root*)	California poppy plant (*Eschscholizia californica*)	Mayapple root/rhizome (*Podophyllum peltatum*)
Calendula flowers (*Calendula officinalis*)	Juniper berries (*Juniperus communis*)	Periwinkle plant (*Vinca rosea*)
Catnip leaves and flowers (*Nepta cataria*)	Ma huang plant (*Ephedra sinica*)	Rauwolfia root (*Rauwolfia serpentaria*)
Chamomile—Roman (*Anthemis nobilis*)	Milk thistle seed (*Silybum marianum*)	Tobacco leaves (*Nicotiana tabacum*)
Chicory root (*Chichorium intybies*)	Mistletoe plant (*Viscien album*)	Wild cherry bark (*Prunus serotina*)
Coltsfoot leaves (*Tussilago farara*)	Motherwort plant (*Leonurus cardiaca*)	
Fenugreek seed (*Trigonella foenum-graecum*)	Mug wort plant (*Artemisia vulgaris*)	
Ginger rhizome (*Zingiber officinale*)	Passion flower leaves (*Passifora incarnata*)	
Gotu kola plant (*Centella asiatica*)	Poke week root (*Phytolacca Americana*)	
Hyssop plant (*Hyssopus officinalis*)	Pulsatilla plant (*Anemore pulsatilla*)	
Mustard seed (*Brassica nigra*)	Senna leaves/pods (*Cassia acutifolia*)	
Nutmeg seeds (*Myristica fragrans*)	Shepard's purse plant (*Capsilla bursa–pastoris*)	
Pennyroyal plant (*Hedeoma pulegroides*)	St. John's wort plant (*Hypericum perforatum*)	
Periwinkle plant (*Vinca rosea*)	Yellow jasmine plant (*Gelsemium sempervirens*)	
Sandalwood wood (*Santalum album*)		
Shepard's purse plant (*Capsella bursa–pastoris*)		
St. John's wort plant (*Hypericum perforatum*)		
Stinging nettles plant (*Urtica* spp.)		
Tansy leaves (*Tanacetum vulgare*)		

Continued

Table 17-2   Drug-Herb Interactions: "Do Not Take Together"—cont'd

Herbs Contraindicated While Breast Feeding

Alkanet root *(Alkanna tinctoria)* H
Aloes dried leaf sap* *(Aloe spp.)* L, G
Basil plant *(Ocimum basilcum)* G
Black cohosh roots/rhizome**(Cimicifuga racemosa)* I
Bladderwrack thallus *(Fucus vesiculosus)* T
Borage leaves *(Borago officinalis)* H
Buckthorn fruit* *(Rhammus catharticus)* L, G
Bugleweed leaves *(Lycopus spp.)* AG
Butterbur rhizome* *(Petasites hybridus)* H
Cascara sagrada bark* *(Rhamnus purshiana)* L, G
Chaparral leaves *(Larrea tridentata, Larrea divaricata)*

Cinchona bark* *(Cinchona spp.)* T

Cocoa seeds *(Theobroma cacao)* S
Coffee seeds* *(Coffea arabica)* S
Cola seeds *(Cola nitida, Cola acuminata)* S
Colocynth fruit pulp* *(Citrullus colocynthis)* L, T
Coltsfoot leaves* *(Tussilago farfara)* H
Comfrey root and leaves* *(Symphytum officinale)* H
Dulse thallus *(Rhodymenia palmetto)* T
Elecampane roots *(Imula helenium)* T
Frangula bark* *(Rhammus frangula)* L, G
Guarana seeds *(Paullinia cupana)* S
Hemp agrimony plant* *(Eupatorium cannabimum)* H
Jasmin flowers *(Jasminum pubescens)* AG

Joe Pye weed root* *(Eupatorium purpureum)* H
Kava root* *(Piper methysticum)* T
Kelp thallus *(Nereocystis luetkeana)* T
Levant wormseed plant* *(Artemisia cina)* T
Licorice root* *(Glycyrrhiza glabra)* T
Life root plant* *(Senecio aureus)* H
Ma huang plant* *(Ephedra sinica)* S
Madder root *(Rubia tinctorum)* G
Male fern rhizome* *(Dryopteris filix-mas)* T
Mate leaves *(Ilex paraguayensis)* S
Meadow saffron corm and seed*
   (Colchicum autumnale) T
Prickly ash bark *(Zanthoxylum americanum,*
   Zanthoxylum clava-herculis) I

Pulsatilla plant* *(Anemone pulsatilla)* I
Queen's root *(Stillingia sylvatica)*
Rhubarb root* *(Rheum palmatum, Rheum officinale)* L, G
Rockweed thallus *(Fucus spp.)* T
Sage leaves* *(Salvia officinalis)* AG
Seaweed thallus *(Laminaria spp.)* T
Senna leaves and pods[a],* *(Cassia spp.)* L, G
Tea leaves *(Camellia sinensis)* S
Tobacco leaves* *(Nicotiana tabacum)* T
Wintergreen leaves* *(Gaultheria procumbens)* T

From Brinker F: *Herb contraindications and drug interactions*, 2nd ed, Sandy, Ore, 2002, Eclectic Medical Publications. With permission from Kuhn M: *Complementary Therapy-Gram* 2:1, 1999, with modifications, 2004.
AG, Antigalactagogue; *G*, Genotoxin; *H*, Hepatic pyrrolizidine; *I*, Irritant; *L*, laxative; *S*, stimulant; *T*, toxic.
[a]Studies indicate that insufficient quantities of the major active metabolite, rhein, from senna are excreted in the breast milk of monkeys or humans to produce a laxative effect. No clinical effect on nursing infants was found when 50 mothers were given laxative doses of standardized senna.

Bibliography for drug/herb interactions

1. Zhou S et al: Predicting pharmacokinetic herb-drug interactions, *Drug Metabol Drug Interact* 20(3):143-58, 2004.
2. Kuhn M, Winston D: Herbal therapies & supplements: a traditional & scientific approach, Philadelphia, 2001, JB Lippincott.
3. Smith M: Drug interactions with natural health products/dietary supplements: a survival guide. Paper presented at Complementary and Alternative Medicine: Implications for Clinical Proactice and State-of-the-Science Symposia; March 12, 2000; Boston.
4. Kuhn M: Complementary therapies for health care providers, Philadelphia, 1999, JB Lippincott.
5. Myers SP, Cheras PA: The other side of the coin: safety of complementary and alternative medicine, *Med J Aust* 181(4):222-225, 2004.

Table **17-2**   **Drug-Herb Interactions: "Do Not Take Together"—cont'd**

6. Lumb AB: Effect of ginger on human platelet function, *Thromb Haemost* 71:110-111, 1994.
7. Buckley MS, Goff AD, Knapp WE. Fish oil interaction with warfarin, *Ann Pharmacother* 38(1):50-52, 2004.
8. Brinker F: Herb and drug contraindication and interaction, ed 2, Sandy, Ore, 2001, Eclectic Institute, Inc.
9. Shader RI, Greenblatt DJ: More on oral contraceptives, drug interactions, herbal medicines, and hormone replacement therapy, *J Clin Psychopharmacol* 20(4):397-398, 2000.
10. Ernst E: Possible interactions between synthetic and herbal medicinal products. Part 1, *Perfusion* 13:4-15, 2000.
11. Brazier NC, Levine MA: Drug-herb interaction among commonly used conventional medicines: a compendium for health care professionals, *Am J Ther* 10(3):163-169, 2003.
12. Ernst E: Interactions between synthetic and herbal medicinal products. Part 2, *Perfusion* 13:60-70, 2000.
13. Fugh-Berman A: Herb-drug interactions, *Lancet* 355(9198):134-138, 2000.
14. Mannel M: Drug interactions with St John's wort: mechanisms and clinical implications, *Drug Saf* 27(11):773-797, 2004.
15. Markowitz JS, DeVane CL: The emerging recognition of herb-drug interactions, with a focus on St. John's wort (Hypericum perforatum), *Psychopharmacol Bull* 35(1):53-64, 2001.
16. Wojcikowski K, Johnson DW, Gobe G: Medicinal herbal extracts-renal friend or foe? Part 1. The toxicities of medicinal herbs, *Nephrology (Carlton)* 9(5):313-318, 2004.
17. Mai I al: Hazardous pharmacokinetic interaction of St. John's wort (Hypericum perforatum) with the immunosuppressant cyclosporine. *Int J Clin Pharmacol Ther* 38(10):500-502, 2000.
18. Mills E et al: Interaction of St. John's wort with conventional drugs: systemic review of clinical trials, *BMJ* 329(7456):27-30, 2004.
19. Piscitelli SC et al: Indinavir concentrations and St. John's wort, *Lancet* 355(9203):547-548, 2000.
20. Johne A et al: Pharmacokinetic interaction of digoxin with an herbal extract from St. John's wort (Hypericum perforatum), *Clin Pharmacol Ther* 66(4):338-345, 1999.
21. Izzo AA: Drug interactions with St. John's wort (Hypericum perforatum): a review of the clinical evidence, *Int J Clin Pharmacol Ther* 42(3):139-148, 2004.
22. Kuhn MA: Herbal remedies: drug-herb interactions, *Crit Care Nurse* 22(2):22-28, 30, 32; quiz 34-35, 2002.
23. Butterweck V et al: Pharmacokinetic herb-drug interactions: are preventive screenings necessary and appropriate? *Planta Med* 70(9):784-791, 2004.
24. Hammerness P et al: Natural Standard Research Collaboration: St. John's wort: a systemic review of adverse effects and drug interactions for the consultation psychiatrist, *Psychosomatics* 44(4):271-282, 2003.
25. Coxeter PD et al: Herb-drug interactions; an evidence based approach. *Curr Med Chem* 11(11):1513-1525, 2004.
26. Patel J et al: In vitro interaction of the HIV protease inhibitor ritonavir with herbal with herbal constituents: changes in P-gp and CYP3A4 activity, *Am J Ther* 11(4):262-277, 2004.
27. Zhou S et al: Pharmacokinetic interactions of drugs with St. John's wort, *J Psychopharmacol* 18(2):262-276, 2004.
28. Sparreboom A et al: Herbal remedies in the United States: potential adverse interactions with anticancer agents, *J Clin Oncol* 15;22(12):2489-2503, 2004.
29. Matthews JM, Etheridge AS, Black SR: Inhibition of human cytochrome P450 activities by kava extract and kava lactones, *Drug Metab Dispos* 30(11):1153-1157, 2002.
30. Anke J, Ramzan I. Kava hepatotoxicity: are we any closer to the truth? *Planta Med* 70(3):193-196, 2004.
31. Ernst E: Cardiovascular adverse effects of herbal medicines: a systemic review of the recent literature, *Can J Cardiol* 19(7):818-827, 2003.
32. Kaye AD, Kucera I, Sabar R: Perioperative anesthesia clinical considerations of alternative medicines, *Anesthesiol Clin North Am* 22(1):125-139, 2004.
33. McCune JS et al: Potential of chemotherapy-herb interactions in adult cancer patients, *Support Care Cancer* 12(6):454-62, 2004.
34. Lyons TR: Herbal medicines and possible anesthesia interactions, *AANA J* 70(1):47-51, 2002.
35. Kligler B: Black cohosh, *Am Fam Physician* 68(1):114-1116, 2003.

The toxic ingredients may be what brings the patient to the ED for treatment.

Social and environmental problems associated with herbal medicines include the whole-sale slaughter of endangered species such as tigers, bears, and rhinoceroses. Certain endangered plant species and their delicate ecosystems likewise are being threatened by the pursuit of natural cures. Medical problems associated with the use of herbal therapies include the following[9-12]:

- Allergic reactions
- Skin rashes
- Elevated liver function tests
- Electrolyte imbalances
- Palpitations
- Hypertension
- Increased bleeding times
- Inhibition of the absorption of prescribed medications
- Displacement of a prescribed drug by the herb (Displacement can increase the adverse effects associated with prescribed medications.)
- Decreased metabolism of a prescribed medication leading to adverse and toxic effects
- An additive effect that increases the level of a prescribed medication

Because so many supplements are available and so many patients take multiple prescribed medications, determining the cause of the problem can be challenging. Herbs come in many forms, such as teas, tinctures, tablets, freeze-dried extracts, capsules, and standardized preparations. Table 17-2 summarizes common drug-herb interactions.[9] Box 17-1 also lists several helpful Web sites.[11]

POPULAR HERBS AND POTENTIAL TOXICITIES

As previously noted, just as there are thousands of prescription medications that can cause toxicity, thousands of herbal preparations can do the same.[12] Comprehensive discussion of each herbal preparation is beyond the scope of this text. Table 17-3 describes some of the most popular herbs and the problems that may be encountered with their use.

References

1. Panel on Definition and Description of CAM: Defining and describing complementary and alternative medicine, *Altern Ther Health Med* 3(2):49-57, 1997.
2. Hageness S, Kreitzer MJ, Kinney ME: Complementary, integrative and holistic care in emergency nursing, *Nurs Clin North Am* 37(1):123-133, 2002.
3. Snyder M, Lindquist R: Issues in complementary therapies: how we got where we are, *Online J Issues Nurs* 6(2):1, 2001.
4. Kreitzer MJ, Jensen D: Healing practices: trends, challenges, and opportunities for nurses in acute and critical care, *AACN Clin Issues* 11(1):7-16, 2000.
5. Klepser TB et al: Assessment of patients' perceptions and beliefs regarding herbal therapies, *Pharmacotherapy* 20(1):83-87, 2000.
6. Fenton MV, Morris DL: The integration of holistic nursing practices and complementary and alternative modalities into curricula of schools of nursing, *Altern Ther Health Med* 9(4):62-67, 2003.
7. Mackenzie ER et al: Ethnic minority use of complementary and alternative medicine (CAM): a national probability survey of CAM utilizers, *Altern Ther Health Med* 9(4):50-56, 2003.
8. Herron M, Glasser M: Use of and attitudes toward complementary and alternative medicine among family practice patients in small rural Illinois communities, *J Rural Health* 19(3):279-284, 2003.
9. Kuhn M: Herbal remedies: drug-herb interactions, *Crit Care Nurse* 22(2):22-30, 2002.

10. Moss TM: Herbal medicine in the emergency department: a primer for toxicities and treatment, *J Emerg Nurs* 24(6):509-513, 1998.
11. Tryens E, Coulston L, Tlush E: Understanding the complexities of herbal medicine, Nursing Spectrum Education/CE. Retrieved August 15, 2003, from http://www.2nursingspectrum.com/CEIself-study_modules/syllabus.html?10=206.
12. Herrara L, Hirshan J: Toxicities of alternative therapies, *Ann Emerg Med* 17(8):1-8, 2003.

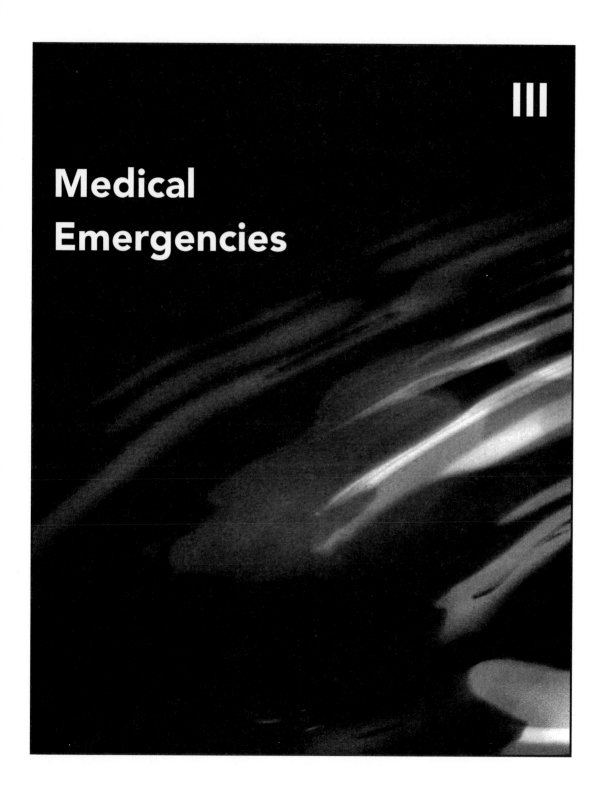

Medical
Emergencies

18

Cardiopulmonary Arrest

Donna S. Gloe, BSN, MSN, EdD, RNBC

For years, cardiovascular disease has been the leading killer of Americans.[1] Myocardial infarction is the major cause of sudden demise, accounting for 1 out of every 5 deaths, with an estimated U.S. mortality of 200,000 to 300,000 per year.[2] Many victims die before receiving medical attention, making it difficult to determine the actual incidence, but about 1 million patients are hospitalized each year with a primary diagnosis of myocardial infarction. Such significant morbidity and mortality rates have prompted a nationwide effort to educate the public about the warning signs of impending myocardial infarction. Community cardiopulmonary resuscitation (CPR) training programs have provided millions of citizens with essential skills to maintain life during the first critical minutes until the arrival of emergency medical services professionals. Even more aggressive efforts have been made to train all health care providers in basic or advanced life support. These programs have greatly improved survival from in-hospital and out-of-hospital cardiac arrest.

BASIC LIFE SUPPORT

Basic life support (BLS), the initial intervention for any type of arrest, can be taught to all levels of personnel from lay providers to highly skilled medical practitioners. The essential components of basic life support involve establishing that the person is unconscious, opening and maintaining an *airway*, initiating rescue *breathing*, and providing *circulatory* assistance when necessary (chest compression). For years, this sequence has been known as the ABCs. With the advent of automated external defibrillators (AEDs), these steps now sometimes are referred to as the ABCDs. In accordance with recent American Heart Association practice changes, lay persons are no longer instructed to perform a pulse check as part of their

Table 18-1 Guidelines for Cardiopulmonary Resuscitation

	Adult	Child	Infant	Neonate
Compression rate (per minute)	100	100	≥100	120
Compression depth	1½-2 inch	1-1.5 inch	½-1 inch	½ to 1 inch
Compression mode	Both hands	Heel of one hand	Apposed thumbs[†]	Apposed thumbs
Compression-to-ventilation ratio	15:2 (1 or 2 rescuers)	5:1 (1 or 2 rescuers)	5:1 (1 or 2 rescuers)	5:1 (1 or 2 rescuers)

From American Heart Association: *Handbook of emergency cardiovascular care,* Dallas, 2002, The Association.
Data from Part 9: Pediatric basic life support, *Circulation* 102(8, suppl):I-253-I-290; Part 3: Adult basic life support, *Circulation* 102(8, suppl): I-22-I-59.
May be performed with ring and middle fingers one fingerwidth below intramammary line if rescuer's hands are too small.

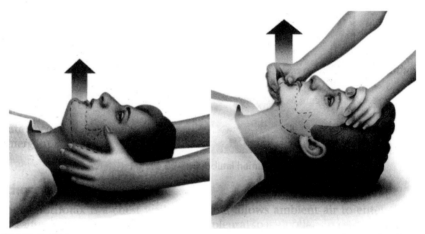

Figure 18-1. A, Jaw thrust. **B,** Chin lift. (From Proehl J: *Emergency nursing procedures,* ed 3, St Louis, 2004, Saunders.)

initial assessment. Lay rescuers should initiate compressions in any unconscious, unresponsive patient who is not breathing and has other signs of circulatory compromise:
- Basic life support is provided to victims of all ages with specific age-related variations. Table 18-1 summarizes basic life support for adults, children, and infants.[3]
- Currently accepted techniques for early airway management in victims of all ages (who are not suspected of having concurrent cervical spine injury) are the jaw thrust (Figure 18-1, *A*) and the chin lift (Figure 18-1, *B*).[4]
- Once unresponsiveness has been verified, the rescuer immediately should call for help. Advanced care such as defibrillation, invasive airway management, and intravenous administration of medications must be initiated as soon as possible.

AUTOMATIC EXTERNAL DEFIBRILLATION

Eighty percent to 90% of adult victims of cardiac arrest are initially in ventricular fibrillation. This rhythm cannot be converted with basic cardiopulmonary resuscitation; defibrillation is the definitive treatment. Because of this, AEDs have become a critical link in the chain

Defibrillator electrode placement

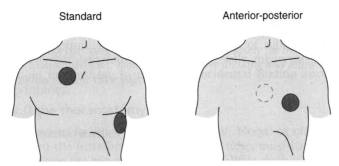

Figure 18-2. Standard and anterior-posterior electrode placement for defibrillation. (From Newberry L, editor: *Sheehy's emergency nursing: principles and practice*, ed 5, St Louis, 2003, Mosby.)

of survival. The earlier this intervention is performed, the greater the odds of survival. The AED is designed for use by laypersons, so rhythm interpretation is not required. A number of brands and models exist on the market, but all work similarly:

- Turn the power on. Sound alerts, lights, and voice prompts guide the rescuer through operation of the device.
- Remove any clothing from the victim's chest and place the two adhesive electrode pads directly on the skin. Electrodes may be placed in the standard (sternal-apical) or anterior-posterior position (Figure 18-2).[5] Most AEDs have a voice prompt or alarm that notifies the user if the electrodes are not attached securely to the chest or if the cables are not properly fastened.
- Stop cardiopulmonary resuscitation, do not touch the victim. The AED cannot analyze the rhythm accurately with cardiopulmonary resuscitation in progress. Several AED models begin analysis as soon as the electrodes are attached, others start after the user pushes the "Analyze" button. In a health care setting, more sophisticated machines can display the rhythm for expert analysis (semiautomatic external defibrillators).
- Direct all rescuers to stand clear. Verify that no one has contact with the patient or stretcher.
- Deliver shocks according to the instructions provided by the AED. All AEDs are programmed to follow the shock sequence recommended by the American Heart Association.[3]

ADVANCED LIFE SUPPORT

For the patient in cardiac arrest, survival depends on early basic life support, early defibrillation, and early interventions for airway and dysrhythmia management. Emergency medical personnel, nurses, respiratory therapists, and physicians can provide advanced life support. Refer to Chapter 19 for a discussion of airway management techniques; Chapter 10 reviews dysrhythmia recognition.

The American Heart Association has standardized the approach to cardiac arrest management with a set of treatment algorithms. These algorithms cover adult, pediatric, and newborn patients. Tables 18-2, 18-3, and 18-4 outline the treatment of ventricular fibrillation/pulseless ventricular tachycardia, pulseless electrical activity, and asystole respectively. Figure 18-3 presents the algorithm for pediatric arrest.[3]

Table 18-2 Pulseless Ventricular Tachycardia/Ventricular Fibrillation

	Airway	Breathing	Circulation	Differential Diagnosis
Basic Life Support				
	Open the airway.	Deliver two slow breaths, and administer oxygen as soon as it is available.	Perform chest compressions.	Ensure availability of monitor/defibrillator. On arrival of AED/monitor/defibrillator, evaluate cardiac rhythm. If PEA or asystole, continue CPR and go to appropriate algorithm. If pulseless VT/VF, shock up to 3 times (200 J, 200 to 300 J, 360 J, or equivalent biphasic energy). • If persistent or recurrent pulseless VT/VF, continue CPR and perform secondary ABCD survey. Reevaluate cardiac rhythm. • If PEA or asystole, continue CPR and go to appropriate algorithm. If return of spontaneous circulation occurs: • Assess vital signs. • Maintain open airway. • Provide ventilation. • Administer medications appropriate for rhythm, blood pressure, and heart rate.
Perform primary ABCD survey. (Correct critical problems *immediately* as they are identified.) Assess responsiveness. Call for help; call for defibrillator.				
Advanced Life Support				
Perform secondary ABCD survey.	Reassess effectiveness of initial airway maneuvers and interventions. Perform invasive airway management.	Assess ventilation. Confirm endotracheal tube placement (or other airway device) by at least two methods. Provide positive pressure ventilation; evaluate effectiveness of ventilations. Secure airway device in place with commercial tube holder (preferred) or tape.	Establish IV access and administer appropriate medications. Epinephrine (Class Indeterminate) 1 mg (1:10,000 solution) IV every 3 to 5 min (Endotracheal dose 2 to 2.5 mg diluted in 10 mL NS or distilled water) Pattern becomes CPR-drug-shock or CPR-drug-shock-shock-shock. or	Search for and treat reversible causes. Defibrillate with 360 J (or equivalent biphasic energy) within 30 to 60 sec.

Consider antiarrhythmics (avoid use of multiple antiarrhythmics because of potential proarrhythmic effects):

- Amiodarone (Class IIb): Initial bolus—300-mg IV bolus diluted in 20 to 30 mL NS or D₅W. Consider repeat dose (150-mg IV bolus) in 3 to 5 min. If defibrillation successful, follow with 1 mg/min IV infusion for 6 hours (mix 900 mg in 500 mL NS), and then decrease infusion rate to 0.5 mg/min IV infusion for 18 hours. Maximum daily dose is 2 g/24 hours IV.

- Lidocaine (Class Indeterminate): 1- to 1.5-mg/kg IV bolus. Consider repeat dose (0.5 to 0.75 mg/kg) in 5 min; maximum IV bolus dose is 3 mg/kg. (The 1.5-mg/kg dose is recommended in cardiac arrest). Endotracheal dose is 2 to 4 mg/kg. A single dose of 1.5 mg/kg is acceptable in cardiac arrest.

- Magnesium (Class IIb if hypomagnesemia present): 1 to 2 g IV (2 to 4 mL of a 50% solution) diluted in 10 mL of D₅W if torsades de pointes or hypomagnesemia

Continued

Table 18-2   **Pulseless Ventricular Tachycardia/Ventricular Fibrillation*—cont'd**

Airway	Breathing	Circulation	Differential Diagnosis
		• Procainamide (Class IIb for recurrent pulseless VT/VF; Class Indeterminate for persistent pulseless VT/VF): 20 mg/min; maximum total dose 17 mg/kg • Consider sodium bicarbonate 1 mEq/kg.	

From Aehlert B: ACLS quick review study guide, St Louis, 2002, Mosby.
AED, Automated external defibrillator; PEA, pulseless electrical activity; CPR, cardiopulmonary resuscitation; VT/VF, ventricular tachycardia/ventricular fibrillation; IV, intravenous; NS, normal saline; D_5W, 5% dextrose in water.

Table 18-3 Pulseless Electrical Activity*

	Airway	Breathing	Circulation	Differential Diagnosis
Basic Life Support				
	Open the airway.	Deliver two slow breaths; administer oxygen as soon as it is available.	Perform chest compressions.	Ensure availability of monitor/defibrillator. On arrival of AED/monitor/defibrillator, perform secondary ABCD survey if rhythm is *not* pulseless VT/VF.
Perform primary ABCD survey. (Correct critical problems *immediately* as they are identified.) Assess responsiveness. Call for help; call for defibrillator.				
Advanced Life Support				
	Reassess effectiveness of initial airway maneuvers and interventions. Perform invasive airway management.	Assess ventilation. Confirm endotracheal tube placement (or other airway device) by at least two methods. Provide positive pressure ventilation; evaluate effectiveness of ventilations. Secure airway device in place with commercial tube holder (preferred) or tape.	Establish IV access. Assess blood flow with Doppler. (If blood flow detected with Doppler, treat using hypotension/shock algorithm.) Administer appropriate medications. Epinephrine 1 mg (1:10,000 solution) IV every 3 to 5 min (Endotracheal dose 2 to 2.5 mg diluted in 10 mL NS or distilled water) If the rate is slow, atropine 1 mg IV every 3 to 5 min to max 0.04 mg/kg (Class IIb). (Endotracheal dose 2 to 3 mg diluted in 10 mL NS or distilled water)	Search for and treat reversible causes (PATCH-4-MD mnemonic). (Fast narrow QRS complex: consider hypovolemia, tamponade, pulmonary embolism, tension pneumothorax; slow wide QRS complex: consider cyclic antidepressant overdose, calcium channel blocker, beta-blocker, or digitalis toxicity.)
Perform secondary ABCD survey. Possible causes of PEA are these (PATCH-4-MD mnemonic): Pulmonary embolism Acidosis Tension pneumothorax Cardiac tamponade Hypovolemia (most common cause) Hypoxia Heat/cold (hypothermia/hyperthermia) Hypokalemia/hyperkalemia (and other electrolytes) Myocardial infarction				

Continued

Table 18-3   Pulseless Electrical Activity*—cont'd

Airway	Breathing	Circulation	Differential Diagnosis
Drug overdose/accidents (cyclic antidepressants, calcium channel blockers, beta-blockers, digitalis)		Consider sodium bicarbonate 1 mEq/kg: • Known preexisting hyperkalemia (Class I) • Cyclic antidepressant overdose (IIa) • To alkalinize urine in aspirin or other drug overdoses (IIa) • Patient that has been intubated and has a long arrest interval (IIb) • On return of spontaneous circulation if long arrest interval (IIb) Consider termination of efforts.	

Table 18-4   Asystole

	Airway	Breathing	Circulation	Differential Diagnosis
Basic Life Support				
Perform primary ABCD survey. (Correct critical problems immediately as they are identified.) Assess responsiveness. Call for help; call for defibrillator. Scene survey: Documentation or other evidence of do not attempt resuscitation order? Obvious signs of death? If yes, do not start/attempt resuscitation.	Open the airway.	Deliver two slow breaths; administer oxygen as soon as it is available.	Perform chest compressions.	Ensure availability of monitor/defibrillator. On arrival of AED/monitor/defibrillator, perform secondary ABCD survey if rhythm is not pulseless VT/VF.
Advanced Life Support				
Perform secondary ABCD survey. Possible causes of asystole (PATCH-4-MD mnemonic): Pulmonary embolism Acidosis Tension pneumothorax Cardiac tamponade Hypovolemia Hypoxia Heat/cold (hypothermia/hyperthermia) Hypokalemia/hyperkalemia (and other electrolytes) Myocardial infarction Drug overdose/accidents (cyclic antidepressants, calcium channel blockers, beta-blockers, digitalis)	Reassess effectiveness of initial airway maneuvers and interventions. Perform invasive airway management.	Assess ventilation Confirm endotracheal tube placement (or other airway device) by at least two methods. Provide positive pressure ventilation; evaluate effectiveness of ventilations. Secure airway device in place with commercial tube holder (preferred) or tape.	Confirm presence of asystole. (Check lead/cable connections; ensure power to monitor is on, correct lead is selected, and gain is turned up; confirm asystole in second lead.) Establish IV access and administer appropriate medications. Epinephrine 1 mg (1:10,000 solution) IV every 3 to 5 min (Endotracheal dose 2 to 2.5 mg diluted in 10 mL NS or distilled water) Atropine 1 mg IV every 3 to 5 min to maximum 0.04 mg/kg (Class IIb) (Endotracheal dose 2 to 3 mg diluted in 10 mL NS or distilled water)	Search for and treat reversible causes (PATCH-4-MD mnemonic). Consider immediate transcutaneous pacing. Consider termination of efforts: • Evaluate the quality of the resuscitation attempt. • Evaluate the resuscitation for atypical clinical features (e.g., hypothermia, reversible therapeutic or illicit drug use). • Does support for cease-effort protocols exist?

Continued

Table 18-4   Asystole—cont'd

Airway	Breathing	Circulation	Differential Diagnosis
		Consider sodium bicarbonate 1 mEq/kg: • Known preexisting hyperkalemia (Class I) • Cyclic antidepressant overdose (IIa) • To alkalinize urine in aspirin or other drug overdoses (IIa) • Patient that has been intubated and has long arrest interval (IIb) • On return of spontaneous circulation if long arrest interval (IIb)	

(From Aehlert B: *ACLS quick review study guide*, ed 2, St Louis, 2002, Mosby.)
*AED, Automated external defibrillator; VT/VF, ventricular tachycardia/ventricular fibrillation; IV, intravenous; NS, normal saline.

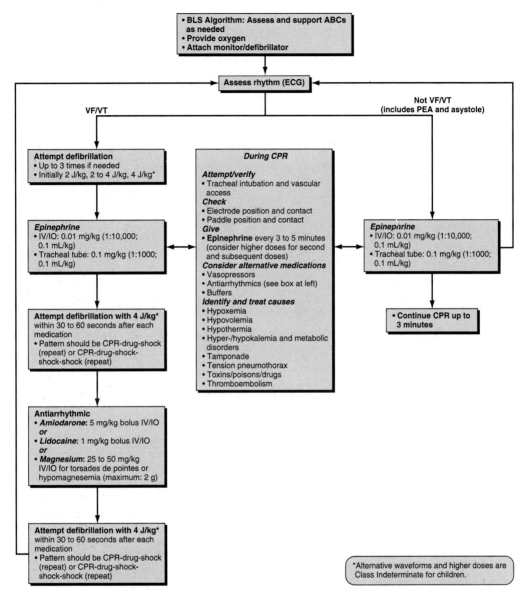

Figure 18-3. Pediatric pulseless arrest pediatric advanced life support treatment algorithm. *BLS,* Basic life support; *ABCs,* airway, breathing, circulation; *ECG,* electrocardiogram; *VF/VT,* ventricular fibrillation/ ventricular tachycardia; *PEA,* pulseless electrical activity; *IV/IO,* intravenous/intraosseus; *CPR,* cardiopulmonary resuscitation. (From AHA guidelines 2000, *Circulation* 102(suppl):1, 2000. with permission.)

Defibrillation

Defibrillation is the definitive treatment for ventricular fibrillation and pulseless ventricular tachycardia. Box 18-1 describes the steps in this procedure. Defibrillation can be performed with traditional paddles; however, hands-free defibrillation pads are faster, safer, and simpler; do not require pressure; and actually have been shown to improve energy delivery.[5] The use of pads also eliminates the need for additional monitoring electrodes. Defibrillation pads come in adult (8 to 12 cm) and pediatric sizes (4.5 cm). Adult pads can be used for up to 50 shocks and provide continuous monitoring for 24 hours. Pediatric pads are designed for infants (<15 kg) and can be used for only 25 shocks. Combination pads with defibrillation and pacing capabilities are also available. These pads provide continuous pacing for 8 hours in adults or 12 hours in children. Importantly, pads are specific to each brand of AED or defibrillator; pads placed in the field may not be compatible with emergency department equipment and must be exchanged.

With use of a traditional monophasic defibrillator, the American Heart Association recommends 360 J of energy for each shock after the first (200 J) and second (300 J) shocks (in adults). Standard monophasic defibrillators provide energy in only one direction, whereas the newer, biphasic defibrillators increase energy delivery by providing bidirectional electrical flow. Consequently, the amount of energy required is lower, generally 150 J rather than the usual 360 J. However, the American Heart Association currently has no standard energy guidelines for biphasic defibrillation; follow the manufacturer's recommendations.

Automatic Implantable Cardioverter-Defibrillators

An automatic implantable cardioverter-defibrillator (AICD) monitors the patient's rhythm and paces or defibrillates according to the programming of the unit. Fast pacing, slow pacing, synchronized cardioversion, and defibrillation are possible depending on the patient's heart rhythm and the type of device. Smaller than a packet of cigarettes, the AICD is implanted in a subcutaneous tissue pocket in the chest or abdomen.

The AICD has the following characteristics:
- Physical contact with the patient when the AICD fires causes a slight tingling sensation that is essentially harmless.
- External defibrillation can be performed in a patient with an AICD, but one must locate the device and not put defibrillation pads or paddles directly over the unit.

Box **18-1** **Steps in Defibrillation**

> Remove nitroglycerin and other ointments or medication patches from the chest. These will create an alternative path for the current.
> Dry the chest if there is excessive moisture from diaphoresis or another source.
> Place defibrillator pads (or paddles) at least 5 inches from a pacemaker or automatic implantable cardioverter-defibrillator.
> Allow at least 1 to 2 inches between pads (or paddles) on infants and children.
> If paddles are used, apply 25 to 30 lb of pressure on the chest to overcome transthoracic resistance.
> Confirm that there is no contact between the patient (or anything touching the patient or stretcher) and the care providers. Contact with the manual resuscitation bag is safe during defibrillation as long as the rescuer touches only the bag.[5]
> Confirm that everyone is "clear" before shocks are delivered.
> Deliver shocks during exhalation to reduce thoracic impedance.[4]
> Unless a return of spontaneous circulation occurs, administer the initial three shocks in rapid sequence.

- Place defibrillation pads anterior-anterior. If this is not effective, try anterior-posterior positioning to improve conduction around the AICD electrodes.[5]
- The AICD can be deactivated with a magnet if necessary.

DIFFERENTIAL DIAGNOSIS IN CARDIOPULMONARY ARREST

Cardiac arrest or near arrest has many causes. Besides myocardial infarction, causes include metabolic disturbances, drugs, and major body system disruptions. Tables 18-5, 18-6, and 18-7

Table **18-5**   **Metabolic Causes of Cardiac Arrest**

Cause	Signs and Symptoms	Intervention	Discussion
Hypoglycemia	Tachydysrhythmias; seizures; loss of consciousness	Dextrose 50%; glucagon intramuscularly if unable to establish intravenous access	Consider this a strong possibility in adults with a history of diabetes. Look for signs of insulin injections or the presence of an insulin pump.
Hyperkalemia	Prolonged Q-T interval; tall, peaked T waves; prolonged P wave; prolonged P-R interval; wide QRS complexes; first-degree heart block; nodal rhythm; idioventricular rhythm; ventricular fibrillation; asystole	Intravenously administered calcium chloride or calcium gluconate; sodium bicarbonate; insulin and glucose; inhaled beta^2-agonists (albuterol)	Condition seen in renal failure (dialysis) patients, in those taking potassium-sparing diuretics, and patients with significant muscle damage (rhabdomyolysis)
Hypokalemia	History of digitalis or diuretic therapy; flattened, inverted T waves; depressed ST segment; U waves; ventricular ectopy	Intravenously administered potassium chloride	U waves are not unique to hypokalemia but indicate the need to check a serum potassium level.
Hypercalcemia	Shortened QT interval; bradycardia; first-, second-, or third-degree heart block; bundle branch block	Hydration and diuresis	May potentiate the effects of digitalis, precipitate digitalis toxicity, and cause hypertension.
Hypocalcemia	Prolonged Q-T interval; torsades de pointes (polymorphic ventricular tachycardia)	Intravenously administered calcium gluconate or calcium chloride	Torsades de pointes is a life-threatening ventricular dysrhythmia that does not respond to the usual treatments for ventricular tachycardia/ventricular fibrillation. May respond to magnesium sulfate, isoproterenol, phenytoin, or overdrive pacing.
Hypermagnesemia	Heart block; asystole	Calcium chloride; saline diuresis; furosemide	Hemodialysis is required for severe cases.
Hypomagnesemia	Premature ventricular contractions; ventricular tachycardia or fibrillation; torsades de pointes	Magnesium sulfate	Dysrhythmias may not respond to the usual drugs. Treat with a magnesium sulfate infusion.

Modified from Newberry L, editor: *Emergency nursing procedures: principles and practice*, ed 5, St Louis, 2003, Mosby.

Table 18-6 Drug-Related Causes of Cardiac Arrest

Cause	Signs and Symptoms	Intervention	Discussion
Antidysrhythmics such as amiodarone, lidocaine, procainamide	Bradycardia, heart block, heart failure, sinus arrest, ventricular fibrillation, ventricular asystole	Discontinue antidysrhythmic agents. Vasopressors, atropine, defibrillation, or pacing may be indicated.	Monitor for electrocardiogram and blood pressure changes.
Beta-blockers such as propranolol, atenolol, labetalol	Cardiac: • Heart blocks • Bradydysrhythmias • Premature ventricular contractions Respiratory: • Bronchospasm	Atropine Aminophylline	Premature ventricular contractions may be rate related.
Calcium channel blockers such as diltiazem, verapamil	Heart failure, bradycardia, atrioventricular block, ventricular fibrillation, asystole	Calcium chloride 10%; use calcium gluconate if acidosis is present.	Pace the patient when other treatments fail.
Digitalis products such as digoxin, digitoxin	First-, second-, and third-degree heart block; ventricular dysrhythmias; asystole	Digoxin immune Fab fragments (Digibind) Intravenously administered magnesium	Digoxin levels will be elevated falsely for up to 2 days after Digibind administration.
Opiates and opioids such as morphine, fentanyl, meperidine, hydromorphone (Dilaudid), heroin	Bradydysrhythmias; heart blocks	Naloxone (Narcan); Nalmefene (Revex)	Street preparations may also contain cocaine, phencyclidine hydrochloride, strychnine, or other potentially lethal adulterants.
Stimulants such as cocaine, amphetamines, phencyclidine hydrochloride, methamphetamines, ecstasy	Tachydysrhythmias; hypertension; myocardial infarction	Benzodiazepines (diazepam, lorazepam) Alpha- and beta-blockers	Consider body packers and continued release of swallowed containers.
Toxins such as carbon monoxide, cyanide	Carbon monoxide: • Tachydysrhythmias • Ventricular ectopy Cyanide: • Cardiovascular collapse	Oxygen and supportive care; hyperbaric oxygenation Cyanide antidote kit; hyperbaric oxygenation; supportive care	Remove patient from the toxin source.
Tricyclic antidepressants such as amitriptyline (Elavil), perphenazine (Triavil, Etrafon), imipramine (Tofranil), doxepin (Sinequan), protriptyline (Vivactil)	Tachydysrhythmias; prolonged Q-T interval; torsades de pointes	Intravenously administered sodium bicarbonate to keep serum pH at 7.5; vasopressors; fluids	Causes direct cardiac toxicity; may cause delayed toxicity in adults.

Table 18-7 Causes of Cardiac Arrest by Body System

System	Cause	Signs and Symptoms	Intervention	Discussion
Cardiac	Acute myocardial infarction	Electrocardiogram: ST segment elevation; T wave inversion; pathological Q waves in zone of infarction; all types of dysrhythmias	IV thrombolysis; IV glycoprotein IIb/IIIa (GP IIb/IIIa) inhibitors; emergency angioplasty or intracoronary stent; emergency coronary artery bypass grafting	The goal of intervention is reperfusion, preservation of myocardium, and minimization of further damage.
	Pericardial tamponade	Decreasing blood pressure; distant/muffled heart sounds; distended neck veins; tachycardia (initially) then bradydysrhythmias or PEA	Aggressive IV fluid boluses; atropine; pericardiocentesis; thoracotomy	Suspect this condition in victims of blunt or penetrating chest trauma and in those with prolonged chest compressions.
Pulmonary	Asthma	Severe bronchospasm causing hypoxia and respiratory acidosis; tachydysrhythmias (especially ventricular fibrillation)	Endotracheal intubation and ventilatory support with minimal volume ventilation; steroids; continuous bronchodilators	Patient will be severely acidotic; consider sodium bicarbonate. May require chest tubes for pneumothorax.
	Pulmonary embolus	Pleuritic chest pain; dyspnea; history of recent surgery, oral contraceptive use, or pregnancy; syncope (initial complaint in 60%); tachydysrhythmias	Good ventilatory support; thrombolysis with rt-PA; thrombectomy (rarely)	Causes acute hypoxia and cor pulmonale leading to tachydysrhythmias, PEA, and asystole.

Continued

Modified from Newberry L, editor: *Emergency nursing: principles and practice*, ed 5, St Louis, 2003, Mosby.
COPD, chronic obstructive pulmonary disease; *IV,* Intravenous; *PEA,* pulseless electrical activity; *rt-PA,* recombinant tissue plasminogen activator.

Table 18-7 Causes of Cardiac Arrest by Body System*—contd

System	Cause	Signs and Symptoms	Intervention	Discussion
	Tension pneumothorax	Severe dyspnea; tachycardia; hypotension; tracheal deviation; asymmetric chest expansion; PEA	Immediate needle decompression and then chest tube insertion	Seen with blunt or penetrating chest trauma; can result from chest compressions (especially in patients with COPD). May occur following central line insertion or after endotracheal intubation and positive pressure ventilation.
Neurologic	Increased intracranial pressure from any cause	Neurogenic respiratory patterns; dilated pupil(s); decerebrate or decorticate posturing; loss of consciousness; wide range of dysrhythmias, especially heart blocks, and bradycardia; widening pulse pressure	Short-term hyperventilation to produce cerebral vasoconstriction, mannitol; positioning (head of bed up, neck aligned); surgery	Symptoms result from damage to the brainstem and autonomic centers. Unless pressure is rapidly reduced, herniation will occur.
Hypovolemic	Any condition causing volume loss: hemorrhage, plasma loss, or extravascular losses	Tachycardia; hypotension; cool, clammy, pale skin; obvious signs of external or internal blood loss; major burns; history of severe vomiting or diarrhea; PEA	IV fluids/blood products; address the cause; surgery	Hypovolemia is a cause of cardiopulmonary arrest that may go unrecognized, especially if volume loss is not obvious.

Box **18-2** **Planning for Cardiac Arrest in Unusual Emergency Department Settings**

Do you have a panic button to call for help in the triage area? How would you respond to a cardiac arrest in your waiting room or outside the building? If you do not have a panic button, how can you call for help? Do you have a special code for overhead announcements? Will your emergency department staff or hospital code team respond outside the building?

Do you have a manual resuscitation bag and personal protective equipment located near wherever it might be needed? At triage? Near the patient bathroom?

Where will you resuscitate the patient?

Do you have an automated external defibrillator available or only a full-function defibrillator? Do you bring the defibrillator to the patient or transport the patient to the resuscitation room?

How do you get a patient out of a car? How do you move the patient to the resuscitation area? Do you have immediate access to a stretcher?

Where is the stretcher kept, who will retrieve it, and what path will the gurney take to the patient?

summarize the possible causes. Interventions listed are in addition to those in the standard treatment algorithms. Familiarity with various causes of cardiac disturbances facilitates the resuscitation process.

SPECIAL CONSIDERATIONS

Each cardiac arrest situation presents its own set of challenges. Management of the patient brought in by an emergency medical services advanced life support unit varies from that of the patient who arrives in the back of a private vehicle or who collapses in the waiting room telephone booth. Practicing a private wide variety of scenarios in mock code drills will help identify issues unique to your practice setting. Questions that should be considered before the event are presented in Box 18-2. Answers to these questions will depend on your emergency department layout, location, and usual practice pattern, but preparation can decrease the chaos and anxiety associated with an actual event.

References

1. American Heart Association: *ACLS provider manual,* Chicago, 2002, The Association.
2. Sgarbossa E: Heart attack. Retrieved July 6, 2003 from http://health.allrefer.com/health/heart-attack-info.html.
3. American Heart Association: *Handbook of emergency cardiovascular care for health care providers,* Chicago, 2002, The Association.
4. Proehl J: *Emergency nursing procedures,* ed 3, Philadelphia, 2004, Saunders.
5. Barnason S: Cardiovascular emergencies. In Newberry L, editor: *Sheehy's emergency nursing: principles and practice,* ed 5, St Louis, 2003, Mosby.

19

Airway Management

Gretta J. Edwards, RN, BS, CEN

One of the most important emergency nursing skills is assessment and management of the patient with an airway emergency. Although many airway disorders exist (see Chapter 20), those discussed in this chapter are related to potentially life-threatening upper airway obstructions.

ASSESSMENT

A rapid primary assessment is indicated for all patients who present with an airway emergency. Initial assessment includes the following:
- Airway patency
  - Drooling, stridor, snoring
  - Obvious obstruction (e.g., blood, vomitus, foreign object)
- Breath sounds
- Respiratory rate and pattern
- Work of breathing
  - Nostril flaring (children), retractions
- Skin color, moisture, and temperature
- Vital signs, including and oxygen saturation (Spo_2) level
- Patient position
- Level of consciousness

HISTORY

The history should include the following:
- Onset and nature of the symptoms
- Past medical history
- History if tobacco use; what type, how much, how long
- Patient's occupation

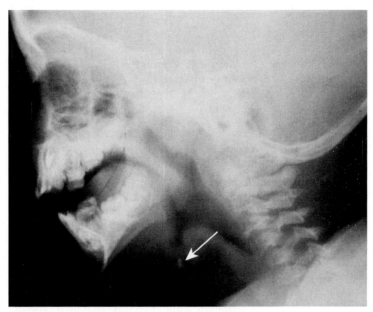

Figure 19-1. Mild epiglottitis. The lateral neck radiograph demonstrates mild epiglottic swelling and thickening of the aryepiglottic folds. (From Zitelli B, Davis H: *Atlas of pediatric physical diagnosis*, ed 4, St Louis, 2002, Mosby.)

- Recent travel history
- Recent exposure to infectious disease

AIRWAY EMERGENCIES

Epiglottitis

Epiglottitis or supraglottitis is a rapidly progressing inflammation of the upper airway that involves the oral cavity, tongue, and epiglottis. This condition, once considered a pediatric disease, is now more common in adults than children because of routine childhood immunizations for *Haemophilus influenzae* type B. When infected, the epiglottis rapidly can become so enlarged that total airway obstruction occurs, requiring intubation or cricothyrotomy. Because agitation may precipitate complete airway closure, it is important keep the patient as calm and quiet as possible. A lateral soft tissue radiograph of the neck will reveal a swollen epiglottis (Figure 19-1). However, direct visualization of the epiglottis using nasopharyngoscopy is replacing radiographic studies as the preferred method of diagnosis. Onset of symptoms is typically swift.

Epiglottitis

Signs and Symptoms

- Anxiety/panic
- Dysphagia
- Drooling
- Dyspnea

- Fever
- Flushing
- Muffled voice
- Sitting forward with the neck extended (sniffing position)
- Sore throat

Interventions

- Allow the patient to assume a position of comfort (upright, leaning forward).
- Provide supplemental oxygen; cool humidified oxygen is optimal.
- Monitor oxygen saturation and cardiac rhythm continuously.
- Obtain airway equipment and a cricothyrotomy tray.
- Keep the patient as calm and quiet as possible.
- Establish intravenous access.
- Administer intravenous antibiotics.
- Facilitate rapid movement to an operating room for intubation by an anesthesiologist (optimal).

Allergic Reactions

An allergic reaction is a hypersensitive response by the immune system to an antigen to which there has been previous exposure. The earlier exposure stimulates the immune system to form antibodies that are activated with subsequent antigen contact. Reactions range from mild to life threatening. Severe reactions (anaphylaxis) may occur suddenly, causing complete airway obstruction within minutes.[1] See Chapter 22 for a discussion of anaphylactic shock. Skin flushing, hives, and urticaria are early signs of an allergic reaction. These symptoms are generally followed by edema of the face, tongue, and oropharynx, nausea, vomiting, and diarrhea. Significant airway swelling requires emergent airway management.

Allergic Reaction

Signs and Symptoms

- Coughing
- Dyspnea
- Facial/upper airway edema
- Flushing
- Hives
- Muffled voice
- Nausea, vomiting, diarrhea
- Sneezing
- Stridor
- Urticaria
- Wheezing

Interventions

- Administer high-flow oxygen.
- Monitor oxygen saturation and cardiac rhythm continuously.
- Obtain airway equipment and a cricothyrotomy tray.
- Establish intravenous access.
- Facilitate early tracheal intubation; do not delay if symptoms are severe or progressive.
- Proceed to surgical airway management if intubation is not possible.
- Administer the following:
- Bronchodilators

- Epinephrine: Subcutaneously for moderate reactions, intravenously for severe reactions
- Antihistamines: Diphenhydramine (Benadryl)
- Corticosteroids
- Histamine$_2$ blockers: Famotidine (Pepcid)

Foreign Body Aspiration

Foreign body aspiration occurs most frequently in children under the age of 9. Symptoms vary widely and may even be delayed depending on the extent of obstruction. Patients may be asymptomatic or exhibit acute airway compromise.

Foreign Body Aspiration

Signs and Symptoms

- Sudden onset of choking or gagging
- Stridor
- Wheezing
- Diminished breath sounds (unilateral or bilateral)
- Dyspnea
- Cough
- Cyanosis
- Sense of impending doom

Interventions

- Rapidly assess airway, breathing, and circulatory status.
- Remove (with suction, fingers, or Magill forceps) any objects visible in the mouth.
- If the patient is moving air, encourage coughing (leaning forward to facilitate expulsion).
- If the patient is moving air, provide supplemental oxygen by any means the patient will tolerate.
- Monitor oxygen saturation and cardiac rhythm continuously.
- Obtain airway equipment and a cricothyrotomy tray.
- If the patient is not moving air, perform abdominal thrusts (chest thrusts in infants).
- Facilitate oral tracheal intubation of the unconscious, nonbreathing patient.
- Direct visualization of the upper airway (with a laryngoscope) may permit foreign body removal.
- If oral intubation is not effective, proceed immediately to a surgical airway.
- Chest and soft tissue lateral neck radiographs can be used to localize objects but should never delay care.

Angioedema

Angioedema (also known as angioneurotic edema) is the development of large welts below the surface of the skin, especially around the eyes and lips. These welts also may affect the hands, feet, and throat. This condition may be hereditary or it may be precipitated by allergen exposure or stress.[2] Use of angiotensin-converting enzyme inhibitors also has been associated with this phenomenon. Although the symptoms are similar to those of an allergic reaction, angioedema is not a true antigen-antibody response, so treatment with antihistamines and corticosteroids is not particularly effective. Angioedema that does not affect the breathing may be uncomfortable, but it is generally harmless and resolves in a few days. Patients with airway compromise require aggressive management because angioedema can cause life-threatening airway obstruction.

Angioedema

Signs and Symptoms

- Abdominal pain
- Facial edema (nose, lips, ears, eyelids)
- Nausea and vomiting
- Stridor
- Urticaria
- Wheals

Interventions

- Provide supplemental oxygen by any means the patient will tolerate.
- Monitor oxygen saturation and cardiac rhythm continuously.
- Establish intravenous access.
- Consider fresh frozen plasma for hereditary angioedema.
- Facilitate early tracheal intubation; do not delay if symptoms are severe or progressive.
- Proceed to surgical airway management if intubation is not possible.
- Stop administration of any angiotensin-converting enzyme inhibitors.

AIRWAY MANAGEMENT

The accepted method of establishing a patient airway in the patient who is not suspected of having concurrent cervical spine injuries is the head tilt/chin lift method. The head is tilted back with one hand while the chin is lifted with the fingers of the other hand. In the patient in whom concurrent injury to the cervical spine is suspected, the jaw thrust maneuver is applied. During this maneuver, the head is kept in a neutral position while the jaw is thrust forward using the fingers of both hands at the angle of the jaw.

COMMON AIRWAY ADJUNCTS

Oxygen

Oxygen therapy is fundamental to the treatment of many serious conditions. Oxygen can be administered by a variety of devices, delivering low or high flow rates (Table 19-1). Patients receiving supplemental oxygen should have continuous saturation monitoring. Potential side effects include dryness of the airways and irritation of the nose, face, or ears.

Oropharyngeal Airway

An oropharyngeal airway is a curved plastic device designed to be inserted over the tongue and into the posterior pharyngeal area (Figure 19-2). The primary use of the oropharyngeal airway is to prevent the tongue from slipping into the posterior pharyngeal area and occluding the airway, but the device also can serve as a bite block in intubated patients. Oropharyngeal airways are recommended for use only in unconscious patients. Because of the risk of aspiration, this device is not appropriate for anyone with an intact gag reflex. These airways come in many sizes. Select one that extends from the corner of the patient's mouth to the tip of the earlobe.[3] An oropharyngeal airway is placed by inserting it upside down with the distal tip against the roof of the mouth. Gently rotate 180 degrees while advancing it into the posterior pharyngeal area. Do not use this technique in children. An alternate method is to use a tongue blade to depress and displace the tongue while inserting the airway right side up. If an oropharyngeal airway is not positioned properly, it actually can cause airway obstruction by pushing the tongue into the throat.

Table **19-1**   **Summary of Oxygen Therapy Devices**

Type of Breathing Device	Oxygen Flow Rate	Oxygen Concentrations	Advantages	Disadvantages
Nasal cannula	2-6 L/min	24%-44%	No rebreathing of expired air	Can only be on patients breating spontaneously; actual amount of inspired oxygen varies greatly
Face mask	5-10 L/min	40%-60%	Higher oxygen concentration than nasal cannula	Not tolerated well by severely dyspneic patients; can only be used on patients who are breathing spontaneously
Partial rebreather mask	8-12 L/min	50%-80%	Higher oxygen concentration than nasal cannula or face mask	Must have tight seal on mask; can only be used on patients breathing spontaneously; actual amount of inspired oxygen varies greatly
Nonrebreather mask	12-15 L/min	85%-100%	Highest oxygen concentration available by mask	Mush have tight seal on mask; do not allow bag to collapse; can only be used on patients breathing spontaneously
Venturi mask	2-12 L/min	24%-50%	Oxygen concentration can be adjusted	Can only be used on patients breathing spontaneously
Pocket mask	10 L/min	50%	Avoids direct contact with patient's mouth; may add oxygen source; may be used on apneic patient; may be used on children; can obtain excellent tidal volume	Rescuer fatigue
Bag-valve-mask	Room air 12 L/min	21% 40%-90%	Quick; oxygen concentration may be increased; rescuer can sense lung compliance; may be used on both apneic and spontaneously breathing patients	Aire in stomach; low tidal volume; difficulty obtaining a leak-proof seal
Oxygen-powered breathing device	100 L/min	100%	High oxygen flow, positive pressure; improved lung inflation	Gastric distension; overinflation; standard device cannot be used in children without special adapter; requires an oxygen source

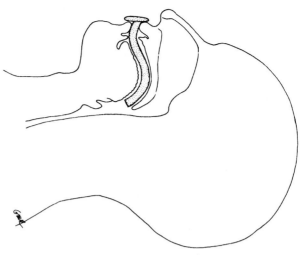

Figure 19-2. Oropharyngeal airway.

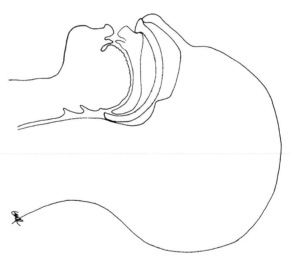

Figure 19-3. Nasopharyngeal airway.

Nasopharyngeal Airway

The nasopharyngeal airway (nasal trumpet, trumpet tube) is a soft rubber catheter about the diameter of the naris (Figure 19-3). Select a size that extends from the patient's nasal opening to the earlobe. Lubricate the nasopharyngeal airway with a water-soluble lubricant or topical anesthetic (e.g., lidocaine jelly 2%) and insert it (bevel toward the septum) into a nostril. Gently push the device into the posterior pharyngeal area (behind the tongue) to a depth approximately level with the base of the ears. If inserted too deeply, the tip can stimulate laryngospasm or enter the esophagus. This airway can be tolerated by alert patients with an intact gag reflex and is particularly useful for tracheal suctioning in the nonintubated patient. Complications include epistaxis, laryngospasm, and vomiting. Because of the potential for nasal and basilar skull fractures, nasopharyngeal airways are contraindicated in patients with facial trauma.

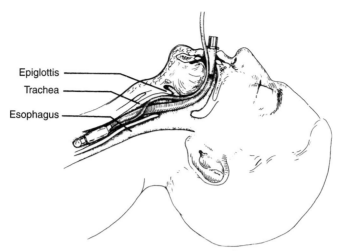

Epiglottis ——

Trachea ——

Esophagus ——

Figure 19-4. Endotracheal tube in place. Note inflated cuff.

Tracheal Intubation

Tracheal tube is passed directly through the mouth or nose into the trachea by way of the vocal cords (Figure 19-4). Tracheal intubation is the most effective means of airway control and aspiration prevention.[3] The standard of care for endotracheal intubation, in any conscious patient, is rapid sequence induction. Rapid sequence induction involves the administration of a series of drugs (oxygen, sedatives, paralytics, and a few supplemental agents) and procedures (cricoid pressure, manual ventilation, suctioning) designed to facilitate intubation. Rapid sequence induction is performed in a standardized, timely, and controlled fashion. Use of this technique minimizes the complications of endotracheal intubation, such as aspiration and airway trauma, and is more comfortable for the patient. Nonetheless, this is not a benign procedure. Once chemically paralyzed, the patient will be unable to breath or maintain an airway. Rapid sequence induction must occur in a smooth, prescribed sequence, often referred to as the seven *P*'s: preparation, preoxygenation, pretreatment, paralysis, placement, placement verification, and postintubation management (Table 19-2). Sedation of the patient before administration of a paralytic agent is critical. Table 19-3 lists medications commonly used in rapid sequence induction.

Alternate Invasive Airways

Endotracheal intubation is the preferred method of airway management in the apneic patient. However, in some settings (e.g., prehospital), practitioners have neither the protocols nor the experience to perform this procedure. Subsequently, alternative airway tools that involve blind (versus directly visualized) tube insertion were developed. These airways have evolved over the years.[4] This category includes devices such as the esophageal obturator airway, the esophageal gastric tube airway, the pharyngotracheal lumen airway, and the Combitube (Kendall Company, Mansfield, MA). Despite their apparent ease of placement, these airways have been associated with significant morbidity, and only the pharyngotracheal lumen and Combitube are used widely today. Potential complications are aspiration, esophageal laceration, and failure to ventilate the correct lumen. If the patient arrives with one of these alternative airways in place, the alternative airway should be exchanged for a tracheal tube as soon as possible. Because emesis often occurs with removal, insert the tracheal tube before cuff deflation and tube withdrawal. The Combitube contains a gastric lumen through which a tube can be inserted for preremoval gastric suctioning.

Table 19-2   **Rapid Sequence Induction**

Time	Step
	Preparation
Zero minus 5-10 minutes	Establish good intravenous access.
	Prepare necessary equipment (bag-valve-mask, suction, tracheal tube, stylet, laryngoscope, tube holder or tape, ventilator).
	Implement continuous cardiac and oxygen saturation monitoring.
	Draw up and label medications.
	Preoxygenation
Zero minus 5 minutes	Preoxygenate with 100% oxygen (by non-rebreather mask or bag-valve-mask).
	(High Pao_2 levels will allow up to 8 minutes of apnea before desaturation occurs.)
	Pretreatment
Zero minus 3 minutes	Administer an appropriate sedating agent (midazolam, fentanyl, etomidate, thiopental, ketamine).
	Give drugs to minimize the effects of intubation such as increased intracranial pressure (lidocaine), bradycardia (atropine), and muscle fasciculations (a small dose of a defasciculating paralytic such as vecuronium, pancuronium, rocuronium).
	Paralysis
Zero	Inject a short-acting neuromuscular blocking agent (succinylcholine, vecuronium, rocuronium, pancuronium).
	Begin (or continue) manual ventilation.
	Placement
Zero plus 45 seconds	Perform the Sellick maneuver (compression of the larynx against the esophagus) to prevent aspiration. Do not release pressure until the tracheal tube cuff has been inflated.
	Intubate the patient and inflate the cuff.
	Placement Verification
	Confirm tube placement by auscultation, chest rise and fall, and a CO_2 detection device.
	Secure the tube.
	Postintubation Management
	Provide additional sedation as needed for ventilator management.
	Administer additional paralytic agents if indicated.
	Obtain a chest radiograph for final verification of placement.

Modified from Hedges JR, Roberts JR, editors: *Procedures in emergency medicine*, ed 4, Philadelphia, 2003, Saunders.

TECHNIQUES FOR MANAGING THE DIFFICULT AIRWAY

Difficulty obtaining an airway can lead to direct airway trauma and morbidity from hypoxia and hypercarbia. Three techniques for establishing an airway when tracheal intubation has failed are described next.

Laryngeal Mask Airway

The laryngeal mask (LMA) airway is a device that is intermediate in design and function between a bag-valve-mask/oropharyngeal airway combination and a tracheal tube (Figure 19-5). The

Table **19-3**   **Rapid Sequence Induction Medications**

Purpose	Medication	Dose	Comments
Sedative	Midazolam	0.1-0.3 mg/kg IV	
Analgesic	Fentanyl	2-3 mcg/kg IV	
Protective agent	Atropine	0.01-0.02 mg/kg (children) 0.5-1 mg IV (adults)	Prevents bradycardia
	Lidocaine	1.5 mg/kg IV	Suppresses cough reflex Blunts intracranial pressure response
Anesthesia	Etomidate	0.2-0.4 mg/kg IV	May cause myotonic or myoclonic activity Reduces bronchospasm; contraindicated in head injury
	Ketamine	1-2 mg/kg IV	Contraindicated in asthma; may cause hypotension and laryngospasm
	Thiopental	2 mg/kg IV	Contraindicated if patient allergic to eggs
	Propofol	0.5-2 mg/kg IV	Contraindicated in hyperkalemia, burns, neuromuscular disease, eye injuries
Paralytic	Succinylcholine	1-2 mg/kg IV	Contraindicated in head and eye injuries, cardiovascular disease
	Pancuronium	0.01 mg/kg IV (defasciculating dose) 0.1 mg/kg IV (paralyzing dose)	
	Rocuronium	0.6-1 mg/kg IV	Contraindicated in head and eye injuries, cardiovascular disease
	Vecuronium	0.01 mg/kg IV (defasciculating dose) 0.1 mg/kg IV (paralyzing dose)	

Modified from Hedges .JR, Roberts JR, editors: *Procedures in emergency medicine*, ed 4, Philadelphia, 2003, Saunders.

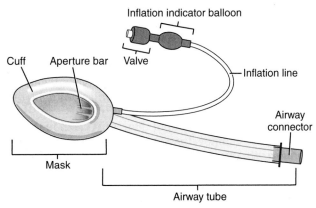

Figure 19-5. Laryngeal mask airway. (From Fultz J, Sturt P: *Mosby's emergency nursing reference*, St Louis, 2005, Mosby.)

LMA provides a safe, swift airway by sealing the outside of the laryngeal inlet with an inflatable cuff. Because laryngeal visualization is not necessary for insertion, the LMA quickly provides an airway when a patent trachea cannot be accessed with an endotracheal tube. Insertion is straightforward but should not be attempted by those without adequate training and insertion protocols. Incorrect positioning can cause obstruction of the airway. LMAs come in infant through adult sizes, as well as disposable and reusable models.

Percutaneous Transtracheal Ventilation

Percutaneous transtracheal ventilation, also known as "needle cricothyrotomy" or "jet insufflation," involves insertion of a large-bore intravenous catheter (10 to 16 gauge) through the cricothyroid membrane into the trachea below the level of the vocal cords. The connector from a size 3.0 endotracheal tube then is inserted into the end of the intravenous catheter and attached to a manual resuscitation bag. This technique is simple and relatively safe to perform and provides rapid access to the airway when the patient cannot be intubated or ventilated by mask (e.g., total upper airway obstruction). However, because the catheter is so narrow, ventilation (especially exhalation) by this method is ineffective and should not be continued for longer than 30 minutes. As an alternative to bagging, the catheter can be connected to a jet ventilator device, attached to a high-pressure oxygen source (Figure 19-6). This device delivers a large volume of oxygen, but few facilities have the necessary equipment readily available.

Surgical Cricothyrotomy

Surgical cricothyrotomy provides rapid entrance into an obstructed airway through an incision to the cricothyroid membrane (Figure 19-7).[5] A cuffed tracheostomy tube is inserted to permit ventilation with a standard resuscitation bag. Cricothyrotomy is the procedure of choice for surgical airway management in an emergency setting. Tracheostomy is a much more complicated, time-consuming, surgical procedure and is not appropriate for emergencies. Several convenient commercial cricothyrotomy kits are currently on the market; these kits contain all the necessary supplies.

VENTILATION

Noninvasive Positive Pressure Ventilation

Noninvasive positive pressure ventilation is an alternative to intubation and mechanical ventilation. Positive pressure is delivered through a tight-fitting oral, nasal, or whole-face mask and reduces the work of breathing. Positive pressure usually is delivered via a continuous positive airway pressure (CPAP) or biphasic positive airway pressure machine (BiPAP), although some standard ventilators are capable of this function. CPAP uses one level of pressure support, whereas BiPAP has different levels of support (peak inspiratory pressure and end-expiratory pressure) for inspiration and expiration. Noninvasive positive pressure ventilation has been used successfully to treat patients with respiratory failure related to chronic obstructive pulmonary disease, asthma, and cardiogenic pulmonary edema. Noninvasive ventilation avoids the complications associated with intubation, such as aspiration and infection, and is more comfortable. Noninvasive positive pressure ventilation is a good alternative for patients who do not wish to be intubated and for those in whom ventilatory assistance is likely to be required for only a few hours. Patients must have an intact airway and must be able to breathe calmly with the machine, but they do not need to be alert. Some patients cannot tolerate the mask. Noninvasive positive pressure ventilation is also unsuitable for those at risk for aspiration and those with large amounts of oral secretions.

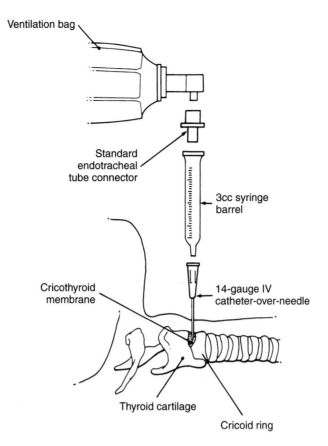

Figure 19-6. A simple setup for translaryngeal ventilation using standard equipment found in any emergency department. This setup is inadequate for adults. High-pressure (50 psi) ventilation systems are optimal. Even with the pressure relief valve on the bag-valve device turned off, only a suboptimal pressure can be developed. However, this technique may be satisfactory in infants and small children. *IV*, Intravenous. (From Roberts JR, Hedges JR: *Clinical procedures in emergency medicine*, ed 4, St Louis, 2004, Saunders.)

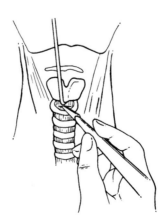

Figure 19-7. The larynx is stabilized with the thumb and middle finger or a tracheal hook (held in the non-dominant hand) while an incision is made in the cricothyroid membrane. (From Roberts JR, Hedges JR: *Clinical procedures in emergency medicine*, ed 4, St Louis, 2004, Saunders.)

Table **19-4** **Troubleshooting Ventilator Alarms**

Alarm	Possible Cause	Intervention
Low exhaled volume	Air leak	Evaluate patient; check connections for leaks; check cuff pressure.
Low airway pressure	Air leak	Evaluate system for leaks.
Low minute ventilation	Low respiratory rate, air leak	Assess patient for change in mental status.
Apnea	Loss of respiratory drive; disconnection from ventilator	Evaluate patient; check connections.
High respiratory rate	Hypoxia; agitation; drug effect; shock	Assess patient; check arterial blood gases; provide reassurance.
High airway pressure	Secretions; kinked tube	Suction secretions; evaluate breath sounds; check for kinks in tube.
High inspiration/expiration ratio	Inspiratory time too long	Adjust ventilator settings.

Mechanical Ventilation

Mechanical ventilation with a standard ventilator is used for a variety of clinical conditions. Goals of ventilation include reversing hypoxemia and respiratory acidosis, relieving respiratory distress and fatigue, preventing or reversing atelectasis, permitting deep sedation and neuromuscular blockade, reducing intracranial pressure, and stabilizing the chest wall. Although mechanical ventilation can be lifesaving, it is associated with numerous complications. Patients who are ventilated mechanically are susceptible to infection, pneumothorax, gastrointestinal disturbances, and cardiovascular compromise related to increased intrathoracic pressure. The patient receiving mechanical ventilation must be monitored carefully for complications related to ventilation, and the ventilator itself should be monitored for problems. Ventilator alarms require prompt attention to prevent life-threatening events (Table 19-4).

Suctioning

Suctioning of oral, nasal, or tracheal secretions often is required to maintain a patent airway. Because suctioning is related to a host of complications, it should be performed only as needed. Suctioning can cause dysrhythmias, airway trauma, hypoxemia, bronchospasm, hemodynamic alterations, and increased intracranial pressure. A closed tracheal suction system attaches directly between the tracheal tube and the ventilator so the secretions can be suctioned from the patient during ventilation. Closed tracheal suction system use minimizes oxygen desaturation during suctioning, eliminates interruption of positive end-expiratory pressure, reduces the incidence of ventilator-associated pneumonias, and is safer for staff (minimizes exposure to body fluids). Because patients receiving high levels of positive end-expiratory pressure are especially prone to desaturate during suctioning, closed suctioning systems are particularly important in this population.

References

1. Hockberger RS, Marx JA, Walls RM, editors: *Rosen's emergency medicine: concepts and clinical practice,* ed 5, St Louis, 2002, Mosby.
2. Hedges JR, Roberts JR, editors: *Procedures in emergency medicine,* ed 4, Philadelphia, 2003, Saunders.
3. Butler KH, Clyne B: Management of the difficult airway: alternative techniques and adjuncts, *Emerg Med Clin North Am* 21:259-289, 2003.
4. Baren JM, Alpern ER, editors: *Emergency medicine pearls,* Philadelphia, 2004, Hanley & Belfus.
5. Stacey KM, Urden LD, Lough ME: *Thelan's critical care nursing: diagnosis and management,* ed 3, St Louis, 2002, Mosby.

20

Respiratory Emergencies

Gretta J. Edwards, RN, BS, CEN

GENERAL ASSESSMENT

Respiratory distress is a common chief complaint in the emergency setting. Rapid and accurate assessment of these patients can prevent potentially life-threatening complications. As with all emergencies, the first priority is to evaluate the patient's airway, breathing, and circulation (ABC) status.

Other pertinent assessment parameters include the following:

- Vital signs, including an oxygen saturation (SpO_2) level
- Peak expiratory flow rate (Compare to standardized charts. What percentile is the patient in?)
- Level of consciousness (altered, fading, or unconscious?)
- Skin color, moisture, and temperature
- Breath sounds (present, absent, diminished, adventitious?)
- Respiratory pattern and rate (tachypneic, bradyneic, irregular?)
- Work of breathing (difficulty inhaling, exhaling, or both?)
- Accessory muscle use (especially sternocleidomastoid neck muscles) in adults
- Retractions (or nasal flaring) in young children
- Position of comfort (Can the patient tolerate lying supine? Is the patient in a tripod position?)
- Speech pattern (How many words can a patient speak before needing to breathe? Phrases? Full sentences?)
- Pursed lip breathing?
- Indicators of a chronic pulmonary problem: Barrel chest, kyphosis, thoracotomy scar, clubbed fingers, nicotine stains on fingers, portable oxygen tank

HISTORY

The history should include the following:
- Establish the onset and nature of the symptoms.
- Obtain a medical history, including previous hospitalizations and intubations for respiratory problems.
- History of tobacco use; what type, how much, how long.
- Patient's occupation.
- Recent exposure to infectious disease.

PULMONARY EMBOLUS

Pulmonary embolus is the third leading cause of death in the United States. In addition, each year an estimated 400,000 cases of pulmonary emboli go undiagnosed, resulting in as many as 100,000 potentially preventable deaths.[1,2] Diagnosis of a pulmonary embolus is difficult because the signs and symptoms are often vague and are similar to those of several other complaints (e.g., myocardial infarction and pneumothorax). A pulmonary embolus occurs when foreign or endogenous material in the venous circulation occludes one or more pulmonary arteries. Most commonly, a pulmonary embolus results from a thrombus that breaks loose from a deep vein in the legs or pelvis. Occlusion of the pulmonary arteries also can occur as a result of a fat, amniotic fluid, or air embolus or intravenous (IV) injection of particulate matter. On occasion, foreign material (such as a bullet) can enter the venous circulation and be transported to the lungs.

Risk Factors

Risk factors for pulmonary embolus include the following:
- Immobility (even of relatively short duration such as a long plane ride)
- History of deep vein thrombosis or previous pulmonary embolus
- Recent trauma associated with vascular injury or limited mobility
- Recent long-bone fracture
- Recent surgery (especially abdominal or pelvic)
- Obesity
- Pregnancy
- Cigarette smoking
- Hypertension
- Stroke
- Thrombophlebitis
- Oral contraceptive use
- Malignancies

Signs and Symptoms

Signs and symptoms of pulmonary embolus vary widely and are related to the size and location of the embolus. Findings tend to be nonspecific and mimic a myriad of other conditions, including pleuritis, myocardial infarction, and panic attack. Just as the body has a clot-forming system, it also has a clot-lysing, fibrinolytic system. Hence even if a clot was initially present, it may be largely dissolved before a definitive diagnosis can be made. Pulmonary emboli are more frequent in women than men and 5 times more common during pregnancy. Lethal pulmonary emboli may occur suddenly with no prodromal signs or symptoms.

The most common signs and symptoms include the following:
- Shortness of breath
- Pleuritic chest pain (usually with a sudden onset)
- Tachypnea
- Tachycardia
- Diaphoresis
- Anxiety, apprehension, restlessness

Additional signs and symptoms that patients who present with a pulmonary embolus may exhibit include the following:
- Fever
- Cough
- Leg pain or swelling
- Crackles or wheezing on auscultation
- Pleural friction rub
- Right bundle branch block with right axis deviation, peaked T waves in limb leads, and depressed T waves in the right precordial leads (V_1, V_2, and V_3)
- Accentuation of pulmonic heart sounds

Patients diagnosed with large pulmonary emboli (>50% occlusion) generally have a high mortality rate. These patients may present with the following:
- Pallor or cyanosis
- Hypotension
- Syncope or decreased level of consciousness
- Hemoptysis
- Signs of right-sided heart failure, including distended neck veins
- Sudden/rapid death

Diagnostic Tests

Diagnostic tests for pulmonary embolus include the following:
- Anterior-posterior and lateral chest radiographs, which are not sensitive for pulmonary embolus but may rule out other conditions such as pneumothorax
- Arterial blood gases
- D-dimer
- Ventilation/perfusion scan
- Ultrasound of the lower extremities and pelvic veins
- Helical (spiral) computed tomography scan
- Magnetic resonance imaging or magnetic resonance angiography
- Pulmonary angiography (invasive, expensive, and time consuming but considered the gold standard for pulmonary embolus diagnosis)

Therapeutic Interventions

Therapeutic interventions for pulmonary embolus include the following:
- Provide supplemental oxygen.
- Monitor oxygen saturation levels.
- Obtain vascular access.
- Administer analgesics as needed.
- Administer nebulized bronchodilators for wheezing.
- Initiate heparin therapy (weight-based bolus followed by continuous infusion); check partial thromboplastin time and International Normalized Ratio (INR) every 4 to 6 hours.
- Consider IV thrombolytic therapy.

SPONTANEOUS PNEUMOTHORAX

A pneumothorax occurs when air enters the pleural space from an opening in the lungs (closed pneumothorax) or the chest wall (open pneumothorax). As air accumulates, the increased pressure (or the loss of negative pressure) causes a partial or even complete collapse of the lung. Spontaneous (nontraumatic) pneumothoraces are closed lung injuries. Primary spontaneous pneumothorax affects patients without known pulmonary disease and usually results from a ruptured congenital pulmonary bleb. The typical patient is a tall, thin male under the age of 40. Spontaneous pneumothoraces caused by a preexisting condition occur most frequently in older men with a history of lung disease such as emphysema. These pneumothoraces are often larger and carry a higher mortality rate.

Signs and Symptoms

Classic signs and symptoms are usually evident with a pneumothorax of 40% or greater. Patients with a small pneumothorax may be relatively asymptomatic.

Common signs and symptoms include the following:

- Sudden onset of pleuritic chest pain (pain with each breath)
- Dyspnea
- Tachypnea
- Cough
- Decreased breath sounds over the affected side
- Cyanosis
- Agitation
- Tympany

Symptoms associated with severe compromise are as follows:

- Subcutaneous emphysema
- Decreased chest excursion on the affected side
- Mediastinal shift
- Distention of neck veins
- Tracheal deviation

Diagnosis

The definitive diagnosis of pneumothorax is made by chest radiograph. However, if symptoms are severe, do not delay therapeutic intervention (chest tube placement) until chest film results are available.

Therapeutic Interventions

The goal of therapy is to reexpand the collapsed lung. Other interventions include the following:

- Monitor oxygen saturation.
- Administer supplemental oxygen.
- Initiate and maintain vascular access.
- Provide analgesia.
- Insert a small-bore chest tube in the upper chest and attach it to a standard water seal chamber or to a Heimlich valve. Generally healthy patients may be discharged from the emergency department with a Heimlich valve in place.
- Bed rest in high Fowler's position.
- Needle thoracostomy is indicated only for tension pneumothorax, a condition rarely associated with spontaneous pneumothorax.

PLEURAL EFFUSION

A pleural effusion is an abnormal collection of fluid in the pleural space. By occupying space in the thoracic cavity, the fluid reduces lung capacity. Pleural effusions may be classified as transudative or exudative. Transudative effusions are caused by systemic factors. Exudative effusions, in which fluid movement is facilitated out of capillaries and into the pleural space, result from increased capillary permeability (Box 20-1).

Signs and Symptoms

Signs and symptoms of pleural effusion include the following:
- Dyspnea
- Cough
- Local or referred pleuritic pain
- Dull, aching chest pain
- Dullness to percussion (on the affected side)
- Decreased breath sounds over the affected area
- Reduced chest wall movement
- Egophony (near the top of fluid line)
- Pleural friction rub
- Signs and symptoms of congestive heart failure, infection, or pleural effusion

Therapeutic Interventions

Obtain anteroposterior and lateral chest radiographs. An effusion will appear as a homogeneously dense opaque area in dependent lung areas. Fluid often will shift with a change in body position.

Other interventions include the following:
- Administer supplemental oxygen if saturation is compromised.
- Provide analgesia.
- Drain pleural fluid by thoracentesis. Liter-sized evacuated (vacuum) bottles, IV tubing, and a needle generally are used for this procedure. Several liters of fluid may be removed. Pleural fluid specimens commonly are sent for cultures and Gram stain.

Box 20-1   Causes of Pleural Effusion

Transudative

After abdominal surgery
Cirrhosis
Congestive heart failure
Pericardial disease
Peritoneal dialysis
Pulmonary embolus

Exudative

Collagen vascular diseases (systemic lupus erythematosus, rheumatoid pleuritis)
Infectious diseases
Neoplastic diseases
Trauma

Data from Lewis SM et al: *Medical-surgical nursing: assessment and management,* ed 5, St Louis, 2000, Mosby.

- If the effusion is large and rapidly accumulating, a chest tube will be inserted.
- Subsequent treatment is based on the underlying cause.
- Improvement in respiratory status may be immediate.

PNEUMONIA

Pneumonia is an acute inflammation of the lung parenchyma caused by an infectious agent, which results in alveolar consolidation. Most cases of pneumonia seen in the emergency department are community-acquired and are generally less virulent than the hospital-acquired variety. Pneumonias are classified as bacterial, viral, mycoplasmal, or fungal. Basically healthy individuals with mild to moderate pneumonia can be discharged. Compromised individuals or anyone who requires continuous supplemental oxygen to maintain saturation levels may require hospital admission.

Risk Factors

Risk factors for pneumonia include the following:
- Smoking
- Recent upper respiratory infection or influenza
- History of pneumonia
- Alcohol abuse
- Underlying cardiovascular disorders
- Underlying pulmonary disorders
- Advanced age (over age 65)
- Altered mental status
- Malnutrition
- Immunocompromised status (drug or disease related)
- Immobility/limited mobility
- Exposure to significant air pollution
- Current endotracheal intubation
- Pneumonia caused by aspiration

Signs and Symptoms

Signs and symptoms of pneumonia include the following:
- Cough (Bacterial pneumonias may be associated with copious purulent sputum.)
- Dyspnea
- Hypoxemia
- Tachypnea
- Tachycardia
- Fever/chills
- Myalgias
- Headache
- Chest pain
- Diaphoresis
- Cyanosis
- Crackles or wheezing
- Apprehension

Therapeutic Interventions

Therapeutic interventions for pneumonia include the following:
- Monitor oxygen saturation levels.
- Administer supplemental oxygen if saturation is compromised.
- Maintain bed rest in a high Fowler's position.
- Provide hydration (oral or IV).
- Obtain chest radiograph.
- Send a complete blood count. Arterial blood gases are necessary only in severe cases.
- Collect blood and sputum cultures. (These may not be ordered for mild to moderate community-acquired pneumonia.)
- Initiate antibiotic therapy appropriate to the causative organism: IV or oral.
- Consider the use of expectorants.
- Nebulize bronchodilators as needed.
- Evaluate the patient's ability to swallow if the pneumonia is caused by aspiration.

PULMONARY EDEMA

The key to patient survival in pulmonary edema is prompt recognition and rapid therapeutic intervention. Cardiogenic pulmonary edema (the most common type) is caused by elevated left-sided heart pressures. Cardiogenic pulmonary edema can result from myocardial infarction, valvular disease, heart failure, or fluid overload. Acute respiratory distress syndrome (ARDS), a form of noncardiogenic pulmonary edema, is the result of damage to the alveolar-capillary membrane. Neurogenic pulmonary edema is associated with significant brain injuries. Regardless of the cause, accumulation of fluid in the alveoli and interstitial space inhibits the exchange of oxygen and carbon dioxide and leads to tissue hypoxia. Normally, the fluid content of the lungs is about 20% of the total volume of the lungs. In acute pulmonary edema, lung fluid content can rise as high as 1000% of normal. The onset of pulmonary edema may be gradual or sudden.

Signs and Symptoms

Signs and symptoms of pulmonary edema include the following:
- Shortness of breath
- Tachycardia
- Tachypnea
- Anxiety, agitation
- Sensation of suffocation
- Chest tightness
- Diaphoresis
- Ashen or cyanotic skin
- Cough
- Orthopnea
- Paroxysmal nocturnal dyspnea
- Cyanosis (central and peripheral)
- Crackles, wheezing, gurgling
- Distended neck veins
- Pink, frothy sputum
- Peripheral edema
- S_3 gallop and decreased heart sounds

Therapeutic Interventions

The goal of pulmonary edema management is to increase oxygenation, decrease cardiac workload, and optimize cardiac function. The following therapeutic interventions will improve circulatory and ventilatory dynamics but may not alter the underlying disease process (e.g., myocardial infarction, head injury, or dysrhythmias). Once the patient's condition is no longer life-threatening, a search must be made for the underlying cause.

Interventions for pulmonary edema include the following:

- Place the patient in a high Fowler's position with the legs dependent (if conscious and able to sit up).
- Administer high-flow oxygen.
- Monitor oxygen saturation and cardiac rhythm (atrial fibrillation is common).
- Check vital signs frequently.
- Establish IV access.
- Obtain a 12-lead electrocardiogram.
- Administer morphine sulfate intravenously to reduce preload, afterload, and anxiety.
- Administer nitroglycerin to reduce preload (contraindicated if the patient is hypotensive).
- Administer furosemide (Lasix) intravenously to decrease intravascular volume and promote vasodilation.
- Place an indwelling urinary catheter to monitor urine output.
- Provide reassurance. These patients are extremely anxious and experience feelings of suffocation and doom. They need verbal support and touch communication.
- Some patients may be extremely diaphoretic and may appreciate an electric fan.

ASTHMA

Asthma is a chronic illness with acute exacerbations characterized by airway hyperreactivity, inflammation, and reversible airflow obstruction (bronchospasm). Asthma affects about 5% of the population of the United States and is the most prevalent chronic childhood disease. Mortality rates for asthma increased 31% from 1990 to 1999 but have recently stabilized.[3] The primary drugs used to treat asthma in the emergency department are oxygen, inhaled beta$_2$-agonists (albuterol), anticholinergic medications (ipratropium bromide) and corticosteroids. Beta$_2$-agonists relax the smooth muscles of the bronchioles and produce bronchodilation, whereas anticholinergic drugs inhibit contraction of bronchial smooth muscle and limit the secretion of mucus. Corticosteroids reduce airway inflammation, inhibit mucous production, and decreases airway swelling and hyperreactivity.

Importantly, all that wheezes is not asthma, and all asthmatics do not necessarily wheeze. Wheezing can be a symptom of other diseases, including chronic obstructive pulmonary disease (COPD), pneumonia, bronchitis, croup, pulmonary embolus, allergic reactions, and heart failure. Wheezing may be absent in acute asthma exacerbations. Some asthmatics, especially children, may have a repetitive cough but no wheeze. Additionally, wheezing disappears with severe bronchospasm because of the lack of air movement. This is an ominous sign and signals the need for immediate intubation. The return of loud wheezing is an indicator of a positive treatment response.

Asthma Triggers

A wide variety of stimulants can precipitate an asthma exacerbation. Common triggers include the following:

- Allergies to food or inhalants (e.g., pollen, latex, mold, or animal dander)
- Exercise

- Cold exposure (breathing cold air, eating ice cream)
- Tobacco smoke
- Upper respiratory infections
- Air pollutants
- Sinusitis, rhinitis
- Medications, especially aspirin and nonsteroidal antiinflammatory drugs
- Food additives

Signs and Symptoms

Signs and symptoms of asthma include the following:
- Wheezing (most commonly expiratory, but also may be inspiratory or *may be absent.*)
- Dyspnea
- Tachypnea
- Tachycardia
- Cough (may be present without wheezing, especially in children)
- Peak expiratory flow rate (PEFR) less than 50% of predicted value
- Use of accessory muscles of respiration, especially sternocleidomastoid muscles in adults
- Retractions and nasal flaring in children
- Chest tightness and hyperresonance on percussion (because of hyperinflation)
- Anxiety or restlessness as a result of catecholamine release and air hunger
- Orthopnea
- Low oxygen saturation
- Diaphoresis
- Halting speech

Therapeutic Interventions

Therapeutic interventions for asthma include the following:
- Allow the patient to maintain a position of comfort.
- Monitor oxygen saturation.
- Provide supplemental oxygen to maintain a high-normal saturation level.
- Administer bronchodilators via a nebulizer or a metered dose inhaler with a spacer.
- Anticholinergics (ipratropium bromide [Atrovent]) frequently are given. The benefit of this therapy in asthma management is questionable, but the therapy is not harmful and some patients seem to have a positive response.
- Measure PEFR before and after interventions. This is the single best determinant of asthma severity and response to treatment.
- Administer corticosteroids. Start steroid therapy early to treat the inflammatory component of asthma. Whether given IV or orally, steroids require about 6 hours to take effect. Bronchodilators only address the bronchospastic component.
- Provide fluid and electrolyte replacement; ensure good hydration. Depending on the duration of the attack, patients may be moderately dehydrated. This contributes to mucous plugging and catecholamine release.

Interventions of Little Benefit

Several interventions, widely used for years, have been shown to add little to the management of the asthma patient:
- *Sputum cultures:* Although many asthmatics produce yellow-green sputum, this is usually an indication of eosinophil activity and not a sign of bacterial infection. Cultures are not warranted unless other signs of infection (e.g., fever, sinusitis, or pharyngitis) exist.

- *Antibiotics:* Because significant bacterial infection is unusual in the asthmatic, antibiotics are generally not indicated.
- *Complete blood count:* This test rarely adds anything to the management of routine asthma except cost. White blood cells are predictably elevated.
- *Chest radiographs:* Asthmatics will have abnormal chest films (air trapping), but nothing is gained therapeutically by documenting this finding unless there is an additional reason to obtain a radiograph, such as suspicion of concomitant pneumonia, pneumothorax, or foreign body aspiration. Intubated patients should have chest films taken.
- *Arterial blood gases:* As with chest radiographs, arterial blood gases in the asthmatic will be abnormal, but in a predictable manner. Following serial PEFR readings and oxygen saturation levels provides more clinically useful data without inflicting this painful procedure on patients. Severe asthmatics (status asthmaticus) and intubated patients may benefit from arterial blood gas measurement.
- *Intravenously administered aminophylline or terbutaline or subcutaneously administered epinephrine:* These agents are less effective and have more side effects than do inhaled beta$_2$-agonists (albuterol). Failure of inhaled bronchodilator therapy is not an indication for parenteral bronchodilators.
- *Sedation:* Asthmatics may be anxious. Anxiety results from hypoxemia and catecholamine release. The cure for anxiety is adequate tissue oxygenation. Sedatives may diminish respiratory drive in the nonintubated patient.

STATUS ASTHMATICUS

Status asthmaticus is a severe asthma exacerbation that does not respond to therapy. Intubation may be required. A history of prior intubation for asthma is a strong predictor of the need for future intubation. Status asthmaticus is associated with a significant mortality rate and must be treated promptly and aggressively.

Signs and Symptoms

Signs and symptoms of status asthmaticus include the following:
- Silent chest: Absent or minimal wheezing, little air movement
- PEFR less than 100 L/min (adults)
- Inability to speak more than a word or two
- Inability to lay flat
- SpO$_2$ less than 90% despite supplemental oxygen
- Pulsus paradoxus greater than 20 mm Hg (because of chest hyperinflation)
- Fatigue, decreasing level of consciousness
- Long expiratory phase
- Hypoxemia, hypercarbia (elevated PcO$_2$), metabolic acidosis
- Increased respiratory rate and accessory muscle use (until the patient becomes fatigued)
- Cyanosis (a late and unreliable sign)

Therapeutic Interventions

Therapeutic interventions for status asthmaticus include the following:
- Monitor SpO$_2$. Measure arterial blood gases as indicated. Hypercarbia is an ominous sign of decompensation. The patient who is still compensating will be *hypo*carbic.

- Provide supplemental oxygen. Unlike the patient with COPD, asthmatics are not normally hypoxic and do not tolerate hypoxia well.
- Administer bronchodilators. Albuterol (via handheld nebulizer or endotracheal tube) may be administered continuously in cases of severe disease.
- Serially measure PEFR as long as the patient is able to cooperate. A patient's inability to perform PEFR testing is an indicator of severe disease.
- Anticholinergics may or may not prove beneficial but usually are tried in status asthmaticus.
- Initiate corticosteroid therapy early in the course of treatment.
- Establish IV access and rehydrate the patient.
- Prepare for possible tracheal intubation. Intubation must be preformed cautiously by a skilled provider. Because patients in status asthmaticus are prone to arrest during intubation, preoxygenate the patient as much as possible and intubate before significant respiratory acidosis occurs.
- Mechanical ventilation is difficult in this population because of severely narrowed airways and massive air trapping. Use small tidal volumes and long expiratory times.
- Heliox, a combination of helium and oxygen, occasionally is used to reduce airflow resistance.
- Intubated patients may require sedation and chemical paralysis.
- Watch closely for pneumothorax development, especially following intubation.
- Occasionally, inhaled general anesthetic agents are used to manage intractable asthma.
- Studies of the effectiveness of IV magnesium administration for status asthmaticus have yielded mixed results, but magnesium generally is considered a benign agent and may be ordered.

ACUTE BRONCHITIS

Acute bronchitis is one of the most common conditions for which persons seek medical care. Bronchitis involves an infection of the upper airways and is characterized by a productive cough. Although the cause of acute bronchitis is usually a viral infection, antibiotics regularly are prescribed, making bronchitis one of the most frequent sources of antibiotic abuse. Multiple studies have shown that the majority of patients with acute bronchitis do not benefit from use of antibiotics. However, older adults and patients with an underlying pulmonary disease (e.g., COPD) are much more likely to have a bacterial infection, and antibiotic therapy may be appropriate.

Signs and Symptoms

Signs and symptoms of acute bronchitis include the following:
- Productive cough
- Dyspnea
- Wheezing
- Generalized, constant chest pain
- Fever
- Hoarseness
- Malaise
- Crackles, wheezing

Therapeutic Interventions

Therapeutic interventions for acute bronchitis include the following:
- Rest
- Bronchodilators (indicated only in the presence of bronchospasm)
- Expectorants
- Fluids (generally oral)
- Aspirin, acetaminophen, or nonsteroidal antiinflammatory drugs
- Reassurance

CHRONIC OBSTRUCTIVE PULMONARY DISEASE

Chronic obstructive pulmonary disease (COPD) is the fourth leading cause of death in the United States.[4] COPD involves a combination of chronic bronchitis, emphysema, and asthma like symptoms such as airflow obstruction and airway hyperreactivity. More than 90% of patients with COPD have a history of smoking. Other causative factors include pollution, industrial inhalants (such as silicon and asbestos), α_1-antitrypsin deficiency, and lower respiratory tract infections during childhood. Chronic obstructive pulmonary disease develops over the course of many years. Patients present to the emergency department with acute exacerbations or when their current level of therapy is no longer adequate.

Nearly all patients with COPD have some combination of chronic bronchitis and emphysema, but most tend to fall into one of two classic patterns: the "blue bloaters" and the "pink puffers." Chronic bronchitis is the most prominent disease process in the blue bloater subgroup. These patients have constant inflammation of the airways, which causes a persistent, productive cough. They usually are obese and have a decreased cardiac output leading to polycythemia, hypoxemia, and right ventricular failure. Blue bloaters retain carbon dioxide, which destroys the usual respiratory drive, leaving the patient dependent on a hypoxic drive. Supplemental oxygen can increase Pao_2 levels, preventing hypoxia and thus blunting the respiratory urge. This can lead to respiratory arrest.

Emphysema results from a loss of alveolar wall mass, producing permanent enlargement of the airspaces. This loss of surface area results in a greatly diminished number of gas exchange units, causing oxygen levels to drop and carbon dioxide (to a lesser degree) to rise. In contrast to the blue bloater, the pink puffer compensates by hyperventilation. The body habitus of the pink puffer is thin, or even cachectic, with a barrel chest and dyspnea appearing early in the disease. To help maximize ventilation, patients with COPD frequently use pursed lip breathing technique and assume a tripod position.

Signs and Symptoms

Signs and symptoms of COPD include the following:
- Dyspnea
- Cyanosis
- Orthopnea
- Productive cough
- Distant breath sounds, wheezes, crackles
- Hyperresonance on percussion
- Pursed lip breathing
- A prolonged expiratory phase of respiration
- Barrel chest
- Clubbing of the fingers

Therapeutic Interventions

Therapeutic interventions for COPD include the following:

- Monitor oxygen saturation. Arterial blood gases may or may not add anything to the management of the patient with COPD.
- Administer oxygen. Patients with COPD often have baseline Pao_2 levels that are minimally acceptable. Unlike the asthmatic, these patients do not require a high normal Spo_2. Titrate supplemental oxygen to maintain a saturation of 90% to 92%. However, *never withhold oxygen from a hypoxic patient.* The most severe life-threatening problem for these patients is hypoxemia. Monitor the pulse oximeter to keep saturation within the target range. Observe the patient carefully for decreased mental status that may signal hypercarbia.
- Administer bronchodilators. Inhaled, short-acting, beta$_2$-agonists (e.g., albuterol) are the first line of defense, but many patients with COPD respond well to nebulized anticholinergics (ipratropium bromide).
- Provide bed rest in a high Fowler's position. However, these patients frequently prefer to sit at the side of the gurney, leaning forward, with their elbows propped on a bedside table (tripod position).
- Initiate and maintain vascular access and provide adequate hydration.
- Monitor for cardiac dysrhythmias.
- If hypoxemia and hypercarbia persist, the patient will need aggressive ventilator support. Unfortunately, once intubated, patients with COPD are difficult to wean from the ventilator. Consider noninvasive positive pressure mask ventilation (continuous positive airway pressure or biphasic positive airway pressure). See Chapter 19 for a discussion of these modalities.
- Patients with COPD often have a list of other medical problems—such as heart failure, dysrhythmias, and pneumonia—that require additional assessment and management.

ACUTE RESPIRATORY DISTRESS SYNDROME

Acute respiratory distress syndrome (ARDS), a form of noncardiogenic pulmonary edema, is an inflammatory syndrome characterized by diffuse alveolar damage that thickens the alveolar walls, causes fluid and protein to leak into the alveoli, and eventually produces alveolar collapse. The precipitating event can be a direct insult to the lung (e.g., aspiration or smoke inhalation) or an indirect injury resulting from a systemic illness (Box 20-2). Progressive atelectasis, increased interstitial and alveolar edema, and significant ventilation-perfusion abnormalities result in progressive hypoxemia and severely decreased lung compliance. Even with aggressive treatment, this disorder is associated with a high mortality rate.

Risk Factors

Risk factors for ARDS include the following:

- Pneumonia
- Sepsis
- Aspiration
- Chemical inhalation
- Multiple trauma
- Massive transfusion
- Chronic alcohol abuse

Box **20-2** Conditions Predisposing to Acute Respiratory Distress Syndrome

Infectious Causes	Metabolic Disorders	Drug-Related
Gram-negative sepsis	Pancreatitis	Dextran 40
Bacterial pneumonia	Uremia	Heroin
Viral pneumonia	Diabetic ketoacidosis	Methadone
Pneumocystis carinii		Salicylates
Tuberculosis	**Inhaled Toxic Agents**	Thiazides
	Oxygen	Propoxyphene
Aspiration	Smoke	Colchicine
Gastric	Toxic gases	
Freshwater and salt water		**Other**
(drowning)	**Hematologic Disorders**	Radiation pneumonitis
Ethylene glycol	Massive blood transfusion	Amniotic fluid emboli
Hydrocarbon fluids	Disseminated intravascular	Increased intracranial pressure
	coagulation	High altitude
Shock	Transfusion reaction	Fluid overload
Septic	Postcardiopulmonary bypass	Eclampsia
Traumatic	or resuscitation	Goodpasture's syndrome
Hemorrhagic		Drug overdose
	Immunologic Reactions	Bowel infarction
Trauma	Drug allergy	Dead fetus
Generalized	Anaphylaxis	
Fat embolism		
Lung contusion		
Multiple major fractures		
Head injury		
Burns		

From Newberry L, editor: *Sheehy's emergency nursing: principles and practice,* ed 5, St Louis, 2003, Mosby.

Signs and Symptoms

Signs and symptoms of ARDS include the following:
- Dyspnea
- Tachypnea
- Tachycardia
- Cyanosis
- Refractory hypoxemia (does not improve significantly with oxygen administration)
- Anxiety, restlessness, agitation
- Accessory muscle use

Therapeutic Interventions

Therapeutic interventions for ARDS include the following:
- Monitor and maintain the patient's airway, breathing, and circulatory status.
- These patients require endotracheal intubation and critical care unit admission.
- Provide mechanical ventilation with a volume-cycled ventilator and positive end-expiratory pressure. Small tidal volumes (6 mL/kg) have been shown to reduce lung damage compared with the much larger (10 to 15 mL/kg) volumes that were once popular.
- Initiate and maintain vascular access.

- Begin careful hydration. Because of their pulmonary status, patients with ARDS will have elevated pulmonary artery pressures even in the presence of hypovolemia. This population may benefit from a pulmonary artery catheter.

INHALATION INJURY

Inhalation injury occurs when smoke, toxic products of combustion, or other noxious fumes are inhaled. Toxic inhalation, not burns, is the leading cause of death in structure fires. The three important components to inhalation injury are (1) asphyxiation, (2) thermal injury, and (3) smoke poisoning. One or more of these conditions may be present.

Asphyxiation occurs when toxic gases displace environmental oxygen. Additionally, once inhaled, carbon monoxide and cyanide prevent the transport and cellular utilization of oxygen. Carbon monoxide exposure is discussed in the following section. Cyanide, which is released from burning synthetic materials, is particularly deadly. Because antidotes for cyanide poisoning exist, early recognition of cyanide inhalation is essential. Symptoms of toxicity include headache, palpitations, giddiness, and dyspnea. Suspect cyanide poisoning with inhalation exposure if the patient has severe dyspnea, a metabolic acidosis, and a normal Pao_2 (oxygen is delivered to the tissues but cannot be used).

Thermal injury (heat damage) generally is limited to the upper airway unless steam was involved. Thermal injury produces erythema, edema, blisters, and charring that can result in rapid and complete airway obstruction. Smoke poisoning is the result of the inhalation of toxic gases. Once in the lungs, these gases damage delicate pulmonary endothelial cells and destroy the cilia, leading to pulmonary edema. Injury severity depends on the length of exposure, the type of chemical(s), and whether the patient was in a confined space at the time of exposure.

Signs and Symptoms

Signs and symptoms of inhalation injury include the following:
- Pain and irritation of the upper airways; burning pain in the throat or chest
- Singed nasal hairs and facial hairs (eyebrows, eyelashes, moustache) if fire was involved
- Facial burns
- Oral and pharyngeal burns, redness, or blistering
- Sputum that contains carbon
- Hypoxemia
- Crackles, wheezing
- Dyspnea
- Restlessness or agitation
- Cough
- Hoarseness (This is an important sign of vocal cord involvement and potential obstruction.)
- Signs of pulmonary edema may appear hours after the exposure
- Cyanide poisoning, which can cause giddiness

Therapeutic Interventions

Therapeutic interventions for inhalation injury include the following:
- Focus on the ABCs.
- Administer oxygen. (Humidified and cooled is optimal but not essential.)
- Initiate and maintain vascular access.

- Monitor arterial blood gas values and oxygen saturation levels.
- Check a carboxyhemoglobin level.
- Admit the patient for observation for 24 to 48 hours. Pulmonary damage may manifest long after initial exposure.
- Perform tracheal intubation or cricothyrotomy if indicated (See Chapter 19.)
- Insert a nasogastric or orogastric tube and attach to suction.
- Provide nebulized racemic epinephrine for upper airway obstruction.
- Administer bronchodilators for lower airway obstruction.
- Use the cyanide antidote kit (contains three drugs, given sequentially) if cyanide poisoning is suspected.

CARBON MONOXIDE POISONING

Carbon monoxide is a colorless, tasteless, odorless gas formed by the burning of organic (carbon-containing) matter. Because carbon monoxide has a 200 to 250 times greater affinity for hemoglobin than does oxygen, hemoglobin molecules quickly become saturated with carbon monoxide and cannot transport oxygen. This leads to tissue hypoxia. Carbon monoxide also shifts the oxyhemoglobin dissociation curve to the left, impairing the ability of hemoglobin to release whatever oxygen molecules it has, further aggravating hypoxia. Fetal hemoglobin has an even greater affinity for carbon monoxide, so a fetus will have a carboxyhemoglobin level about 30% higher than that of the mother. Carbon monoxide poisoning may occur in isolation, as in the case of a malfunctioning furnace, or can be mixed with other toxic gases (e.g., in a structure fire). Smoking and exposure to automobile exhaust elevate baseline carboxyhemoglobin levels as high as 10% to 15%. Symptoms worsen as carboxyhemoglobin levels increase. Table 20-1 summarizes the symptoms of carbon monoxide poisoning.

Therapeutic Interventions

Therapeutic interventions for carbon monoxide poisoning include the following:
- Administer high-flow oxygen. Oxygen is the antidote for carbon monoxide. Give it early and aggressively.

Table 20-1   Symptoms of Carbon Monoxide Poisoning

Carboxyhemoglobin Level (%)	Symptoms
5-10	Headache
	Dizziness
10-20	Headache
	Nausea, vomiting
	Loss of coordination
	Flushed skin
	Dyspnea
20-30	Confusion
	Lethargy
	Visual disturbances
	Angina
30-60	Dysrhythmias
	Seizures
	Coma
≥60	Cherry red skin
	Death

- Facilitate endotracheal intubation as needed (e.g., patients with seizures or loss of consciousness).
- Monitor cardiac rhythm.
- Monitor carboxyhemoglobin levels.
- When carbon monoxide toxicity is suspected, do *not* use a pulse oximeter. This device *measures the percent* of hemoglobin molecules that are saturated, *not what they are saturated with* (oxygen versus carbon monoxide).
- Draw an arterial blood gas sample to check a *measured* saturation level (SaO_2). Assess this number, along with the carboxyhemoglobin level, and then compare with the SpO_2. If the SaO_2 and SpO_2 are similar, it is safe to use the pulse oximeter.
- Hyperbaric oxygen therapy is highly effective but logistically complicated. Few facilities have a hyperbaric oxygen chamber available, so intrafacility transfer, with all of its attendant complications, is required. Fortunately, when one is breathing 100% oxygen, the half-life for the elimination of carbon monoxide from the body is 50 to 70 minutes. This means that carboxyhemoglobin actually may be lowered to acceptable levels in less time than it would take to complete a transfer to a hyperbaric unit. Additionally, the patient may require burn unit admission, which is not necessarily at the same facility as the hyperbaric oxygen chamber.

HIGH-ALTITUDE PULMONARY EDEMA

High-altitude pulmonary edema (HAPE) is the most common cause of death related to altitude. Early recognition and treatment significantly improve outcome. HAPE typically occurs 2 to 4 days after rapid ascent to an altitude above 8000 feet. The condition also is seen in patients who normally live at high altitudes, travel to sea level for 2 weeks or more, and then return home. Symptoms are usually worse at night. HAPE is a form of non-cardiogenic pulmonary edema. Although the exact cause remains unclear, it appears to be related to increased pulmonary artery pressures that occur in response to significant elevation.

Signs and Symptoms

Signs and symptoms of HAPE include the following:
- Dyspnea at rest
- Cough; may be productive of pink, frothy sputum
- Weakness, fatigue, exercise intolerance
- Chest tightness or congestion
- Tachypnea
- Tachycardia
- Crackles, wheezing
- Confusion
- Cyanosis

Treatment

Treatment for HAPE includes the following:
- The most effective treatment is descent to lower altitude. This usually reverses the disease process.
- Provide high-flow oxygen to maintain normal saturation levels.

- Keep the patient warm.
- Pressurize the patient in a portable, inflatable, hyperbaric chamber commonly used wilderness situations (e.g., Gamow bag).
- Administer nifedipine and morphine to dilate the pulmonary vasculature.
- Provide bed rest.
- Consider administration of acetazolamide (There are no documented studies that confirm the effectiveness of this treatment).[2]

SUBMERSION INJURY

Drowning accounts for about 3700 deaths in the United States each year.[5] When a victim is unexpectedly submerged, air hunger eventually develops, causing an involuntary gasp with aspiration of water, which triggers laryngospasm (wet drowning). However, in 10% to 20% of drownings, severe laryngospasm actually prevents the aspiration of water (dry drowning). Both seawater and freshwater produce significant pulmonary damage, causing hypoxia and loss of surfactant. Contaminants such as mud, algae, and chlorine can obstruct or damage the smaller airways and increase the risk of infection. Although submersion in cold water slows the progression of hypoxic brain injury, these victims also may require treatment for hypothermia. To qualify as a true cold water drowning, water temperature must be near freezing, not simply chilly. Conversely, patients who drown in hot tubs generally have poorer outcomes. When assessing a patient with a submersion injury, one also must consider precipitating factors. Seizures, head or cervical trauma, cardiac arrest, stroke, drug or alcohol intoxication, scuba diving injuries, and child abuse can be the proximate cause of a submersion injury.

Risk Factors

Risk factors for submersion injury include the following:
- Lack of supervision
- Inability to swim
- Risk-taking behaviors
- Alcohol use
- Underlying medical conditions

Signs and Symptoms

Findings associated with near drowning vary widely and are related directly to the extent of hypoxic injury:
- History of immersion
- Progressive dyspnea
- Wheezing
- Crackles
- Cough (sometimes with pink, frothy sputum)
- Tachycardia
- Chest pain
- Mental confusion
- Coma
- Cyanosis
- Respiratory or cardiac arrest

Therapeutic Interventions

Therapeutic interventions for submersion injury include the following:
- Start high-flow oxygen, endotracheal intubation, and advanced life support as indicated.
- Establish vascular access.
- Immobilize the cervical spine if there is a possibility of injury.
- Monitor arterial blood gases and oxygen saturation.
- Check core body temperature; warm the patient as needed.
- Add positive end-expiratory pressure (intubated patients) to reinflate collapsed alveoli.
- Suction fluids and secretions from intubated patients as needed. If frequent suctioning is required, use a closed suction system.
- Elevate the head of the stretcher if the cervical spine has been cleared.
- Correct acid-base imbalances.
- Consider prophylactic adminstration of antibiotics.
- Administer bronchodilators as needed.
- Insert a nasogastric or orogastric tube to decompress the stomach. Vomiting is common.
- Consider central venous pressure monitoring, an arterial pressure line, or a pulmonary artery catheter to monitor volume, cardiac, and pulmonary status.
- Admit patients for a minimum of 24 hours of observation.

References

1. Newberry L, editor: *Sheehy's emergency nursing: principles and practice,* ed 5, St Louis, 2003, Mosby.
2. Hockberger RS, Marx JA, Walls RM, editors: *Rosen's emergency medicine: concepts and clinical practice,* ed 5, St Louis, 2002, Mosby.
3. Baren JM, Alpern ER, editors: *Emergency medicine pearls,* Philadelphia, 2004, Hanley & Belfus.
4. Palm KH, Decker W: Acute exacerbations of chronic obstructive pulmonary disease, *Emerg Med Clin North Am* 21(2):331-352, 2003.
5. Center for Disease Control and Prevention: Water-related injuries: fact sheet. Retrieved September 15, 2004, from http://www.cdc.gov/ncipc/factsheets/drown.htm.

21

Cardiac Emergencies

Donna S. Gloe, BSN, MSN, EdD, RNBC

Chest pain is the chief patient complaint in a variety of serious cardiac emergencies. Any time the heart or great vessels are in jeopardy, health care providers must evaluate the problem rapidly and begin treatment. Often this must be done without the benefit of a detailed assessment or an in-depth history. This chapter presents essential elements of cardiac assessment, outlines a number of serious cardiovascular conditions, and describes their emergency treatment.

CHEST PAIN ASSESSMENT

To assess chest pain, do the following:
- Use the PQRST mnemonic to gather information about the pain (see Table 7-4; *Provoke/palliates, Quality, Radiates, Severity, Time*). A recently published mnemonic, CHEST PAIN, includes assessment of history and risk factors (Table 21-1).
- Assess vital signs, oxygen saturation, and skin color, temperature, and moistness.
- Examine a rhythm strip for the presence of dysrhythmias. Leads II or MCL_1 are preferred.
- Obtain a brief history and evaluate the patient's cardiac risks (Box 21-1). The presence of multiple risk factors significantly increases the likelihood of a cardiac event.
- Table 21-2 discusses differential diagnoses to consider in patients who complain of chest pain.
- Note current medication use, including prescription, over-the-counter, and herbal therapies.
- Identify other symptoms, including dyspnea, neck vein distention, diaphoresis, nausea, and vomiting.
- Consider noncardiac causes of chest pain such as esophageal disease, recreational drug use, pulmonary conditions, and anxiety disorders. Table 21-3 highlights etiologic factors related to the differential diagnosis of chest pain.

Text continued on p. 333

Table **21-1**   **CHEST PAIN Mnemonic for Chest Pain Assessment**

Letter	Trigger words	Assessment
C	Commenced when?	When did the pain start? Was onset associated with anything specific? Exertion? Activity? Emotional upset?
H	History/risk factors	Do you have a history of heart disease? Is there a primary relaive (parent/sibling) with early onset and/or early death related to heart disease? Do you have other risk factors, e.g., diabetes, smoking, hypertension, or obesity?
E	Extra symptoms?	What else are you feeling with the pain? Are you nervous? Sweating? Is your heart racing? Are you short of breath? Do you feel nauseated? Dizzy? Weak?
S	Stays/radiates	Does the pain stay in one place? Does it radiate or go anywhere else in the body? Where?
T	Timing	How long does the pain last? How long has this episode lasted? How many minutes? Is the pain continuous or does it come and go? When did it become continuous?
P	Place	Where is your pain? Check for point tenderness with palpation.
A	Alleviates	What makes the pain better? Rest? Changing position? Deep breathing?
	Aggravates	What makes the pain worse? Exercise? Deep breathing? Changing positions?
I	Intensity	How intense is the pain? Rate the pain from 0 to 10.
N	Nature	Describe the pain. (*Listen for descriptors such as sharp, stabbing, crushing, dull, burning, elephant sitting on my chest.*) Do not suggest descriptors.

From Newberry L, Barret G, Ballard N: A new mnemonic for chest pain assessment, *J Emerg Nurs* 31:84–85.

Box **21-1**   **Cardiac Risk Factors: Patient Characteristics and High-Risk Behaviors**

Aging
Cocaine or stimulant use
Diabetes
Emotional stress
Hyperlipidemia
Hypertension
Immediate family history

Lack of exercise
New onset of fatigue within the past month (particularly in women)
Obesity
Previous myocardial infarction, angina, cardiac surgery, or peripheral vascular disease
Smoking

Table 21-2   Differential Diagnosis of Chest Pain

Cause	Onset of Pain	Characteristics of Pain	Location of Pain
Acute myocardial infarction	Sudden onset; lasts more than 30 min to 1 hr	Pressure, burning, aching, tightness, choking	Across chest; may radiate to jaws and neck and down arms and back
Angina	Sudden onset; lasts only a few minutes	Ache, squeezing, choking, heaviness, burning	Substernal; may radiate to jaw and neck and down arms and back
Dissecting aortic aneurysm	Sudden onset	Excruciating, tearing	Center of chest; radiates into back; may radiate to abdomen
Pericarditis	Sudden onset or may be variable	Sharp, knifelike	Retrosternal; may radiate up neck and down left arm
Pneumothorax	Sudden onset	Tearing, pleuritic	Lateral side of chest
Pulmonary embolus	Sudden onset	Crushing (but not always)	Lateral side of chest
Hiatal hernia	Sudden onset	Sharp, severe	Lower chest; upper abdomen
Gastrointestinal disturbance or cholecystitis	Sudden onset	Gripping, burning	Lower substernal area, upper abdomen
Degenerative disk (cervical or thoracic spine) disease	Sudden onset	Sharp, severe	Substernal; may radiate to neck, jaw, arms, and shoulders
Degenerative or inflammatory lesions of shoulder, ribs, scalenus anterior	Sudden onset	Sharp, severe	Substernal; radiates to shoulder
Hyperventilation	Sudden onset	Vague	Vague

From Newberry L, editor: *Sheehy's emergency nursing: principles and practice*, ed 5, St Louis, 2003, Mosby.

History	Pain Worsened by	Pain Relieved by	Other
Age 40 to 70 yr; may or may not have history of angina	Movement, anxiety	Nothing; no movement, stillness, position, or breath holding; only relieved by medication (morphine sulfate)	Shortness of breath, diaphoresis, weakness, anxiety
May have history of angina; precipitating circumstances; pain characteristic; response to nitroglycerin	Lying down, eating, effort, cold weather, smoking, stress, anger, worry, hunger	Rest, nitroglycerin	Unstable angina occurs even at rest
Nothing specific, except that pain is usually worse at onset		Nothing	Blood pressure difference between right and left arms, murmur of aortic regurgitation
Short history of upper respiratory infection or fever	Deep breathing, trunk movement, maybe swallowing	Sitting up, leaning forward	Friction rub, paradoxic pulse over 10 mm Hg
None	Breathing	Nothing	Dyspnea, increased pulse, decreased breath sounds, deviated trachea
Sometimes phlebitis Deep vein thrombosis Recent surgery	Breathing	Not breathing	Cyanosis, dyspnea, profound anxiety, hypoxemia, cough with hemoptysis
May have none	Heavy meal, bending, lying down	Bland diet, walking, antacids, semi-Fowler position	
May have none	Eating, lying down	Antacids	
May have none	Movement of the neck or spine, lifting, straining	Rest, decreased movement	Pain usually on outer aspect of arm, thumb, or index finger
May have none	Movement of arm or shoulder	Elevation and arm support to shoulder postural exercises	
Hyperventilation, anxiety, stress, emotional upset	Increased respiratory rate	Slowing of respiratory rate	Be *sure* hyperventilation is from nonmedical cause

Table 21-3   Etiologic Factors To Be Considered in the Differential Diagnosis of Chest Pain

Etiologic factors	P Precipitating/Palliating	Q Quality	R Radiating/Region	S Severity/Symptoms	T Time/Temporal
Ischemic/angina	Precipitating factors: Effort-related activity, large meals, emotional stress Palliation: Ceases with activity abatement, relief with nitroglycerin, relief with rest	Tightness, burning, deep, constrictive	Retrosternal, area affected the size of the palm of the hand Pain may radiate to left shoulder, left hand (e.g., especially the fourth and fifth fingers), epigastrium trachea, larynx Never involves region above the level of the eye	Associated symptoms: Profuse diaphoresis, weakness, shortness of breath, nausea, vomiting	Gradual onset of pain builds up to maximum pain intensity; usually anginal pain lasts 1-5 min
Myocardial infarction	Precipitating factors: effort-related activity, large meals, emotional stress	Severe chest pain	Chest pain; may have radiation of pain to back, jaw, or left arm	Associated symptoms: Palpitations, dyspnea, diaphoresis, nausea, vomiting, dizziness, weakness, sense of impending doom	Usually pain has lasted 30 min or more
Acute pericarditis	Precipitating factors: May occur after AMI; also may be related to viral, collagen, or vascular disorders	Chest pain may be due to severe and crushing type of pain	Anterior chest pain with radiation to the neck, arms, or shoulders; pain may be intensified by deep inspiration	Associated symptoms: Fever (i.e., between 101° and 102° F [38.3° and 38.9° C]); pericardial friction rub; electrocardiogram; ST segment elevation in all leads except V_1 and aV_R	May be hours to days
Dissecting aortic aneurysm	Sudden onset	Severe, ripping, tearing type of pain	Anterior and posterior chest Often radiates from anterior chest to intrascapular region or to abdomen Pain may move with progression of aortic dissection	Associated symptoms: Dyspnea, tachypnea, CHF (i.e., because of aortic regurgitation caused by dissection); also, CVA, syncope, paraplegia and pulse loss associated with dissecting aneurysm	Sudden onset

Condition	Precipitating factors / Palliation	Quality	Location	Associated symptoms	Timing
Esophageal disorders (esophageal reflux, esophageal spasm)	Precipitating factors: often triggered by exercise or by food (large meal, spicy foods, acidic foods, cold foods) or ethanol intake	Burning or pressurelike pain; May be severe	May radiate to neck, ear, jaw, or lower abdomen	Associated symptoms: Dysphagia, aspiration	Minutes to days
Cocaine induced	Precipitating factors: cocaine use; Palliation: Relieved with nitroglycerin	Severe pain	Substernal location, with radiation to both arms	Associated symptoms: Tachycardia, palpitations, diaphoresis, nausea, dizziness, syncope, dyspnea	Occurs from 1 to 6 hr after cocaine use
Postoperative coronary artery bypass graft (CABG) after harvest of internal mammary artery (IMA)	Precipitating factors: use of IMA for graft of CABG patient	Mild to severe chest pain, burning, prickling, and dull type of sensations	Anterior chest; may radiate over entire chest wall and particularly over the site of the graft; may radiate to neck or axilla	Associated symptoms: Numbness, tenderness on palpation of the sternum, hyperesthesia along the incisional line, delayed healing of the sternum	Persistent type of pain; Shooting-type pain may last for several seconds and occur several times per day
Mitral valve prolapse	Palliation: Relief in recumbent position, no relief with nitroglycerin	Dull and aching; although also may be sharp	Nonretrosternal chest pain	Associated symptoms: Systolic murmur, unexplained dyspnea, weakness, midsystolic (apical) click	Onset may be sudden or recurrent; May last for a few seconds, or be persistent for days
5-Fluorouracil (FU) therapy	Precipitating factors: following infusion of 5-FU; Palliation: relief with nitroglycerin	Mild to severe pain	Central chest pain; radiates to left shoulder and left arm	Associated symptoms: Nausea, vomiting, tachycardia, hypertension	Occurs several days after intravenous bolus or infusion of 5-FU; No chest pain between treatment
Spontaneous pneumothorax	COPD, chronic asthma	Sharp or stabbing; described as moderate to severe	Usually pain of entire lung region (hemithorax); may rediate to back and neck	Associated symptoms: Decreased or absent breath sounds; pneumothorax per chest radiograph	Continuous pain until treated

Continued

Table 21-3 Etiologic Factors To Be Considered in the Differential Diagnosis of Chest Pain—cont'd

Etiologic factors	P Precipitating/Palliating	Q Quality	R Radiating/Region	S Severity/Symptoms	T Time/Temporal
Tachydysrhythmias	Precipitating factors: Anxiety, digitalis toxicity, exercise, organic heart disease Palliation: Terminated by antidysrhythmics, direct current shock, vagal maneuvers	Sharp, stabbing type of chest pain May have palpitations, "skipped beats"	Precordial chest pain	Associated symptoms: Weakness, fatigue, lethargy, palpitations, dizziness, vertigo	Paroxysmal in onset Lasts briefly to hours
Anxiety disorders	May have history of depression or anxiety	Pain may be vague, diffuse; may be further described as disabling	Anterior chest and abdomen	Associated symptoms: Dyspnea, fatigue, anorexia	Variable; often continuous for hours to days
Monosodium glutamate	Occurs with ingestion of food high in monosodium glutamate	Burning type of chest pain	Retrosternal chest pain	Associated symptoms: Facial pain, nausea, vomiting	Occurs shortly after meals up to several hours after meal
Musculoskeletal	Precipitating factors: pain with inspiration or with musculoskeletal movement	Generalized aching stiffness with point tenderness, swelling	Tenderness of the anterior chest wall	Persistent chest pain without relief with rest	

From Newberry L, editor: *Sheehy's emergency nursing: principles and practice,* ed 5, St Louis, 2003, Mosby.
AMI, Acute myocardial infarction; *CHF,* congestive heart failure; *CVA,* cerebrovascular accident; *COPD,* chronic obstructive pulmonary disease.

RHYTHM ASSESSMENT

Modern bedside monitors and telemetry units provide multiple lead viewving options. Available configurations include three-lead, four-lead, and five-lead systems (Figures 21-1 and 21-2). A combination of leads II, MCL_1, and MCL_6 provide the best differentiation of QRS complex morphology.[1] Additionally, some monitoring systems are capable of continuous ST segment evaluation, which is particularly useful in patients with ongoing chest pain whose initial electrocardiogram was nondiagnostic.

The majority of bedside monitors now come with critical alarms for ventricular fibrillation, ventricular tachycardia, and asystole. Most also have default alarms for ventricular ectopy, ST segment elevation, and ST segment depression. Adjust the alarm settings to fit the patient's clinical situation per institution protocol.

Standard 12-Lead Electrocardiogram

With six limb leads (Figure 21-3) and six precordial leads (Figure 21-4), the 12-lead electrocardiogram acquires 12 different views of the electrical activity of the heart and records them on standardized electrocardiogram paper or in a computer system. Changes in the normal electrocardiogram occur when the electric signal encounters myocardial damage or ischemia (Figure 21-5). The site of damage determines the location of the abnormal waveform on the electrocardiogram tracing. Figures 21-6, 21-7, 21-8, and 21-9 illustrate electrocardiogram changes associated with anterior, inferior, lateral, and posterior myocardial infarctions (MIs) respectively.

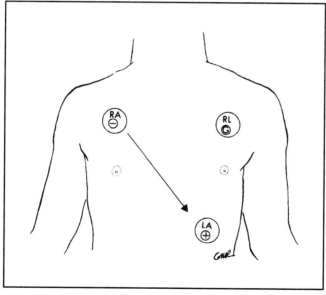

Figure 21-1. Three-lead monitoring system.

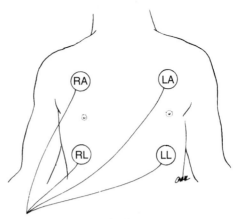

Figure 21-2. Four-lead monitoring system.

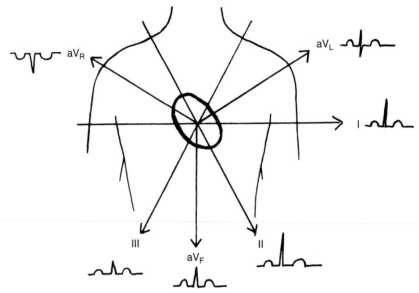

Figure 21-3. Six limb leads.

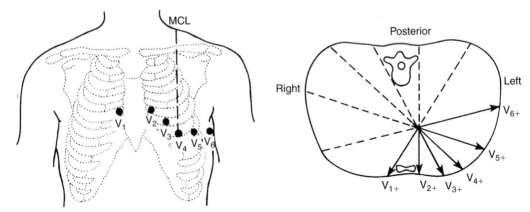

Figure 21-4. Precordial leads. (From Newberry L, editor: *Sheehy's emergency nursing: principles and practice*, ed 5, St Louis, 2003, Mosby.)

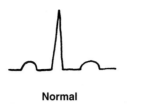

Normal

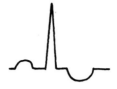

Ischemia
T wave inversion
(intramural ischemia)
Decreased blood supply
ST Segment depression
(subendocardial ischemia)

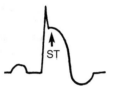

Injury
Acute or recent;
the more elevated
the ST segment,
the more recent
the injury

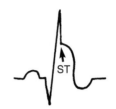

Infarct
Significant Q wave
greater than 0.04 seconds
wide and greater than
25% of the associated
R wave
Indicates myocardial
necrosis

Figure 21-5. Acute electrocardiogram changes.

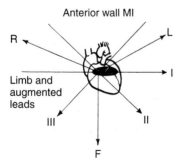

Anterior wall MI

R

L

I

Limb and
augmented
leads

III

II

F

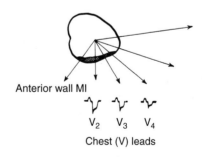

Anterior wall MI

V₂ V₃ V₄

Chest (V) leads

Figure 21-6. Anterior myocardial infarction *(MI)*. (From Newberry L, editor: *Sheehy's emergency nursing: principles and practice,* ed 5, St Louis, 2003, Mosby.)

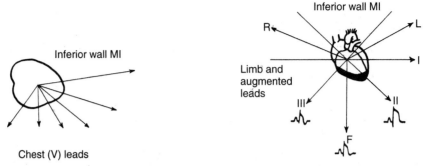

Figure 21-7. Inferior myocardial infarction *(MI)*. (From Newberry L, editor: *Sheehy's emergency nursing: principles and practice*, ed 5, St Louis, 2003, Mosby.)

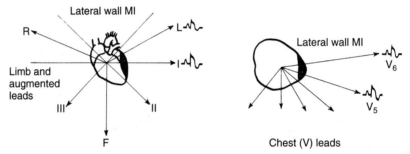

Figure 21-8. Lateral myocardial infarction *(MI)*. (From Newberry L, editor: *Sheehy's emergency nursing: principles and practice*, ed 5, St Louis, 2003, Mosby.)

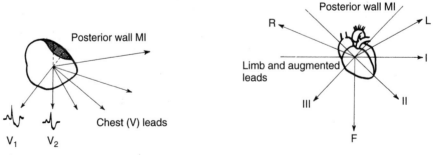

Figure 21-9. Posterior myocardial infarction *(MI)*. (From Newberry L, editor: *Sheehy's emergency nursing: principles and practice*, ed 5, St Louis, 2003, Mosby.)

Additional Leads

Three additional views provided by a 15-lead electrocardiogram are used to identify right ventricular infarction. An 18-lead electrocardiogram is indicated when there is ST depression in the precordial leads. These additional views have proved useful for identifying the presence of a posterior wall infarction.

Leads Placement

The emergency nurse should keep the following in mind for lead placement:
- Attempt to maintain the patient's modesty. Explain what you are doing.
- If necessary, remove excess hair to ensure good skin contact. Rub the skin with an alcohol pad to remove dry flakes and hair particles.
- Ascertain that there is sufficient conduction medium (gel) between the electrode and the patient; avoid placing electrodes over large muscle masses.
- Before beginning, confirm that all leads are placed correctly. A common mnemonic used to guide correct lead placement is "Green and white are on the right, Christmas trees (red and green) below the knees."
- Do not allow lead wires to touch anything metal; this will produce 60-cycle interference. If interference occurs, check for loose leads, leads or wires in contact with metal, and interference from other electrical equipment.
- If the patient is being admitted, mark the location of the chest leads to facilitate consistent daily electrocardiograms.
- Confirm that the correct patient name, medical record number, date, and time appear on the electrocardiogram.
- Examine the electrocardiogram for changes related to acute ischemia, injury, or previous infarction (refer to Figure 21-5 for interpretation information).
- Note any axis deviation on the electrocardiogram. Deviation to the left or right is associated with conduction abnormalities and other conditions (Figure 21-10).

ACUTE CORONARY SYNDROMES

Acute coronary syndromes refer to a continuum of disease processes that include unstable angina, non–ST segment elevation MI (non-STEMI), and ST segment elevation MI (STEMI). Non-STEMI entails subendocardial or intramural wall damage, whereas STEMI involves full-thickness myocardial necrosis.[2] Sudden cardiac death can result from either condition. Recognition and early intervention are critical for patient survival. Non-STEMI usually is related to intermittent occlusive thrombosis, whereas unstable angina occurs from partial occlusion by an atherosclerotic plaque. Patients with non-STEMI and those with unstable angina are at significant risk for progression to STEMI.[3]

Unstable Angina

Ischemic chest pain (angina) occurs when myocardial oxygen demand exceeds the available supply. This occurs most commonly following atherosclerotic changes in the coronary arteries. Three types of angina are recognized: stable, unstable, and variant (also called Prinzmetal angina). Table 21-4 lists the differential angina diagnoses. Figure 21-11 illustrates common sites for anginal pain.

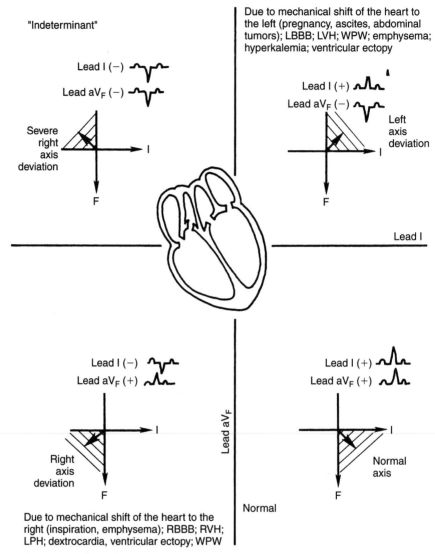

"Indeterminant"

Due to mechanical shift of the heart to the left (pregnancy, ascites, abdominal tumors); LBBB; LVH; WPW; emphysema; hyperkalemia; ventricular ectopy

Lead I (−)

Lead aV$_F$ (−)

Severe right axis deviation

F

Lead I (+)

Lead aV$_F$ (−)

Left axis deviation

F

Lead I

Lead I (−)

Lead aV$_F$ (+)

Right axis deviation

F

Lead aV$_F$

Lead I (+)

Lead aV$_F$ (+)

Normal axis

F

Normal

Due to mechanical shift of the heart to the right (inspiration, emphysema); RBBB; RVH; LPH; dextrocardia, ventricular ectopy; WPW

Figure 21-10. Patterns of axis deviation and associated conditions. *LBBB,* Left bundle branch block; *LVH,* left ventricular hypertrophy; *WPW,* Wolfe-Parkinson-White syndrome; *RBBB,* right bundle branch block; *RVH,* right ventricular hypertropy; *LPH,* left posterior hemiblock.

Myocardial Infarction

Myocardial infarction is a localized, ischemic necrosis of the myocardium caused by severe narrowing or complete obstruction of one or more coronary arteries. Occlusion may be caused by a thrombus, spasm, or hemorrhage. The size and location of the infarction depend on which coronary artery is affected and where the artery is blocked (Table 21-5, p. 341). The extent and depth of necrosis determine whether the ST segment will be elevated (STEMI) or not (non-STEMI).[4] The incidence of MI increases with age. However, cases of MI (unrelated to

Table 21-4   **Comparison of Characteristics of Angina**

Characteristic	Stable Angina	Unstable Angina	Prinzmetal Angina
Location of pain	Substernal; may radiate to the jaw, neck, and down arms or back	Substernal; may radiate to the jaw, neck, and down arms or back	Substernal; may radiate to the jaw, neck, and down arms and back
Duration of pain	1-15 min	Occurs progressively more frequently with episodes lasting as along as 30 min	Occurs repeatedly at about the same time of day. Episodes tend to cluster between midnight and 8 AM.
Pain characteristics	Commonly referred to as an aching, squeezing, choking, heaving, or burning discomfort	Same as stable angina, but more intense	Distinctly painful
Severity of pain	Generally severity is the same as previous episodes	The severity, duration, or frequency of events increases over time	Extremely severe
Other symptoms	None for most patients	Diaphoresis, weakness, S_3 or S_4 heart sound, pulsus alternans, transient pulmonary crackles	Diaphoresis, weakness, S_3 or S_4 heart sound, pulsus alternans, transient pulmonary crackles
Pain worsened by	Exercise, activity, eating, cold weather, reclining	Exercise, activity, eating, cold weather, reclining	Occurs at rest
Pain relieved by	Rest, nitroglycerin, isosorbide	Rest, nitroglycerin, and isosorbide may provide only partial relief	Nitroglycerin may be helpful
Electrocardiogram findings	Transient ST segment depression that disappears with pain relief	Patients often have ST segment depression or T wave inversion but the electrocardiogram may be normal	Episodic ST segment elevation with pain. ST segment returns to baseline when the pain subsides. Patients are prone to develop ventricular dysrhythmias.
Additional characteristics	Most common in middle-aged and elderly males and postmenopausal females.	Most common in middle-aged and elderly males and postmenopausal females; often referred to as preinfarction angina	Generally occurs in younger patients; thought to result from coronary artery spasm

recreational drugs such as cocaine) have been reported in patients as young as 17. (Refer to Box 21-1 for a review of cardiac risk factors.)

Clinical findings

Pain related to an MI typically begins suddenly and can last from several minutes to several days. The pain classically is localized in the substernal area with radiation to the jaw or down the arm. Careful investigation of complaints of chest discomfort is always prudent, paying particular attention to the patient's presenting story, medical history, and cardiac risk factors. Variant presentations are common, especially in women. Myocardial infarction can be associated with atypical symptoms such as toothache, fatigue, gastrointestinal upset, or other sensations of discomfort. Elderly patients may have dyspnea as their primary complaint and

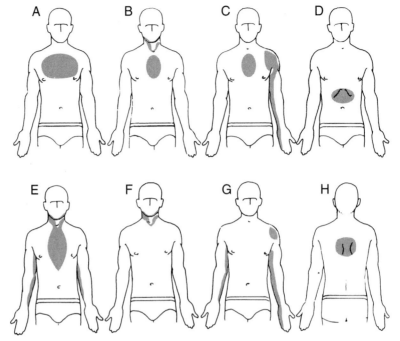

Figure 21-11. Common sites for anginal pain. **A,** Upper part of chest. **B,** Beneath sternum, radiating to neck and jaw. **C,** Beneath sternum, radiating down left arm. **D,** Epigastric. **E,** Epigastric, radiating to neck, jaw, and arms. **F,** Neck and jaw. **G,** Left shoulder. **H,** Intrascapular. (From Urden LD, Stacy KM, Lough ME: *Thelan's critical care nursing: diagnosis and management,* ed 4, St Louis, 2002, Mosby).

diabetics may have minimal pain. Myocardial infarction pain cannot be reproduced with chest palpation and is unrelated to inspiration or expiration.

Signs and symptoms

Signs and symptoms of myocardial infarction include the following:
- Pain frequently is described as crushing, sharp, or burning or as a pressure, tightness, or choking. Patients also may describe the feeling of "something sitting on my chest."
- Pain may be localized to the substernal area or epigastrium or may radiate to the left side of the neck, intrascapular area, jaw, arm, elbow, or wrist. Some patients may experience pain in the right arm or the right side of the neck.
- Pain is usually continuous and lasts more than 30 minutes. Myocardial pain has a circadian variation. The incidence peaks between 6 AM and noon, usually occurring within 2 to 3 hours of rising.[2]
- Associated symptoms include diaphoresis, nausea, vomiting, dyspnea, orthopnea, weakness, dizziness, syncope, and palpitations.
- The patient may experience a sense of impending doom.
- Blood pressure is usually decreased.
- Heart rate is generally elevated except in inferior MI, in which bradycardia is typical.
- Pallor or a dusky appearance may be present.
- Peripheral edema forms as a result of decreased cardiac output and increased venous pressure.
- Heart sounds vary depending on the physiologic status of the myocardium but a fourth heart sound is common.

Table **21-5**   **Coronary Arteries in Myocardial Infarction**

Right Coronary Artery	*Left Coronary Artery*

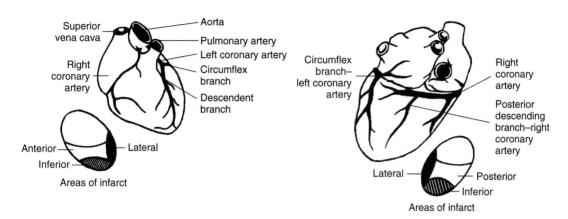

Right Coronary Artery

Supplies the following:
  Right atrium
  Right ventricle
  Inferior/diaphragmatic surface of left ventricle
  Sinoatrial node (55%)
  Atrioventricular node (90%)
  Bundle of His
Block causes the following:
  Infarction of posterior or inferior wall of left ventricle
  Right ventricle infarction
  In inferior myocardial infarction (leads II, III, aV_F), anticipate second-degree heart block or Mobitz type I block (Wenckebach).

Left Coronary Artery

Left circumflex branch

Supplies the following:
  Left atrium
  Lateral wall of left ventricle
  Sinoatrial node (45%)
  Atrioventricular node (10%)
  Posterior/inferior division of left bundle
Block causes the following:
  Lateral wall infarction
  Posterior wall infarction (near base)
  In lateral wall myocardial infarction and electrocardiogram changes seen in leads I, AV_L, and V_5 and V_6.

Left anterior descending branch

Supplies the following:
  Anterior wall of left ventricle
  Interventricular septum
  Bundle of His
  Right bundle
  Posterior/inferior division of left bundle
  Apex of left ventricle
Block causes the following:
  Infarction of anterior wall of left ventricle
  Effect on papillary muscle (which attaches to mitral valve)
  In anterior myocardial infarction (leads V_2, V_3, V_4), anticipate second-degree heart block, Mobitz type II block, or third-degree block.

From Newberry L, editor: *Sheehy's emergency nursing: principles and practice*, ed 5, St Louis, 2003, Mosby.

Table 21-6   Cardiac Markers for Acute Myocardial Infarction

Cardiac Marker	Initial Elevation After Acute Myocardial Infarction	Mean Peak Time	Time to Return to Baseline
Myoglobin	1-4 hours	6-7 hours	18-24 hours
Troponin-I (cTn 1) (cardiac specific)	3-12 hours	10-24 hours	3-7 days
Troponin-T (cTn T) (cardiac specific)	3-12 hours	12-48 hours	10-14 days
Creatine kinse-MB (CK-MB)	4-12 hours	10-24 hours	48-72 hours
CK-MB subforms: MB1 & MB2	1-6 hours	18 hours	Unkown
Lactate dehydrogenase (LDH)	8-12 hours	24-48 hours	10-14 days
*LDH-1/LDH-2 ration >0.76 is significantly associated with acute myocardial infarction			

Therapeutic interventions

Time is a critical factor in the management of the patient with an MI. Chest pain protocols (or chest pain pathways) effectively have helped many emergency departments standardize their approach to the patient with MI. Treatment begins with early recognition. Obtain an electrocardiogram within 5 minutes of arrival, collect blood for essential laboratory tests, and rapidly determine the need for fibrinolytic therapy, percutaneous coronary interventions, or surgery.

Cardiac markers

Serum marker studies are a crucial component of MI care. The time a marker peaks and the time it returns to baseline provide information essential to early identification and management of the patient with MI (Table 21-6). Advances in cardiac care continue to identify more sensitive biomarkers. Currently, troponin I is the most widely used measure of cardiac damage but CK-MB (creatine kinase myocardial-bound) and myoglobin also may be assessed.

Albumin cobalt binding is a promising new marker. This study identifies MI-related protein structural changes by evaluating the amount of cobalt bound to albumin. Albumin cobalt binding can be used along with troponin I to identify MI patients. The test was cleared for marketing in 2003 but is not yet widely available.

Medications

The American Heart Association recommends the mnemonic *MONA* (morphine, oxygen, nitroglycerin, and aspirin) as a guide to MI medication administration (Table 21-7). Of the four MONA medications, aspirin is the most underrated. Early aspirin ingestion has been shown to significantly decrease 1-year mortality in patients with unstable angina.[5] Aspirin also reduces the risk of infarction.

Other medications routinely given to the patient with MI include anticoagulants, beta-blockers, fibrinolytics, angiotensin-converting enzyme inhibitors, and glycoprotein IIb/IIIa inhibitors. In general, every patient with MI should receive a beta-blocker and an anticoagulant, unless specific contraindications are present. Fibrinolysis is appropriate for STEMI patients and for those with a new onset left bundle branch block, as long as no contraindications exist and the patient presents within the appropriate time frame. Non-STEMI patients and STEMI patients who do not qualify for fibrinolytic therapy are started on glycoprotein IIb/IIIa inhibitors. See the following sections for further discussion of cardiac pharmacotherapy.

Table 21-7   **MONA Medications for the Patient With Myocardial Infarction**

Medication	Dose	Comments
Morphine Sulfate	2-4 mg IV push given slowly over 1 to 5 min. Repeat every 5-30 min; titrate to effect. No maximum dose.	The drug of choice for ischemic chest pain. Also reduces preload and decreases myocardial oxygen demand. Hold for significant hypotension.
Oxygen	4 L/min via nasal cannula	Adjust to maintain adequate oxygen saturation.
Nitroglycerin	*Sublingual tablets:* 0.3-0.4 mg; repeat as needed every 5 min for up to 3 doses. *Sublingual spray:* Spray for 0.5 to 1 sec (provides 0.4 mg per dose). Repeat as needed every 5 min for up to 3 doses. Do not shake the container before spraying because this affects the dose delivered. *Intravenous:* Give patient bolus with 12.5 to 25 mcg followed by and infusion of 10 to 20 mcg/min. Titrate to pain relief.	Establish IV access before giving nitroglycerin to a patient who has never previously received it. Monitor BP before and after nitroglycerin administration. Limit SBP changes to a 10% decrease in the patient with MI who is normotensive or a 30% decrease if hypertensive. Hold further doses for an SBP ≤90 mm Hg. Limit SBP changes to a 10% decrease in the patient with MI who is normotensive or a 30% decrease if hypertensive. Hold further doses for an SBP ≤90 mm Hg. Maximum IV dose is 200 mcg/min. Drug concentration should not exceed 400 mcg/mL. Side effects include hypotension, tachycardia, ischemia, and headache. Avoid giving nitroglycerin to patients with right ventricular infarction, hypotension, severe bradycardia, or severe tachycardia. Nitroglycerin is contraindicated in patients who have taken sildenafil citrate (Viagra) or vardenafil (Levitra) within 24 hr. May interfere with the anticoagulant effect of heparin; monitor activated partial thromboplastin time and prothrombin time (international normalized ratio).
Aspirin	160 to 325 mg orally. Chew for faster absorption.	Administer as soon as possible after chest pain starts. The antiplatelet activity of aspirin decreases mortality after acute MI. Do not give to patients hypersensitive to salicylates. Patients on daily aspirin therapy can receive an additional tablet safely at chest pain onset.

From American College of Cardiology, American Heart Association: ACC/AHA guidelines for the evaluation and management of chronic heart failure in the adult. Retrieved November 11, 2003, from www.acc.org/clinical/guidelines/failure/iii_assessment.htm
IV, Intravenous; *BP,* blood pressure; *SBP,* systolic blood pressure; *MI,* myocardial infarction.

Anticoagulant therapy

Anticoagulants do not affect existing clots but inhibit further thrombin formation (Table 21-8). These drugs are indicated for all patients with MI and are used along with fibrinolytic agents to prevent reocclusion of the affected vessel. Heparin and aspirin are given to patients with ST segment depression and unstable angina. Heparin is available in unfractionated (standard) and low-molecular-weight (newer) forms. Protamine sulfate, the antidote for unfractionated heparin, does not reverse the effects of low-molecular-weight heparins. However, because these agents are not administered as continuous drips, overdose is unusual.

Table 21-8 **Anticoagulant Therapy for the Patient With Myocardial Infarction**

Medication	Dose	Comments
Heparin, unfractionated (standard heparin)	Give a 60 units/kg IV bolus (maximum bolus of 5000 units). Follow with an infusion of 12 units/kg/hr (maximum 1000 units/hr) for patients >70 kg.	Obtain a baseline aPTT, PT-INR, and RBC Maintain aPTT at 1.5 to 2 times the control. Maintain PT-INR between 2 and 3. Never give concurrently with other heparin products. Do not give if the platelet count is <100,000 mm³ Overdose can be reversed with protamine sulfate.
Dalteparin (Fragmin) Enoxaparin (Lovenox)	1 mg/kg bid subcut for 2-8 days. Given concurrently with aspirin.	These agents are low-molecular-weight heparins. Contraindicated in those with hypersensitivity to pork. Protamine sulfate does not reverse the effects of these agents.
Desirudin	0.1 mg/kg IV bolus followed by an infusion of 0.1 mg/kg/hr for 72 hr.	Used for patients with history of heparin-induced thrombocytopenia.
Lepirudin	0.4 mg/kg IV bolus followed by an infusion of 0.15 mg/kg/hr for 72 hr.	Used for patients with history of heparin-induced thrombocytopenia.

IV, Intravenous; *aPTT*, activated partial thromboplastin time; *PT-INR*, prothrombin time (International Normalized Ratio).

Table 21-9 **Beta-Blocker Therapy for the Patient With Myocardial Infarction**

Medication	Dose
Esmolol (Brevibloc)	0.5 mg/kg bolus over 1 min followed by a continuous infusion at 0.5 mg/kg/min. Maximum dose is 0.3 mg/kg/min. Titrate to effect. The half-life is short (2-9 min).
Metoprolol (Lopressor)	5 mg slow intravenous (IV) push. Repeat as needed at 5-min intervals to a total of 15 mg. Give 25-50 mg PO within 15 min of the last IV dose (unless contraindicated). Oral dose is 50 mg bid for 24 hr; then increase to 100 mg bid.
Propranolol (Inderal)	0.1-mg/kg slow IV push, divided into three equal doses, at 2- to 3-min intervals. Do not infuse faster than 1 mg/min. Repeat after 2 min if necessary.
Atenolol (Tenormin)	5 mg IV over 5 min, wait 10 min, and then give second 5-mg dose over 5 min. In 10 min (if tolerated well) start 50 mg PO and then 50 mg PO bid. Oral dose is 100 mg daily.
Labetalol (Normodyne)	10 mg IV push over 1-2 min. May repeat or double labetalol dose every 10 min to a maximum of 150 mg. Another option is to give the initial dose as a bolus and then start a labetalol infusion at 2-8 mg/min.

Beta-blocker therapy

Beta-blockers decrease morbidity and mortality after acute MI by reducing the incidence of ventricular fibrillation and by lowering myocardial oxygen demand (Table 21-9). Heart rate, systemic arterial pressure, and myocardial contractility decrease in response to beta-blocker therapy. The incidence of reinfarction and recurrent ischemia drop as well. These drugs are contraindicated in patients with heart rates less than 60 beats/min, a systolic blood pressure of less than 100 mm Hg, moderate to severe left ventricular failure, heart block, severe chronic obstructive pulmonary disease, or asthma. Side effects include atrioventricular block, symptomatic bradycardia, and hypotension.

Fibrinolytic therapy

Fibrinolytic agents are given to dissolve coronary thrombi, restore blood flow to the myocardium, and halt further evolution of the infarction process. These agents prevent myocardial necrosis, reduce ischemia, limit infarct size, and improve left ventricular function. Indications for fibrinolytic therapy are acute chest pain indicative of MI of less than 12 hours' duration, electrocardiographic evidence of ST segment elevation, or new left bundle branch block. Absolute contraindications to fibrinolysis include previous hemorrhagic stroke, any stroke or cerebrovascular event within 1 year, active internal bleeding (excluding menses), and suspected aortic dissection. Fibrinolytic drugs may be used cautiously in cases of pregnancy, hypertension (blood presssure greater than 180/110 mm Hg), trauma within the last 2 to 4 weeks, and internal bleeding within the past month. Table 21-10 reviews currently approved fibrinolytic agents. Once a mainstay of therapy, the role of fibrinolysis in MI treatment is diminishing as the early use of percutaneous coronary interventions becomes more common.

Angiotensin-converting enzyme inhibitors

Angiotensin-converting enzyme ACE inhibitors are important adjuncts in the treatment of large or anterior wall MIs, heart failure without hypotension, and prior MI (Table 21-11). ACE inhibitors reduce mortality and improve left ventricular function in most post-MI patients by preventing adverse left ventricular remodeling, delaying progression of heart failure, and decreasing recurrent MI and sudden death.

These agents provide the greatest benefit to patients with the following:
- Suspected MI
- ST segment elevation in two or more anterior precordial leads
- Hypertension
- Clinical heart failure without hypotension (in patients not responding to digitalis or diuretics)
- Clinical signs of acute MI with left ventricular dysfunction
- A left ventricular ejection fraction of less than 40%

ACE inhibitors are contraindicated in pregnancy (may cause fetal injury or death) and in individuals with angioedema or hypersensitivity to ACE inhibitors. Reduce the dose in patients with renal failure (creatinine greater than 3 g/dL). Avoid these agents in persons with bilateral renal artery stenosis. Watch for hypotension, which is especially pronounced following the initial dose and in volume-depleted patients. ACE inhibitors generally are started when fibrinolytic therapy is complete and blood pressure has stabilized.

Glycoprotein IIb/IIIa inhibitors

Glycoprotein IIb/IIIa inhibitors are given to limit platelet aggregation and reduce the risk of further thrombus development that occurs despite aspirin and heparin therapy (Table 21-12). These agents are indicated in patients with unstable angina or acute phase non-STEMI and in those undergoing percutaneous coronary interventions. Glycoprotein IIb/IIIa inhibitors are contraindicated in patients with bleeding disorders or an increased risk of significant bleeding. Adverse reactions include hypotension, thrombocytopenia, and hemorrhage (including intracranial bleeding).

Dysrhythmia management

Prophylactic dysrhythmia therapy is no longer recommended for the patient with MI. Treatment is indicated only for life-threatening dysrhythmias. Rhythms that require intervention include symptomatic bradycardia, atrial fibrillation, ventricular ectopy, ventricular tachycardia, ventricular fibrillation, and asystole. See Chapter 10 for a discussion of each rhythm. For information regarding dysrhythmia treatment, refer to the algorithms in Chapter 18.

Table 21-10 Comparison of Fibrinolytic Agents

Agent	Action	Dose	Comments
Streptokinase (Streptase, Kabikinase)	Exogenous plasminogen activator; not clot specific	*IV:* 1.5 million units IV over 1 hr *Intracoronary:* 10,000 to 30,000 units; followed by maintenance infusion of 2000 to 4000 units/min until thrombolysis occurs (e.g., 150,000 to 500,000 units total)	Half-life in plasma is 18 min; has a prolonged effect on coagulation because of depletion of fibrinogen, which persists for 18-24 hr; antibodies to the drug may be present in persons who have been exposed to *Streptococcus* infection resulting in allergic reactions (e.g., rash, fever, or chills); patients should not be retreated with streptokinase for a period of 2 wk to 1 yr after initial administration because of secondary resistance to development of antibodies
Anistreplase (Eminase)	Inactivated derivative of thrombolytic enzyme synthesized from streptokinase and lysoplasminogen; promotes thrombolysis after activation within the body	*IV:* 30 units over 2-5 min; dilute only with 5 mL sterile water	Do not give to patients who are allergic to streptokinase; may not be as effective as usual when administered more than 5 days after the previous dose or after streptokinase therapy or streptococcal infection; discard if not used within 30 min of mixing
Alteplase (Activase, Activase rt-PA)	Proteolytic enzyme; direct activator of plasminogen; high degree of clot specificity	*IV:* 15 mg IV bolus over 1-2 min; then 50 mg over 30 min; then 35 mg over 60 min	Half-life in plasma is 5-7 min; may cause sudden hypotension; inline IV filters can remove as much as 47% of the drug
Reteplase (Retavase)	Activates the conversion of plasminogen to plasmin; high degree of clot specificity	*IV:* 10 units over 2 min; then repeat 10 units in 30 min after initiation of first bolus	Give normal saline fluid before and after administration of reteplase. Reconstitute just before administration and use within 4 hr after reconstituting
Tenecteplase (TNKase)	Activates clot-bound plasminogen to plasmin	*IV:* 30-50 mg bolus over 5 sec. Dosing based on patient weight: <60 kg = 30 mg TNKase ≥60 to <70 kg = 35 mg TNKase ≥70 to <80 kg = 40 mg TNKase ≥80 to <90 kg = 45 mg TNKase ≥90 mg = 50 mg TNKase	More fibrin specificity and less incidence of bleeding than alteplase

From Newberry L, editor: *Sheehy's emergency nursing: principles and practice,* ed 5, St Louis, 2003, Mosby.
IV, Intravenous.

Table 21-11   Angiotensin-Converting Enzyme Inhibitor Therapy for the Patient With Myocardial Infarction

Medication	Dose
Captopril	Administer 6.25 mg PO; advance to 25 mg tid and then 50 mg tid as tolerated.
Enalapril	Administer 2.5 mg PO, and titrate to 20 mg PO bid.
	Intravenous dosing: 1.25 mg initially over 5 min and then 1.25-5 mg every 6 hours.
Lisinopril	Administer 5 mg within 24 hr of onset of symptoms. Give 5 mg after 24 hr, 10 mg after 48 hr, and then 10 mg once daily for 6 wk.
Ramipril	Administer 2.5 mg PO, and titrate to 5 mg PO bid as tolerated.

Table 21-12   Overview of Glycoprotein IIb/IIIa Inhibitors

Glycoprotein IIb/IIIa Inhibitor	Dosage	Potential Side Effects
Abciximab (ReoPro)	0.25 mg/kg over 10-60 min 0.125 mg/kg/min for 12 hr	Potential for increased bleeding, hypotension, bradycardia, nausea and vomiting, diarrhea
Eptifibatide (Integrilin)	180 mcg/kg over 1 to 2 min 2 mcg/kg/min for up to 72 hr	Potential for increased bleeding, hypotension
Tirofiban (Aggrastat)	0.4 mcg/kg/min for 30 min 0.1 mcg/kg/min for 12-24 hr	Potential for increased bleeding, nausea, bradycardia

From Newberry L, editor: *Sheehy's emergency nursing: principles and practice,* ed 5, St Louis, 2003, Mosby.

Percutaneous Coronary Interventions

A variety of invasive techniques now are used for the acute phase management of patients with MI. *Percutaneous coronary interventions* is the generic term applied to a number of nonsurgical procedures for revascularizing myocardial tissue. Under sterile conditions in a catheterization laboratory, a steerable catheter is threaded through a femoral artery sheath into the occluded coronary vessel. The catheter tip is positioned at the site of stenosis. An angiogram is performed to determine the extent and location of occlusion. Atherosclerotic plaques are identified and removed or are flattened against the arterial wall (angioplasty). During the procedure, a stent can be placed to ensure the artery remains open. Patients who are acceptable candidates for percutaneous coronary interventions must be identified quickly; the goal for door-to-reperfusion time is 90 ± 30 minutes. Consequently, availability of these procedures is limited to patients in facilities with invasive coronary services and to those geographically situated near such a facility.

HEART FAILURE

The term *heart failure* has replaced the older term *congestive heart failure* because many patients do not have volume overload on their initial examination. Heart failure is characterized by dyspnea, fatigue, and fluid retention. However, not all symptoms are present in all patients. Onset can be gradual or sudden and occurs when the heart can no longer produce sufficient cardiac output at normal filling pressure to meet metabolic demands. This typically happens when the left ventricular ejection fraction drops to less than 40%.

Table 21-13 **Stages of Heart Failure**

Phase	Characteristics/Description
A	The patient is at risk for developing heart failure. No cardiac structural abnormalities are present.
B	The patient has a structural abnormality of the heart but no symptoms of heart failure.
C	The patient has past or current symptoms of heart failure associated with structural changes of the heart.
D	The patient has end-stage disease and requires specialized treatment such as mechanical ventilation, continuous infusion of inotropic agents, cardiac transplant, or hospice care.

From American College of Cardiology, American Heart Association: ACC/AHA guidelines for the evaluation and management of chronic heart failure in the adult. Retrieved November 11, 2003, from www.acc.org/clinical/guidelines/failure/iii_assessment.htm
IV, Intravenous; *BP,* blood pressure; *SBP,* systolic blood pressure; *MI,* myocardial infarction.

Table 21-14 **Causes of Heart Failure by Type**

Type	Cause
Left ventricular failure	Systemic hypertension, aortic stenosis, aortic regurgitation, mitral regurgitation, cardiomyopathy, bacterial endocarditis, myocardial infarction
Right ventricular failure	Mitral stenosis, pulmonary hypertension, bacterial endocarditis on the right side of the heart, right ventricular infarction
Biventricular failure	Left ventricular failure, cardiomyopathy, myocarditis, dysrhythmias, anemia, thyrotoxicosis

Four distinct phases of heart failure have been identified (Table 21-13) Treatment is determined by the stage of the disease at the time of presentation.[6] Coronary artery disease is responsible for about two thirds of all cases of heart failure. Heart failure is characterized as left ventricular failure, right ventricular failure, or biventricular failure. Table 21-14 identifies causes associated with each type. Box 21-2 lists conditions and events that precipitate heart failure. Left ventricular failure produces pulmonary edema, whereas right ventricular failure is associated with an enlarged liver. Regardless of the type, the ultimate result of heart failure is fluid overload and decreased tissue perfusion. Heart failure is the most common reason for hospital admission among the elderly; 6% to 10% of patients over the age of 65 have been diagnosed with heart failure.[7]

Signs and Symptoms

Signs and symptoms of heart failure include the following:
- Bilateral crackles, wheezes
- Cough
- Cyanosis
- Dependent edema, anasarca, ascites
- Distended neck veins
- Dyspnea on exertion
- Exercise intolerance
- Frothy pulmonary secretions
- Gallop rhythms (S_3 and S_4)

Box **21-2** **Precipitating Conditions or Events Associated With Acute Heart Failure**

Acquired immunodeficiency syndrome	Increased intracranial pressure
Pneumothorax	Infective endocarditis
Administration of a cardiac depressant or salt-retaining drug	Intracranial tumors
	Myocardial infarction
Anemia	Oxygen toxicity
Bradycardia (<30 beats/min)	Pericardial disease
Cardiomyopathies	Physical, environmental, or emotional stress
Coronary artery disease	Pulmonary embolus
Development of a second form of heart disease	Reduction or cessation of a medication
Drugs: methotrexate, busulfan, hexamethonium, nitrofurantoin	Respiratory distress syndrome
	Systemic infection
Dysrhythmias	Tachycardia (>180 beats/min)
Fever of any cause	Uremic pneumonia
Fluid overload, accidental or intentional	Valvular heart disease
Hypertension (systemic or pulmonary)	Viral myocarditis
Hyperthyroidism	

- Hemoptysis
- Hepatomegaly
- Nausea, anorexia, bloating, constipation
- Nocturia
- Orthopnea
- Palpitations
- Paroxysmal nocturnal dyspnea
- Pulmonary edema
- Tachycardia
- Tachypnea
- Weakness
- Weight gain

Patient Assessment

Assessment of the patient with heart failure includes the following:
- Obtain vital signs, including oxygen saturation.
- Place the patient on a cardiac monitor.
- Auscultate the lungs and heart.
- Evaluate for associated symptoms (see the foregoing list).
- Obtain a medical history and perform a focused physical examination.
- Draw a complete blood count sample to identify infection or anemia.
- Monitor electrolyte levels; hyperkalemia and hyponatremia can occur with severe failure.
- Check blood urea nitrogen and creatinine; these may be elevated with severe heart failure.
- Draw a sample for a C-reactive protein test.
- Measure a B-type natriuretic peptide level. This test also is referred to as *brain* natriuretic peptide (Box 21-3).
- Obtain a 12-lead electrocardiogram and a chest radiograph.
- Monitor cardiac biomarkers to determine whether MI is the cause of the heart failure.

Box **21-3**   B-Type Natriuretic Peptide

The cardiac ventricles are the major source of B-type natriuretic peptide.
B-type natriuretic peptide is a useful marker for the diagnosis of heart failure.
Plasma B-type natriuretic peptide levels correlate with the level of left ventricular dysfunction.
Plasma B-type natriuretic peptide level greater than 100 pg/mL indicates left ventricular dysfunction or symptomatic heart failure.
B-type natriuretic peptide can be used to differentiate dyspnea caused by heart failure from primary pulmonary diseases.

From American College of Cardiology, American Heart Association: ACC/AHA guidelines for the evaluation and management of chronic heart failure in the adult. Retrieved November 11, 2003, from www.acc.org/clinical/guidelines/failure/iii_assessment.htm
IV, Intravenous; *BP,* blood pressure; *SBP,* systolic blood pressure; *MI,* myocardial infarction.

Further Therapeutic Interventions for Acute Heart Failure

Other therapeutic interventions for acute heart failure include the following:
- Treat precipitating conditions such as anemia, atrial fibrillation, hypertension, valvular disorders, or MI.
- Provide high-flow oxygen. Anticipate intubation.
- Establish intravenous access.
- Give morphine sulfate (a venous vasodilator) to decrease preload, relieve anxiety, and minimize hyperventilation.
- Insert an indwelling urinary catheter.
- Give a rapid-acting loop diuretic (e.g., furosemide) to reduce preload. Repeat at the same dose (or double the initial dose) if there is insufficient response within 15 to 30 minutes.
- Initiate digoxin therapy for patients with rapid atrial fibrillation, severe heart failure, or an ejection fraction less than 30%.
- Consider a continuous infusion of sodium nitroprusside (Nipride) to aid vasodilation in hypertensive patients.
- Give ACE inhibitors to decrease preload and afterload. Begin at a low dose to prevent hypotension; titrate rapidly upward as needed.
- Initiate a dopamine infusion for severe hypotension.
- Start a continuous infusion of dobutamine (Dobutrex) to increase cardiac contractile force in patients with refractory heart failure.
- Treat significant tachydysrhythmias and bradydysrhythmias.

MALIGNANT HYPERTENSION

Blood pressure is derived from a combination of cardiac output and peripheral vascular resistance; in hypertension either or both of these components is elevated. In recent years the criteria for adult hypertension have been lowered. Table 21-15 gives the current guidelines. Complications related to uncontrolled hypertension include renal failure, heart disease, and stroke. Patients with chronic hypertension—and those without a previously recognized problem—can develop acute hypertension. Acute hypertension is subclassified as malignant hypertension, hypertensive emergency, or hypertensive urgency.[7] Refer to Chapter 45 for a discussion of hypertension in the pregnant patient.

Malignant hypertension is defined as a sudden and precipitous increase in blood pressure. Patients can have retinopathy, heart failure, renal compromise, and encephalopathy. Immediate intervention is required.

Table **21-15**   **Classification of Hypertension in Adults**

Blood Pressure Classification	Systolic Blood Pressure (mm Hg)		Diastolic Blood Pressure (mm Hg)
Normal	<120	and	<80
Prehypertension	120-139	or	80-89
Hypertension	140-159	or	90-99
Stage 2 hypertension	≥160	or	≥100

Data from Franco V, Opcril S, Carretero OA: Hypertensive therapy. I, *Circulation* 109:2953.8, 2004.

Hypertensive emergency involves a significant elevation in blood pressure that must be treated within an hour to prevent end organ damage.

Hypertensive urgency is a substantial blood pressure elevation that should be treated within 24 hours of presentation.

Signs and Symptoms

Signs and symptoms of malignant hypertension include the following[9]:
- Altered level of consciousness
- Chest pain
- Dizziness
- Epistaxis
- Headache
- Heart failure
- Hematuria and oliguria
- Presence of S_3 and S_4
- Seizures
- Tinnitus
- Visual complaints
- Retinopathy

Therapeutic Interventions

Therapeutic interventions for malignant hypertension include the following[8]:
- Send laboratory studies: Complete blood count, electrolytes, blood urea nitrogen, creatinine, and urinalysis.
- Obtain a 12-lead electrocardiogram and a chest radiograph.
- An echocardiogram may be done to assess left ventricular function.
- Administer a rapid-acting intravenous antihypertensive such as labetalol, esmolol, fenoldopam, or nicardipine. Avoid nitroprusside in extreme crisis because of the potential for toxicity.
- The aim of therapy is to reduce pressure by 30% within 30 minutes rather than normalize.

ACUTE PERICARDITIS

Acute pericarditis occurs more often in adults than in children. The cause can be infectious, structural, pharmacologic, or idiopathic (Table 21-16). Chest pain associated with pericarditis occurs suddenly, ranges from mild to severe, and increases with activity. Characteristic pericarditis pain is aggravated by lying flat or on the left side and by coughing or deep inspiration. Neither rest nor nitroglycerin relieves the pain, but sitting up, leaning forward, and

Table 21-16   **Causes of Pericarditis**

Category	Discussion
Idiopathic	May follow a viral or febrile illness but the cause is often never established.
Viral	Echovirus, coxsackievirus, adenovirus, varicella, Epstein-Barr, cytomegalovirus, hepatitis B, human immunodeficiency virus
Bacterial	Staphylococcus, Streptococcus, *Haemophilus*, Salmonella, Legionella, *Mycobacterium tuberculosis*
Fungal	*Candida*, Aspergillus, *Histoplasma capsulatum*, *Coccidioides immitus*
Parasitic	*Entamoeba histolytica*, *Toxoplasma gondii*, Echinococcus
Neoplasms	Lung, breast, lymphoma, leukemia, melanoma, radiation therapy
Drugs	Procainamide, hydralazine, dantrolene, fibrinolytic agents
Connective tissue disease	Systemic lupus erythematosus, rheumatoid arthritis, scleroderma
Others	Uremia, hemodialysis, myocardial infarction, chest trauma, aortic dissection, pancreatitis, irritable bowel syndrome

taking antiinflammatory agents may help. The most common clinical finding is a pericardial friction rib. The friction rub, best heard at the sternal border, makes a grating, scraping, or leathery scratching sound.

Signs and Symptoms

Signs and symptoms of acute pericarditis include the following:
- Chest pain that occurs suddenly and is associated with deep inspiration; described as sharp, stabbing, or knifelike. Pain occasionally radiates to the neck, arms, or back.
- Fever and chills, usually improved after the first day
- Diaphoresis
- Dyspnea and cough
- Tachycardia or other dysrhythmias
- A pericardial friction rub that increases when the patient leans forward. The sound is triphasic, associated with ventricular systole, ventricular diastole, and atrial systole. The rub is usually transient and may change over time.
- Malaise
- Decreased blood pressure if effusion is present
- Electrocardiogram changes occur in 90% of patients with pericarditis, but it is important to note that, unlike MI, there are no reciprocal changes in opposing leads. Changes vary throughout the course of pericarditis. In the acute phase, look for ST segment elevation (1 to 3 mm) with tall peaked T waves (present in all leads except aV_R and V_1).

Therapeutic Interventions

Therapeutic interventions for acute pericarditis include the following:
- Treat the underlying cause (e.g., infection, MI, or rheumatoid arthritis).
- Obtaining a chest radiograph may help establish the cause (e.g., tuberculosis, effusion, or aortic dissection).
- Initiate oxygen saturation and cardiac rhythm monitoring.
- Treat discomfort and anxiety with sedation, analgesia, nonsteroidal antiinflammatory drugs, position of comfort, and bed rest.
- Start corticosteroid therapy.
- An echocardiogram can detect and determine the amount of pericardial effusion.
- A pericardectomy may be performed for constrictive pericarditis.

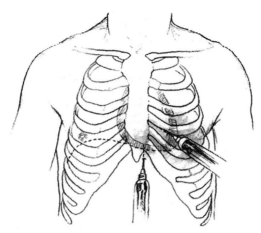

Figure 21-12. Pericardiocentesis. (From Newberry L, editor: *Sheehy's emergency nursing: principles and practice*, ed 5, St Louis, 2003, Mosby.)

Cardiac Tamponade

Cardiac tamponade results when blood or effusion fluid collects in the minimally distensible pericardial sac and compresses the heart. Compression prevents adequate ventricular filling during systole and emptying during diastole, producing a critical decrease in cardiac output. Trauma is the most common cause of cardiac tamponade seen in emergency departments. However, infectious, neoplastic, and iatrogenic causes also can produce tamponade. A significant potential exists for tamponade following certain invasive cardiac procedures such as catheterization or coronary artery bypass grafting. Cardiac tamponade also can occur in association with dissection of the aorta near the root.

Early recognition and immediate intervention are crucial to prevent cardiac arrest as tamponade worsens and output drops. Immediate treatment for acute cardiac tamponade includes pericardiocentesis (Figure 21-12). This procedure can be performed readily in the emergency department using a prepackaged kit or by simply attaching a spinal needle to a large syringe. Increasing the intravascular volume with a rapid fluid bolus is a temporizing measure that will raise filling pressures on the right side of the heart and briefly augment cardiac output.

The severity of signs and symptoms depends on the rate of fluid accumulation, the degree of pericardial compliance, and the patient's intravascular volume. An initial (but transient) hypertensive state can exist as decreased cardiac output causes compensatory vasoconstriction and increased peripheral vascular resistance. Patients can develop profound shock with as little as 100 mL of fluid in the pericardial sac. The three classic signs of cardiac tamponade, collectively referred to as Beck's triad, are hypotension, muffled heart sounds, and distended neck veins.

Signs and Symptoms

Signs and symptoms of cardiac tamponade include the following:
- Cold, clammy skin
- Muffled heart sounds
- Pulsus paradoxus (>10 mm Hg drop in systolic blood pressure during inspiration)
- Restlessness, weakness
- Decreased arterial pressure, decreased systolic blood pressure, narrow pulse pressure
- Tachycardia and a weak, thready pulse
- Elevated central venous pressure and distended neck veins
- Loss of the apical cardiac impulse

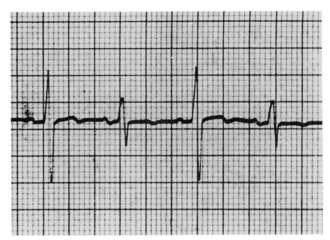

Figure 21-13. Electrical alternans. (From Newberry L, editor: *Sheehy's emergency nursing: principles and practice,* ed 5, St Louis, 2003, Mosby.)

- Shock
- A widened cardiac silhouette on chest radiograph. The heart can assume a "water bottle" shape. (This finding is more common with slowly developing effusions than with acute tamponade.)
- Electrical alternans (Figure 21-13)
- Cyanosis, increased respiratory rate, dyspnea, orthopnea, air hunger
- Low voltage on electrocardiogram tracings
- Hamman's crunch

THORACIC AORTIC DISSECTION

Ninety percent of cases of aortic dissection involve patients with a long-standing history of systemic hypertension[9] and a preexisting aortic aneurysm. This condition is seen more often in males than in females and usually occurs in the sixth or seventh decade of life. Causes of thoracic dissection associated with younger patients include trauma, pregnancy, and Marfan syndrome. Dissection occurs when a violation of the intimal layer of the aorta allows blood to leak between the medial and adventitial layers. The dissection can extend above or below the initial tear. Figure 21-14 illustrates different types of dissections.

Dissection occludes nearby vessels that branch off the aorta, including coronary, carotid, spinal, mesenteric, and renal arteries. Rupture of the dissection into the pericardial sac leads to pericardial tamponade. Rupture into the chest cavity causes massive hemothorax and exsanguination.

Chest pain occurs in 90% of patients with dissection. This pain is described as sudden, excruciating, tearing, and moving from anterior to posterior. Symptoms may be confused with those of myocardial infarction, back pain, pericarditis, or peptic ulcer.

Signs and Symptoms

Signs and symptoms of thoracic aortic dissection include the following:
- A mass effect (compression by the expanding aorta) can cause dysphagia, hoarseness, and airway compromise.[7]

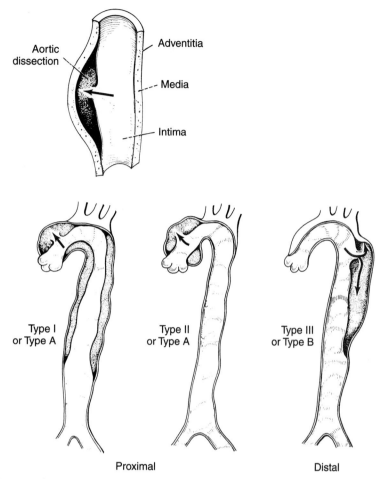

Figure 21-14. Aortic dissection. (From Urden LD, Stacy KM, Lough ME: *Thelan's critical care nursing: diagnosis and management*, ed 4, St Louis, 2002, Mosby.)

- Pericardial friction rub
- Widened mediastinum on chest radiographs
- Altered level of consciousness, syncope, and coma
- Aortic insufficiency murmur (type II)
- Apprehension, sense of impending doom
- Diaphoresis, pallor, peripheral cyanosis
- Dyspnea, orthopnea
- Hemiplegia caused by carotid obstruction
- Hypertension or hypotension can occur.
- Nausea and vomiting
- Oliguria as a result of renal artery occlusion
- Palpable pulsations at the left sternoclavicular joint
- Paraplegia caused by spinal cord ischemia
- Shock

- Tachycardia
- Unequal or absent pulses, generally pulses are absent *unilaterally*.
- Variable left- and right-sided blood pressures. Significant side-to-side differences may be present depending on the location of the dissection and the vessels affected.
- Hamman's crunch

Therapeutic Interventions

Therapeutic interventions for thoracic aortic dissection include the following:
- Allow the patient to assume a position of comfort.
- Provide supplemental oxygen; titrate to saturation level.
- Insert a minimum of two large-bore intravenous catheters (14 or 16 gauge) with an isotonic solution infusing to keep the veins open.
- Send a specimen to type and crossmatch a minimum of 6 units of packed red blood cells.
- Draw a cardiac marker sample to rule out MI.
- Obtain a 12-lead electrocardiogram. Although ST segment elevation is unusual, 10% to 20% of aortic dissection patients show changes consistent with an MI.
- Get a chest radiograph to identify a widened mediastinum.
- An echocardiogram is helpful for identification of the dissection.
- Angiography, computed tomography, and magnetic resonance imaging also may be obtained if the patient's condition permits.
- Control pain with intravenous adminstration of morphine.
- Use beta-blockers to decrease blood pressure, heart rate, and left ventricular contractility. Labetalol (Normodyne) is the preferred drug because of its beta$_1$ and beta$_2$ receptor blocking action.
- Start a nitroprusside (Nipride) infusion at 0.3 to 10 mg/kg per minute, titrate to a systolic blood pressure of 120 mm Hg. *Do not start nitroprusside therapy before beginning beta-blocker therapy,* or the heart rate can increase, potentially extending the dissection.
- Surgery is indicated for acute dissections of the ascending aorta or when medical therapy fails with other types of dissection.

References

1. Proehl J: *Emergency nursing procedures,* ed 3, Philadelphia, 2004, Saunders.
2. Jordan KS, editor: *Emergency nursing core curriculum,* ed 5, Philadelphia, 2000, Saunders.
3. American Heart Association: *Handbook of emergency cardiovascular care for healthcare providers,* Dallas, 2002, The Association.
4. Barnason S: Cardiovascular emergencies. In Newberry L, editor: *Sheehy's emergency nursing: principles and practice,* ed 5, St Louis, 2003, Mosby.
5. O'Rourke R, Fuster V, Alexander R: *Hurst's the heart manual of cardiology,* ed 10, New York, 2001, McGraw-Hill.
6. American College of Cardiology, American Heart Association: ACC/AHA guidelines for the evaluation and management of chronic heart failure in the adult. Retrieved November 11, 2003, from www.acc.org/clinical/guidelines/failure/iii_assessment.htm.
7. Ferri F: *Ferri's Clinical advisor: instant diagnosis and treatment, 2000 edition,* St Louis, 2000, Mosby.
8. Emergency medicine. In Graber M, Lanternier ML, editor: Graber M: *University of Iowa Family Practice Handbook,* ed 4, St Louis, 2001, Mosby.
9. Urden LD, Stacy KM, Lough ME: *Thelan's critical care nursing: diagnosis and management,* ed 4, St Louis, 2003, Mosby.

22

Shock

Cheri Kommor, RN, CEN

Shock is a complex syndrome that results when tissue oxygenation or nutrient delivery are insufficient to maintain the metabolic needs of the cell.[1] Most commonly, this state is due to inadequate tissue perfusion but also results when the cells are unable to use available oxygen (e.g., cyanide toxicity). Prolonged periods of inadequate oxygen delivery cause cellular hypoxia and accumulation of toxic metabolites that damage tissue and initiate a cascade of events leading to multiple organ dysfunction. Structures crucial to cellular oxygen delivery are the heart, lungs, blood, and vascular system.

Failure of any one of these components produces shock. Without treatment, this process progresses to the death of cells, tissues, organs, and—ultimately—the entire organism. Early intervention is essential to interrupt this cascade of events. However, management of shock can be difficult, and mortality is high. Appropriate therapeutic intervention requires identifying whether the problem is related to limited volume, pump failure, pulmonary failure, or vascular dilation.

Shock is characterized by its underlying cause and pathophysiology. Shock most often is categorized into four basic types: hypovolemic, cardiogenic, distributive and obstructive.[2] The goal of therapy for all shock types is the restoration of adequate tissue oxygenation while preventing cellular necrosis and organ system failure.

SHOCK CLASSIFICATIONS

A brief overview of shock classifications follows. For a more complete description, see the following sections.

Hypovolemic

Hypovolemia is the most common cause of shock. This state is caused by a significant reduction in whole blood or plasma volume. Traumatic bleeding, hemorrhage from other causes (e.g., gastrointestinal bleeding or abdominal aneurysm rupture), severe burns (resulting in plasma loss), or general dehydration (as a consequence of excessive vomiting, diarrhea, polyuria, or profuse diaphoresis) can produce hypovolemic shock.[3]

Cardiogenic

Cardiogenic shock results from a loss of myocardial contractility, leading to inadequate cardiac output. The heart can fail to be an effective pump in cases of myocardial infarction, cardiac contusion, tamponade, myocarditis, papillary muscle rupture, severe dysrhythmias, valvular disease, or cardiomyopathy.

Distributive

Distributive shock occurs when venous pooling, occlusion of the microvascular, or poor blood flow distribution limit tissue oxygenation. Three types of distributive shock are septic, anaphylactic, and neurogenic.

Septic shock

Septic shock is the most common form of distributive shock. This state is produced by an overwhelming infection that causes cellular destruction, microvascular occlusion, and systemic vasodilation. The subsequent inadequate tissue perfusion, third spacing, and altered cellular metabolism affect multiple organs.

Anaphylactic shock

Anaphylactic shock is an acute, severe allergic reaction stimulated by a profound antibody response to an antigen. This reaction causes histamine release, increased capillary permeability, vasodilation, smooth muscle contraction, angioedema, and bronchoconstriction.

Neurogenic shock

Neurogenic shock results from a loss of sympathetic tone, which interferes with the ability of the body to vasoconstrict and produces massive vasodilation. This state leads to severe hypotension and unopposed vagal response that can cause bradycardia. Neurogenic shock is associated with acute spinal cord disruption from traumatic injuries above the level of T6. Spinal anesthesia causes a temporary loss of sympathetic tone that produces a similar but transitory state.[3] Likewise, profound hypoglycemia (insulin shock) and vasovagal syncope (fainting) involve inhibition of sympathetic outflow from the vasomotor center of the medulla, causing loss of vasomotor regulation.

Obstructive

Obstructive shock is a form of indirect pump failure; the heart itself is fine, but an external force decreases cardiac output and inhibits pump function. Obstructive shock is caused by anything that compresses the heart (cardiac tamponade, tension pneumothorax, or massive hemothorax) or obstructs blood outflow (massive pulmonary embolus, pulmonary hypertension, or severe aortic stenosis).

PATHOPHYSIOLOGY OF SHOCK

Shock Stages

Regardless of the underlying cause, the basic pathophysiology of shock consists of inadequate oxygen delivery at the cellular level, causing acidosis and subsequent organ dysfunction. Symptoms follow a predictable cascade of events through initial, compensatory, progressive, and refractory stages. The speed of progression and clinical manifestations seen at each stage vary by patient. Optimal therapy requires early identification of shock type and rapid intervention. The following pathophysiologic mechanisms are described according to each stage of shock.[2]

Initial/Early Stage

In this phase, signs of poor tissue oxygenation are subtle:
- Possible decrease in mean arterial pressure (MAP), typically no more than 5 to 10 mm Hg
- Drop in cardiac output (about 15%)
- Reduced tissue perfusion and oxygen delivery to the cells
- Slight rise in heart rate above the patient's baseline level
- Shift from aerobic to anaerobic metabolism
- Increased lactic acid production

Compensatory Stage

The body activates a number of mechanisms in an attempt to restore cardiac output and preserve vital organ function. Table 22-1 highlights prominent compensatory mechanisms. This phase is characterized by the following:
- A decrease in MAP of 10 to 15 mm Hg
- A further drop in cardiac output (15% to 30%)

Table 22-1   Compensatory Mechanisms in Shock

Compensatory Mechanism	Effect on Body
Sympathetic nervous system (SNS) stimulation	A drop in blood pressure stimulates receptors in the aortic arch and carotid bodies to activate the SNS.
	Epinephrine and norepinephrine are released, causing an increase in heart rate, cardiac contractility, and diastolic blood pressure.
	Selective vasoconstriction redistributes blood to the heart and brain.
Activation of the renin-angiotensin-aldosterone mechanism	Renin is stimulated by a decrease in renal blood flow. This causes the secretion of angiotensin I.
	Angiotensin I circulates and is converted to angiotensin II in the lungs.
	Angiotensin II causes vasoconstriction and release of aldosterone from the adrenals.
	Aldosterone increases sodium and water reabsorption in the tubules, producing a drop in urine output. This results in increased vascular tone, intravascular volume, blood return to the heart, cardiac output, and blood pressure.
Antidiuretic hormone release	Antidiuretic hormone is secreted by the posterior pituitary in response to hypovolemic states.
	This hormone causes renal reabsorption of sodium and water and limits urine output.
	The result is an increase in intravascular volume, cardiac output, and urine specific gravity.
Intracellular fluid shifts	In response to intravascular volume depletion, fluid shifts from the interstitial and intracellular spaces to the intravascular space.
	This shift augments intravascular volume, blood return to heart, cardiac output, and blood pressure.
	These fluid shifts produce cellular dehydration and profound thirst (if the patient is awake).

- Activation of compensatory mechanisms:
  - Tachypnea (>20 breaths/min)
  - Tachycardia (>100 beats/min)
  - Decreased urinary output (<30 mL/hr)
  - Vasoconstriction (to shunt blood to vital organs)

Progressive Stage

Once shock reaches the progressive stage, compensatory mechanisms are no longer able to maintain adequate tissue perfusion. The emergency nurse should look for the following[2]:

- Hypoperfusion of vital organs
- Sustained decreases in MAP of greater than 20 mm Hg (from the patient's baseline)
- Cardiac output reduction (by 30% to 40%)
- An increased heart rate (may be >150 beats/min) with a weak, thready pulse
- Reduced myocardial oxygenation and contractility
- Ischemia of nonessential organs such as the kidneys, intestines, and skin
- Increased capillary permeability

Refractory Stage

The refractory (or irreversible) phase of shock indicates progression to cellular, tissue, and organ death. Signs include the following:

- Multiple system organ failure
- Profound hypoperfusion
- Severe hypoxemia
- Renal shutdown
- Clotting abnormalities (disseminated intravascular coagulation)
- Intractable circulatory failure
- Profoundly negative arterial base deficit

Throughout the four stages of shock, each of the vital organ systems of the body is affected. Box 22-1 lists the effects of shock on various organs.

Box 22-1 Effects of Shock on Various Body Organs

Heart

↓ Coronary perfusion
↓ Pump function
↓ Stroke volume
↓ Cardiac output
↓ Blood pressure

Brain

↓ Blood flow to the brain
↓ Brain function
↓ Level of consciousness

Lungs

↓ Oxygenation
↑ Respiratory rate
↓ Gas exchange
↑ CO_2 retention
↑ Anaerobic metabolism

Liver

↑ Glycogenolysis[4]
↑ Blood glucose levels
↓ Hepatic blood flow
↑ Hepatic ischemia
↑ Acidosis

Kidneys

↓ Renal blood flow
↑ Vasoconstriction
Release of antidiuretic hormone
↓ Urine output
Renal failure

TYPES OF SHOCK

Hypovolemic Shock

Hypovolemia results from a loss of whole blood, plasma, or fluid and electrolytes. Figure 22-1 illustrates the pathway of hypovolemic shock development.

The following are common causes of hypovolemic shock:

- *Traumatic hemorrhage:* Long bone or pelvic fractures, solid organ rupture, major vessel disruption, open wounds
- *Nontraumatic hemorrhage:* Gastrointestinal bleeding, ruptured aortic aneurysm, ruptured ectopic pregnancy, posterior epistaxis, obstetric hemorrhage, disseminated intravascular coagulation

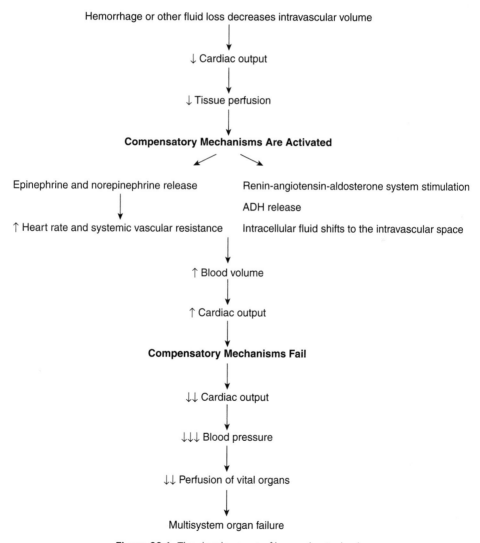

Figure 22-1. The development of hypovolemic shock.

- Fluid shifts: Peritonitis, massive crush injuries, severe burns
- Nonblood fluid loss: Severe diarrhea or vomiting, excessive diaphoresis
- Urinary fluid loss: Diabetic ketoacidosis, diabetes insipidus, diuretic abuse

Table 22-2 estimates potential blood volume losses associated with common traumatic injuries.

Early identification and treatment of hypovolemic shock are essential to good patient outcomes. Age and preexisting health conditions also affect the potential for recovery. Classically, hemorrhagic shock is categorized based on the percent of volume depletion. Table 22-3 lists typical physiologic responses according to the degree of blood loss.[5]

Clinical presentation in hypovolemic shock is related to the amount and rate of actual volume loss and includes the following signs and symptoms:

- Tachycardia (Classes II to IV)
- Hypotension (Classes III and IV)
- Orthostatic blood pressure (BP) changes from lying to sitting or standing (a drop in systolic BP greater than 20 mm Hg or a heart rate increase greater than 20 beats/min)
- Narrowing pulse pressure (Pulse pressure = Systolic BP − Diastolic BP) (Classes II to IV)
- Tachypnea (Classes II to IV)
- Altered mental status, restlessness, anxiety, dizziness, and lethargy caused by decreased cerebral perfusion. Patients with a 40% blood loss will lose consciousness.
- Decreased central venous pressure and pulmonary artery wedge pressures
- Reduced stroke volume, cardiac output, and tissue perfusion
- Drop in renal perfusion with decreased urinary output (Classes II to IV)
- Extreme thirst (early sign)

Table 22-2 Estimated Blood Loss by Site of Injury

Injury	Estimated Blood Loss (mL)
Pelvic fracture	3000
Femur fracture	1000
Tibial fracture	650
Intraabdominal injury	2000
Thoracic injury	2000

Table 22-3 Physiologic Response According to the Degree of Blood Loss (70-kg Patient)

	Class I	Class II	Class III	Class IV
Blood loss	0-15% (<750 mL)	15%-30% (750-1500 mL)	30%-40% (1500-2000 mL)	>40% (>2000 mL)
Heart rate	<100	100-120	120-140	>140
Blood pressure	Normal	Normal	Decreased	Decreased
Pulse pressure	Normal or increased	Decreased	Decreased	Decreased
Mental status	Slightly anxious	Moderately anxious	Confused, lethargic	Unconscious
Respirations	14-20 min	20-30 min	30-40 min	>35 min
Urine output	>30 mL/hr	20-30 mL/hr	5-15 mL/hr	<5 mL/hr
Capillary refill	<2 sec	>2 sec	>4 sec	No filling noted
Skin	Cool/pink	Cold/pale	Cold/moist	Cyanotic/mottled

From Newberry L, editor: *Sheehy's emergency nursing: principles and practice*, ed 5, St Louis, 2003, Mosby.

- Rapid, thready pulse
- Cool, clammy skin
- Delayed capillary refill

  Management of the patient in hypovolemic shock is directed toward preventing further fluid losses and restoring circulating volume. Interventions include the following:

- Support the patient's airway, breathing, and circulation.
- Administer oxygen via a nonrebreather mask to the conscious patient. Endotracheally intubate unconscious patients.
- Monitor oxygen saturation with continuous pulse oximetry. Obtain arterial blood gas measurements as indicated. Keep arterial base deficit less than –6.
- Control bleeding if possible (e.g., dressings, direct pressure, splints, and rapid surgical intervention)
- Initiate intravenous (IV) isotonic crystalloid infusion.
  - Cannulate two or more veins with large-bore IV catheters (14 to 16 gauge in adults).
  - Isotonic crystalloids are administered at a 3:1 ratio (300 mL of crystalloid for every 100 mL of blood loss).[6]
  - Lactated Ringer's solution, normal saline, and Plasmalyte are examples of isotonic crystalloids.
  - Isotonic solutions increase intravascular volume and help maintain electrolyte balance.[2] (See Chapter 8.)
  - Lactated Ringer's solution is the crystalloid most commonly used for initial hydration.[4] The solution contains electrolytes and an alkalizing agent, which counteracts metabolic acidosis (as long as liver function is intact).
  - Infusing warmed fluids helps minimize hypothermia and subsequent metabolic acidosis.[6]
- Replace hemorrhagic losses with blood products if the patient remains symptomatic after 3 to 4 L of crystalloids.[5]
- Type-specific and crossmatched blood is preferred.
- In cases of severe loss, use O-negative blood until a type and crossmatch are complete. (Males and women beyond childbearing age may be given O-positive blood.)
- Consider autotransfusion of chest blood. (See Chapter 37.)
- The use of vasopressor agents in patients with acute volume depletion is not appropriate. If the patient remains hypotensive, look for sites of fluid loss, correct the underlying problem, and give more fluids (crystalloids or blood products).
- Monitor the patient for any sign of complications associated with infusion of blood products and crystalloids. Table 22-4 summarizes these complications.
- Prepare the patient for diagnostic studies and surgical interventions.
- Insert an indwelling urinary catheter, and track urine output.
- Place the patient on a cardiac monitor. Check for dysrhythmias.
- Monitor hemodynamic status. (See Chapter 11.)
- Keep the patient warm using blankets, warming lights, or convection heaters (e.g., Bair Hugger [Arizant Healthcare, Eden Prairie, Minn]).
- Consider using a pneumatic antishock garment for splinting pelvic and lower extremity fractures associated with significant blood loss.[7]
- Insert a gastric tube to reduce gastric distention, which is associated with vomiting and aspiration. Distention can stimulate the vagus nerve, causing bradycardia.

Cardiogenic Shock

The pump failure caused by cardiogenic shock results in the inability of the heart to forcibly eject sufficient blood to meet the tissue oxygenation needs of the body. Cardiogenic shock

Table **22-4**   **Complications of Blood Product and Crystalloid Replacement**

Problem	Cause	Comments
Hypothermia	Crystalloids and banked blood transfused without warming.	Hypothermia inhibits efforts to reverse metabolic acidosis and aggravates coagulopathies.
Hyperkalemia	Lysis of red blood cells causes potassium release. Potassium levels are particularly high in banked blood.	Monitor serum potassium levels. Observe for dysrhythmias and peaked T waves.
Hypocalcemia	The citrate anticoagulant used in banked blood binds free serum calcium.	Check serum calcium level after infusion of about 10 units of blood. Give calcium chloride or calcium gluconate as needed.
Acidosis	The pH of banked blood is 7.1 (acidotic).	Monitor arterial pH. Observe for dysrhythmias.
Alkalosis	The citrate in banked blood is converted by the liver to bicarbonate (alkalotic).	Monitor arterial pH, especially in patients with hepatic dysfunction.
Clotting disorders	Most clotting factors have been removed from packed red blood cells.	Perform clotting studies. Transfuse fresh frozen plasma, platelets, and cryoprecipitate as needed.
Intravascular debris	Banked blood contains debris as a result of processing.	Always infuse blood through a blood filter. Some evidence supports the use of microfilters.

is associated with a high mortality rate, often leading to death within 24 hours. This form of shock may be caused by acute conditions such as myocardial infarction, penetrating trauma, myocardial rupture, dysrhythmias, or pericardial tamponade. Cardiogenic shock also can result from progressive conditions such as myocarditis or a cardiomyopathy. When myocardial damage occurs, portions of the myocardium become dysfunctional. If the damaged area is large (>40% of the ventricle), cardiac output decreases significantly. When cardiac output is reduced, blood pressure drops, tissue perfusion is inadequate, and shock quickly follows. Figure 22-2 illustrates the pathophysiology of cardiogenic shock. Clinical manifestations of this condition resemble those seen in patients with acute myocardial infarction and include the following:

- Chest pain, diaphoresis, nausea, vomiting, syncope
- Electrocardiogram changes indicative of myocardial ischemia, injury, or infarction
- Cardiac dysrhythmias
- Elevated cardiac biomarkers
- Shallow, rapid respirations
- Hypoxemia
- Decreased myocardial contractility
- Muffled heart tones
- S_3 or S_4 heart sounds
- Reduced cardiac output (<4 L/min or a cardiac index <2.2 L/min)
- Decreased level of consciousness (anxiety, restlessness, lethargy, unconsciousness)
- Pale, cool, clammy skin
- Minimal urine output
- Metabolic acidosis
- Signs of left ventricular failure
  - Pulmonary edema caused by incomplete emptying of the left ventricle
  - Diffuse crackles and wheezes
  - Decreased peripheral pulses
  - Hypotension

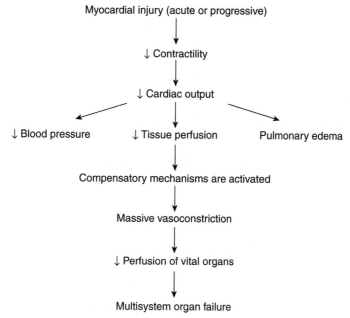

Figure 22-2. The development of cardiogenic shock.

- Signs of right ventricular failure
  - Jugular venous distension
  - Peripheral edema
  - Hepatomegaly

Management of the patient in cardiogenic shock focuses on reducing cardiac workload and improving myocardial contractility. Interventions include the following:

- Support the patient's airway, breathing, and circulation.
- Intubate as necessary.
- Correct preload problems.
  - *Decreased preload:* Increase central venous pressure, pulmonary artery wedge pressure, and pulmonary artery diastolic pressure by administering intravenous fluids. (See Chapter 11.)
  - *Increased preload:* Decrease central venous pressure, pulmonary artery wedge pressure, and pulmonary artery diastolic pressure with vasodilatory agents or diuretics.
- Correct afterload problems.
  - *Decreased afterload:* Increase blood pressure and systemic vascular resistance with vasopressors.
  - *Increased afterload:* Decrease blood pressure and systemic vascular resistance wth vasodilatory agents.
- Support myocardial contractility and cardiac output.
  - Inotropic medications such as dopamine and dobutamine increase contractility and improve systolic BP.
  - An intraaortic balloon pump is a percutaneously placed diastolic assist device designed to increase cardiac output, maximize oxygen delivery, improve blood flow to the coronary arteries, and decrease myocardial oxygen consumption.
- Administer nitroglycerin intravenously to diminish myocardial pain, increase coronary perfusion, reduce preload and afterload, decrease left ventricular filling pressures,

and improve cardiac output. However, use nitroglycerin cautiously in hypotensive patients.

- Give morphine sulfate to reduce pain and anxiety, ease respiratory effort, minimize pulmonary edema, and decrease afterload.
- Use sodium nitroprusside (IV drip) to decrease afterload (use cautiously in patients with hypotension).
- Administer diuretics (furosemide) to reduce preload, reverse pulmonary edema, and improve cardiac output.
- Give a beta-blocker to decrease the heart rate and increase cardiac filling time.
- Assist with insertion of a pulmonary artery catheter and arterial line to guide fluid administration and drug titration.
- Administer antidysrhythmic agents and initiate cardiac pacing as indicated.
- Obtain an echocardiogram to quantify left ventricular wall defects, calculate the ejection fraction, and evaluate valve function.
- Prepare the patient for coronary interventions such as percutaneous transluminal coronary angioplasty or coronary artery bypass graft surgery.

Distributive Shock

This type of shock is characterized by an abnormal distribution of intravascular volume as a result of decreased sympathetic tone, pooling of blood in venous and capillary beds, and increased vascular permeability. The three categories of distributive shock are septic, anaphylactic, and neurogenic.[2]

Septic shock

Septic shock, the most common form of distributive shock, results from the inflammatory response of the body to an overwhelming systemic infection. Septic shock usually is caused by gram-negative bacteria (*Pseudomonas aeruginosa, Escherichia coli,* or *Klebsiella pneumoniae*). Gram-positive bacteria, yeast, fungi, and viruses also have been cited as causes. The source of infection varies widely and may be an indwelling urinary catheter, severe burn, pneumonia, or postpartum complication. Other risk factors for septic shock include immunosuppression, large open wounds, implanted devices, and gastrointestinal ischemia. Once sepsis progresses to septic shock, mortality is 40% to 90%.[5] As with so many conditions, death from sepsis is more common in the very young and the very old.

Once they enter the circulation, gram-negative bacteria discharge endotoxins. The toxins trigger release of histamine, prostaglandins, and other chemical mediators, causing massive vasodilation, increased capillary permeability, and redistribution of fluid into the interstitium. The resulting inadequate tissue perfusion, third spacing of fluid, and altered cellular metabolism affect multiple organs. Figure 22-3 illustrates the development of septic shock.

Signs and symptoms of septic shock fall into two phases: (1) the early, hyperdynamic, or warm phase and (2) the late, hypodynamic, or cold phase when compensation fails. Clinical findings associated with each phase are as follows:

Hyperdynamic Phase (Early, Warm Shock)

- The patient is febrile.
- The skin appears flushed, and petechiae may be present.
- Cardiac output is significantly elevated.
- Systemic vascular resistance is low due to vasodilation.
- The patient is tachycardic and tachypneic.

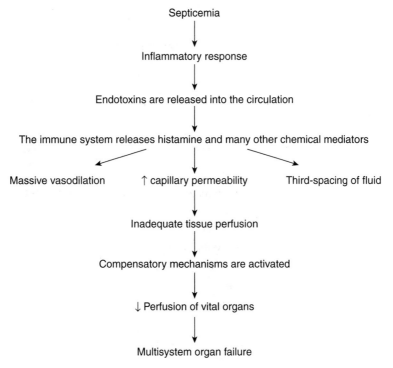

Septicemia

↓

Inflammatory response

↓

Endotoxins are released into the circulation

↓

The immune system releases histamine and many other chemical mediators

Massive vasodilation   ↑ capillary permeability   Third-spacing of fluid

↓

Inadequate tissue perfusion

↓

Compensatory mechanisms are activated

↓

↓ Perfusion of vital organs

↓

Multisystem organ failure

Figure 22-3. The development of septic shock.

- Systolic blood pressure is near normal, but diastolic pressure is low (widened pulse pressure).
- Mental status changes include agitation, anxiety, or malaise.

Hypodynamic Phase (Late, Cold Shock)

- Body temperature is subnormal.
- Respirations are rapid and shallow.
- Cardiac output is low.
- Hypotension and tachycardia are present.
- Systemic vascular resistance is increased because of profound vasoconstriction.
- Inadequate tissue perfusion causes the skin to be cool, pale, and mottled.
- Renal hypoperfusion decreases urinary output (<30 mL/hr).
- Serum lactate levels are elevated, reflecting anaerobic metabolism and lactic acidosis.
- Mental status changes include lethargy and coma.

Management of the patient in septic shock is directed toward identifying and correcting the initiating infectious event, establishing and maintaining adequate tissue perfusion, and restoring normal cellular function. Interventions include the following:
- Support the patient's airway, breathing, and circulation.
- Provide supplemental oxygen to maintain a Pao_2 greater than 60 mm Hg; intubate as necessary.[6]

- Restore intravascular volume with intravenously administered crystalloids.
- Identify and remove potential sources of infection (e.g., retained foreign bodies, retained placenta, or abscesses).
  - Debride wounds and necrotic tissue.
  - Remove existing invasive devices (e.g., indwelling urinary catheters, ventriculoperitoneal shunts, or long-term vascular access devices).
- Obtain blood and wound cultures before initiating antibiotic therapy. However, do not delay antibiotics in patients in whom cultures cannot be obtained after multiple attempts.
- Begin timely antibiotic administration.
  - A combination of an aminoglycoside and a third-generation cephalosporin usually is ordered initially.[6]
  - Therapy is modified as infectious organisms are identified.
  - Use aminoglycosides cautiously in the elderly and in other patients with renal insufficiency.
  - Antibiotics may exacerbate symptoms initially as dying bacteria release even more endotoxins.
- Closely monitor the patient's hemodynamic status.
- Consider administration of drotrecogin alfa (Xigris), a new agent for the treatment of sepsis.
- Anticipate insertion of an arterial line to track blood pressure changes (see Chapter 11).
- Administer an antipyretic agent to warm hypothermic patients with a body temperature above 38° C (100.4° F).
- Positive inotropic medications (e.g., dobutamine) may be given to increase cardiac contractility and output.
- After initial volume replacement, consider vasopressor use to constrict dilated blood vessels.

Anaphylactic shock

Anaphylactic shock is a life-threatening antigen-antibody hypersensitivity reaction resulting from reexposure to an antigen. Common allergens include certain foods, food additives, insect venoms, drugs, latex, and iodine contrast dyes. In a sensitized individual, antigen exposure triggers the release of a variety of mediators that exert their effects on the vascular and pulmonary systems. Massive vasodilation and increased capillary permeability redistribute fluid into the interstitial space causing profound hypovolemia and vascular collapse. Fluid leaking into the alveoli produces pulmonary congestion. Angioedema causes progressive airway obstruction and subsequent respiratory arrest. Figure 22-4 outlines the development of anaphylactic shock. Symptoms of anaphylaxis are acute, sudden, and rapidly progressive. The emergency nurse should look for the following:

- Respiratory difficulty
  - Stridor
  - Airway obstruction
  - Bronchospasm
  - Wheezing
- Hypoxia
- Hypotension
- Tachycardia
- Urticaria
- Angioedema
- Pruritus
- Warm, dry skin that later becomes cool and pale
- Abdominal pain and diarrhea

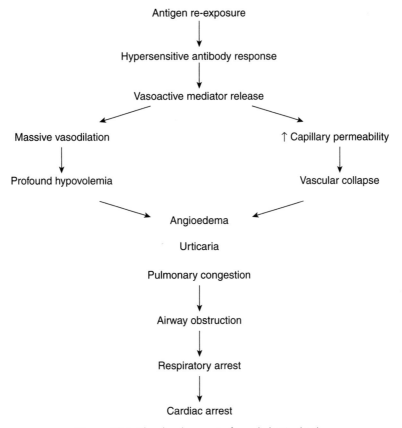

Figure 22-4. The development of anaphylactic shock.

- Chest tightness, dysrhythmias, and cardiac irritability
- Respiratory and cardiac arrest

Management of the patient in anaphylactic shock is directed toward maintaining a patent airway and counteracting the anaphylactic reaction. Interventions include the following:

- Aggressively support the patient's airway, breathing, and circulation.
- Provide high-flow oxygen. Airway obstruction can develop rapidly, so early intubation is indicated.
- Establish IV access and administer crystalloids to treat hypotension.
- Give epinephrine intravenously. This promotes vasoconstriction, dilates the bronchioles, and inhibits further release of mediators.
  - The IV dose is 0.1 to 0.5 mL of a 1:10,000 solution given by slow IV push. Repeat in 5 to 15 minutes as necessary.[7]
  - Patients with milder reactions (not in shock) can be treated with subcutaneously administered epinephrine, 0.2 to 0.3 mL of 1:1000 solution.
  - Propranolol (Inderal) should be available in the event of persistent epinephrine-induced hypertension and tachycardia.
- Administer a nebulized bronchodilator (albuterol) for bronchospasm.
- Give diphenhydramine (Benadryl), a histamine$_1$ blocker, and famotidine (Pepcid), a histamine$_2$ blocker, to decrease circulating histamine levels.

- Steroids such as methylprednisolone (Solu-Medrol) are used to limit the inflammatory response.
- Cricothyrotomy may be required for severe airway compromise.

Neurogenic shock

Neurogenic shock is caused by decreased sympathetic tone following spinal cord injury, spinal anesthesia, or vasomotor center depression from head trauma. This condition also can result from the use of certain adrenergic-blocking agents (such as doxazosin [Cardura] or terazosin [Hytrin]) that impair nerve impulse transmission and decrease sympathetic tone.[2] Neurogenic shock is associated with dilation of the arterioles and venules, producing a relative hypovolemia and hypotension. Unlike hypovolemic shock, in which volume is lost, in neurogenic shock vascular volume remains in the circulation but must travel through a highly dilated vasculature. This results in arterial and venous pooling. The combination of low blood pressure and loss of sympathetic tone contributes to two significant clinical findings unique to neurogenic shock: bradycardia and warm, dry, flushed skin. Figure 22-5 illustrates the neurogenic shock pathway. Other clinical manifestations include the following:

- Hypotension (systolic BP <90 mm Hg or 30 mm Hg less than baseline)
- Tachypnea
- Full, regular pulses
- Paraplegia or quadriplegia (in patients with spinal cord damage)
- Pale, cool, clammy skin above the level of the lesion
- Poikilothermy (a body temperature that varies with environmental temperature)
- Priapism (in male patients)

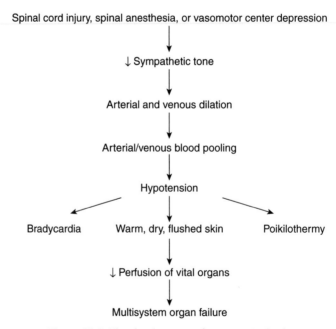

Figure 22-5. The development of neurogenic shock.

- Loss of sensation, motor function, or reflexes below the level of a spinal cord disruption
- A decreased level of consciousness because of hypotension or brain injury
- Normal urine output (initially)

Management of the patient in neurogenic shock is primarily supportive. Interventions include the following:

- Support the patient's airway, breathing, and circulation.
- Place the patient in a supine position. Blood pressure will drop if the head of the bed is elevated.
- Institute spinal immobilization measures in patients with a suspected cord or vertebral injury and assist with spinal realignment and stabilization with tongs or a halo ring device.
- Give crystalloids intravenously to expand intravascular volume.
- Intravenously administered vasopressors may be used to help constrict the vasculature and increase BP.
- In patients with a recent (less than 8 hours old) spinal cord injury, high-dose intravenously administered methylprednisolone (Solu-Medrol) may be given. However, use is associated with a number of significant complications, and little evidence exists to support this practice.
- Give atropine intravenously for symptomatic bradycardia.
- Warm or cool the patient as needed to maintain a normothermic core temperature.

Obstructive Shock

Obstructive shock is a form of pump failure that occurs as a result of forces external to the heart: an outflow obstruction or an increased resistance to ventricular filling. Massive pulmonary emboli, coarctation of the aorta, or aortic stenosis may cause obstruction to blood outflow. Pericardial tamponade, tension pneumothorax, and high levels of positive end-expiratory pressure result in increased resistance to ventricular filling. Regardless of the cause, the end result is a reduction in cardiac output and inadequate tissue perfusion. Clinical manifestations of obstructive shock depend on the cause. Management focuses on relieving the source of obstruction and providing basic supportive care, including the following:

- Support the patient's airway, breathing, and circulation.
- Administer high-flow oxygen; intubate as necessary.
- Establish IV access.

Symptoms and specific interventions associated with various causes of obstructive shock are addressed individually.

Pulmonary embolism

Signs and symptoms

- Dyspnea
- Tachypnea
- Chest pain
- Anxiety
- Hypoxemia

Interventions

- Administer an anticoagulant to the patient (heparin drip).
- Consider administration of a fibrinolytic agent (rt-PA, streptokinase).
- In rare instances, surgical embolectomy is performed.

Coarctation of the aorta

Signs and symptoms

- Hypertension of the upper extremities with hypotension in the lower extremities

Interventions

- Prepare the patient for an aortogram, cardiac catheterization, and surgical intervention (aortic grafting).
- IV access
- Oxygen

Aortic stenosis

Signs and symptoms

- Chest pain
- Dyspnea
- Cyanosis
- Syncope
- Hypoxemia
- Cough
- Mental status changes

Interventions

- Prepare the patient for cardiac catheterization and surgical intervention (valve replacement).
- IV access
- Oxygen
- Supportive treatment of symptoms

Pericardial tamponade

Signs and symptoms

- Elevated central venous pressure
- Cyanosis
- Distended neck veins
- Decreased cardiac output
- Hypotension
- Muffled heart sounds
- Electrical alternans
- Hamman's crunch

Interventions

- Immediate pericardiocentesis is required, followed by surgical intervention (cardiac repair or creation of a pericardial window).
- IV access
- Oxygen

Tension pneumothorax

Signs and symptoms

- Decreased central venous pressure
- Reduced cardiac output
- Hypotension
- Hypoxemia
- Severe shortness of breath
- Jugular vein distention
- Tracheal deviation
- Mediastinal shift
- Unilateral chest hyperexpansion
- Absent breath sounds on affected side

Interventions

- Immediate needle thoracostomy to relieve the tension (Insert the needle in the second intercostal space, at the midclavicular line.)
- Chest tube placement

CONCLUSION

Although shock has many causes, the common denominator in all shock states is an inability to meet the demand for oxygen in the body. Treatment involves measures to increase cardiac output and tissue perfusion to improve oxygen delivery. Prompt diagnosis and intervention are crucial for reducing the high overall morbidity and mortality associated with shock states.

References

1. Jacobs B, Hoyt K: *Trauma nursing core course,* ed 5, Des Plaines, Ill, 2000, Emergency Nurses Association.
2. Brewer C, Chavez JA: Stopping the shock slide, *RN* 65(9):30-34, 2002.
3. Vary TC, McLean B, Van Rueden KT: Shock and multiple organ dysfunction syndrome. In McQuillan KA et al: *Trauma nursing from resuscitation through rehabilitation,* ed 3, St Louis, 2002, Saunders.
4. Puntillo KA, Schell HM: *Critical care nursing secrets,* ed 1, Philadelphia, 2001, Hanley & Belfus.
5. Newberry L, editor: *Sheehy's emergency nursing: principles and practice,* ed 5, St Louis, 2003, Mosby.
6. Bartley MK, Mower-Wade DM, Chiari-Allwein JL: Shock, do you know how to respond? *Nursing 2000* 30(10):34-39, 2000.
7. Saunderson-Cohen S: *Trauma nursing secrets,* ed 1, Philadelphia, 2002, Hanley & Belfus.

23

Neurologic Emergencies

Kathy M. Dolan, RN, MS, CEN

A wide variety of neurologic disorders can bring a patient to the emergency department (ED). Severity ranges from minor discomfort to life-threatening conditions requiring emergent medical or surgical intervention. Several common neurologic emergencies are discussed in this chapter. Neurologic disorders associated with acute injury are presented in Chapters 35 and 36.

HEADACHE

Headache is not a diagnosis per se but rather a symptom of some underlying disorder. A patient may have the first headache ever experienced, exacerbation of a chronic condition, or a significant change in the nature of the pain. Headache can be caused by a long list of extracranial conditions such as hypoglycemia, acidosis, uremia, drugs, and ear infections. Identification and treatment of the underlying problem will resolve these headaches. Intracranial causes of headache include vascular disorders, hypertension, inflammation, temporal arteritis, hemorrhage, tumors, and trauma.[1] Table 23-1 summarizes the characteristics of various headache types.

Headache Types

Tension headache

Tension headaches usually occur in times of physical or emotional stress. Tension headache pain is described as dull, tight, or constricting. Pain is typically nonpulsating and bilateral and is located in the frontal or occipital regions. Interventions focus on identifying and treating the causal factor(s). Tension headaches usually respond to mild analgesics such as nonsteroidal antiinflammatory agents. Severe tension headaches may be indistinguishable from migraines, and stronger drugs are necessary.

Traumatic headache

Traumatic headaches are a sequela of minor and severe head injuries. Local tissue damage from trauma can lead to muscle contraction and tension on the extracranial vasculature. Concussions and contusions may be followed by intermittent headaches that persist for months. Intracerebral bleeds generally are accompanied by a severe headache of sudden onset. Refer to Chapter 35 for further discussion of intracerebral hemorrhage.

Temporal arteritis

Temporal arteritis produces severe, unilateral, throbbing frontotemporal pain. Palpation of the temporal area causes great discomfort. Pain may involve the neck and jaw. Loss of vision can also occur because of ischemic optic neuritis. Steroids should be given immediately to prevent visual loss. Patients with temporal arteritis are usually over 50 years old and have a history of polymyalgia rheumatica.[1] A biopsy is required for definitive diagnosis.

Vascular headaches

Migraines and cluster headaches are two types of vascular headaches.

Cluster headaches

Fortunately, cluster headaches are rare and short-lived. Unlike most other headache types, cluster headaches are more common in men. Believed to be caused by dysfunction of the trigeminal nerve, these headaches are characterized by intense unilateral pain in the orbital or temporal region that lasts 15 to 180 minutes. The headaches tend to occur in clusters—that is, daily on the same side of the face for several weeks—before going into remission. Associated findings include ipsilateral conjunctival injection, lacrimation, nasal congestion, rhinorrhea, and facial swelling.[2]

Migraine headaches

Migraine presentation can vary considerably between patients, and several types of migraine have been classified. Most migraines are not spontaneous but instead occur in response to a variety of environmental, emotional, hormonal, food, and medication triggers (Table 23-2). Helping patients identify their trigger(s) is key to preventing or minimizing future attacks.

Headache Assessment

Emergency department management of the patient with headache focuses on assessment and initial treatment of symptoms. Although extremely painful and debilitating, migraines and other common headaches are benign and eventually will resolve, even without treatment. However, a headache also can be an indication of a serious underlying disorder. The individual who has never experienced a headache, has atypical headache pain, or has "the worst headache of my life" requires thorough evaluation. The PQRST mnemonic (*P*rovokes/palliates, *Q*uality, *R*adiates, *S*everity, *T*ime) can be used to guide the patient interview. (See Table 7-4.) The following are other subjective and objective considerations:
- Is this the first headache (or the first of its type) ever experienced?
- When did the headache start?

Table 23-1   **Characteristics of Various Types of Primary Headaches**

Headache	Patient Population	Family History	Aura	Quality (Pain)
Migraine without aura	Onset age: 6-25 yr Female-to-male 3:1 but 1:1 at extremes of age	Positive	No	Begins as a dull, penetrating pain that progresses to moderate or severe throbbing pain
Migraine with aura	As above	As above	Yes	Throbbing
Tension type	Any age or gender		No	Dull, squeezing, nonthrobbing and not exacerbated by routine activity
Cluster	Age 20-40 Male-to-female 9:1	Occasionally positive	Uncommon (6%)	Boring
Subarachnoid hemorrhage	80% of patients are aged 40-65 years	Yes	No	Throbbing, severe
Chronic paroxysmal hemicrania	33 years Female-to-male 2:1	Absent	No	Severe

Data from Martin CO: Neurology. In Graber MA, Laternier ML, editors: *University of Iowa family practice handbook*, ed 4, Iowa City, 2001, University of Iowa.

Table 23-2   **Migraine Headache Triggers**

Category	Examples
Environmental	Changes in weather, season, or barometric pressure; bright or unusual colors; sun glare; flickering lights; television; tobacco, including secondhand smoke
Emotional/hormonal	Stress; anxiety; fatigue; altered sleep cycles; menstruation; pregnancy; hypoglycemia; intense physical exertion, including sexual activity
Food	Alcohol, especially red wine; aged cheeses; chocolate; monosodium glutamate; caffeine; coffee; aspartame
Medications	Cimetidine, nifedipine, theophylline

- Is there a history of trauma (long ago or recent)?
- Is this headache associated with nausea or vomiting?
- Are there signs of meningeal irritation (e.g., stiff neck, photophobia, or fever)?
- Have there been personality changes or unusual behaviors since onset of the headache?
- Is there memory loss or confusion related to the headache?
- Has the patient had any recent infections?
- Are there visual changes? Blurring? Diplopia? Hemianopia?
- Have there been any new neurologic deficits?
- Has blood pressure been elevated? For how long?

Location	Duration	Behavior During Headache	Associated Symptoms
Unilateral or bilateral	6-48 hr	Reclusive, supine in darkened room	Nausea, vomiting, photophobia, phonophobia
Unilateral	3-12 hr	As above	Visual prodrome, nausea, vomiting, photophobia, phonophobia
Diffuse bilateral	30 min to 7 days		Depression
Unilateral, especially orbit, severe, boring, tearing like a "hot poker in the eye"	15-120 min	Agitated, pacing, rocking, moaning, crying	Ipsilateral tearing, Horner's syndrome, nasal stuffiness, hemifacial sweating
Variable	Variable		May have focal neurologic symptoms or decreased level of consciousness, but may be alert with nonfocal examination
Severe, sharp, boring, throbbing, unilateral, orbital, supraorbital, or temporal pain always on the same side; unilateral, orbital, or temporal	1-40 attacks a day lasting 2-25 min No periods of remission		Conjunctival injection, ptosis lacrimation, rhinorrhea, and relieved with indomethacin (Indocin)

- Does the patient have a history of emotional or psychiatric problems?
- What medications (prescription, OTC, herbals) is the patient currently taking? *Not* taking? (This includes drugs for treatment of this headache event.)
- Has the patient ever had a seizure? When? What kind?

Therapeutic Interventions

Therapeutic interventions for headache include the following:
- Nonsteroidal antiinflammatory drugs can be given orally (e.g., ibuprofen) or parenterally (ketorolac).
- Provide relief of nausea and vomiting with antiemetics such as metoclopramide (Reglan), ondansetron (Zofran), chlorpromazine (Thorazine), and prochlorperazine (Compazine). These agents are highly effective. When these agents are given intravenously, some patients also obtain headache relief. When considering administration of droperidol, it is important to remember that it can cause QT prolongation.
- Manage vascular headache pain with dihydroergotamine or serotonin inhibitors such as sumatriptan (Imitrex).
- Cluster headaches may be treated with calcium channel blockers (e.g., verapamil) and with antiseizure medications such as divalproex (Depakote), topiramate (Topamax), and gabapentin (Neurontin).
- Use narcotic analgesics if headache-specific agents are ineffective.
- Consider a computed tomography scan to rule out life-threatening causes (e.g., subarachnoid hemorrhage).

ALTERED LEVEL OF CONSCIOUSNESS

Level of consciousness (LOC) is affected by structural abnormalities, metabolic imbalances, medications, and injury. A few of the many causes of alteration in LOC are traumatic brain injury, alcohol and other drug intoxications, diabetes mellitus, stroke, seizures, hypoglycemia, and subarachnoid hemorrhage. The clinical presentation of patients with an altered LOC ranges from mildly confused to completely unresponsive. Thorough assessment is required to intervene in potentially lethal situations. A simple tool used to identify the cause of altered LOC is the AEIOU-TIPS mnemonic (Box 23-1).

Ascertain the patient's presenting neurologic status by examining the pupils and calculating a Glasgow Coma Scale (GCS) score (see Table 7-8). Possible GCS scores range from 15 (best) to 3 (worst). A patient with a GCS score of 8 or less is considered severely altered (comatose). A score of 9 to 12 indicates moderate abnormality; those who score 13 to 15 are considered only mildly altered.[3]

Unconsciousness

Unconsciousness is defined as a lack of awareness of self or of anything surrounding oneself, despite application of various stimuli. Causes of unconsciousness can be categorized as structural, metabolic, toxic, or psychiatric (Table 23-3). Assessment of the patient who is unconscious or who has an altered LOC must be done concurrently with emergent interventions for

Box **23-1**   **AEIOU-TIPS for Assessment of the Patient With Altered Level of Consciousness**

A	Alcohol (acute intoxication, withdrawal)
E	Epilepsy (or any seizure), environmental conditions (hypothermia, heatstroke)
I	Insulin (too much or too little)
O	Oxygen underdose or overdose
U	Uremia (or other metabolic disorders)
T	Trauma, toxicity, tumors, thermoregulation
I	Infection, ischemia
P	Psychiatric, poisoning
S	Stroke, syncope (or other neurologic/cardiovascular cause)

Table **23-3**   **Differential Diagnosis for Coma**

Category	Differential Diagnosis
Structural	Abscess, aneurysm, hematoma, hemorrhage, inflammation (meningitis, encephalitis), subarachnoid hemorrhage, stroke, trauma, tumor
Metabolic	Cardiac arrest, decreased cardiac output, elevated serum ammonia, fluid/electrolyte imbalance, hepatitis, hepatic dysfunction, hypoglycemia, hypothermia, hypothyroidism, seizure, vitamin deficiencies
Toxicity	Alcohols, anticholinergics, benzodiazepines, carbon monoxide, cyanide, opiates, salicylates, sedatives, tricyclic antidepressants, gamma hydroxybutyrate (GHB)
Psychiatric	Hysteria, malignant catatonia, psychogenic unresponsiveness

airway, breathing, and circulation. Box 23-2 lists various assessment points for the unconscious patient.

Therapeutic Interventions

Therapeutic interventions for altered LOC include the following:
- Protect the patient from further deterioration.
- Support the patient's airway, breathing, and circulation.
- Provide supplemental oxygen and titrate to oxygen saturation levels. Anticipate tracheal intubation if the patient is unable to maintain adequate oxygenation or ventilation.
- Patients with a GCS score of 8 or less generally require tracheal intubation for airway protection regardless of their ability to oxygenate and ventilate.
- Evaluate vital signs for indications of shock or hypothermia.
- Measure blood glucose to identify hypoglycemia. Inject 50 mL of dextrose 50% (D_{50}) intravenously (IV) if the patient is hypoglycemic.
- Give thiamine 50 to 100 mg IV before D_{50} infusion if alcohol abuse is suspected (to prevent the development of Wernicke-Korsakoff psychosis).
- Obtain serum electrolyte levels, a complete blood count, a 12-lead electrocardiogram, toxicologic screens, a urinalysis, and chest radiographs (as indicated by the patient's history and condition).

Box **23-2** **Assessment of the Unconscious Patient**

General

Temperature (hypothermia or hyperthermia)
Pulse (bradycardia, tachycardia, ectopy)
Respirations (abnormal rate or pattern)
Blood pressure (hypotension or hypertension)
Oxygen saturation (hypoxemia)
Skin signs (color, temperature, moistness)
Pupils (size, equality, reactivity, nystagmus)
Breath odor (ketones, ethanol, other)
Petechiae (systemic infection)
Lung sounds (absent, adventitious)
Trauma (obvious injury)
Incontinence

Specific

Deep tendon reflexes (hyporeflexive or hyperreflexive)
Posturing and tone (flexion/extension, rigidity/flaccidity)
Paralysis (unilateral or bilateral, upper or lower extremities)
Babinski's reflex
Battle sign
Hemotympanum
Raccoon eyes
Meningeal irritation (Brudzinski's or Kernig's signs)
Tongue lacerations (from seizures)
Track marks (substance abuse)
Burns on the roof of the mouth (inhalant abuse)
Implanted medication pumps (insulin or intrathecal drugs)

- Administer naloxone (Narcan) 0.4 to 2 mg IV to patients with suspected opiate toxicity.
- Consider flumazenil (Romazicon) administration, 0.2 mg IV, for patients with suspected benzodiazepine toxicity.
- Immobilize the spine and obtain spinal radiographs if trauma is suspected.
- Facilitate a computed tomography scan of the head if focal neurologic findings or signs of trauma are present.
- Perform and document serial neurologic examinations including a Glasgow Coma Scale score and pupillary evaluation.

SEIZURES

A seizure is an episode of abnormal electrical activity in the brain. Like a headache, a seizure is a symptom rather than a disease. The three most common seizure categories are generalized, focal, and status epilepticus. Seizure frequency is slightly higher in males than in females, with a peak incidence in those over age 65 years.[4]

Seizures may be caused by hypoxia, head trauma, tumors, vascular disorders, metabolic abnormalities, drug toxicities, birth defects, or infection. Idiopathic seizures (no identifiable cause) are not unusual. Critical information related to seizure assessment includes (1) what happened immediately before the seizure, (2) any history of recent or long past head trauma, and (3) what drugs or other substances the patient has consumed (including over-the-counter, recreational, and herbal agents) or failed to take (missed medications).

Seizure Types

Generalized tonic-clonic

Tonic-clonic seizures, formerly referred to as grand mal seizures, involve a sudden loss of consciousness and organized muscle tone, accompanied by extensor muscle spasms, apnea or irregular respirations, and bilateral clonic movements. Once the seizure ends, the patient fades into a postictal state characterized by muscle relaxation, deep breathing, and depressed LOC.

Febrile seizures

Febrile seizures are a type of tonic-clonic seizure. They occur as a single seizure, without focal features. Febrile seizures, triggered by a rapid rise in body temperature, typically last less than 15 minutes. Most incidents occur in patients less than 5 years of age as a result of neurologic system immaturity. Treatment is directed at protecting the patient from injury, lowering the fever, and managing any underlying infectious conditions.

Partial seizures

Clinical manifestations of a partial (focal) seizure may be sensory, motor, or autonomic. Obsolete names for this type of seizure include Jacksonian, psychomotor, and minor motor. Focal brain lesions—such as tumors, abscesses, infarctions, or scars—cause partial seizures. Seizure activity is usually unilateral, does not produce loss of consciousness, and is not considered life threatening. Single seizures, lasting less than 5 minutes, rarely require pharmacologic therapy. Medications for long-term control of partial seizures include carbamazepine (Tegretol), phenytoin (Dilantin), gabapentin (Neurontin), and sodium valproate (Depakene).

Seizure Management

Emergency department management of the patient who is having a seizure (or presents following a recent seizure) focuses on (1) assessment of airway, breathing, and circulatory status; (2) immediate control of any current seizure activity; and (3) investigation of possible causes.

Therapeutic Interventions

Therapeutic interventions for seizures include the following:
- Protect the airway but never force any object into the patient's mouth.
- Administer oxygen as needed to maintain saturation.
- Safeguard the patient from injury.
- Measure the blood glucose level.
- Administer naloxone (Narcan) 0.4 to 2 mg and/or D_{50} 50 mL IV if narcotic toxicity or hypoglycemia are potential causes.
- Give benzodiazepines (diazepam, lorazepam) intravenously to control unresolved seizures. Intravenously administered anticonvulsants, such as phenytoin (Dilantin) or phenobarbital, are appropriate once seizures have been controlled.
- Draw and send therapeutic drug level sample for any anticonvulsant agents the patient may be taking.
- Consider intravenously administered fosphenytoin (Cerebyx) for short-term control of generalized convulsive status epilepticus. Monitor the electrocardiogram, blood pressure, and respirations continually during infusion and for 10 to 20 minutes after the infusion is complete.

Status Epilepticus

The patient in status epilepticus experiences a series of consecutive seizures or one continuous seizure that does not resolve spontaneously and is unresponsive to traditional treatment. This situation is a medical emergency that requires immediate intervention. With multiple or continuous seizures the patient does not have an opportunity to recover between events. The resulting acidosis, hypoglycemia, hypercalcemia, muscle damage, and autonomic dysfunction are associated with significant morbidity and mortality.

Therapeutic interventions

Therapeutic interventions for status epilepticus include the following:
- Open and clear the airway.
- Provide oxygen as needed to maintain saturation. Consider tracheal intubation if the seizure is prolonged.
- Establish IV or intraosseous access.
- Identify and treat the cause as soon as possible.
- Administer naloxone (Narcan) 0.4 to 2 mg IV if narcotic toxicity is a potential cause.
- Infuse dextrose 50%, 50 mL if the patient is hypoglycemic. (First give thiamine 50 to 100 mg IV to alcoholic patients.)
- Initiate anticonvulsant therapy:
  - Benzodiazepines (diazepam, lorazepam, midazolam): IV, intraosseously, or per rectum until seizures are controlled.
  - Fosphenytoin sodium (Cerebyx): 20 mg phenytoin equivalents (PE)/kg IV infused at 100-150 mg PE/min. Unlike phenytoin, fosphenytoin may be diluted in 5% dextrose in water or normal saline. Orders for fosphenytoin must always be written in PE units.

Cardiac monitoring and observation for hypotension are essential. Fosphenytoin may be given intramuscularly.

- Phenytoin (Dilantin): 18 to 20 mg/kg IV. Do not inject intramuscularly. Always mix and infuse phenytoin with normal saline, *not* a dextrose-containing solution. Place the patient on a cardiac monitor. Give the drug slowly; do not exceed an infusion rate of 50 mg/min.
- Phenobarbital: 130 mg IV every 10 to 15 minutes (up to 1 g) as needed (adult dose).
- Consider general anesthesia if status epilepticus does not respond to any of these medications.
- Paralytic agents will stop muscle activity but do nothing to control brain activity, so seizures will continue despite lack of external evidence.

STROKE

Strokes are categorized based on their cause: ischemic or hemorrhagic. Early identification of the type is critical because appropriate treatment of one classification can be lethal for the other. Risk factors for stroke include hypertension, bacterial endocarditis, hyperlipidemia, prosthetic heart valves, diabetes mellitus, collagen disorders, smoking, oral contraceptive use, cardiac disease, recent neck trauma, and atrial fibrillation.[5]

Triage of the patient with a possible stroke must be immediate, accompanied by rapid assessment and intervention. Several prehospital stroke scales are available. The two most widely used are the Cincinnati Stroke Scale (Table 23-4) and the Los Angeles Prehospital Stroke Screen (Box 23-3).[6,7] These instruments help identify the patient with a probable stroke and are used by many ED as a quick triage tool.

The most validated tool for determining stroke severity is the National Institutes of Health Stroke Scale. Table 23-5 highlights selected components of the scale. Refer to the American Stroke Association Web site *(www.strokeassociation.org)* or other references to view the complete

Table **23-4**   **Cincinnati Stroke Scale**

Parameter	Action	Results	Discussion
Facial droop	Ask patients to show their teeth or smile.	*Normal:* Both sides of the face move equally. *Abnormal:* One side of face does not move as well as the other.	
Arm drift	Have the patient close both eyes and raise the arms out straight for 10 seconds.	*Normal:* Both arms drift downward to the same extent, or the arms do not move at all (other findings, such as grip, may be helpful). *Abnormal:* One arm does not move, or one arm drifts downward compared with the other.	If any one of these three signs is abnormal, there is a 72% probability of a stroke.
Abnormal speech	Ask the patient to say, "You can't teach an old dog new tricks."	*Normal:* Patient uses words correctly without slurring. *Abnormal:* Patient slurs words, uses the wrong words, or is unable to speak.	

From Kothari R et al: *Acad Emergency Med* 1997, pp 986-990. With permission from the Society for Academic Medicine.

Box **23-3** Los Angeles Prehospital Stroke Screen

Criteria

Answer *yes, no,* or *unknown* to the following:
Age greater than 45 years?
No history of seizures or epilepsy?
Symptom duration less than 24 hours?
At baseline the patient is not wheelchair bound or bedridden.
Fingerstick glucose is between 60 and 400 mg/dL.
Obvious asymmetry (right vs. left) in any of the following three examination categories (must be unilateral):
- Facial smile/grimace: Equal or droop
- Grip: Equal, weak grip, or no grip
- Arm strength: Equal, drifts down, or falls rapidly

Discussion

The Los Angeles Prehospital Stroke Screen (LAPSS) is used for evaluation of noncomatose patients with acute, nontraumatic, neurologic complaints.
- The LAPSS is positive if the answer to the first 6 items is *yes.*
- Ninety-three percent of stroke patients have a positive LAPSS.
- The patient still can be having a stroke even when the LAPSS is negative.

Modified from Kidwell C et al: Identifying stroke in the field: prospective validation of the Los Angeles Prehospital Stroke Screen, *Stroke* 31:71-76, 2003.

Table **23-5** National Institutes of Health Stroke Scale

Component	Assessment Points
Level of consciousness	
1a. Level of consciousness questions	What is the month? What is your age?
1b. Level of consciousness commands	Open and close mouth.
	Grip and release the evaluator's hand.
Best gaze	Test horizontal eye movements only.
Visual fields	Test upper and lower quadrant visual fields.
Facial palsy	Patient shows teeth or raises eyebrows and closes eyes.
Motor arm	Check for drift.
Motor leg	Check for drift.
Limb ataxia	Perform finger-nose-finger and heel-shin tests on both sides.
Sensory	Elicit sensation or grimace to pinprick.
Best language	Ask patient to describe what is happening in a picture.
Dysarthria	Ask patient to read or repeat words from a list.
Extinction and inattention	Does the patient attend to both sides of the body?

scale. The American Stroke Association website also has a free, online National Institutes of Health Stroke Scale tutorial. The patient's stroke score is measured at the time of presentation, 2 hours after arrival, following interventions or significant changes in status, and 24 hours after admission.

Hemorrhagic Stroke

Hemorrhagic strokes are subclassified as intracerebral, subarachnoid, or cerebellar. Hemorrhagic stroke occurs suddenly; the patient typically experiences acute pain with or without changes in LOC. Intracerebral and cerebellar bleeds usually are related to hypertension. Subarachnoid hemorrhages are associated more commonly with trauma or aneurysms. Patients with an aneurysmal subarachnoid hemorrhage typically have the "worst headache of my life." Anticoagulants and fibrinolytic therapy are *contraindicated* in patients with hemorrhagic stroke.

Ischemic Stroke

Ischemic events account for 80% to 85% of all strokes.[8] These strokes occur when a local thrombus or embolus occludes a cerebral artery. Emboli generally originate in the heart or large arteries following atrial fibrillation, myocardial infarction, or surgery. Symptom onset is sudden. Stroke caused by thrombosis develops more gradually and, like myocardial infarction, frequently occurs in the early morning hours. Thrombosis is often the cause of transient ischemic attacks. Risk factors for ischemic stroke include hypertension, advanced age, diabetes, smoking, and elevated serum lipid levels. Ischemic strokes are categorized as transient, reversible, stroke in evolution, and completed stroke (Table 23-6).

Signs and Symptoms

Signs and symptoms of stroke include the following:
- Headache, vertigo, ataxia
- Nausea and vomiting
- Sudden neurologic deficits: Sensory, motor, or cognitive
- Unequal pupil size
- Hemiparesis
- Receptive or expressive dysphasia
- Dysphagia (difficulty swallowing) and drooling

Table 23-6   Stroke Classification

Type	Description
Transient ischemic attack (TIA)	A neurologic deficit of less than 12 hours in duration. Most last only 5 to 30 minutes. A transient ischemic attack may be a prodrome to stroke. The attack is caused by an embolus or local thrombosis. Symptoms resolve when the occlusion dislodges or dissolves (partially or completely).
Reversible ischemic neurologic deficit	Stroke symptoms last between 24 hours and several weeks. The patient has mild, minimal, or no permanent deficits.
Stroke in evolution	Symptoms last longer than 24 hours with progressive neurologic deterioration. Residual deficits are present.
Completed stroke	Permanent neurologic damage occurs.

- Dysarthria (speech disturbances)
- Facial droop
- Abnormal flexion or extension
- Sleepiness
- Coma (occasionally)

Therapeutic Interventions

Therapeutic interventions for stroke include the following:
- Support the patient's airway, breathing, and circulatory status.
- Obtain bedside blood glucose level. Do not give dextrose unless the patient is hypoglycemic.
- Obtain basic laboratory studies (electrolytes, complete blood count, prothrombin time [international normalized ratio], and activated partial thromboplastin time).
Initiate cardiac monitoring to evaluate for concurrent myocardial infarction.
- Correct dysrhythmias.
- Give labetalol (Normodyne) IV to keep blood pressure less than 185 mm Hg systolic and less than 110 mm Hg diastolic.
- Facilitate a rapid head computed tomography scan (without contrast) to determine whether the stroke is ischemic or hemorrhagic and to identify any other intracranial cause of symptoms (e.g., tumor, subdural hematoma, or intracerebral hemorrhage).
- Complete a fibrinolytic therapy checklist to determine whether the patient meets inclusion criteria for fibrinolytic therapy.
- Fibrinolytic therapy with Intravenous recombinant tissue plasminogen activator (alteplase [Activase]) is only appropriate for patients with ischemic stroke in whom symptom onset is known to be less than 3 hours before the time of drug administration (Box 23-4).
- If the patient is not eligible for fibrinolytic therapy, begin heparin anticoagulation. (Heparin is not started for 24 hours in patients who received fibrinolytic therapy.)
- Watch for signs of internal and external bleeding, particularly intracranial hemorrhage.

Box **23-4** **Fibrinolytic Therapy for Ischemic Stroke**

Medication
Alteplase
Total dose is 0.9 mg/kg intravenously (IV).
Maximum IV dose is 90 mg.
Bolus is 10% of the total dose, given IV over 1 minute.
Remainder of the total dose is given IV over 60 minutes.
Administration
Intravenous administration
Must be started within 3 hours of symptom onset.
Intraarterial administration
May be given up to 6 hours after symptom onset.
Dose is given by the radiologist.
Requires cannulization of the femoral or brachial artery.

Data from Hazinski MF, Cummins RO, Field JM, editors: *2000 Handbook of emergency cardiovascular care for healthcare providers,* Dallas, 2000, The Association.

NEUROMUSCULAR DISORDERS

Guillain-Barré Syndrome

Guillain-Barré syndrome is an acute paralytic disease that decreases myelin in the nerve roots and peripheral nerves. About half of all patients with Guillain-Barré syndrome experience a mild febrile illness several weeks before the onset of symptoms. Risk factors for this ascending paralytic condition include infection with human immunodeficiency virus, cytomegalovirus, or hepatitis B; pregnancy; and Hodgkin's lymphoma.[4]

Signs and symptoms

Signs and symptoms of Guillain-Barré syndrome include the following:
- A tingling sensation in the hands and feet that may be present for hours or weeks before diagnosis
- Difficulty walking, climbing stairs, or getting up from a chair
- Severely diminished superficial and deep tendon reflexes (particularly the lower extremities)
- Symmetrical paralysis, usually beginning in the lower extremities, that gradually ascends to the respiratory muscles
- Respiratory insufficiency
- Urinary retention
- Postural hypotension

Therapeutic interventions

Therapeutic interventions for Guillain-Barré syndrome include the following:
- Support the patient's airway, breathing, and circulatory status.
- Tracheal intubation and mechanical ventilation are required for any patient with a severe presentation.
- Assess for alternative causes of neuropathy such as heavy metal poisoning, diabetes, vitamin B_{12} deficiency, myasthenia gravis, multiple sclerosis, amyotrophic lateral sclerosis, and botulism.
- Provide general supportive care until the condition spontaneously resolves, generally weeks after onset.

Myasthenia Gravis

Myasthenia gravis is a defect of neuromuscular transmission. Onset is generally in persons in their 20s and 30s. This condition occurs more frequently in females than in males and may have a familial connection. Many commonly prescribed drugs—such as antibiotics, psychotropic drugs, and antidysrhythmic drugs—can precipitate a myasthenic crisis. The hallmark of myasthenia gravis is weakness, particularly of the ocular, facial, and neck muscles or of the upper extremities. Patients in myasthenic crisis can experience fatal respiratory paralysis.

Signs and symptoms

Signs and symptoms of myasthenia gravis include the following:
- Increasing fatigue
- Delayed recovery of muscle strength after exercise
- Weak eye muscles, visual changes, and diplopia (but *not* pupillary changes)
- An abnormal smile because of weak facial and jaw muscles

- Dysphagia (difficulty swallowing), weak pharyngeal muscles
- Inability to handle oral secretions
- Possible aspiration

Therapeutic interventions

Therapeutic interventions for myasthenia gravis include the following:
- Support the patient's airway, breathing, and circulatory status.
- Tracheal intubation and mechanical ventilation are required for patients with a severe presentation.
- A wide variety of medications, particularly pyridostigmine bromide (Mestinon), are used for ongoing management of myasthenia gravis.
- Symptoms of myasthenic crisis and cholinergic crisis (too much pyridostigmine bromide) are similar. To differentiate between the two, administer edrophonium chloride (Tensilon), an anticholinesterase inhibitor, in a Tensilon challenge. If symptoms improve, the test is considered positive, indicating the patient is in myasthenic crisis.
- Treat myasthenic crisis with neostigmine (Prostigmin) 1 mg IV.

MISCELLANEOUS NEUROLOGIC EMERGENCIES

Shunt Problems

Ventricular shunts decrease intracranial pressure by diverting cerebrospinal fluid from the lateral ventricles to the torso (thorax or abdomen). Complications related to shunts are infection and shunt malfunction. Malfunction occurs when the shunt becomes obstructed by debris, blood clots, or brain tissue. Obstruction also results if the shunt ends become disconnected or malpositioned. Regardless of the underlying problem, the patient usually has an altered LOC because of increased intracranial pressure. If the problem develops rapidly, the patient experiences acute changes; if the problem develops over time, changes in LOC occur gradually. Infection generally is associated with fever; malfunction is not.

Therapeutic Interventions

Therapeutic interventions for shunt problems include the following:
- Determine the patient's neurologic status at the time of ED presentation.
- Elicit a history of acute or gradual LOC changes.
- Early signs of increased intracranial pressure include headache and nausea progressing to projectile vomiting, lethargy, and coma.
- Identify other neurologic findings such as ataxia, incontinence, and pupillary changes.
- Look for signs of infection including fever and meningeal irritation (stiff/painful neck, headache, photophobia).
- Treatment includes lumbar puncture or shunt tapping to aspirate cerebrospinal fluid. If infection is suspected, send cultures and institute antibiotic therapy.
- Surgical intervention is required for obstructed, fractured, or malpositioned catheters.

References

1. Jordan KS, editor: *Emergency nursing core curriculum,* ed 5, Philadelphia, 2000, Saunders.
2. Denny CJ, Schull MJ: Headache and facial pain. In Tintinalli JE, Kelen GD, Stapczynski JS, editors: *Emergency medicine: a comprehensive study guide,* ed 6, New York, 2004, McGraw-Hill.
3. Engel J: *Pediatric assessment: pocket guide series,* ed 4, St Louis, 2002, Mosby.

4. Ferri F: *Ferri's clinical advisor: instant diagnosis and treatment, 2000 edition,* St Louis, 2000, Mosby.
5. Hazinski MF, Cummins RO, Field JM, editors: *2000 Handbook of emergency cardiovascular care for healthcare providers,* Dallas, 2000, American Heart Association.
6. Kothari R et al: Cincinnati Prehospital Stroke Scale: reproducibility and validity, *Ann Emerg Med* 33:373-378, 1999.
7. Kidwell C et al: Identifying stroke in the field: prospective validation of the Los Angeles Prehospital Stroke Screen, *Stroke* 31:71-76, 2000.
8. Newberry L, editor: *Sheehy's emergency nursing: principles and practice,* ed 5, St Louis, 2003, Mosby.

24

Abdominal Pain

Anita Johnson, BSN, RN, and Terri Roberts, RN, BSN

Abdominal pain is a frequent complaint among patients who seek care in the emergency department. Those experiencing abdominal pain may be suffering from a minor illness or a life-threatening event. This abdominal pain may be a symptom of an acute process or a chronic condition. Abdominal pain is one of the most common presenting complaints among school-aged children and adolescents. Because pain is a symptom, not a diagnosis, interventions are directed toward identifying the cause of pain and treating the source.

TYPES OF ABDOMINAL PAIN

Abdominal pain is classified as visceral, somatic, or referred.

Visceral Pain

The stretching of a hollow viscus causes visceral pain. Patients describe this sensation as "cramping" or "gas pain." Pain waxes and wanes and usually is centered around the umbilicus or below the midline of the abdomen. Visceral pain is diffuse and difficult to localize on examination. Autonomic responses to this pain include diaphoresis, nausea, vomiting, decreased blood pressure, tachycardia, and spasm of the abdominal wall muscles. Many inflammatory conditions begin with visceral pain symptoms, including the following[1]:
- Appendicitis
- Cholecystitis
- Pancreatitis
- Intestinal obstruction

Somatic Pain

Somatic abdominal pain results from bacterial or chemical irritation of abdominal nerve fibers. This pain is sharp and intense and routinely is localized to a particular area. Associated findings include involuntary guarding and rebound tenderness.[1]

Table 24-1   Potential Sources of Referred Abdominal Pain by Location

Problem Area	Pain Referred to
Fluid collection under the diaphragm	Top of the shoulder
Ruptured peptic ulcer	Back
Pancreas	Midline back or directly through to back
Biliary tract	Around the right side to the scapula
Dissecting or ruptured aneurysm	Lower back and thighs
Renal colic	Groin and external genitalia
Appendix	Right lower quadrant or epigastrium
Uterine disorders	Lower back
Rectal disease	Lower back

From Thomas D et al: *Common chief complaints in core curriculum for pediatirc emergency nursing*, Sudbury, Mass, 2003, Jones & Bartlett.

Box **24-1**   **Chronic Conditions Associated With Severe Abdominal Pain**

Crohn's disease
Irritable bowel syndrome
Peptic ulcers
Reflux esophagitis
Regional enteritis
Ulcerative colitis

Box **24-2**   **Extraabdominal Conditions That May Present as Abdominal Pain**

Empyema	Pneumothorax
Hip joint disease	Rheumatic fever
Myocardial infarction	Sickle cell anemia
Pleurisy	Spinal tumor
Pneumonia	

Referred Pain

Referred pain is pain experienced some distance from its point of origin. Referred pain may be sharp and localized or characterized as a distant ache. Table 24-1 summarizes potential sources of referred abdominal pain by location.[1] Box 24-1 lists chronic conditions associated with significant abdominal pain. Box 24-2 gives examples of extraabdominal conditions in which abdominal pain may be the chief complaint.

The emergency nurse must appreciate that each individual will react differently to pain. Multiple factors including age and culture influence how individuals express pain. Patients' reports of pain need to be accepted, and treatment must be individualized. (See Chapter 14.)

ASSESSMENT OF THE PATIENT WITH ABDOMINAL PAIN

Initial evaluation of the patient with abdominal pain begins with an airway, breathing, and circulatory assessment. On completion of the primary survey, a focused assessment is done. Table 24-2 summarizes abdominal pain assessment.

Table **24-2**   **PQRST Assessment of Abdominal Pain**

Component	Description
Provocation	What makes pain better? Worse? Position? Vomiting?
Quality or character	What does pain feel like? Burning? Tight? Crushing? Tearing? Pressure? Cramping?
Radiation, location, referral	Where does pain radiate? Where is it most intense? Where does it start?
Severity	How severe is pain on a scale of 0 to 10?
Time	When did pain start? When did it end? How long did it last?

From Newberry L, editor: *Sheehy's emergency medicine: principles and practice*, ed 5, St Louis, 2003, Mosby.

Subjective Data

History

Obtain a chief complaint and thorough history of the present illness. The PQRST mnemonic, is an easy tool to remember; in addition, it includes all of the necessary components for a complete assessment (see Table 24-2).

Vomiting

Common causes of nausea and vomiting are gastroenteritis, acute gastritis, pancreatitis, or an obstruction located high in the intestines. Intractable vomiting and vomiting of feces is an indication of intestinal obstruction. Bloody emesis is suggestive of gastritis or peptic ulcers. Abdominal pain that precedes vomiting is characteristic of appendicitis.
Assess for the following:
• Blood, bile, fecal matter
• Onset, frequency, duration

Intestinal symptoms

Acute abdominal conditions often are associated with bowel content changes (Table 24-3). Assess for the following:
• Gastrointestinal bleeding (upper or lower)
• Diarrhea
• Constipation
• Changes in stool color, consistency, or frequency

Urinary tract symptoms

Pathologic processes involving the urinary tract may be the source of abdominal pain (Table 24-4). For additional information, on disorders of the urinary tract, refer to Chapter 30. Assessment of urinary symptoms includes the following:
• Hematuria
• Dysuria
• Urinary frequency
• Costovertebral angle tenderness

Gynecologic symptoms

Most gynecologic symptoms indicate a primary gynecologic problem such as pelvic inflammatory disease, ruptured ectopic pregnancy, ruptured ovarian cyst, endometriosis, fibroids, or ruptured corpus luteum. Vaginal bleeding is associated with dysmenorrhea, abortion, ruptured ectopic pregnancy, placental problems, or one of many other gynecologic or obstetric disorders. (See Chapter 45.)

Table 24-3   Causes of Abnormal Stools

Description	Possible Cause
Diarrhea	Inflammatory disease
Constipation (or no flatus)	Dehydration, paralytic ileus, intestinal obstruction
Clay-colored stool	Biliary obstruction
Melena (black tarry stool)	High intestinal bleeding
Bright red blood	Lower intestinal bleeding
Bloody diarrhea	Amebic dysentery, Crohn's disease, ulcerative colitis

Table 24-4   Causes of Urinary Tract Symptoms

Symptom	Possible Cause
Burning on urination	Urinary tract infection
Pain on urination	Obstruction somewhere in urinary tract
Hematuria	Urinary tract infection or renal colic

Age-related factors

Intussusception is unusual in persons over the age of 2 years. Intestinal obstructions are rare in those under age 40. Appendicitis occurs most frequently in individuals between the ages of 5 and 45.

Historical data

As part of the subjective assessment, a general medical history should elicit the following information:
- Past and present diseases
- Previous surgeries
- Current medications
- Allergies
- Immunization status
- Alcohol, tobacco, or other drug use
- Recent foreign travel

Objective Assessment

Physical examination

The patient's position of choice and overall physical appearance can offer important clues to diagnosis.

Vital signs

Consider the following factors related to vital signs:
- Body temperature in patients with abdominal pain is often initially normal but rises as the disease progresses. Temperature elevation is characteristic of peritonitis or any condition associated with fulminant infection.
- An increased heart rate is common.
- Rapid respirations may indicate acute abdominal infection such as pancreatitis or peritonitis.
- When peritonitis is present, respirations may be shallow with little abdominal wall motion.
- Hypotension strongly suggests an acute surgical condition (Box 24-3).

Box **24-3**   **Abdominal Conditions That May Require Surgical Intervention**

Appendicitis	Peritonitis
Bowel infarction	Ruptured ectopic pregnancy
Bowel obstruction	Ruptured or dissecting intraabdominal
Cholecystitis	aneurysm
Diverticulitis	Salpingitis
Massive gastrointestinal bleed	Solid organ injury
Pancreatitis	Ureteral stone
Perforation of a hollow viscus	

Abdominal assessment

Perform an abdominal assessment in the following sequence:
1. Inspection
2. Auscultation
3. Percussion
4. Palpation

Inspection

Observe the patient's abdomen for the following[2]:
- Distention, flatness, symmetry, and contour
- Pulsating masses
- Signs of trauma
- Umbilical inflammation, infection, protrusion, bruising
- Striae, scars, discoloration, lesions
- Uterine enlargement
- Diastasis rectus (separation of the left and right sides of the rectus abdominis muscle)

Auscultation

Bowel sounds are difficult to assess in the emergency care setting because it takes 3 to 5 minutes of auscultation to establish the absence of bowel sounds. All four quadrants of the abdomen should be auscultated:
- Absent or decreased bowel sounds may indicate peritonitis or paralytic ileus.
- Vascular sounds, such venous hums or bruits, are abnormal findings.
- Fetal heart tones can be auscultated at about 20 weeks' gestation (12 weeks by Doppler ultrasound).

Percussion

Percussion is done over all four quadrants:
- Tympany occurs over air masses (stomach, intestines).
- Dull sounds are normal over solid organs or tumors.
- Check for pain with percussion of the costovertebral angle.

Palpation

Palpate the abdomen as gently as possible. Be sure to observe the patient's face during this examination for clues to the level of pain. Remember to palpate tender areas last. Check for the following:
- Spasm
- Tenderness
- Masses
- Ascites

Diagnostic studies

Several laboratory tests, radiographic studies, and endoscopic procedures are used commonly on patients complaining of abdominal pain.

Blood

- Complete blood count (CBC) with differential
- Serum electrolytes, including calcium and magnesium
- Liver function studies
- Serum amylase, lipase
- Sickle cell screen
- Toxicologic screen
- *Helicobacter pylori* testing
- Type and crossmatch
- Coagulation studies
- Human chorionic gonadotrophin (serum pregnancy test)

Stool

- Occult blood (Hemoccult)
- Ova and parasites
- Enzyme-linked immunosorbent assay
- White blood cells, mucus, protein
- Cultures

Urine

- Urinalysis
- Cultures
- Toxicologic screen
- Human chorionic gonadotrophin (urine pregnancy test)

Other

- Vaginal cultures
- Ureteral cultures

Imaging studies

- Upright chest
- Abdominal flat plate (kidney, ureter, bladder)
- Abdominal cross-table lateral
- Posteroanterior upright chest (to detect thoracic involvement)

Special studies to diagnose cause of abdominal pain[3]

- Barium enema
- Intravenous urography or cystography
- Intravenous cholangiography
- Upper gastrointestinal series (barium swallow)
- Angiography
- Nuclear scanning
- Esophagoscopy, gastroscopy, or esophagogastroduodenoscopy (EGD)
- Sigmoidoscopy, proctoscopy, colonoscopy
- Esophageal manometry
- Abdominal paracentesis
- Peritoneal lavage

- Local wound exploration
- Ultrasonography
- Computed tomography (CT)
- Magnetic resonance imaging

COMMON ABDOMINAL EMERGENCIES

Esophagitis

Esophagitis is an inflammation of the hiatal esophagus caused by the regurgitation of gastric acids and often is accompanied by a hiatal hernia or gastric ulcer. Esophagitis also may result from ingestion of a caustic substance such as a strong acid or alkali.[3]

Signs and symptoms

- Steady, substernal pain that increases with swallowing
- Occasional vomiting
- Weight loss
- Upper gastrointestinal bleeding
- Foul breath

Diagnostic studies

- Barium swallow studies
- Endoscopy
- EGD

Therapeutic interventions

- Bland diet
- Antacids
- Proton pump–inhibiting drugs (e.g., lansoprazole and omeprazole) or histamine (H_2) blockers (e.g., famotidine and ranitidine)
- Surgery to correct anatomic defects, if present
- If esophagitis is caused by caustic ingestion, perform the following:
  - Airway, breathing, and circulatory support as indicated
  - Dilation of the esophagus
  - Antibiotic administration

Patient/family education and discharge instructions

- Avoid caffeine, tobacco, ethanol, milk, and carbonated beverages.
- Avoid foods containing peppermint or spearmint.
- Avoid eating or drinking for 2 hours before bedtime.
- Consume a low-fat diet.
- Sleep with the head of the bed elevated (upper legs of the bed can be put on bricks).

Esophageal Obstruction

The most common cause of esophageal obstruction in children is an ingested foreign body. Obstruction in adults is usually due to a bone or food bolus.

Signs and symptoms

- History of foreign body ingestion
- Patients complain of "something stuck in my throat"
- Difficulty swallowing
- Drooling
- Subcutaneous emphysema of the neck (if esophageal perforation has occurred)

Diagnostic studies

- Chest radiographs
- Neck radiographs

Therapeutic interventions

- If the object does not have sharp edges and can pass into the stomach, it usually will proceed through the intestines without difficulty.
- Intravenously administered glucagon relaxes esophageal smooth muscles and allows passage into the stomach.
- Esophagoscopy is used to retrieve the object.

Mallory-Weiss Syndrome

This syndrome is caused by violent retching and vomiting that is not synchronized with gastric regurgitation. Esophageal tearing occurs producing bleeding at the gastroesophageal junction.[3-5]

Signs and symptoms

- History of retching with vomiting of normal gastric contents, followed by hematemesis

Diagnostic studies

- CBC
- Type and screen or crossmatch
- EGD

Therapeutic interventions

- Support of the patient's airway, breathing, and circulation
- Supplemental oxygen
- Lactated Ringer's solution or normal saline solution by intravenous (IV) line
- Blood replacement as indicated
- Endoscopy to cauterize bleeding vessels
- Surgical repair
- Balloon tamponade with a Sengstaken-Blakemore or Minnesota tube should be avoided unless other efforts have failed.

Patient/family education and discharge instructions

- Limit alcohol intake.

Boerhaave's Syndrome

Boerhaave's syndrome refers to small tears of the esophagus that result from forceful vomiting and retching. These tears are caused by distention of the esophagus associated with heavy lifting, seizures, blunt trauma, and childbirth.

Signs and symptoms

- Retrosternal chest/esophageal pain that worsens with swallowing
- Bloody expectoration once the patient has cleared the vomitus
- Possible massive bleeding and shock if tears are severe

Diagnostic tests

- Chest radiograph
- CT
- Emergency endoscopy

Therapeutic interventions

- Support of the patient's airway, breathing, and circulation
- Supplemental oxygen
- Lactated Ringer's solution or normal saline solution by IV
- Blood replacement as indicated
- Antibiotic therapy (the thoracic cavity is contaminated by esophageal contents)
- Close observation
- Surgical repair if bleeding is heavy and uncontrolled

Upper Gastrointestinal Bleeding

Upper gastrointestinal bleeding is defined as any bleeding proximal to the ligament of Treitz. Bleeding peptic ulcers account for two thirds of all upper gastrointestinal bleeds. The source of bleeding is granulation of the ulcer, which erodes into a vessel during the healing process.[4]

Signs and symptoms

- Possible history of chronic alcohol ingestion
- Epigastric tenderness
- Hematemesis
- Melena (blood and stomach acids mixed with stool)
- Possible shock
- Jaundice, hepatomegaly, and liver enlargement (in patients with liver failure)

Diagnostic studies

- Endoscopy
- CBC
- Type and cross match

Therapeutic interventions

- Support of the patient's airway, breathing, and circulation
- Supplemental oxygen

- Lactated Ringer's solution or normal saline solution by IV
- Blood transfusion
- Saline lavage through a large nasogastric or orogastric tube to determine whether bleeding is ongoing or has stopped
- Surgery if bleeding is uncontrolled and the patient shows signs of shock
- Bed rest

Bleeding Esophageal Varices

Patients with liver disease are at high risk for the development of esophageal varices. Portal hypertension causes collateral vessels to form between the stomach and the systemic veins of the lower esophagus. Rupture of these vessels can be rapidly fatal. Variceal rupture is the leading cause of death in more than one third of cirrhotic patients.[3,4]

Signs and symptoms

- Massive bleeding from the upper gastrointestinal tract
- History of chronic alcohol ingestion or portal hypertension
- Hematemesis
- Melena
- General deterioration in mental or physical status
- Signs of shock

Diagnostic studies

Laboratory

- Liver function studies
- CBC
- Type and crossmatch
- Coagulation studies

Imaging

- Endoscopy
- Ultrasound
- Abdominal CT scan

Therapeutic interventions

- Support of the patient's airway, breathing, and circulation
- Supplemental oxygen
- Lactated Ringer's solution or normal saline solution by IV
- Blood replacement as indicated
- Nasogastric tube to suction
- Saline lavage through a large nasogastric or orogastric tube to determine whether bleeding is ongoing or has stopped.
- Drug therapy: Somatostatin or octreotide (to decrease portal pressure by relaxing mesenteric vascular smooth muscle) *or* vasopressin and nitroglycerin by IV (this combination is associated with more complications)
- Balloon tamponade with a Sengstaken-Blakemore or Minnesota tube (Figure 24-1);
- Indwelling urinary catheter
- Endoscopy and injection sclerotherapy
- Surgical repair

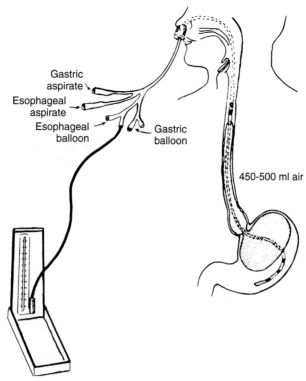

Gastric
aspirate

Esophageal
aspirate

Esophageal
balloon

Gastric
balloon

450-500 ml air

Figure 24-1. Diagram of a Minnesota tube in a patient. (From Roberts JR, Hedges JR: *Clinical procedures in emergency medicine,* ed 4, Philadelphia, 2004, Saunders.)

Gastritis

Gastritis is an inflammation of the gastric mucosa. Gastritis can occur as a result of hyperacidity, ingestion of a gastric irritant, bile reflux, or shock.[3,4]

Signs and symptoms

- Epigastric pain
- Nausea and vomiting
- Gastric mucosal bleeding
- Epigastric tenderness on palpation
- Headache
- Anorexia
- Hiccuping
- Diarrhea

Diagnostic studies

- Endoscopy
- Upper gastrointestinal series
- Biopsy
- *H. pylori* testing
- Serum electrolytes

- CBC
- Amylase, lipase
- Kidney function tests (BUN and creatinine)

Therapeutic interventions

- Nothing by mouth
- Nasogastric tube to suction
- IV rehydration
- Antiemetics
- Anticholinergic medications
- Analgesic agents
- Antibiotics (to treat *H. pylori* infection as indicated)
- Proton pump–inhibiting drugs (e.g., lansoprazole and omeprazole) or histamine (H_2) blockers (e.g., famotidine and ranitidine)
- Antacids

Patient/family education and discharge instructions

- Make dietary modifications.
- Promote rest.
- Reduce stress.

Peptic Ulcer

A peptic ulcer can occur in the stomach or the duodenum. These ulcers most commonly are related to hyperacidity.[3]

Signs and symptoms

- Burning pain in the epigastric region, usually occurring early in the morning and just before meals
- Pain is relieved by antacids, bland foods, or vomiting
- Symptoms intensify during stressful periods when gastric acid production is increased
- Loss of appetite
- Weight loss
- Vomiting
- Constipation or diarrhea
- Hematemesis
- Tarry stools

Diagnostic studies

- Endoscopy
- Upper gastrointestinal series (barium contrast study)
- *H. pylori* testing
- Type and cross match
- Stool examination for occult blood
- CBC
- Liver enzymes

Therapeutic interventions

- Nasogastric tube to perform intermittent suction for severe vomiting
- Fluid and electrolyte replacement as needed
- Proton pump–inhibiting drugs (e.g., lansoprazole and omeprazole) or histamine (H_2) blockers (e.g., famotidine and ranitidine)
- Antibiotics (to treat *H. pylori* infection as indicated)
- Bland diet
- Antacids
- Surgical repair

Age/developmental considerations

- Peptic ulcers occur most frequently in persons between the age of 40 and 60 years.
- Toddlers and young children with peptic ulcers may complain of generalized abdominal pain.

Cholecystitis

Cholecystitis is an inflammation of the gallbladder that may be exacerbated by the presence of gallstones.

Signs and symptoms

- Sudden onset of epigastric pain that radiates to the right upper quadrant (especially following ingestion of fried or greasy foods)
- Localized pain on palpation, with rebound tenderness
- Pain referred to the right subclavicular area
- Anorexia
- Nausea and vomiting
- Low-grade fever: 38° C (100.4° F)
- Mild jaundice
- Murphy's sign (inability to take deep breaths during palpation beneath right costal arch below hepatic margin)[3]

Diagnostic studies

- Ultrasound
- Radioisotope cholescintigraphy
- Abdominal CT
- Flat and upright radiographs of abdomen
- CBC

Therapeutic interventions

- Nasogastric tube
- Lactated Ringer's or normal saline solution by IV
- Antibiotics
- Analgesics
- Antiemetics
- Possible surgery (cholecystectomy)

Age/developmental considerations

The incidence of cholecystitis is highest in women at midlife, overweight individuals, and any patient over the age of 40.

Pancreatitis

Two general types of pancreatitis are acute and chronic. Acute pancreatitis usually is caused by excessive ethanol ingestion or by a gallstone that blocks the pancreatic duct, trapping digestive enzymes in the pancreas. Acute pancreatitis may resolve spontaneously or it may progress to a severe, life-threatening condition. About 80,000 cases of pancreatitis occur in the United States each year; about 20% of these are considered severe. Chronic pancreatitis occurs when digestive enzymes slowly destroy the pancreas and surrounding tissues, generally following years of alcohol abuse. This results in an inability to digest fats, proteins, and carbohydrates properly. Insulin production also is affected. Hemorrhagic pancreatitis is an emergent condition in which digestive enzymes have eroded through a major abdominal vessel.[6]

Signs and symptoms

- Severe upper abdominal pain that radiates through to the back
- Epigastric tenderness
- Nausea and vomiting
- Low-grade fever
- Hypotension
- Signs of shock (tachycardia, hypotension)
- Abdominal distention
- Foul-smelling, fatty stool

Diagnostic studies

Laboratory

- Serum amylase, lipase
- Serum electrolytes, including calcium and magnesium
- CBC
- Liver function tests
- Blood glucose

Imaging

- Abdominal radiographs
- Ultrasound (for gallstones)
- Abdominal CT (for critically ill patients)
- Chest radiographs

Therapeutic interventions

- Support of the patient's airway, breathing, and circulation
- Supplemental oxygen
- Lactated Ringer's solution or normal saline solution by IV
- Blood replacement as indicated

- Nasogastric tube to low intermittent suction
- Analgesics
- Antiemetics
- Antibiotics (for necrotizing pancreatitis)
- Possible hospital admission
- Possible surgery

Patient/Family Education and Discharge Instructions

- Eliminate alcohol and caffeine consumption

Incarcerated Hernia

A hernia is the protrusion of a bowel loop (or other abdominal contents) through the abdominal musculature, but not through the skin. If the blood supply to the hernia is good, no urgent care is required. Incarcerated hernias have a compromised blood supply and are a medical emergency. Hernias most commonly are found in the inguinal, femoral, and umbilical regions.

Signs and symptoms

- Obvious area of herniation
- Pain at the site
- Nausea and vomiting
- Abdominal distention

Therapeutic interventions

- If the hernia is not incarcerated, an attempt may be made to reduce it manually.
- If incarceration is present, surgical repair is required.

Appendicitis

Appendicitis occurs as a result of obstruction of the appendiceal lumen, which decreases blood supply. This results in distention and ischemia, which, if untreated, may progress to necrosis and perforation. Appendicitis affects both ages and sexes; however, it is most commonly found in males between the ages of 10 to 30 years. It is estimated that approximately 6% of the total population will develop appendicitis.

Signs and Symptoms

- Abdominal pain or cramping
  - Rovsing's sign (pain in right lower quadrant of abdomen that intensifies with palpation on the left lower quadrant)
  - Pain that is localized to the right lower quadrant of the abdomen at McBurney's point
  - Rebound tenderness (late sign)
- Anorexia, nausea, vomiting
- Guarding
- Pyrexia (finding is more common after perforation occurs)
- Elevated WBC count

Diagnostic Studies

Laboratory

- CBC
- Urinalysis (to rule out urinary tract infection)

Imaging

- Ultrasound
- Abdominal CT

Therapeutic interventions

- Prepare patient for surgical intervention (laparoscopy)
- Infuse intravenous crystalloids to maintain hydration.
- Maintain NPO status.
- Administer antiemetics, analgesics, antibiotics, and antipyretics.
- Insert nasogastric tube.

Intestinal Obstruction

Intestinal obstructions are caused by a variety of conditions, including fecal impaction, hernias, adhesions, tumors, paralytic ileus, intussusception, regional enteritis, volvulus, gallstones, abscesses, or hematomas. A primary mechanical obstruction or a secondary obstruction may be caused by an inflammatory condition or nervous system disorder. The immediate complication of intestinal obstruction is dehydration. Other potential complications include infarction, bowel perforation, and infection.[4]

Signs and symptoms

- Nausea and vomiting (fecal material)
- Crampy pain that is wavelike and colicky
- Borborygmi (loud, rumbling bowel sounds)
- Abdominal distention
- Constipation
- Rectal blood and mucus, without fecal matter or flatus
- Dehydration
- Diffuse abdominal tenderness and rigidity

Diagnostic studies

- CBC
- Serum electrolytes
- Kidney function tests (BUN and creatinine)
- Serum amylase
- Abdominal radiographs
- Colonoscopy

Therapeutic interventions

- IV rehydration with lactated Ringer's or normal saline solution
- Nasogastric tube to low intermittent suction
- Maintain NPO status

- Antibiotics
- Indwelling urinary catheter
- Rectal tube
- Possible surgical repair

Patient/family education and discharge instructions

- High-fiber diet with plenty of water
- Watch for signs of infection after surgery

Lower Gastrointestinal Bleeding

Bleeding from the large bowel or rectum usually is caused by ulcerative colitis, tumors, polyps, cecal ulcers, ruptured hemorrhoids, or a ruptured diverticula. Bleeding is usually modest; however, life-threatening hemorrhage may occur.

Signs and symptoms

- Bright red blood from the rectum

Diagnostic studies

- Colonoscopy
- CBC

Therapeutic interventions

- Fluid and blood replacement by IV as indicated
- Control the bleeding (depending on the source)
- Possible surgical repair

Irritable Bowel Syndrome

Irritable bowel syndrome is characterized by abdominal discomfort and changes in stool frequency or consistency: chronic or recurrent diarrhea, constipation, or both. Pain is usually in the lower abdomen (although location and intensity vary) and is described as crampy or as a generalized ache with superimposed periods of abdominal cramps. Sharp, dull, gaslike, or nondescript pains are also common. Pain and discomfort usually are relieved with a bowel movement.[4,5]

Signs and symptoms

- Constipation, diarrhea, or both
- Abdominal pain
- Abdominal distention/bloating
- Anorexia
- Nausea and vomiting

Diagnostic studies

- Erythrocyte sedimentation rate
- CBC
- Hemoccult test
- Barium enema
- Colonoscopy, sigmoidoscopy

Therapeutic interventions

- Analgesics
- Antidiarrheals
- Anticholinergics
- Antidepressants

Patient/family education and discharge instructions

- Make dietary modifications.
- Fluids should not be taken with meals; this results in distention.

Ulcerative Colitis

Ulcerative colitis is a recurrent ulcerative and inflammatory disease of the mucosal and sub-mucosal layers of the colon and rectum.[3]

Signs and symptoms

- Anorexia
- Nausea and vomiting
- Abdominal cramps
- An urgent need to defecate
- Frequent stools (usually more than 20 per day)
- Bloody diarrhea
- Rectal bleeding
- Weight loss
- Weakness

If the colon is perforated, the following also may occur:

- Fever
- Tachycardia
- Generalized signs of shock and sepsis

Diagnostic studies

Laboratory

- CBC
- Stool sample
- Serum albumin

Imaging

- Abdominal series
- Abdominal CT scan
- Magnetic resonance imaging
- Abdominal ultrasound

Endoscopic

- Sigmoidoscopy
- Colonoscopy

Therapeutic interventions

- Normal saline or lactated Ringer's solution by IV
- Antibiotics

- Corticosteroids
- Analgesics
- Antidiarrheals/antiperistaltics
- Surgical repair
- Hospital admission

Cultural considerations

The incidence of ulcerative colitis is highest among Caucasians and persons of Jewish heritage.

Patient/family education and discharge instructions

- Diet modification
- Medications
- Ostomy teaching if surgery was performed

Toxic Megacolon

Toxic megacolon is a severe dilation of the colon associated with colitis.[4,6]

Signs and symptoms

- Abdominal distention and pain
- Vomiting
- Fatigue
- Fever
- Explosive diarrhea
- A quiet abdomen
- Possible shock

Therapeutic interventions

- IV fluid rehydration
- Antibiotics
- Corticosteroids
- Nasogastric tube to low intermittent suction
- Surgical repair
- Hospital admission

References

1. Newberry L: Gastrointestinal emergencies. In Newberry L, editor: *Sheehy's emergency nursing: principles and practice,* ed 5, St Louis, 2003, Mosby.
2. Cummings S, Cummings P: Abdominal emergencies. In Jordan KS, editor: *Emergency nursing core curriculum,* ed 5, Philadelphia, 2000, WB Saunders.
3. Smeltzer SC, Bare BG: *Brunner and Suddarth's textbook of medical-surgical nursing,* ed 10, Philadelphia, 2004, Lippincott.
4. Kidd PS, Sturt PA, Fultz J: *Mosby's emergency nursing reference,* ed 2, St Louis, 2000, Mosby.
5. Marx J, Hockberger R, Walls R, editors: *Rosen's emergency medicine: concepts and clinical practice,* ed 5, St Louis, 2002, Mosby.
6. Lewis T: Pancreatitis. In Hayden SR et al, editors: *Rosen and Barkin's 5-minute emergency medicine consult,* ed 2, Philadelphia, 2003, Lippincott Williams & Wilkins.

25

Hematologic and Immunologic Emergencies

Christopher Schmidt, APRN, BC, MSN, CEN, ENP, CDR, NC, USN and Jeffery S. Johnson, NC, USN, RN, MSN, CEN

The number of patients presenting to emergency departments (EDs) with hematologic and immunologic emergencies is increasing because of better treatment and enhanced longevity of persons with these conditions. Several pathologic processes directly affect the blood and the organs that produce blood. The three most commonly encountered by emergency nurses are sickle cell disease and crisis, hemophilia, and anemia. Patients with leukemia and lymphoma experience specific immunologic emergencies—related to their disease and its treatment—that must be identified and managed. As a result of the dramatic increase in transplant survival, a growing number of organ recipients are being evaluated in EDs for transplant-related complications.

HEMATOLOGIC DISORDERS

Sickle Cell Disease

Sickle cell disease is a congenital hemolytic anemia that occurs primarily, but not exclusively, in those of West African descent. Defective hemoglobin molecules cause red blood cells to assume a sickled configuration instead of their usual jelly doughnut shape (Figure 25-1).

An individual with one sickle cell gene possesses the sickle cell trait, but the disease remains clinically inactive. In contrast, a person who inherits two sickle cell genes has sickle cell disease. Early childhood diagnosis and effective treatments have substantially improved the prognosis for individuals with this disease.[1,2]

Sickle cell crisis (vasoocclusive crisis)

Sickled cells carry normal amounts of hemoglobin. However, the cells tend to clump together because of their distinct shape. Clumping increases blood viscosity, resulting in capillary

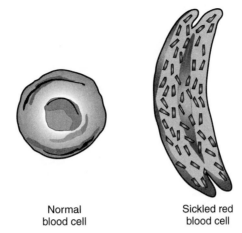

Normal
blood cell

Sickled red
blood cell

Figure 25-1. Defective hemoglobin molecules cause red blood cells to become sickle shaped. (Reprinted with permission from Klasco RK, editor: CareNotes™ System, Greenwood, Colo [Vol 30 exp 3/2004], Thomson MICROMEDEX).

obstruction by limiting the diameter of the vessel. Decreased circulation, edema formation, tissue ischemia, and severe pain ensue (Figure 25-2). Sickle cell crisis occurs more frequently at night and is associated with a number of precipitants (Box 25-1). If the ischemic state is not corrected, local tissue necrosis soon follows, which can lead to organ dysfunction.

Signs and symptoms

- History of sickle cell disease
- Episodic pain in the most common sites:
  - In children: Hands, feet, abdomen (abdominal pain is similar to appendicitis)
  - In adults: Long bones, large joints, spinal column[2-4]
- Weakness
- Pallor

Results of diagnostic studies

- Elevated reticulocyte count
- Sickled cells on smear
- Leukocytosis
- Thrombocytosis
- Decreased hemoglobin and hematocrit

Therapeutic interventions

- Analgesia
  - Acetaminophen or codeine for mild to moderate pain
  - Ketorolac (Toradol) or morphine sulfate for moderate to severe pain
- Supplemental oxygen
- Intravenous rehydration ($D_{5.45}$ normal saline)
- Patients may require blood transfusion if they are significantly anemic.
- Antibiotics (if infection is present)

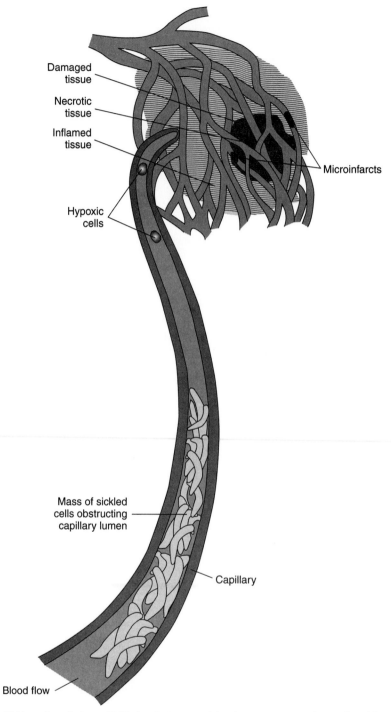

Figure 25-2. Sickle cell pathology. Sickled cells increase blood viscosity, impede capillary blood flow, and can cause tissue and organ ischemia and necrosis. (From *Atlas of pathophysiology*, Philadelphia, 2002, Springhouse.)

Box **25-1** **Sickle Cell Crisis Precipitants**

Cold ambient temperature High altitude Infection	Metabolic or respiratory acidosis Stress

- Local application of heat to areas of pain
- Warm environment
- Emotional support[4]

Age/developmental considerations

- Infants and young children with sickle cell disease may experience hand-foot syndrome.
- Incidence of ischemic stroke is increased in children with sickle cell anemia.
- Disease has a significant psychological influence on patients because of altered body image, frequently missed days of school or work, sexual problems, depression, and fear of a shortened life span.

Complications

- Recurrent crisis
- Chronic hemolytic anemia, transient aplastic crisis
- Frequent infections: Pneumonia, meningitis, osteomyelitis
- Cholelithiasis and cholecystitis
- Delayed sexual maturation, priapism
- High incidence of spontaneous abortion, perinatal mortality, maternal mortality
- Renal failure
- Bone disease (particularly infarction leading to avascular necrosis of the femoral head)
- High-output cardiac failure
- Autosplenectomy
- Pulmonary embolus
- Cor pulmonale
- Chronic skin ulcers
- Jaundice, hepatomegaly, hepatic infarction
- Coma, death[2-4]

Patient/family education and discharge instructions

- Apply warm, moist heat to affected areas to reduce pain and swelling.
- Keep the patient well hydrated.
- Get bed rest, as needed.
- Exercise regularly.
- Avoid high altitudes or flying in a nonpressurized aircraft. Low partial oxygen pressures may precipitate a crisis.
- Limit exposure to cold. Cover skin and maintain warmth in winter months. Avoid skin chilling by air-conditioning in summer months.
- Seek medical care for the following:
  - Shortness of breath
  - Weakness or fatigue

- Chest, abdominal, or back pain
- Swelling of the hands, feet, or joints[3,4]
- Patients considering reproduction may benefit from genetic counseling.
- Acute chest syndrome (ACS) is the leading cause of death in this population.

HEMOPHILIA

Hemophilia is a congenital coagulation disorder usually caused by a lack of one of two essential circulating plasma proteins: factor VIII or factor IX. It is an inherited sex-linked disease found primarily in males. Hemophilia produced by a factor VIII deficiency is referred to as hemophilia A, or classic hemophilia. This form is responsible for 85% of the 20,000 hemophilia cases in the United States. A factor IX deficiency is called hemophilia B, or Christmas disease. An estimated 14% of patients with hemophilia have this chromosomal defect.[4,5]

Despite their etiologic differences, the clinical presentations of hemophilia A and B are similar. These conditions are characterized by bleeding into the soft tissues, muscles, and weight-bearing joints (knees, elbows, and ankles). Bleeding also can occur in the oral or nasal mucosa, the urinary system, the gastrointestinal tract, or the central nervous system (usually following trauma).[6] Hemophilia typically is diagnosed in infancy, but some mild cases go undetected until childhood or adolescence.

Factors VIII and IX are proteins normally found in the plasma. Clotting factors circulate in an inactive form until stimulation of the clotting cascade initiates factor activation, such as occurs when a cut or bruise is sustained. Factors in the cascade are activated, in a domino-like fashion, until fibrinogen becomes fibrin and a clot finally is formed. Any one factor inactivated or removed from the sequence impedes or deters proper clot formation. Hemophilia severity depends on the extent of factor function in each individual patient. Figure 25-3 depicts the clotting cascade system. A majority of patients with hemophilia A produce factor VIII, but it either is entirely nonfunctional or operates below normal capacity. Typically, patients seeking emergency care are well aware of their disease and have years of experience managing it. Their arrival at the ED usually indicates failure of standard home therapy.

Symptoms are not always evident in the early stages of hemorrhage. Hence if indicated by history, treatment should be initiated immediately. Episodes of hemarthrosis resulting from type A or B hemophilia are usually self-limiting because the joint capsule can distend only to a certain point before bleeding is eventually tamponaded.

Von Willebrand's Disease

A third type of bleeding disorder (nonhemophilia) is von Willebrand's disease. This condition results from a decrease in von Willebrand's factor, a plasma protein necessary for platelet function. The disease is manifested by mucocutaneous bleeding, easy bruising, menorrhagia, and gastrointestinal bleeding. Treatment is similar to that for hemophilia and may involve administration of plasma or desmopressin acetate (DDAVP). Cryoprecipitate also can be administered, but it generally is reserved for emergency situations in which more specific agents are unavailable.[7] Definitive treatment for hemophilia and von Willebrand's disease involves rapid factor replacement. Table 25-1 describes hemophilia types. Table 25-2 lists dosing guidelines for factor replacement.

Signs and symptoms

- Bleeding into soft tissue, muscles, body cavities, or joint capsules
- Paresthesia that progresses to nerve injury, following a compressing hematoma

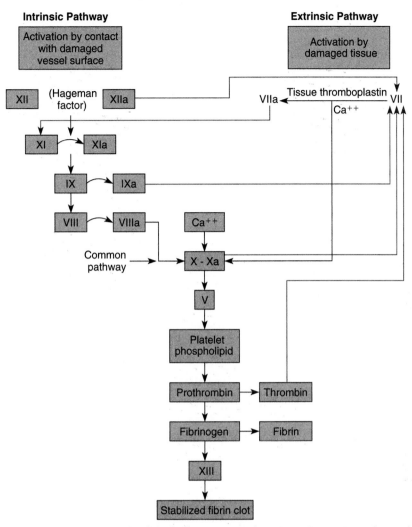

Figure 25-3. The coagulation cascade of the body. (From Huether SE, McCance KL: *Understanding pathophysiology,* ed 2, St Louis, 2000, Mosby.)

Table **25-1**   **Hemophilia Types**

Type	Missing Factor	Indications for Treatment
Type A	Factor VIII	Bleeding into joints or muscles; open wounds
Type B (Christmas disease)	Factor IX	requiring repair; heavy or persistent bleeding; history of trauma that could result in internal bleeding; injury to the head, neck, mouth, tongue, face, or eyes; planned invasive or surgical procedures

Table **25-2**   Factors VIII and IX Replacement Guidelines

Severity	Percent (%)	Treatment and Dosing
Normal	50-100	For patients with normal or low normal levels, treatment usually is not indicated.
Low normal	25-49	
Mild hemophilia	6-24	Type A: For mild cases, desmopressin 0.3 mcg/kg may be tried. Otherwise, recombinant factor VIII is the treatment of choice. Each unit given should raise the factor level by ~2%.
Moderate hemophilia	1-5	
Severe hemophilia	<1	
		Type B: Give recombinant factor IX. Each unit given should raise the factor level by ~1%.
		Give enough factor (VIII or IX) to increase the level to a minimum of 25% of normal.

- Hematuria
- Altered mental status, confusion, irritability, and coma caused by intracranial bleeding
- Shock resulting from profound blood loss

Diagnostic studies

- Complete blood count (CBC)
- Bleeding time (prolonged in 15% to 20% of patients)
- Partial thromboplastin time (elevated), prothrombin time (international normalized ratio) and platelet count (usually normal)
- Factor VIII level (low in hemophilia A)
- Factor IX level (low in hemophilia B)

Therapeutic interventions

- Immobilize, elevate, apply ice, and place a light pressure dressing on the site of injury.
- Administer recombinant clotting factors VIII or IX. Factor replacement is the preferred treatment for hemophilia A and B.
- Transfuse fresh or fresh frozen plasma if clotting factors are not available.
- Give desmopressin acetate (DDAVP). This drug stimulates release (but not formation) of factor VIII, making it useful for mild bleeding episodes.
- Cryoprecipitate transfusion was the treatment of choice for hemophilia A in the past. Clotting factor administration now is considered safer.
- Aspirate joints to relieve pain and remove blood.
- Observe patients closely for further bleeding.[5,6]

Cultural considerations

Certain patients may not consent to transfusion of blood products based on religious beliefs (e.g., Jehovah's Witnesses).

Patient/family education and discharge instructions

- If a joint was involved, suggest range-of-motion exercises and limited weight bearing.
- Patients considering reproduction may benefit from genetic counseling.

Table **25-3**   **Anemias**

Type	Causes
Microcytic hypochromic	Iron deficiency; impaired globin synthesis; chronic blood loss
Macrocytic normochromic	Deficiencies of vitamin B_{12} or folic acid; chemotherapy
Normocytic normochromic	Acute blood loss; hemolysis; chronic diseases or infections; various endocrine and renal disorders

Box **25-2** **Signs and Symptoms of Acute and Chronic Anemias**

Acute	Chronic
Cool, clammy skin	Changes in level of consciousness
Decreased blood pressure	Chest pain
Decreased level of consciousness	Congestive heart failure
Decreased urine output	Dizziness
Increased thirst	Fatigue (especially with exertion)
Narrowing pulse pressure	Headache
Postural hypotension	Irritability
Tachycardia	Pallor
Tachypnea	Shortness of breath

- Watch for indications of significant blood loss:
  - Persistent bleeding despite hemorrhage control measures such as direct pressure and elevation
  - Pale, cool skin
  - Feeling faint or fatigued
  - Shortness of breath
- Obtain hematologic and orthopedic follow-up as necessary.

Anemias

Anemia is defined as a hemoglobin count of less than 50% of the normal value. At sea level the normal hematocrit ranges from 40% to 52% in men. Standard values for women[8] are between 35% and 47%. Anemia may present acutely or chronically. Several types of anemia exist, and cause varies (Table 25-3). Management depends on the clinical presentation as determined by the acuteness of onset and the severity of symptoms.[9]

The emergency nurse must remember that during an acute bleeding episode, hemoglobin and hematocrit remain normal until hemodilution occurs. As a result, hemoglobin and hematocrit are poor early indicators of acute bleeding. Box 25-2 lists clinical signs and symptoms associated with chronic and acute anemias.

Diagnostic studies

Anemia can be diagnosed based on history and the following:
- Orthostatic vital signs
- CBC abnormalities
- Reticulocyte count
- Wright's stain[4]

Therapeutic interventions

The primary goal of anemia therapy is to identify and treat the underlying cause of blood loss, blood cell destruction, or reduced red cell production. However, in patients who are significantly hypovolemic, do the following first:

- Provide supplemental oxygen.
- Place one or more large-bore intravenous catheters.
- Initiate fluid resuscitation with normal saline or lactated Ringer's solution.
- Type and crossmatch.
- Transfuse blood components as indicated.[3,8,9]

Age/developmental considerations

Elderly patients are at increased risk for aplastic anemia because of extensive prescription medication use.

Patient/family education and discharge instructions

- Seek medical care for unusual bleeding or bruising (e.g., gum bleeding, epistaxis, and minor wounds that bleed extensively).
- Avoid nonsteroidal antiinflammatory drugs and aspirin.
- Control bleeding with direct pressure. Ice may be applied to vasoconstrict vessels and slow blood loss.
- Seek medical care immediately for shortness of breath, lightheadedness, weakness, or chest pain.

HEMATOLOGIC MALIGNANCIES

Leukemia

Leukemia is a group of disorders of the blood and the blood-producing organs. Leukemia is caused by malignant proliferation of the white blood cell precursors known as "blasts." Bone marrow failure is a predominant characteristic of the disease because leukemic cells inhibit normal erythrocyte and platelet production, which potentiates anemia and suppresses immune function.[3] Vascular organs affected by leukemic cells include the spleen, liver, and lymph nodes. White blood cell counts as high as 100,000 cells/mm^3 have been recorded in leukemic patients.[10]

Leukemia is classified according to the type of leukocyte produced and the progression of the disease (Table 25-4). Symptoms vary depending on the type and course. Leukemia may be lymphogenous (malignant cells are generated in lymphoid tissue) or myelogenous (cancerous

Table 25-4   Classifications of Leukemia

Type and Abbreviation	Cause
Acute lymphoblastic (or lymphocytic) (ALL)	Accumulation of immature lymphocytes
Acute myelogenous (AML)	Accumulation of immature myeloid cells
Chronic lymphocytic (CLL)	Accumulation of mature-appearing neoplastic lymphocytes
Chronic myelogenous (CML)	Accumulation of immature granulocytes

Data from Barudi M: Leukemia. In Dambro M, editor: *Griffith's 5-minute clinical consult 2003*, ed 11, Philadelphia, 2003, Lippincott Williams & Wilkins; Leukemia and Lymphoma Society: Facts 2003. Retrieved September 20, 2003 from http://www.leukemia-lymphoma.org; Lymphoma Information Network: Treatment therapy, Retrieved September 20, 2003 from http://www.Lymphomainfo.net.

cells are produced within bone marrow). Acute courses of leukemia have a rapid onset and are characterized by an enormous proliferation of immature cells. In such cases, patient life expectancy may be as brief as 6 months. In contrast, chronic leukemia is characterized by excessive production of mature leukocytes in the periphery and the bone marrow. Chronic disease develops much more slowly and life expectancy is considerably longer.[3,11] Leukemia affects men nearly twice as often as women; 30% of leukemia cases occur in children.

Signs and symptoms

- Fever
- Fatigue, weakness, and lethargy
- Bleeding (e.g., bruising, petechiae, purpura, gum bleeding, and epistaxis)
- Pallor
- Anorexia, vomiting, weight loss
- Bone pain
- Lymphadenopathy
- Headache, visual disturbances
- Hepatomegaly, splenomegaly
- Opportunistic infections (fungal, viral, or bacterial)[10-12]

Diagnostic studies

- CBC with differential, coagulation studies, serum chemistries
- Lumbar puncture for analysis of cerebrospinal fluid if neurologic findings are present
- Definitive diagnosis (not usually performed in the emergency department):
  - Bone marrow aspiration and biopsy
  - Chromosome studies of peripheral blood or bone marrow

Therapeutic interventions

- Intravenous hydration to maintain an adequate urine output
- Blood product transfusion as needed
- Broad-spectrum antibiotic therapy and pan-cultures (i.e., blood, urine, and sputum cultures) if the patient is febrile or neutropenic[10-12]
- Protective isolation
- Hospital admission, transfer, or outpatient follow up for the following:
  - Systemic chemotherapy
  - Bone marrow transplantation

Patient/family education and discharge instructions

- Use a soft-bristle toothbrush to avoid gum bleeding.
- Protect against contact with infected persons or contaminated items.
- Avoid taking nonsteroidal antiinflammatory drugs and aspirin.
- Patients already taking certain chemotherapy medications will be photosensitive; avoid open sunlight or wear sunscreen.

Lymphoma

The term *lymphoma* encompasses a multitude of malignant neoplasms that directly affect the lymphoid tissue and lymphatic system. These systems are responsible for defending the body against invading pathogens. Lymphomas constitute 10% to 12% of childhood cancers and rank as the third most common childhood malignancy.[11,12]

Lymphomas are classified in a variety of ways. According to the revised European-American lymphoma (REAL) classification, lymphomas are differentiated by the type of cells that proliferate, their appearance, and their genetic makeup (stage).[13] In addition, these diseases may be categorized as slow growing or devastatingly aggressive.

Hodgkin's disease

Hodgkin's disease accounts for 14% of malignant lymphomas. This condition is characterized by painless enlargement of the lymph nodes, spleen, and other lymphoid tissue. Enlargement occurs because of the replication of lymphocytes, histocytes, eosinophils, and (specifically) Reed-Sternberg giant cells. Hodgkin's disease affects more men than women. In 2003 an estimated 7600 new cases of Hodgkin's disease occurred.[13] Fortunately, the overall incidence has decreased since 1973. Treated aggressively, this disease is curable in 80% of patients. Left untreated, the disease is usually fatal. The Epstein-Barr virus has been identified as a possible causative factor.

Non-Hodgkin's lymphoma

Non-Hodgkin's lymphoma is much more prevalent than the Hodgkin's variety. This group of diseases involves cancerous growth of the B or T cells of the lymphoreticular system. There are 29 different non-Hodgkin's lymphoma types, making it the fifth most common cancer in the United States.[14] The incidence of non-Hodgkin's lymphoma has increased more than 80% since 1973; in 2003 an estimated 53,400 cases were diagnosed.[13] The rising incidence of non-Hodgkin's lymphoma has been attributed to the aging population, a growing number of patients treated with chemotherapy or radiation therapy, rising numbers of persons taking immunosuppressive medications, and the epidemic of acquired immunodeficiency syndrome.[11,13] Prognosis depends on the cell type, the stage of the disease, and the treatment modalities used. With aggressive intervention, cure rates can be as high as 65% to 90%, especially in children.[14]

Non-Hodgkin's lymphoma can start as a localized tumor (within an organ) and then metastasize systemically, via the lymphatic system, to distant nonlymphoid tissues. Disease in sites other than the lymph nodes makes diagnosis difficult. The initial clinical presentation may be similar to a viral infection or cat scratch fever.[11,12] Gastrointestinal symptoms can mimic peptic ulcer disease. The number of individuals with human immunodeficiency virus (HIV) and non-Hodgkin's lymphoma is on the rise. These patients suffer predominately central nervous system effects.[15]

Risk factors

- History of chemotherapy or radiation therapy
- Advanced age
- HIV infection
- Occupational risks:
  - Farm workers: Pesticide and herbicide exposure
  - Painters and mechanics: Solvent and organic chemical exposure (e.g., benzene)
  - Other: Petroleum, rubber, and plastic industry workers
- Medications:
  - Immunosuppressive medications
  - Nonsteroidal antiinflammatory drugs[16]

Signs and symptoms

- Fatigue, malaise
- Fever, cough, night sweats*
- Anorexia, weight loss*
- Pruritus*
- Splenomegaly, hepatomegaly
- Painless lymphadenopathy; a firm, palpable mass

Diagnostic studies

- CBC, serum electrolytes, liver function tests, erythrocyte sedimentation rate
- Hepatitis profile
- HIV testing (if risk factors are present)
- Computed tomography scans of the affected area (brain, abdomen, chest, pelvis)[11,12,14,17]

Therapeutic interventions

- Protective isolation
- Basic supportive care as indicated by the patient's condition
- Antibiotics if infection is present
- Hospital admission, transfer, or outpatient follow up for the following:
  - Chemotherapy or radiation therapy
  - Blood or bone marrow stem cell transplantation
  - Immunosuppressive therapy

Patient/family education and discharge instructions

- Use a soft-bristle toothbrush to avoid gum bleeding.
- Chemotherapy and radiation inhibit immune function. Avoid persons with contagious conditions and be aware of signs of infection.
- Chemotherapy and radiation inhibit sperm production. Males may want to consider sperm banking.

Complications

- Upper airway obstruction
- Superior vena cava syndrome
- Hypercalcemia
- Malignant pericardial effusion with tamponade
- Acute spinal cord syndrome
- Disseminated intravascular coagulation[14]

IMMUNE SUPPRESSION

Patients who are immunosuppressed for whatever reason can become neutropenic (neutrophil count <1500 cells/mm³), making it difficult for them to fend off infection. The immunosuppressed patient is susceptible to viral, fungal, protozoal, and bacterial infections, especially

---

*Pruritus, fever, night sweats, and weight loss occur in 40% of patients with Hodgkin's disease. These findings are less common features of non-Hodgkin's lymphoma.[11,12]

Box **25-3 Conditions Affecting Immunosuppression**[19]

Advanced age
Chronic alcohol consumption
Damaged B or T cell immune function
Diabetes
End-stage renal failure
Hematologic malignancies
Hepatic disease
Infection (e.g., human immunodeficiency virus)
Long-term cytotoxic chemotherapy
Major burns
Pharmacological agents, including transplant immunosuppressants (e.g., cyclosporine)
Radiation therapy
Splenic impairment or splenectomy

Data from Lowery D, Wright D: The organ transplant patient. In Marx J, Hockberger R, Walls R, editors: *Rosen's emergency medicine: concepts and clinical practice*, ed 5, St Louis, 2002, Mosby.

gram-negative bacteria. Transplant patients in particular are predisposed to invasion by organisms normally held at bay by an intact immune system. Febrile neutropenic patients warrant immediate medical attention and require pan-cultures, antibiotic therapy, and hospital admission. Although less common, a severely neutropenic patient may be unable to mount a febrile response. These individuals also warrant emergent evaluation and treatment.[3,18] Many factors can trigger immune suppression or an immunocompromised state (Box 25-3).

Signs and Symptoms

- Weakness, malaise
- Dyspnea
- Chest and abdominal pain
- Fever (fever may not be present in extremely immunosuppressed individuals)
- "Toxic" appearance
- Shock[18]

Diagnostic Studies

- Basic blood studies (CBC, chemistries, coagulation tests)
- Cultures (blood, stool, urine, wound, sputum, cerebrospinal fluid)
- Inflammatory markers: Erythrocyte sedimentation rate, C-reactive protein (Erythrocyte sedimentation rate increases after several days, whereas C-reactive protein rises within hours.)
- HIV (if risk factors are present)
  - HIV-positive patients should have their viral load and CD4 counts checked. (Elevated viral loads and low CD4 levels make patients more susceptible to infection.)
- Imaging studies as indicated to identify sites of infection (chest radiograph, computed tomography of the head, thorax, abdomen, or pelvis)

Therapeutic Interventions

- Protective isolation
- Intravenous rehydration
- Broad-spectrum antibiotic therapy

Box 25-4 Immunosuppressive Agents Used by Organ Transplant Patients

Anti-CD3 monoclonal antibody (OKT3)
Azathioprine
Corticosteroids
Cyclosporine
Mycophenolate (mofetil, MMF, CellCept)
Tacrolimus

Data from Lowery D, Wright D: The organ transplant patient. In Marx J, Hockberger R, Walls R, editors: *Rosen's emergency medicine: concepts and clinical practice,* ed 5, St Louis, 2002, Mosby.

- Do not check temperatures per rectum in a neutropenic patient. Rectal probe–induced microtrauma to the mucosa can predispose patients to invasion by their own gut flora.[3,18]

Patient/Family Education and Discharge Instructions

- Teach HIV-positive patients to learn and remember their viral load and CD4 counts. Knowing these numbers will greatly assist future health care providers.
- Avoid anyone who might be acutely infectious.
- Return immediately in the event of chest pain, fever, shortness of breath, weakness, light-headedness, or vomiting.

Transplant Rejection

Since the first successful heart transplant in 1967, the number of transplant patients has grown significantly. Organs routinely transplanted include the heart, lungs, liver, pancreas, and kidneys. (See Chapter 16.) Evolving surgical techniques, advanced immunosuppressive agents, improved organ preservation, careful tissue matching, and effective antirejection therapies have contributed to increased survival after transplantation.[19,20]

A fear of rejection and potential life-threatening complications are common concerns experienced by organ recipients who seek emergency care. Transplant patients may suffer from acute or chronic organ rejection, infection, or drug toxicity from the use of immunosuppressive medications.[19,20] Because transplant patients must take immunosuppressants continually, their normal inflammatory processes are blunted (Box 25-4). This often makes symptoms of even significant medical insults subtle. An organ recipient's ability to mount a fever is blunted, and pain response may be diminished as well because of decreased innervation. Therefore any transplant patient presenting for care must be seen urgently, even if complaints are vague.[20]

Infection is the leading cause of death in transplant patients. Infection may occur immediately after transplantation or months after surgery. These patients have a lifelong increased susceptibility to infection from viral (e.g., cytomegalovirus, hepatitis B virus, hepatitis C virus, HIV), bacterial (e.g., *Mycobacterium tuberculosis, Pseudomonas,* other gram-negative bacteria), fungal (e.g., *Cryptococcus* and *Histoplasma capsulatum*), and protozoal organisms. Exposure to infectious agents can occur before the transplant procedure, during hospitalization (nosocomial), or in the community following discharge.[19,20]

Types of Rejection

Rejection may be hyperacute, acute, or chronic:
- *Hyperacute:* Occurs intraoperatively, immediately following organ attachment. ABO incompatibility and antibodies are the causative factors.

- *Acute:* Occurs weeks to several months after transplantation. The body identifies the organ as foreign tissue and seeks to destroy it. Onset can begin immediately if immunosuppressive therapy is stopped.
- *Chronic:* A low-grade immunologic response that may occur years following transplantation.

Signs and Symptoms

- Low-grade fever
- Fatigue
- Dyspnea
- Abnormal breath sounds
- Peripheral edema
- Jugular vein distention
- Pericardial friction rub
- Decreased electrocardiogram voltage
- Dysrhythmias
- Cardiomegaly
- Hypotension
- Vascular collapse[20]

Diagnostic Studies

- CBC, coagulation studies, transaminase levels, serum chemistries
- 12-lead electrocardiogram
- Determination of immunosuppressive drug levels (e.g., cyclosporine)
- Culture as indicated (blood, urine, sputum, wound site, cerebrospinal fluid)
- Radiographic imaging to identify sites of infection (chest radiograph, computed tomography scans)

Therapeutic Interventions

- Consult the patient's transplant team immediately to obtain assistance with management of this difficult patient population. If unable to contact the patient's transplant service, seek guidance from your regional transplant team.
- Differentiate between rejection and infection. Febrile patients require aggressive management, including pan-cultures and broad-spectrum intravenous antibiotic therapy.
- Isolate the patient from anyone with an active infection.[19,20]

Patient/Family Education and Discharge Instructions

- Follow-up with your transplant team to ensure adherence to protocols.
- Always take prescribed immunosuppressive medications as directed.
- Because of immunosuppressant use, normal symptoms of infection or rejection may not be experienced. Contact your specialist for questions or concerns.
- Return immediately in the event of chest pain, shortness of breath, fever, malaise, fatigue, vomiting, or confusion.

References

1. Dart B: A voice of hope rings out in the Senate, *Atlanta Journal-Constitution* 2003. Retrieved September 20, 2003 from http://www.ajc.com/living/content/living/0603/13keone.html.
2. Holmes H, editor: *Atlas of pathophysiology,* Springhouse, Pa, 2002, Springhouse Lippincott Williams & Wilkins.
3. Lombardo D: Hematologic emergencies. In Newberry L, editor: *Sheehy's emergency nursing: principles and practice,* ed 5, St Louis, 2003, Mosby.
4. Marett B: Blood disorders. In Sheehy S, Lenehan G, editors: *Manual of emergency care,* ed 5, St Louis, 1999, Mosby.
5. Coyne M, Lusher J: Guidelines for emergency care of patients with hemophilia, *Emerg Med* 32:69-77, 2000.
6. Bowman P: Hemophilia. In Dambro M, editor: *Griffith's 5-minute clinical consult 2003,* ed 11, Philadelphia, 2003, Lippincott Williams & Wilkins.
7. Eberest M: Hemophilias and Von Willebrand's disease. In Tintinalli J, Kelen G, Stapczynski J, editors: *Emergency medicine: a comprehensive study guide,* ed 5, New York, 1999, McGraw-Hill.
8. Hamilton G, Janz T: Anemia, polycythemia, and white blood cell disorders. In Marx J, Hockberger R, Walls R, editors: *Rosen's emergency medicine: concepts and clinical practice,* ed 5, St Louis, 2002, Mosby.
9. Binder L: Anemia. In Harwood-Nuss A, Wolfson A, editors: The clinical practice of emergency medicine. Retrieved September 20, 2003 from http://pco.ovid.com/lrppco/index.html.
10. Barudi M: Leukemia. In Dambro M, editor: *Griffith's 5-minute clinical consult 2003,* ed 11, Philadelphia, 2003, Lippincott Williams & Wilkins.
11. Leukemia and Lymphoma Society: Facts 2003. Retrieved September 20, 2003 from http://www.leukemia-lymphoma.org.
12. Lymphoma Information Network: Treatment therapy, Retrieved September 20, 2003 from http://www.Lymphomainfo.net.
13. National Cancer Institute: Surveillance, Epidemiology and End Results (SEER) Program 1975-2000, Bethesda, Md, 2003, The Institute.
14. Johnston JM: Non-Hodgkin's lymphoma. Retrieved September 20, 2003 from http://www.imedicine.com/wc.dll.
15. Fertikh D, Brooks M: Brain lymphoma. Retrieved September 20, 2003 from http://www.imedicine.com.
16. Cerhan J et al: Association of aspirin and other non-steroidal anti-inflammatory drug use with incidence of non-Hodgkin's lymphoma, *Int J Cancer* 106:784-788, 2003.
17. Gajra A: B-cell lymphoma. Retrieved September 21, 2003 from http://www.imedicine.com.
18. Langdorf M, Burns M: The immunocompromised patient. In Marx J, Hockberger R, Walls R, editors: *Rosen's emergency medicine: concepts and clinical practice,* ed 5, St Louis, 2002, Mosby.
19. Lowery D, Wright D: The organ transplant patient. In Marx J, Hockberger R, Walls R, editors: *Rosen's emergency medicine: concepts and clinical practice,* ed 5, St Louis, 2002, Mosby.
20. Zavotsky K, Sapienza J, Wood D: Nursing implications for ED care of patients who have received heart transplants, *J Emerg Nurs* 27:33-39.

26

Metabolic Emergencies

Lisa M. Pruner, MS, RN

Disruption in the production, supply, or utilization of hormones or electrolytes can result in a medical emergency that requires prompt assessment, diagnosis, correction, and identification of the precipitating cause.

DIABETIC EMERGENCIES

Diabetes mellitus is a chronic condition in which the body is unable to metabolize glucose—the primary energy source of the cell—because of a lack of effective insulin. Two major types of diabetes mellitus occur. Type I (formerly called insulin-dependent diabetes or juvenile-onset diabetes) is due to an absolute insulin deficiency. Type II (previously referred to as non–insulin-dependent diabetes or adult-onset diabetes) is characterized by insulin resistance, increased hepatic glucose release, impaired glucose storage, and eventual insulin deficiency. Type II is the more prevalent form. The goals of diabetes management are to decrease macrovascular and microvascular complications, balance food intake with energy expenditure, and ensure a sufficient amount of insulin (endogenous or exogenous) to maintain blood glucose levels at or near normal. When these goals are not achieved, a diabetic crisis occurs.

Hypoglycemic Emergencies

Hypoglycemia is the most common acute complication of diabetes and the most frequent side effect of insulin and oral hypoglycemic agent use. To prevent or reduce long-term vascular complications, the 2003 American Diabetes Association Practice Recommendations stress strict glycemic control aimed at keeping glucose at near-normal levels. As increasing numbers of diabetic patients follow these intensive therapy regimens, the number of hypoglycemic patients seen in emergency departments (EDs) is likely to rise. Severe hypoglycemia requires medical intervention, whereas mild and moderate hypoglycemia are generally self-treated conditions.

Normal blood glucose levels range from 80 to 120 mg/dL (4.4 to 6.6 mmol/L). *Hypoglycemia* is defined as a blood glucose level less than 50 mg/dL (2.8 mmol/L) or less than 40 mg/dL in infants. Symptoms of hypoglycemia may be present at higher blood glucose levels (>50 mg/dL) in individuals whose serum glucose values normally run high but have dropped precipitously.[1] Persons taking sulfonylureas and meglitinides for their diabetes are also prone to hypoglycemia. When used alone biguanides, alpha-glucosidase inhibitors, and thiazolidinediones usually do not cause hypoglycemia. Particularly at risk for hypoglycemia are patients with type I diabetes who are on intensive insulin therapy regimens and those with type II diabetes taking a long-acting oral hypoglycemic agent such as chlorpropamide (Diabinese).[2,3]

Causes

- Too much insulin (includes accidental and intentional overdoses of insulin or oral hypoglycemic agents)
- Sulfonylurea potentiation
- Increased exercise or activity
- Insufficient food intake
- Alcohol consumption

Signs and symptoms

In mild hypoglycemia, adrenergic symptoms are the predominant findings. However, these symptoms are masked in patients with long-standing diabetes, beta-blocker ingestion, or alcoholism. This "hypoglycemic unawareness," a result of autonomic neuropathy, eliminates an individual's ability to recognize the following early signs and symptoms of hypoglycemia:

- Shaking
- Sweating
- Tachycardia
- Hunger
- Pallor
- Tingling of the lips
- Anxiety
- Palpitations
- Restlessness

Moderate hypoglycemia is characterized by neuroglycopenic symptoms as a result of insufficient glucose to the brain:

- Behavioral changes, irritability
- Inability to concentrate, confusion
- Headache
- Drowsiness
- Slurred speech
- Weakness, staggering gait
- Blurred vision

Severe hypoglycemia is a medical emergency that, if left untreated, will result in the following:

- Seizures
- Coma

- Permanent neurologic damage
- Death

Therapeutic interventions

Treatment of hypoglycemia in the conscious patient

- Recognize the symptoms.
- Measure the serum glucose level. A fingerstick blood glucose test (performed with a light-reflectance meter) is adequate to begin treatment if the equipment is functioning properly and the operator is trained adequately.
- Obtain a laboratory analysis of serum glucose for confirmation of the meter reading. However, do not delay treatment while awaiting laboratory results if the patient is symptomatic.
- Administer 15 g of a rapid-acting carbohydrate (Box 26-1).
- If the serum glucose level does not improve within 10 minutes, administer a second 15-g dose of carbohydrates orally. (Sympathetic nervous system symptoms should resolve quickly, but neurogenic symptoms may continue for an hour or more even if blood glucose levels are greater than 100 mg/dL.)
- Increases in serum glucose are often temporary following oral carbohydrate administration (usually lasting less than 2 hours). A snack or meal eaten soon after blood glucose begins to rise will decrease the risk of recurrent hypoglycemia.

Treatment of hypoglycemia in the semiconscious or unconscious patient

- Measure the blood glucose level (as previously discussed).
- Administer 50% dextrose, 25 to 50 mL intravenously (IV).
- Consider continuous infusion of 5% dextrose in water (D_5W) or 10% dextrose in water ($D_{10}W$) to maintain serum glucose within the normal range.
  Or (if IV access is not readily available):
- Administer glucagon 1 mg intramuscularly (0.5 mg in children ages 3 to 5 years; 0.25 mg in children less than 3 years).
- If there is no improvement in 20 minutes, repeat the same glucagon dose.
- Once the patient can swallow, give 20 g of carbohydrates by mouth to restock depleted glycogen stores and to prevent recurrence of hypoglycemia.

Box 26-1 Treatment of Hypoglycemia

Each of the following contains 15 g of carbohydrates:
  1 cup of milk
  1 small tube of glucose gel
  10 jelly beans
  3 glucose tablets
  8 small sugar cubes or 4 tsp of sugar
  1/2 cup regular soda (Avoid in patients with renal failure.)
  1/2 cup orange juice (Avoid in patients with renal failure.)
  1/3 cup apple juice
  1/2-oz box of raisins
  3 tsp of honey or syrup
  8 Lifesaver candies
  1 small tube of cake frosting

- Vomiting is common following the administration of glucagon; position the patient to avoid aspiration.
- Glucagon may not be effective if liver glycogen stores have been depleted.
- Serially monitor serum glucose levels, vital signs, and neurologic status frequently.

Following successful hypoglycemia treatment, it is helpful for patients to reflect on possible causes to prevent future episodes. Recalling recent insulin doses, injection times, food intake, activities, and special circumstances may help to identify the cause of hypoglycemia. Frequent or prolonged bouts of hypoglycemia contribute to permanent neurologic damage. Early recognition of symptoms and prompt treatment is essential. Advise diabetic patients to wear identification such as a MedicAlert necklace or bracelet.[1,2,4,5] Table 26-1 describes characteristics of common insulins.[6]

Table 26-1 Types of Insulin: Onset, Peak, and Duration of Action

Type	Brand Names	Onset	Peak	End	Color
		Number of hours following subcutaneous administration*			
Rapid-Acting Analogs					
Insulin lispro	Humalog	1/4	1/2-11/2	6-8	Clear
Insulin aspart	Novolog	1/4	1/2-11/2	3-5	Clear
Short-Acting Analogs					
Regular insulin	Regular Humulin R Novolin R Ilentin II	1/2-1	2-5	8-12	Clear
Intermediate-Acting Analogs					
NPH (isophane insulin suspension)	Humulin N Novolin N Iletin II NPH	1-11/2	4-12	24	Cloudy
Insulin zinc suspension Humulin L	Novolin L Lente Ilentin II	1-21/2	7-15	18-24	Cloudy
Long-Acting Analogs					
Insulin zinc suspension, extended	Humulin U Ultralente	4-8	10-30	>36	Cloudy
Insulin glargine	Lantus	1	No peak	24	Clear

Data from American Diabets Association: Position statement: insulin administration, *Diabetes Care* 26(suppl 1): S121-S122; Eisenbarth G, Polonsky K, Buse J: Type 1 diabetes mellitus. In Larson P et al, editors: *Williams textbook of endocrinology*, ed 10, Phiadelphia, 2003, Saunders; Kazlauskaite R, Fogelfeld L: Insulin therapy in type 2 diabetes, *Dis Month* 46:392-411, 2003; McCorminck, M, Quinn L: Treatment of type 2 diabetes mellitus: pharmacology and intervention, *J Cardiovasc Nurs* 16:63-66, 2002; and White J, Campbell K, and Yarborough P: Pharmacologic therapies. In Franz M: *Core curriculum for diabetes*, ed 4, Chicago, 2001, American Association of Diabetes Educatros.
*These times are approximate and are based on biosynthetic human insulin. Animal insulins tend to have slightly longer action times. Individual variations in insulin absorption and action may be caused by many factors, including dose, injection technique, injection site, insulin temperature, exercise following injection, and insulin antibodies. When mixing two types of insulin, always draw clear regular insulin into the syringe first. If mixing regular insulin with Humulin L, Novolin L, or Lente Ilentin II, the mixture should be injected immediately. Do not shake Lantus (insulin glargine) before administration or mix it with any other insulin.[6]

Reactive Hypoglycemia

Reactive, or postprandial, hypoglycemia occurs in response to a meal. This condition occurs in persons who do not have diabetes. Onset is generally 1 to 2 hours after eating.

Causes

- Altered gastrointestinal motility after gastric surgery
- Fructose intolerance
- Impaired glucose tolerance
- Insulinoma
- Idiopathic

Therapeutic interventions

- Administer glucose orally.
- Refer patients for further workup to determine the cause of their condition and to develop a treatment plan.

Hyperglycemic Emergencies

Diabetic ketoacidosis

Diabetic ketoacidosis (DKA) accounts for 80% to 90% of hyperglycemic emergencies. This condition is an acute diabetic complication and in some cases may be the initial presentation of new-onset diabetes (particularly type I). DKA results from an inadequate amount of available insulin and is characterized by profound dehydration, electrolyte losses, ketonuria, and acidosis. When insulin is unavailable to transport glucose into the cells, the liver metabolizes fatty acids into ketone bodies. This accumulation of ketones produces metabolic acidosis.

Diabetic ketoacidosis usually is limited to type I diabetic patients, but under conditions of extreme stress, it may occur in those with type II diabetes. A 6% to 10% mortality is associated with DKA as a result of the precipitating cause, the DKA itself, or treatment complications.[1,4,7,8]

Causes

- New-onset diabetes
- Inadequate insulin dosing or omission of insulin doses
- Illness or infection in a known diabetic patient (this is the most common cause of DKA)
- Myocardial infarction
- Stroke
- Trauma
- Surgery
- Steroid use
- Pancreatitis
- Pregnancy
- Emotional stress

Signs and symptoms

- Anorexia, nausea, vomiting
- Polyuria, polydipsia
- Blurred vision
- Abdominal pain, diminished bowel sounds

- Tachycardia, orthostatic hypotension
- Poor skin turgor, dry mucous membranes
- Weakness, drowsiness
- Mental status ranges from normal to comatose
- Acetone on the breath (fruity-smelling breath)
- Kussmaul respirations (rapid, deep breathing)
- Hypothermia
- Hyporeflexia
- Ketonuria, glucosuria
- Hyperglycemia (>250 mg/dL)
- pH less than 7.3
- Serum bicarbonate less than 15 mEq/L

Differential diagnosis
- Alcoholic ketoacidosis
- Hyperglycemic hyperosmolar nonketotic coma
- Starvation ketosis
- Uremia
- Lactic acidosis
- Toxic ingestion

Diagnostic studies
- Obtain a serum glucose level. If this cannot be done rapidly, give unconscious diabetic patients 25 g of dextrose (50% dextrose solution) intravenously. Hypoglycemia is the most common cause of altered mental status in persons with diabetes; giving this small amount of additional glucose is not harmful to patients with DKA.
- Use dipstick to test urine for glucose and ketones. Send a urinalysis (infection is a frequent precipitant of DKA).
- Draw and send blood for serum glucose determination, complete blood count with differential, electrolytes, arterial blood gases, blood urea nitrogen (BUN), creatinine, phosphate, and amylase.
- Obtain a chest radiograph, 12-lead electrocardiogram, and blood cultures as indicated.
- Additional studies may be needed to identify the underlying cause.

Therapeutic interventions
The treatment goals for DKA are fluid and electrolyte replacement, reversal of ketonemia and hyperglycemia, and identification of the precipitating cause. Although the condition requires emergent intervention, correction that occurs too rapidly may result in cerebral edema, hypoglycemia, or hypokalemia.[1,8]

Replace fluids
- Volume losses in DKA can be extensive. Total body fluid deficits average 6 L (adults) or 100 mL/kg of body mass.
- Restore intravascular volume and renal perfusion. Begin fluid replacement before initiating insulin therapy or electrolyte replacement.
- Administer normal saline at 1 L/hr for 1 to 2 hours and then 100 to 500 mL/hr (adults). For children, replace 20 mL/kg of body mass in the first hour. More aggressive fluid replacement is indicated if the patient is in hypovolemic shock.
- Switch to 0.45% saline (4 to 14 mL/kg per hour) if hypovolemia has been reversed and the serum sodium level is still high or normal.
  - If the sodium concentration is low, continue normal saline administration.

- Aim to replace half of the estimated volume lost over 12 to 24 hours.
- Strictly monitor intake and output. Incorporate urinary losses into fluid replacement calculations.
- Use cautious fluid replacement in the elderly and in patients with renal or cardiac disease.

Administer insulin

- Insulin therapy is required to reverse ketogenesis.
- Insulin by IV is recommended; intramuscularly or subcutaneously administered insulin is absorbed erratically in the presence of hypovolemia.
- The treatment of choice for moderate to severe DKA is regular insulin by continuous IV infusion. Give an IV bolus of 0.1 unit of regular insulin per kilogram of body mass and then start a continuous IV infusion at 0.1 unit/kg per hour. Remember to prime the tubing and discard the first 30 to 50 mL of the insulin/normal saline solution because insulin binds to plastic.
- Individuals with mild DKA may receive an insulin bolus of 0.4 unit/kg of body mass. Half of the dose is given IV, the other half is administered intramuscularly or subcutaneously. Subsequent doses may be subcutaneous or intramuscular, but the subcutaneous route is less painful and just as effective as intramuscular route.
- Measure serum glucose hourly.
- Expect a 65 to 125 mg/hr decline in the serum glucose level.
- Double the hourly insulin infusion dose if the serum glucose level has decreased by less than 50 mg/dL after 1 hour of therapy. Continue to double the insulin dose until a consistent 50 to 70 mg/dL hourly reduction in glucose levels is achieved.
- When serum glucose falls to 250 mg/dL, change the IV fluid to a dextrose-containing solution (e.g., $D_5W/0.45\%$ saline) and decrease the insulin dose to 0.05 to 0.1 unit/kg per hour IV (or to 5 to 10 units subcutaneously every 2 hours) to maintain a serum glucose level of 150 to 200 mg/dL. Too rapid a decrease in serum glucose will increase the risk of cerebral edema.
- Insulin therapy must be continued aggressively until ketogenesis is halted.
- Ketogenesis is considered reversed when the serum glucose is less than 200 mg/dL, the anion gap is less than or equal to 12 mEq/L, venous pH is greater than 7.3, and the serum bicarbonate level is greater than or equal to 18 mEq/L.
- To calculate an anion gap, add the serum bicarbonate and serum chloride levels and then subtract this number from the serum sodium level [Anion gap = $Na^+ - (HCO_3 + Cl^-)$]. A normal anion gap is 12 ± 2 mEq/L.
- Depending on the insulin type, subcutaneous insulin therapy must be initiated 1 to 4 hours before discontinuation of the IV insulin infusion so as to avoid recurrence of hyperglycemia and ketogenesis.

Replace electrolytes

- Measure serum electrolytes at the time of patient arrival and every 2 to 4 hours thereafter.
- In most cases the serum potassium level initially will be elevated. Fluid resuscitation, insulin therapy, and acidosis correction reduce extracellular potassium levels.
- Once serum potassium is less than 5 mEq/L, begin IV potassium replacement to keep blood levels between 4 and 5 mEq/L. If the initial serum potassium is less than 3.3 mEq/L, delay insulin therapy and start potassium replacement immediately.
- Begin potassium replacement only after it has been established that the patient has adequate urine output and is not in renal failure.
- Phosphate replacement also may be necessary.
- Sodium bicarbonate can be given IV if the arterial pH is less than or equal to 7.

Monitor for complications

- Hypoglycemia
- Cerebral edema
- Dysrhythmias
- Pulmonary congestion

Follow-up

- Identify the precipitating cause of DKA and treat the underlying problem.
- Hospital admission usually is indicated.
- If DKA resulted from poor diabetes management, additional patient and family education is needed.

Hyperosmolar hyperglycemic nonketotic coma

Hyperosmolar hyperglycemic nonketotic coma (HHNC) accounts for 10% to 20% of hyperglycemic emergencies and is associated with a 20% to 60% mortality.[9] This condition is an acute complication of type II diabetes (frequently undiagnosed). Clinical findings include dehydration, extreme hyperglycemia, electrolyte imbalances, hyperosmolarity, and altered mental status. In contrast to DKA, acidosis is not present in the patient in HHNC (Table 26-2). The high mortality rate of HHNC is related to advanced patient age, diagnostic delays, failure to treat the condition aggressively, and the presence of severe underlying conditions. Elderly patients, especially those with mental impairment or debilitating conditions, are at increased risk. As the population ages, HHNC likely will be seen more frequently in the future. Potential complications of treatment include cerebral edema, systemic hypoperfusion, cerebral infarction, and hypokalemia.

Causes

Illnesses

- Chronic renal insufficiency, uremia
- Vomiting or severe diarrhea
- Acute viral illnesses

Table 26-2   Comparison of Diabetic Ketoacidosis and Hyperosmolar Hyperglycemic Nonketotic Coma Patient Presentations

Feature	*Diabetic Ketoacidosis*	*Hyperosmolar Hyperglycemic Nonketotic Coma*
Patient's age	Usually <40 years	Usually >60 years
Duration of symptoms	Usually <2 days	Usually >5 days
Glucose level	Usually <600 mg/dL	Usually >800 mg/dL
Sodium level	Likely to be low or normal	Likely to be normal or high
Potassium level	High, normal, or low	High, normal, or low
Bicarbonate level	Low	Normal
Ketone bodies	At least 4+ in a 1:1 dilution	<2+ in a 1:1 dilution
pH	Low, usually <7.3	Normal
Serum osmolality	Usually <350 mOsm/kg	Usually >350 mOsm/kg
Cerebral edema	Often subclinical, occasionally clinical	Rapid glucose decline increases the risk.
Prognosis	3%-10% mortality	20%-60% mortality
Subsequent course	Ongoing insulin therapy usually is required.	Insulin therapy often is not required.

- Gram-negative infections: pneumonia, sepsis, urinary tract infection
- Gastrointestinal bleeding
- Myocardial infarction
- Pulmonary embolism
- Subdural hematoma
- Stroke
- Pancreatitis
- Major burns
- Heat stroke

Medications

- Thiazide diuretics
- Steroids and other immunosuppressive agents
- Phenytoin
- Propranolol
- Cimetidine

Other causes

- Total parenteral nutrition
- Tube feeding without sufficient free water
- Renal dialysis
- Recent cardiac surgery

Signs and symptoms

- Mental status ranges from drowsy to unresponsive
- Seizures
- Dehydration
- Hyperglycemia (>600 mg/dL)
- Hyperosmolality (>300 mOsm/kg). Serum osmolality may be calculated as follows:
  Osmolality (mmol/L) = (Serum sodium × 2) + (Blood glucose/18) + (BUN/2.8)
- Absent or minimal serum ketones
- pH greater than 7.3
- Serum bicarbonate greater than 20 mEq/L

Differential diagnosis

- DKA
- Alcoholic ketoacidosis
- Lactic acidosis
- Other causes of altered mental status

Diagnostic studies

- Serum glucose, electrolytes, BUN, and creatinine levels
- Complete blood count with differential
- Urinalysis
- Arterial blood gases
- Other studies as indicated to determine the underlying cause

Therapeutic interventions

The goals of HHNC treatment are rehydration, correction of electrolyte imbalances, serum glucose reduction, and identification of the precipitating cause.[8]

Replace fluids

- The average fluid deficit in patients in HHNC is 9 to 12 L.
- Begin fluid resuscitation with normal saline. Give 1 L over the first hour to restore blood pressure and urine output. (Patients in hypovolemic shock require more volume replacement.)
- Use caution when rehydrating the elderly and persons with renal or cardiac disease.
- Switch to 0.45% saline at 5 to 15 mL/kg per hour if the serum sodium level is normal or high. Continue normal saline at 5 to 15 mL/kg per hour if sodium is low.
- Insert an indwelling urinary catheter to strictly monitor intake and output. Incorporate urinary losses into fluid replacement calculations.
- When the blood glucose drops to 300 mg/dL, change to a dextrose-containing IV solution such as D_5W/0.45% saline. Adding dextrose to IV fluids reduces the risk of cerebral edema associated with rapid decreases in serum glucose levels.

Administer insulin

- The goal of insulin therapy in patients in HHNC is to reduce serum glucose levels by 100 to 200 mg/dL per hour.
- Patients who are acidotic, hyperkalemic, or in renal failure require IV insulin therapy.
- Give an IV bolus of regular insulin, 0.15 units/kg. Then start a continuous regular insulin infusion at 0.1 units/kg per hour. Anticipate a decrease in serum glucose of greater than or equal to 50 mg/dL in the first hour of therapy. If this reduction is not achieved, double the hourly insulin dose until a consistent decline of 100 to 200 mg/dL per hour is maintained. When the serum glucose level reaches 300 mg/dL, reduce the continuous insulin infusion to 0.05 to 0.1 units/kg per hour.
- Monitor serum glucose levels hourly. Check serum chemistries every 2 to 4 hours until the patient is stable.
- In some cases of HHNC, insulin is not necessary; fluid replacement alone is adequate to reduce serum glucose levels.

Replace electrolytes

- After adequate urine output is documented, begin potassium replacement at 20 to 30 mEq/L of IV fluid.
- If potassium is less than 3.3 mEq/L, delay insulin therapy until hypokalemia has been corrected.
- Check the potassium level every 2 hours until the patient is stable.

Follow-up

- Critical care admission is indicated.
- Identification and treatment of the precipitating cause is essential.

PITUITARY EMERGENCIES

Diabetes Insipidus

Neurogenic diabetes insipidus occurs when antidiuretic hormone (ADH) is produced in insufficient quantities by the hypothalamus or is not released by the posterior pituitary gland. In nephrogenic diabetes insipidus, adequate amounts of ADH are produced and released, but the renal tubules are unresponsive to the hormone. This renders the kidneys unable to concentrate urine appropriately, and excessive amounts of dilute urine are excreted. Diabetes insipidus may be a temporary or a permanent condition, depending on the amount of hypothalamic secretory tissue remaining and the extent of renal impairment.[10]

Nephrogenic diabetes insipidus does not respond to ADH replacement therapy. The disease must be treated with dietary sodium and protein restrictions, thiazide diuretics, and nonsteroidal antiinflammatory drugs. Although the names are similar, diabetes insipidus has no association with diabetes mellitus.

Causes

Neurogenic
- Tumors of the hypothalamus or pituitary region
- Head injury
- Surgical brain trauma
- Ischemia or infection of the hypothalamus or pituitary
- Meningitis, encephalitis
- Cerebral aneurysm
- Drugs: Phenytoin, lithium

Nephrogenic
- Polycystic kidney disease
- Pyelonephritis
- Sickle cell disease
- Sarcoidosis
- Familial genetic disorders

Signs and symptoms
- Weight loss, fatigue
- Polydipsia, polyuria (5 to 20 L/day)
- Urine specific gravity less than 1.005
- Urine osmolality less than 300 mOsm/kg
- Serum osmolality greater than 295 mOsm/kg
- Serum sodium greater than 145 mEq/L

Therapeutic interventions
- Evaluate for possible causes.
- Begin fluid replacement. Rehydrate orally if the patient is asymptomatic and the total body water deficit is not extreme. In severe cases, replace volume loss with hypotonic IV fluids (e.g., 0.45% saline).
- Too rapid volume correction can cause cellular edema.
- Closely monitor intake, output, and neurologic status.
- Replace ADH with the following:
  - Aqueous pitressin (IV or subcutaneous)
  - Lysine vasopressin spray (nasal)
  - Desmopressin acetate (DDAVP)

Syndrome of Inappropriate Antidiuretic Hormone Secretion

The syndrome of inappropriate antidiuretic hormone (SIADH) secretion results when abnormal amounts of antidiuretic hormone (ADH) are released from the pituitary, producing water intoxication. Hyponatremia and hypotonicity characterize this syndrome. The syndrome is more common in the elderly.[10]

Causes

- Head trauma
- Infections: Brain abscesses, meningitis, human immunodeficiency virus, pneumonia
- Stroke, cerebral aneurysm, other central nervous system disorders
- Malignancies
- Hypoxia
- Positive pressure ventilation
- Adrenal insufficiency
- Pain, stress
- Drugs: Oral hypoglycemic agents, psychotropics, antineoplastic agents, general anesthetics, narcotics

Signs and symptoms

- Headache, fatigue
- Confusion, decreased level of consciousness, seizures
- Nausea, vomiting
- Diminished deep tendon reflexes
- Weight gain without edema
- Dilutional hyponatremia
- Decreased plasma osmolality
- Increased urine osmolality, sodium, and specific gravity

Therapeutic interventions

- Treatment is determined by symptom severity and the extent of hyponatremia.
- If the patient is asymptomatic, water intake simply may be restricted to 500 to 1000 mL/day.
- Give IV normal saline or oral salt tablets.
- Symptomatic patients who have severe hyponatremia require IV hypertonic saline (3% to 5%) and furosemide (Lasix). Recheck serum sodium levels every 1 to 2 hours.
- Overly aggressive sodium correction can cause intracellular dehydration.
- Closely monitor intake, output, and neurologic status.

THYROID EMERGENCIES

Thyroid hormones affect almost every organ system. Severe thyroid dysfunction, both hypothyroid and hyperthyroid states, are medical emergencies.

Thyroid Storm (Hyperthyroid Crisis)

"Thyroid storm," a hyperthyroid crisis, most commonly occurs in previously undiagnosed hyperthyroid patients in situations of acute stress. If not promptly identified and treated, this condition progresses to exhaustion, cardiac failure, and death in as little as 2 hours. Untreated, hyperthyroid crisis carries a mortality of 20% to 60%. Thyroid storm is 4 times more likely to occur in women than in men. Patients typically have elevated levels of triiodothyronine T_3, thyroxine T_4, and free thyroxine (free T_4), with decreased thyroid-stimulating hormone (TSH) levels.[9]

Causes

- Stress
- Manipulation of the thyroid gland
- Severe drug reactions
- Surgery
- Trauma
- Myocardial infarction
- Infection
- DKA
- Embolism

Signs and symptoms

- Flushing, diaphoresis, hyperthermia
- Anxiety, tremors, agitation, psychosis, decreased level of consciousness
- Nausea, vomiting
- Tachydysrhythmias, cardiac failure
- Tachypnea, pulmonary edema
- Hypertension
- Abdominal pain
- Muscle weakness
- Exophthalmos (in patients with chronic hyperthyroidism)
- Hepatomegaly
- Hypercalcemia
- Hyperglycemia
- Metabolic acidosis

Therapeutic interventions

Care of the patient with thyroid storm involves identification and treatment of the underlying cause, thyroid hormone level reduction, and emergent management of systemic manifestations such as hyperthermia and cardiac dysrhythmias.

Therapeutic interventions for thyroid storm include the following:
- Administer supplemental oxygen.
- Begin fluid and electrolyte replacement.
- Provide continuous cardiac monitoring.
- Reverse hyperthermia.
- Treat the precipitating cause.
- Closely monitor intake and output, as well as respiratory, neurologic, and cardiac status.
- Give acetaminophen (not aspirin) to reduce hyperthermia.
- Administer a beta-blocking agent to counteract sympathetic hyperstimulation (use with extreme caution in patients with asthma or heart failure).
- Consider digoxin by IV for cardiac failure.
- Initiate antithyroid drugs.
- Administer propylthiouracil.
- Administer methimazole.
- Give iodine: Sodium iodide, potassium iodide, or Lugol's solution.
- Administer corticosteroids and B vitamins.
- Ensure that fluid and calorie intake are adequate to meet the patient's increased metabolic demands.

Myxedema Coma (Hypothyroid Coma)

Myxedema coma is a rare but serious hypothyroid emergency. Generally, myxedema coma results from a new stress in patients with preexisting hypothyroidism. This disorder occurs most often in older patients with underlying pulmonary or vascular disease. Respiratory failure is the usual cause of death from myxedema coma; mortality is 30% to 80%.[9]

Causes

- Infection
- Heart failure
- Drugs: Amiodarone, interferon, general anesthesia, sedatives, antidepressants, narcotics (there is an increased sensitivity to opioids in this population)
- Trauma, surgery
- Exposure to cold temperatures
- Stress

Signs and symptoms

- Thyroxine level is decreased; TSH is elevated.
- Fatigue, lethargy, impaired mentation, stupor, seizures, coma
- Hypothermia without shivering
- Bradycardia
- Hypoventilation
- Hypotension
- Hyponatremia
- Hypoglycemia
- Fluid retention
- Dry skin
- Respiratory or metabolic acidosis
- Goiter

Therapeutic interventions

- Tracheal intubation and mechanical ventilation are indicated for patients with significant hypoventilation.
- Begin gentle rehydration and sodium replacement.
- Provide passive warming.
- Treat infections aggressively.
- Identify and treat any underlying causes.
- Initiate IV thyroid hormone replacement (levothyroxine, thyroxine).
- Administer glucocorticoids.

Thyroiditis

Thyroiditis generally is characterized by anterior neck pain that appears gradually or suddenly following an upper respiratory infection (usually viral).[9]

Signs and symptoms

- Pain in the neck, especially when the head is turned
- Increased neck pain with swallowing

- Firm or nodular thyroid
- Hoarse voice
- Fever, malaise
- Tachycardia

Therapeutic interventions

- Aspirin or acetaminophen
- Bed rest
- Antibiotics (if a nonviral infection is suspected)
- Propranolol (Inderal)
- Glucocorticoids
- Possible thyroid surgery

ADRENAL EMERGENCIES

The adrenal cortex (outer portion of the adrenal gland) produces glucocorticoids (cortisol), which largely control metabolism. The cortex also produces mineralocorticoids (aldosterone), which contribute to fluid and electrolyte balance. The adrenal medulla (inner core of the adrenal gland) secretes the autonomic nervous system stimulants epinephrine and norepinephrine.

Acute Adrenal Insufficiency

Acute adrenal insufficiency (adrenal crisis, addisonian crisis) results from a sudden decrease in cortisol and aldosterone levels. This acute, life-threatening condition most commonly occurs in individuals with preexisting chronic adrenal insufficiency (Addison's disease) and often is triggered by an acute illness or stressor. Primary adrenal insufficiency is rare and usually is related to adrenal gland destruction. Symptoms occur when significant portions of the glands are destroyed. Secondary adrenal insufficiency (suppression of adrenal hormone release) is much more common. Long-term glucocorticoid use (hydrocortisone, prednisone) causes adrenal gland suppression, primarily reducing cortisol production. Consequently, abrupt discontinuation of supplemental steroids may precipitate acute adrenal crisis.[9]

Causes

- Stress, infection, or trauma in individuals with preexisting chronic adrenal insufficiency
- Direct injury, infection, hemorrhage, or infarction of the adrenal glands
- Malignancies with metastasis to the adrenals
- Abrupt withdrawal of glucocorticoid therapy
- Adrenalectomy
- Pituitary necrosis
- Head injury with pituitary or hypothalamic injury

Signs and symptoms

- Anorexia, nausea, vomiting, diarrhea, abdominal cramping, weight loss
- Fatigue, weakness, irritability, lethargy, confusion, and disorientation progressing to coma
- Dehydration, azotemia
- Hypotension, hypovolemic shock
- Tachycardia
- Headache

- Fever
- Hyponatremia, hypoglycemia, hypochloremia
- Hyperkalemia (in patients with primary adrenal insufficiency)
- Truncal obesity, moon face (in patients with a history of long-term steroid use)
- Hyperpigmentation, particularly of the knuckles, axilla, gums, and the creases of the hands
- Amenorrhea

Therapeutic interventions

- Begin fluid and electrolyte replacement.
- Treat hyperkalemia.
- Initiate continuous cardiac monitoring.
- Obtain serum electrolytes, glucose, creatinine, cortisol, and adrenocorticotropic hormone levels.
- Identify and treat underlying causes.
- Administer hydrocortisone by IV.
- Critical care admission usually is indicated.

Pheochromocytoma

Pheochromocytoma is a tumor (usually benign) of the chromaffin cells in the adrenal medulla. These tumors stimulate excessive catecholamine secretion (especially norepinephrine) and produce active peptides. The hallmark of this condition is extreme hypertension, which may be persistent or paroxysmal.[9]

Signs and symptoms

- Hypertension
- Headache, visual disturbances
- Fatigue, anxiety, mental status changes
- Diaphoresis
- Pallor
- Tremor
- Palpitations, chest pain
- Abdominal pain
- Tachyarrhythmias

Therapeutic interventions

- Control the hypertensive crisis with an IV alpha-blocking agent (phentolamine) or nitroprusside (Nipride).
- Maintain a normal volume status.
- Observe for cardiac dysrhythmias and treat as indicated.
- Prepare the patient for surgery (tumor removal).

ELECTROLYTE DISORDERS

Electrolytes, ions that conduct electrical current, are essential for proper cellular functioning and maintenance of fluid and acid-base balance. An excess or deficit of any vital electrolyte can result in a life-threatening crisis. Refer to Table 26-3 for a summary of cardiovascular changes associated with major electrolyte disturbances.[10]

Table 26-3   Common Cardiovascular Rhythm Changes from Major Electrolyte Disturbances

Electrolyte	Rhythm Changes	Typical Levels Associated With Cardiac Disturbances
Calcium: Normal—total serum Ca⁺⁺, 8.5-10 mg/dL; free serum Ca⁺⁺, 4.5-5.5 mg/dL		
Hypocalcemia	Prolonged ST segment and Q-T interval Inverted T waves Reduced cardiac contractility (hypotension) Diverse dysrhythmias (bradycardia, VT, asystole)	Ionized Ca⁺⁺ <3.2 mg/dL
Hypercalcemia	Shortened ST segment and Q-T interval Inverted T waves with decreased amplitude Atrial and ventricular dysrhythmias Increased cardiac contractility (hypertension) Cardiac standstill or arrest	Total Ca⁺⁺ >14 mg/dL
Magnesium: Normal— 1.3-2.1 mEq/L		
Hypomagnesemia	Changes are similar to those of hypokalemia Increased P-R interval, QRS complex duration, Q-T interval Broad, flat, or inverted T waves ST segment depression Hypotension Atrial and ventricular dysrhythmias (PACs, PVCs, SVT, VF, torsade de pointes)	Usually <1 mEq/L
Hypermagnesemia	Signs are similar to those of hyperkalemia Hypotension Bradycardia Prolonged QRS, P-R interval, and Q-T interval Heart blocks progressing to cardiac arrest	3-7 mEq/L 12-15 mEq/L 15-20 mEq/L
Phosphorus: Normal— 2.5-4.5 mg/dL		
Hypophosphatemia	Changes are similar to those of hypercalcemia Reduced cardiac contractility (hypotension) Atrial and ventricular dysrhythmias Further reductions in contractility lead to decreased coronary artery perfusion and ischemia followed by an increase in dysrhythmia severity.	Moderate, <2.5 mg/dL Severe, <1.0 mg mg/dL >4.5 mg/dL

Condition	ECG/Clinical Changes	Level
Hyperphosphatemia	Changes are similar to those of hypocalcemia	
	Tachycardias	
Potassium: Normal—3.5-5 mEq/L		
Hypokalemia	ST segment depression	Usually <3 mEq/L
	Inverted T waves (waves flatten as the level rises)	
	Hypotension	
	Ventricular ectopy	
Hyperkalemia	Tall, peaked, tented T waves	6.0-6.5 mEq/L
	Shortened Q-T interval	
	Increased P-R interval and QRS complex duration	
	P wave prolongation with decreased amplitude	
	P waves disappear	Usually >8 mEq/L
	T waves and QRS complexes merge	
	Bradycardia or AV block	
	Progression to VF or asystole	Usually >10-11 mEq/L
Sodium: Normal—135-145 mEq/L	Not typically a direct cause of rhythm changes	
	Abnormal levels involve fluid shifts and signs of hypovolemia/hypervolemia with tachycardia or bradycardia.	

Data from Baran D: Disorders of mineral metabolism. In Irwin R, Rippe J, editors: *Intensive care medicine*, ed 5, Philadelphia, 2003, Lippincott; Black R: Disorders of plasma sodium and plasma potassium. In Irwin R, Rippe J, editors: *Intensive care medicine*, ed 5, Philadelphia, 2003, Lippincott; Gibbs M, Wolfson A, Tayal V: Electrolyte disturbances. In Marx J, Hockberger R, Walls R, editors: *Rosen's emergency medicine: concepts and clinical practice*, ed 5, St. Louis, 2002, Mosby; Guzman J, Krause J: Hypocalcemia: hypercalcemia. In Kruse J, Fink M, Carlson R, editors: *Saunders' manual of critical care*, Philadelphia, 2003, Saunders; Guzman J, Krause J: Hypocalcemia: hypomagnesemia. In Kruse J, Fink M, Carlson R, editors: *Saunders' manual of critical care*, Philadelphia, 2003, Saunders; Kee J, Paulanka B: *Handbook of fluid, electrolyte, and acid-base imbalances*, New York, 2000, Delmar; Kruse J: Hypokalemia. In Kruse J, Fink M, Carlson R, editors: *Saunders' manual of critical care*, Philadelphia, 2003, Saunders; Kruse J: Hyperkalemia. In Kruse J, Fink M, Carlson R, editors: *Saunders' manual of critical care*, Philadelphia, 2003, Saunders; Layton A, Bernards W, Kriby R: Fluids and electrolytes in the critically ill. In Civetta J, Taylor R, Kirby R, editors: *Critical care*, ed 2, Philadelphia, 1992, Lippincott; Marino P: *The ICU book*, ed 2, Philadelphia, 2000, Lippincott; Metheny N: *Fluid and electrolyte balance: nursing considerations*, ed 4, Philadelphia, 2000, Lippincott; Rice R: Magnesium, calcium, and phosphate imbalances: their clinical significance, *Crit Care Nurs* May/June, pp 90-112, 1983; Singer G: Fluid and electrolyte management: potassium. In Carey C, Lee H, Woeltje K, editors: *The Washington manual of therapeutics*, Philadelphia, 1998, Lippincott; and Stark J: The renal system. In Alspach J: *Core curriculum for critical care nursing*, Philadelphia, 1998, Saunders.

VT, Ventricular tachycardia; *PACs*, premature atrial contractions; *PVCs*, premature ventricular contractions; *SVT*, supraventricular tachycardia; *VF*, ventricular fibrillation; *AV*, atrioventricular.

Calcium Disturbances

About 45% of calcium in the blood is physiologically available for cellular needs. This portion is referred to as "active," "free," or "ionized" calcium. Another 40% is bound to serum protein (primarily albumin) and is not physiologically active. The remaining calcium (about 15%) is combined with other electrolytes. Changes in blood pH alter the amount of ionized calcium. As blood pH rises, more calcium binds with serum proteins, thus decreasing free calcium levels. As pH decreases, less calcium is protein-bound and ionized calcium levels rise. Likewise, when serum protein drops, total serum calcium also decreases. Understanding these relationships allows clinicians to identify signs and symptoms of calcium disorders.[10]

Hypocalcemia

Hypocalcemia is an unusual diagnosis in the emergency setting. The condition is uncommon and generally is related to a chronic disorder such as parathyroid hormone deficiency or impairment. However, hypocalcemia occurs in about 20% of individuals with gram-negative bacterial sepsis and also in patients following massive transfusion of banked blood. The protein binding of ionized calcium that occurs with acute hyperventilation causes a quickly reversible form of hypocalcemia.[10]

Causes

- Impaired absorption: small bowel resection, Crohn's disease, malnutrition
- Increased renal loss: renal failure, diuretics
- Alkalosis (usually hyperventilation syndrome)
- Pancreatitis
- Multiple blood transfusions
- Hypomagnesemia

Signs and symptoms

Clinical findings in patients with hypocalcemia depend on actual calcium levels and the severity of ionized calcium loss.

Signs and symptoms of hypocalcemia include the following:
- Numbness and tingling (mouth, hands, feet)
- Muscle cramps
- Nausea, vomiting, diarrhea, abdominal pain
- Hyperactive reflexes
- *Chvostek's sign:* contraction of the facial muscles when the facial nerve is tapped against the bone, anterior to the ear
- *Trousseau's sign:* Occlusion of the brachial artery (with an inflated blood pressure cuff) for 3 minutes results in carpal spasm.
- Tetany
- Hypotension
- Laryngeal spasm with stridor
- Dysrhythmias, T wave inversion
- Seizures
- Abnormal blood clotting (bleeding, bruises, petechiae)
- Pathologic bone fractures

Therapeutic interventions

Acute
- Identify and treat the underlying cause.

- Administer a 10% calcium gluconate solution IV over 10 to 15 minutes (rapid administration can cause hypotension). Calcium chloride may be substituted, but infiltration of this drug causes local tissue necrosis.
- Institute seizure precautions.
- Monitor vital signs, cardiac function, and respiratory status.
- Minimize external stimulation.
- Administer calcifediol.

Chronic
- Begin ergocalciferol therapy.
- Give vitamin D orally.
- Increase dietary calcium intake.
- Provide oral calcium supplementation.

Hypercalcemia

Hypercalcemia is usually a complication of a malignancy but also may be caused by hyperparathyroidism, thiazide diuretics, hypervitaminosis D, hyperthyroidism, Addison's disease, or renal failure. Overingestion of calcium for osteoporosis prevention should be considered a cause. This condition is rarely acute. The goal of hypercalcemia treatment is to identify the underlying cause and reduce serum levels. Calcium level reduction usually can be accomplished by rehydration.[10]

Signs and symptoms
- Nausea, vomiting, constipation
- Thirst, dehydration from polyuria
- Dry nose, itching
- Dysrhythmias, shortened Q-T interval
- Weakness
- Postural hypotension
- Elevated BUN
- Confusion, lethargy, coma

Therapeutic interventions
- Administer normal saline by IV at 200 to 500 mL/hr until euvolemia is achieved.
- Furosemide (Lasix) may be given to prevent fluid overload and promote renal elimination of calcium. *Caution:* Furosemide and thiazide diuretics can worsen hypercalcemia unless adequate amounts of saline are administered.
- Give sodium bicarbonate, hydrocortisone, and calcitonin.
- Dialysis may be required in severe cases of hypercalcemia.
- Hospital admission and continuous cardiac monitoring are indicated if levels are extremely elevated and the patient is symptomatic.

Magnesium Disturbances

Hypomagnesemia

Dietary magnesium is consumed primarily in green vegetables. Magnesium is absorbed in the small bowel and is excreted by the kidneys. The enzyme systems that control cell membrane permeability, muscle contraction, oxidative phosphorylation, and fat and nucleic acid synthesis are activated by magnesium.

Decreased serum magnesium levels result from poor dietary intake, especially when magnesium needs are increased, such as during pregnancy, lactation, or growth spurts. Chronic alcohol abuse, malabsorption syndromes, nasogastric suctioning, vomiting, diarrhea, bowel resection, or excess renal losses also can cause hypomagnesemia. Other disorders associated with this condition are parathyroid diseases, hyperthyroidism, sepsis, diuretic abuse, and DKA treatment. Hypomagnesemia also should be considered in patients who have received massive transfusions of citrated blood, those with acute pancreatitis, and persons who recently underwent cardiopulmonary bypass surgery. Drug-induced hypomagnesemia can be caused by administration of cisplatin and nephrotoxic agents such as aminoglycosides and amphotericin B.[10]

Signs and symptoms

- Anorexia, nausea, vomiting, diarrhea
- Tremors, leg cramps, muscle fibrillation, hyperreflexia, ataxia, tetany
- Positive Chvostek's and Trousseau's signs (see Hypocalcemia)
- Hypertension
- Vertical nystagmus
- Insomnia, apathy, confusion, psychosis, hallucinations, altered mental status
- Dysrhythmias: paroxysmal supraventricular tachycardia, prolonged P-R and Q-T intervals, ventricular tachycardia, ventricular fibrillation, torsades de pointes
- Laryngeal stridor

Therapeutic interventions

- Monitor for cardiac dysrhythmias.
- Administer magnesium orally if levels are mildly depleted.
- Give magnesium replacement by IV (or deep intramuscular injection) to symptomatic patients and those with greatly reduced levels.
- Supplemental magnesium is excreted readily in the urine, necessitating repeated doses. Long-term replacement therapy often is required.
- Hospitalization generally is indicated for magnesium levels less than or equal to 1 mEq/L.
- Monitor electrolyte levels, vital signs, and respiratory and neurologic status over time.
- Institute seizure precautions.

Hypermagnesemia

Hypermagnesemia is an uncommon but life-threatening condition associated with severe fluid loss or renal failure. The cause of this condition is usually iatrogenic, resulting from excessive administration of magnesium-containing products such as antacids, enemas, and dialysate solution or from lithium overdose. Hypermagnesemia also may be seen in patients with DKA, Addison's disease, viral hepatitis, and hypothermia and in those receiving magnesium therapy for pregnancy-induced hypertension.[10]

Signs and symptoms

Mild (3 to 5 mEq/L)

- Bradycardia
- Hypotension
- Nausea, vomiting
- Muscular weakness, decreased deep tendon reflexes (DTRs)
- Red, warm, diaphoretic skin

Moderate (5 to 10 mEq/L)

- Prolonged P-R interval, Q-T interval, and QRS complex duration
- Loss of DTRs
- Paralysis
- Decreased level of consciousness

Severe (>10 mEq/L)

- Third-degree heart block
- Respiratory muscle paralysis
- Asystole

Therapeutic interventions

- Initiate continuous cardiac monitoring.
- Identify and treat the underlying cause.
- Halt further magnesium intake.
- Administer fluids and diuretics by IV to enhance excretion (if renal function is normal).
- For levels greater than 5 mEq/L, give 5 mL of a 10% calcium chloride solution over 30 seconds. This dose may be repeated. Watch carefully for tissue infiltration.
- Levels greater than or equal to 5 mEq/L usually require hospitalization.
- Consider renal dialysis with a magnesium-free dialysate.
- Monitor electrolyte levels, vital signs, and respiratory and neurologic status over time.

Phosphorus Disturbances

Hypophosphatemia

In human beings, 80% to 85% of the phosphate in the body is contained in the bones and teeth, and 15% to 20% is intracellular. Food products are the main source of phosphate, which is excreted by the kidneys. This ion plays an essential role in cellular structure and function, glycolysis, oxygen delivery, and maintenance of serum calcium levels. Hypophosphatemia is more common in patients with chronic alcohol abuse, diabetes, chronic bowel disease, or severe burns. Phosphorus levels drop when the electrolyte is lost through the intestines or kidneys or when sepsis, respiratory alkalosis, epinephrine administration, or hepatic failure cause intracellular phosphate shifts. In patients with chronic obstructive pulmonary disease or asthma, hypophosphatemia can be a reversible cause of respiratory muscle hypocontractility and impaired tissue oxygenation. Clinical signs appear when serum phosphorus is less than 2 mg/dL and becomes life threatening when levels dip below 1 mg/dL.[10]

Signs and symptoms

Moderate decrease

- Weakness, tremors, muscle pain
- Tingling of the fingers and circumoral area
- Joint stiffness, pain in the bones, fractures
- Anorexia
- Confusion
- Chest pain

Severe decrease

- Hemolytic anemia
- Anisocoria (unequal pupils)

- Impaired oxygen delivery
- Paralysis
- Seizures, coma, death

Therapeutic interventions

- Decrease the intake of substances such as phosphorus-binding antacids.
- In cases of mild to moderate hypophosphatemia, replace phosphorus orally with 1 to 3 g per day by giving skim milk or Neutra-Phos.
- If the condition is severe or the patient is symptomatic, phosphorus replacement by IV is required. *Caution:* Phosphorus replacement by IV can lead to a rapid decrease in serum calcium levels.

Hyperphosphatemia

Hyperphosphatemia is a serum phosphorus level greater than 4.5 mg/100 mL. This electrolyte abnormality is most commonly due to poor renal phosphorus excretion but occasionally is caused by phosphorus moving from the intracellular to the extracellular space as a result of cellular tissue destruction (e.g., rhabdomyolysis). Other causes include endocrine diseases such as acromegaly or hypoparathyroidism and excessive intake of phosphate-containing laxatives or enemas.[10]

Signs and symptoms

- Anorexia, nausea, vomiting
- Pruritus
- Muscle weakness, tetany
- Tachycardia
- Calcium phosphate deposition in the joints, muscles, kidneys, and blood vessels

Therapeutic interventions

- Administer a phosphate-binding agent such as magnesium or a calcium-containing antacid.
- Decrease dietary intake of phosphorus.
- If hyperphosphatemia is severe, dialysis may be required.

Potassium Disturbances

As the primary intracellular ion, potassium is responsible for muscle depolarization and neurologic function.

Hypokalemia

Hypokalemia is defined as a serum potassium level less than 3.5 mEq/L. This condition results from excess potassium excretion in the urine (diuresis) or feces (diarrhea or malabsorption). Additional causes include metabolic alkalosis, insulin therapy, and inadequate potassium intake. Trauma patients may experience short-term hypokalemia because of elevated serum epinephrine levels.[10]

Signs and symptoms

- Fatigue, muscle weakness (mostly noted in the legs), leg cramps
- Nausea, vomiting, anorexia, paralytic ileus
- Polydipsia

- Decreased reflexes, central nervous system irritability, paresthesias, paralysis
- Flattened or inverted T waves, ST segment depression
- Dysrhythmias (premature ventricular contractions, atrial tachycardia, nodal tachycardia, ventricular tachycardia, ventricular fibrillation)
- Hypotension
- Respiratory or cardiac arrest

Therapeutic interventions

- Monitor closely for dysrhythmias; treat as indicated.
- Correct mild hypokalemia with increased dietary potassium or oral supplements.
- Never give potassium intramuscularly.
- Intravenous replacements must be diluted and given slowly; never give a potassium bolus to patients.
- Typically, IV replacement therapy involves 40 mEq of potassium chloride infused over 4 hours (adjusted to actual replacement needs). In emergent situations, as much as 15 mEq/hr can be administered.
- Potassium IV infusion is irritating to the veins. Check peripheral sites frequently and consider giving lidocaine before infusion. Administration through a large vein or a central line improves patient comfort.
- Monitor serum potassium levels and other pertinent electrolytes.
- Measure hourly urine output. Hold supplemental potassium in oliguric patients.
- Consider switching the patient to a potassium-sparing diuretic.
- A coexisting magnesium deficiency makes it more difficult to correct hypokalemia.

Hyperkalemia

Hyperkalemia (serum potassium level >5 mEq/L) may be caused by an insulin deficiency, major crush injuries, electrical burns, extensive thermal burns, severe acidosis, increased potassium intake, Addison's disease, overuse of potassium-containing salt substitutes, or digoxin toxicity.[10]

Signs and symptoms

- Irritability, anxiety
- Muscle weakness (early sign) progressing to paralysis starting in the legs
- Abdominal cramping, hyperactive bowel sounds, diarrhea
- Decreased reflexes
- Paresthesias of the face and hands
- Dysrhythmias
- Tall, tented T waves progressing to a widened QRS complex, a prolonged P-R interval, and then ventricular fibrillation or asystole
- Respiratory and cardiac arrest

Therapeutic interventions

- Identify and treat any underlying causes.
- Several therapeutic options exist for the management of hyperkalemia. The severity of the condition dictates the number of therapies used. Interventions are aimed at increasing excretion and cellular uptake of potassium.
- Slowly administer 10 mL IV of a 10% calcium chloride solution (or 20 mL IV of 10% calcium gluconate). This helps protect cardiac cells from potassium-induced irritability but does not actually decrease potassium levels. Calcium chloride has a rapid onset of action that lasts for 30 to 60 minutes. Calcium chloride is especially useful in hyperkalemic dialysis patients, particularly those in cardiac arrest situations.

- Give nebulized albuterol (Proventil, Ventolin) 2.5 mg mixed with 3 mL isotonic saline over 10 minutes.
- Slowly administer sodium bicarbonate by IV, one to three ampules (44 mEq/ampule), over 20 to 30 minutes. This causes the cells to absorb potassium. The onset of action is immediate and lasts 1 to 2 hours.
- Infuse insulin and glucose by IV. This combination drives potassium intracellularly. Give one ampule of $D_{50}W$ (50 mL) and 10 units of regular insulin. Monitor serum glucose levels and observe the patient closely for hypoglycemia.
- Administer sodium polystyrene sulfonate (Kayexalate), a cation exchange resin, orally or by rectal enema. Onset of action is slow, making this drug a poor choice for the initial treatment of life-threatening hyperkalemia.
- In patients with adequate renal function, administer 40 mg furosemide (Lasix) and normal saline by IV (100 mL/hr) to promote diuresis and potassium loss.
- Institute hemodialysis if potassium levels are life threatening, especially in patients with renal failure who are unable to excrete excess potassium.

Sodium Disturbances

Hyponatremia

A serum sodium level of less than 135 mEq/L is considered hyponatremia. This condition occurs with an actual decrease in the amount of extracellular sodium or an increase in the extracellular fluid volume, resulting in dilutional hyponatremia. Sodium loss can be caused by diuretic use, vomiting, severe burns, lack of dietary sodium, and intracellular sodium shifts. Conditions causing extracellular fluid accumulation include heart failure, hepatic failure, excess ADH secretion, and hyperglycemia.[10]

Signs and symptoms

The severity of clinical findings depends on the serum sodium level and the extent of cerebral cell edema.

Signs and symptoms of hyponatremia include the following:
- Headache
- Tremors
- Cool, clammy skin
- Lethargy, confusion, seizures, coma

Therapeutic interventions
- Identify and treat any underlying cause.
- In conscious patients, begin with conservative therapies such as water restriction and oral sodium replacement.
- Treat hyponatremia cautiously. Aggressive correction is dangerous and is associated with pituitary damage.
- For severe hyponatremia, consider slow IV sodium replacement, with a 3% to 5% saline solution, followed by diuretics to promote water excretion.
- Replace coexisting electrolyte losses.
- Monitor for neurologic changes.
- Severe, symptomatic hyponatremia usually requires intensive care unit admission.

Hypernatremia

Hypernatremia is defined as a serum sodium level greater than 145 mEq/L. This condition can result from an increase in total sodium or a decrease in body water. Fluid decrease is the most common cause. Volume depletion may occur as a result of urinary losses, fever, hyperventilation, water deprivation, diarrhea, or excessive perspiration.

An increased serum sodium level causes water to move from the intracellular space to the extracellular space in an attempt to achieve osmotic equilibrium. The resulting cellular dehydration produces central nervous system depression and (occasionally) intracerebral hemorrhage.[11]

Signs and symptoms

- Thirst
- Fatigue, lethargy, confusion, coma

Therapeutic interventions

- To avoid cerebral edema, treat the underlying condition and slowly restore serum sodium levels to normal.
- If water loss is the cause, begin gradual hypotonic fluid replacement with oral water ingestion or D_5W or a $D_5W/0.45\%$ saline solution by IV.

References

1. Farhat D: Disorders of glucose, *Top Emerg Med* 23(4):27-43, 2001.
2. Cryer P, Childs B: Negotiating the barrier of hypoglycemia in diabetes, *Diabetes Spectrum* 15(1): 20-27, 2002.
3. McCormick M, Quinn L: Treatment of type 2 diabetes mellitus: pharmacologic intervention, *J Cardiovasc Nurs* 16(2):55-67, 2002.
4. American Diabetes Association: Position statement: hyperglycemic crisis in patients with diabetes mellitus, *Diabetes Care* 26(S1):S109-S117, 2003.
5. Cydulka R, Siff J: Diabetes mellitus and disorders of glucose homeostasis. In Marx J, Hockberger R, Walls R, editors: *Rosen's emergency medicine: concepts and clinical practice,* ed 5, St Louis, 2002, Mosby.
6. American Diabetes Association: Insulin administration, *Diabetes Care* 26(Suppl 1):S111-S124, 2003.
7. Eisenbarth G, Polonsky K, Buse J: *Type 1 diabetes mellitus.* In Larson P, Kronenburg H, editors: William's textbook of endocrinology, ed 10, Philadelphia, 2003, Saunders.
8. Umpierrez G, Murphy M, Kitabchi A: Diabetic ketoacidosis and hyperglycemic hyperosmolar syndrome, *Diabetes Spectrum* 15(1):28-36, 2002.
9. Sabatine M: *Pocket medicine,* Philadelphia, 2000, Lippincott.
10. Melmed S et al: *William's textbook of endocrinology,* ed 10, Philadelphia, 2003, Saunders.
11. Kee J, Paulanka B: *Handbook of fluid, electrolyte, and acid-base imbalances,* New York, 2000, Delmar.

27

Alcohol Emergencies

Gwen Barnett, RN

Acute alcohol intoxication and other alcohol-induced problems may culminate in a medical emergency. Acute intoxication and acute withdrawal can be life threatening.

Whenever possible, obtain a thorough history:

1. When was the patient's last drink?
2. How much did the patient drink? (Remember that it is the *amount* of alcohol and not the type that affects blood ethanol level.)
3. How much does the patient usually drink each day? How much each week?
4. When did the patient last eat?
5. Is the patient taking any drugs (over-the-counter, recreational, prescription, or nutritional supplements)? Specifically ask about disulfiram (Antabuse) and metronidazole (Flagyl).
6. Does the patient have any other medical or psychiatric conditions?
7. Did the patient consume only ethanol or were toxic alcohols involved (methanol, isopropanol, or ethylene glycol)?

ACUTE INTOXICATION

Acute intoxication is caused by consumption of a large amount of alcohol over a short period of time. The amount of ethanol required to produce acute intoxication varies widely and depends on the patient's drinking frequency, the amount of food consumed with the alcohol, and the physiologic tolerance of the drinker (Table 27-1). Before determining that a patient is "just drunk," the emergency nurse must identify any other illnesses or injuries contributing to the patient's condition such as head trauma, diabetic ketoacidosis, hypothermia, or drug overdose.[1]

Table **27-1**   **Blood Alcohol Levels and Associated Signs and Symptoms (70-kg Person)**

Percent	Signs and Symptoms
0.05	Few symptoms, particularly in experienced drinkers
0.10	Giddy; decreased muscle coordination; decreased inhibitions
0.15	Decreased sensory awareness; slurred speech; vertigo; ataxia; elevated pulse rate; diaphoresis
0.20	Severely diminished sensory awareness; greatly reduced reaction to stimuli; inability to walk; nausea and vomiting
0.30	Confusion; stupor
0.40	No response to stimuli; decreased deep tendon reflexes; hypotension, tachycardia; cool, clammy, moist skin; seizures
0.50	Death from respiratory arrest caused by inhibition of the medullary respiratory center

Signs and Symptoms

Signs and symptoms of acute intoxication include the following:
- Aspiration (common)
- Decreased muscle coordination
- Dehydration, hypovolemia
- Hypoglycemia
- Hypotension
- Hypothermia or hyperthermia
- Lactic acidosis
- Nausea, vomiting, abdominal pain
- Respiratory depression
- Tachycardia, dysrhythmias

Therapeutic Interventions

Therapeutic interventions for acute intoxication include the following:
- Ensure the patient has a secure airway; aspiration is a major cause of death in the acutely intoxicated. Initial assessment should include airways breathing, circulation (ABCs).
- Administer supplemental oxygen as needed.
- Initiate continuous cardiac monitoring.
- Draw and send laboratory studies: Ethanol level, electrolytes, complete blood count, glucose.
- Obtain fingerstick glucose.
- Warm or cool the patient to maintain normothermia.
- Obtain a chest radiograph to check for aspiration, if indicated.
- Decontaminate the stomach with gastric lavage and administer activated charcoal if indicated for other drug toxicity (not indicated for ethanol because of the rapid absorption of alcohol).
- Control seizures with diazepam (Valium).
- Intravenously infuse 5% dextrose in water, lactated Ringer's solution, or 5% dextrose in normal saline in patients who are hypovolemic or ketotic.
- Give dextrose 50% and thiamine 100 mg to prevent Wernicke-Korsakoff syndrome (Box 27-1).
- In cases of severe intoxication, consider renal dialysis, especially in patients who have ingested toxic alcohols.
- Replace electrolytes as needed.

Box **27-1** Wernicke-Korsakoff Syndrome

Wernicke-Korsakoff syndrome involves two distinct processes. This condition occurs in thiamine-deficient patients if glucose is administered before the patient receives thiamine therapy. Thirty percent to 80% of the alcohol-dependent population has a thiamine deficiency. Symptoms may be permanent but can be reversed partially with thiamine-replacement therapy. Administration of 100 mg of thiamine (per day) to all alcohol intoxicated or withdrawing patients can prevent Wernicke-Korsakoff syndrome.

Wernicke's Encephalopathy

Gait ataxia
Mental confusion
Nystagmus
Ophthalmoplegia

Korsakoff's Syndrome

Confabulation
Mental confusion

ALCOHOLIC SEIZURES

Alcoholic seizures, or "rum fits," are seizures that occur in chronic alcoholics, generally following 8 to 36 hours of abstinence. This condition typically consists of one to three generalized, tonic-clonic seizures over a 6-hour period. A severely decreased blood alcohol level, hypoglycemia, or electrolyte imbalances can precipitate these seizures. Without intervention, patients may progress to delirium tremens.

Therapeutic Interventions

Therapeutic interventions for alcoholic seizures include the following:
- Support and protect the patient's airway, breathing, and circulation.
- Provide supplemental oxygen as needed.
- Monitor arterial blood gases (if indicated).
- Control seizures with benzodiazepines.
- Give dextrose 50% for hypoglycemia
- Administer dextrose, thiamine, and naloxone intravenously (to rule out opioid toxicity).
- Use of anticonvulsants is controversial.

ALCOHOL WITHDRAWAL

In chronic alcoholics, withdrawal will begin 6 to 48 hours after a reduction or cessation of ethanol intake. This condition lasts 2 to 7 days.[2]

Minor Withdrawal

Minor withdrawal begins within 24 hours of cessation or reduction of alcohol consumption.

Signs and symptoms

Signs and symptoms of minor withdrawal include the following:
- Hangover
- Headache
- Insomnia, hyperalertness, irritability, anxiety
- Nausea, vomiting
- Tachycardia, hypertension
- Tremor, mild ataxia

Therapeutic interventions

Therapeutic interventions for minor withdrawal include the following:
- Rest
- Aspirin
- Rehydration

Major Withdrawal

Severe cases of alcohol withdrawal occur in chronic alcoholics 24 hours to 5 days after cessation or reduction of alcohol consumption.

Signs and symptoms

Signs and symptoms of major withdrawal include the following:
- Anorexia, nausea, vomiting
- Anxiety, irritability, disorientation, decreased level of consciousness, delirium, seizures
- Diaphoresis, hyperthermia
- Hallucinations (auditory and visual)
- Slight lateral nystagmus, photophobia
- Tachycardia, hypertension
- Tremor, ataxia, hyperreflexia

Therapeutic interventions

Therapeutic interventions for major withdrawal include the following:
- Support and protect the patient's airway, breathing, and circulation.
- Replace fluids and electrolytes as indicated.
- Administer thiamine and multivitamins intravenously.
- Sedate patients with benzodiazepines (diazepam or lorazepam).
- Give dextrose 50% for hypoglycemia.
- Provide reassurance and reorientation as needed.

DELIRIUM TREMENS

Delirium tremens (DT) occurs after a severe drop in the amount of ethanol consumed by an alcoholic, usually starting on the third day without alcohol. DT is an acute medical emergency. Untreated, this condition is associated with a 10% to 15% mortality. Death typically results from hyperthermia or peripheral vascular collapse.[1]

Signs and Symptoms

Signs and symptoms of delirium tremens include the following:
- Diaphoresis, hyperthermia
- Gross tremors
- Hypotension, tachycardia, dysrhythmias
- Incontinence
- Increasing agitation, confusion, hallucinations (auditory, tactile, and visual)
- Mydriasis (widely dilated pupils)
- Seizures
- Tachypnea

Therapeutic Interventions

Therapeutic interventions for delirium tremens include the following:
- Provide careful airway management.
- Give haloperidol (Haldol).
- Administer chlordiazepoxide (Librium).
- Manage seizures and protect seizing patients by padding gurney rails.
- Rehydrate with fluids intravenously; replace electrolytes as needed.

DISULFIRAM REACTIONS

Disulfiram (Antabuse) is a drug given in some alcohol detoxification programs. This agent is designed to cause an acute, unpleasant, physiologic reaction when taken with foods or medications containing alcohol. This includes cough syrups, fermented vinegar, and even inhaled rubbing alcohol or aftershave.

Signs and Symptoms

Signs and symptoms of disulfiram reaction include the following:
- Chest and abdominal pain
- Conjunctival reddening
- Decreased level of consciousness
- Flushing of the face, chest, and neck
- Headache
- Hypotension
- Perspiration
- Severe nausea and vomiting (begins 5 to 15 minutes following contact with alcohol) that may continue for 6 to 12 days
- Tachycardia, tachypnea
- Vertigo

Therapeutic Interventions

Therapeutic interventions for disulfiram reaction include the following:
- Support and protect the patient's airway, breathing, and circulation.
- Initiate intravenous infusion of normal saline.
- Consider ascorbic acid administration.

- Treat with diphenhydramine (Benadryl) or chlorpheniramine.
- Provide antiemetics as needed.

References

1. Schaider J et al, editors: *Rosen and Barkin's 5-minute emergency medicine consult,* ed 2, Philadelphia, 2003, Lippincott Williams & Wilkins.
2. Lombardo D: Substance abuse. In Newberry L, editor: *Sheehy's emergency nursing: principles and practice,* ed 5, St Louis, 2003, Mosby.

28

Toxicologic Emergencies

Tamara Gentry , RN, BSN

Toxicology is the science of poisons and their effects on living organisms. According to the American Association of Poison Control Centers (AAPCC), in the year 2002 more than 2.3 million toxic exposures were reported nationwide. More than half of these cases involved children under the age of 6. Exposures can be occupational, environmental, recreational, or therapeutic. The vast majority of poisonings are unintentional, relatively mild, and do not require emergency services. Toxic exposures occur through inhalation, ingestion, injection, or contact with skin and mucous membranes. Treatment in a health care facility is required by about 25% of those who contact a poison control center. Only 14% of these are admitted to a critical care unit.[1]

Because most patients with a poison exposure will have no significant problems, it is important to be able to recognize those at greatest risk for serious complications and death. Consider persons in the following categories as "red flag" patients:

- Adults: The older the patient, the more likely to die.
- Pharmaceuticals: Pharmaceutical agents are generally more toxic than are plants, household chemicals, and recreational drugs.
- Polypharmacy: Patients exposed to multiple substances are at increased risk for death.
- Intentional poisonings: Persons who intentionally expose themselves to toxic substances are considerably more likely to suffer adverse events than are those with accidental exposures.
- Altered mental status or other severe symptoms on presentation: Patients who are already significantly compromised on emergency department arrival are more likely to have a poor outcome.

Table 28-1 lists diagnostic clues for identifying unknown toxins.
Obtain an exposure history:

- To what substance or substances was the patient exposed?
- When did the exposure occur? Is this an acute or chronic exposure?

Table 28-1   Diagnostic Clues in Unknown Exposures

Metabolic Acidosis (MUDPILES)	Radiopaque Medications (CHIPE)	Breath Odor
Methanol	Chloral hydrate	**Alcohol:** ethanol, chloral hydrate, phenols
Uremia	Heavy metals	**Acetone:** acetone, salicylates, isopropyl alcohol
Diabetic ketoacidosis	Iron	**Bitter almond:** cyanide
Paraldehyde	Phenothiazines	**Coal gas:** carbon monoxide
Isoniazid, iron	Enteric-coated tablets	**Garlic:** arsenic, phosphorus, organophosphates
Lactic acidosis		**Nonspecific:** Consider inhalant abuse.
Ethanol, ethylene glycol		**Oil of wintergreen:** methylsalicylates
Salicylates, sympathomimetics		

Urine Color

Red: hematuria, hemoglobinuria, myoglobinuria, pyrvinium (Vanquin), phenytoin (Dilantin), phenothiazines, mercury, lead, anthocyanin (a food pigment found in beets and blackberries)
Brown-black: hemoglobin pigments, melanin, methyldopa (Aldomet), cascara, rhubarb, methocarbamol (Robaxin)
Blue/blue-green: amitriptyline (Elavil), methylene blue, triamterene (Dyazide), Clorets gum, *Pseudomonas*
Brown/red-brown: Porphyria, urobilinogen, nitrofurantoin (Macrodantin), furazolidone (Furadantin), metronidazole (Flagyl), aloe, seaweed
Orange: rifampin, phenazopyridine (Pyridium), sulfasalazine (Azulfidine)

From Dart R et al, editors: *The 5 minute toxicology consult*, Philadelphia, 2000, Lippincott Williams & Wilkins.

- What was the route of exposure?
- Are there currently any signs or symptoms of poisoning?
- How much of the substance is involved?
- Was the exposure accidental or intentional?
- Does the patient have a history of toxic exposures?
- What treatment was rendered before arrival of emergency medical services?
- How old is the patient?
- What is the patient's medical history (especially cardiac, hepatic, psychiatric, and renal disorders)?
- Are there any psychological, social, or environmental risk factors involved?
  Treatment goals for the poisoned patient are as follows:
- Limit further absorption.
- Enhance excretion.
- Administer the appropriate antidote (if one is available).
- Give basic and advanced supportive care (physiologic and psychological) as needed.
- Provide education to patients, families, and significant others to prevent future incidents.
  Basic and advanced supportive care for toxic exposure patients include the following:
- Support the patient's airway, breathing, and circulation; airway protection is critical in patients with an altered mental status.
- Provide supplemental oxygen as needed.
- Establish intravenous access and infuse lactated Ringer's solution or normal saline solution.
- Give naloxone (Narcan) 0.4 to 2 mg intravenously (IV), endotracheally, intramuscularly, subcutaneously, intraosseously, or sublingually if the patient has a potential opioid exposure.
- Check a blood glucose level, and infuse dextrose 50% at 50 mL (25 g) IV as needed to maintain normoglycemia.

- Administer 50 to 100 mg thiamine IV to patients with suspected chronic alcohol abuse.
- Initiate continuous cardiac monitoring and obtain 12-lead electrocardiograms as indicated.
- Monitor urinary output.
- Draw arterial blood gases as indicated.
- Serial monitoring of electrolyte levels, vital signs, and respiratory, cardiac, and neurologic status.

POISON INFORMATION

The science of toxicology is evolving rapidly, and practices routinely change as better interventions are identified. Because it is difficult for individual practitioners to keep current, poison control centers have assumed a vital role in the identification and management of toxic emergencies. Poison control centers are located throughout the United States. Poison control center experts help clinicians assess patients and can suggest current management practices. These centers have access to POISINDEX and other toxocology databases that are updated regularly. Poison center contact should be made (by an emergency department physician or nurse) for each poisoned patient (Box 28-1). This allows poison control centers to track patients and gather demographic and statistical information.

THERAPEUTIC INTERVENTIONS FOR POISONINGS AND OVERDOSES

Gastrointestinal Decontamination

Decontamination of the digestive system can be done in several ways, including by induced emesis; gastric lavage; administration of activated charcoal, multiple doses of activated charcoal cathartics; and whole-bowel irrigation.

Induced emesis

Although once a mainstay of care, the role of syrup of ipecac in the management of the poisoned patient has significantly decreased in recent years. The AAPCC reports that syrup of ipecac was used in only 0.6% of poisonings in 2002, down from over 13% in 1983.[1] In their 1997 position paper, the American Academy of Clinical Toxicology and the European Association of Poison Centres and Clinical Toxicologists ("the Academy") stated unequivocally that "there is no evidence from clinical studies that ipecac improves the outcome of poisoned patients and its routine administration ... should be abandoned."[2] Syrup of ipecac is only marginally effective at emptying the stomach, its use is associated with numerous contraindications and complications, and emesis can delay charcoal administration significantly. Nonetheless, this drug still is being given by some emergency medical services systems and hospitals throughout the United States. Table 28-2 gives syrup of ipecac dosages.

Box **28-1** **Nationwide Poison Control Center Phone Number**

1-800-222-1222

Table **28-2**   **Syrup of Ipecac Dosages**

Age	Ipecac	Follow with Fluids
1 year old	10 mL	15 mL/kg
1 to 12 years old	15 mL	4 to 6 oz
>12 years old	30 mL	6 to 8 oz

Gastric lavage

Gastric lavage is moderately more effective than ipecac-induced emesis for the removal of ingested substances if a large-bore (Ewald) tube is used along with adequate fluid volumes and frequent repositioning. Lavage has the additional advantage of allowing the instillation of activated charcoal without delay. However, the Academy's position is that "gastric lavage should not be employed routinely in the management of poisoned patients ... There is no certain evidence that its use improves ... outcome and it may cause significant morbidity."[3] Although there is a paucity of data that support this technique, gastric lavage theoretically may benefit the following patient populations:
• Symptomatic patients who present within 1 hour of ingestion.
• Symptomatic patients who have ingested an agent that slows gastrointestinal motility.
• Patients who have ingested a sustained-release medication.
• Patients who have taken massive or life-threatening amounts of a substance.

Like induced emesis, to be of any benefit, gastric lavage should be initiated within 1 hour of ingestion. Complications of this procedure include accidental tracheal intubation, aspiration, decreased oxygenation during the procedure, and stomach or esophageal perforation.

To perform gastric lavage, do the following:
1. Protect the patient's airway.
    a. Intubate the patient's trachea before lavage if there is central nervous system (CNS) depression or an absent gag reflex.
    b. Have suction readily available.
2. Select the proper size of gastric tube. The tube must be large enough for whole pills and pill clumps to be removed.
    a. *Adults:* Use a 36 to 40 French Ewald tube, inserted via the oral route.
    b. *Children:* Use a 24 to 32 French tube (provided it is large enough for the ingested pills to pass easily).
3. Lubricate the tube with a water-soluble lubricant.
4. Have cooperative patients sit upright and take sips of water while swallowing the tube.
5. Advance the tube to the stomach.
6. Auscultate over the epigastrium while forcing air into the tube to confirm gastric placement.
7. Secure the tube with tape.
8. Place the patient in a left lateral position with the head dependent (if there are no contraindications to this position).
9. Lavage with warmed tap water or normal saline solution (adults, 150 to 200 mL; children, 10 mL/kg).
10. Allow the fluid to return by gravity or suction.
11. Repeat the lavage process only until the returned fluid is clear. Prolonged lavage can result in electrolyte disturbances.
12. Send a sample of the gastric aspirate and any pill fragments to the laboratory for analysis if the ingested substance is unknown.

Box **28-2** **Substances** *Not* **Absorbed by Activated Charcoal**

Caustics
Heavy metals (lead, zinc, mercury)
Hydrocarbons
Iron preparations
Lithium
Toxic alcohols

Data from Criddle L: Toxicologic emergencies. In Newberry L, editor: *Sheehy's emergency nursing: principles and practice,* ed 5, St Louis, 2003, Mosby.

13. Instill activated charcoal (as ordered) and then remove the tube. Lavage tubes are uncomfortable and they stimulate the gag reflex. If continued gastric access is necessary (e.g., for repeated charcoal doses) insert a standard oral or nasal gastric tube.

Activated charcoal

Over the last decade, extensive research has indicated that the use of activated charcoal alone is equivalent or even superior to other poisoning treatment modalities and combinations. Given by mouth or gastric tube, activated charcoal has the advantage of being minimally invasive and easy to administer, and it can be given safely to children and adults. Activated charcoal absorbs and binds most commonly ingested substances. Despite these benefits the Academy's position on activated charcoal is that "single-dose activated charcoal should not be administered routinely ... [it] may be considered if a patient has ingested a potentially toxic amount of a poison (which is known to be adsorbed by charcoal) up to 1 hour previously."[4]

The sole use of activated charcoal for gastric decontamination has not achieved universal acceptance, and many institutions still combine activated charcoal with gastric emptying procedures. Cases of adverse events associated with activated charcoal administration (primarily aspiration) are few, but their prevalence is increasing as the use of activated charcoal grows.

Specific contraindications to use of activated charcoal include the following:
- Ingestion of a corrosive agent
- Decreased or absent bowel sounds (relative contraindication)
- Toxins not bound by charcoal (Box 28-2).[5]

Recommendations for the administration of activated charcoal are as follows:
- Activated charcoal should not be administered until ipecac-induced emesis has subsided (usually 60 to 90 minutes after the patient last vomited).
- Alert, cooperative patients can drink activated charcoal through a straw.
- Activated charcoal is gritty but not particularly unpleasant tasting. Flavoring (e.g., cherry syrup or chocolate syrup) makes the charcoal more palatable and does not decrease its effectiveness.
- Small, intermittent doses may reduce vomiting.
- Shake the activated charcoal mixture (slurry) thoroughly to eliminate clumping.
- More dilute slurries are easier to drink or pass through a gastric tube, particularly tiny pediatric tubes.
- In patients with an altered mental status, aggressively protect the airway (tracheal intubation) before administration of activated charcoal. Visualization of the epiglottis is difficult *after* activated charcoal has been vomited. Aggressive suctioning of aspirated charcoal appears to improve patient outcome.
- A standard-sized Salem sump tube is adequate for activated charcoal instillation.

Box **28-3** **Indications for Multiple-Dose Activated Charcoal**

Evidence-Based	Frequently Used
Carbamazepine	Digoxin
Dapsone	Phenytoin
Phenobarbital	Salicylates
Quinine	Sustained-release preparations
Theophylline	Tricyclic antidepressants

- Securely anchor gastric tubes to prevent retraction from the stomach to the esophagus.
- Reconfirm appropriate gastric tube placement immediately before administration of activated charcoal.

Multiple-dose activated charcoal

For a few poisonings, multiple dose ("multi-dose" or "repeated dose") activated charcoal has been shown to enhance total body clearance and drug elimination. The Academy's position is that "multiple-dose activated charcoal should be considered only if a patient has ingested a life-threatening amount of dapsone, carbamazepine, phenobarbital, quinine, or theophylline."[6] Nonetheless, multidose activated charcoal commonly is used for other susbstances as well (Box 28-3).

When multiple doses of activated charcoal are indicated, repeat activated charcoal administration every 2 to 6 hours. Give adults 20 to 50 g; children should receive half that amount. Studies have indicated that gastric suctioning before repeating an activated charcoal dose helps avoid gastric distention.

Cathartics

Cathartics such as magnesium sulfate, magnesium citrate, sodium citrate, or sorbitol have long been added to activated charcoal to enhance gastrointestinal elimination of poisons. However, overuse of cathartics causes diarrhea, nausea and vomiting, abdominal pain, increased magnesium levels, electrolyte imbalances, and hypovolemia. Cathartics should not be given if bowel sounds are absent. Never administer cathartics to children less than 1 year of age; cases of fatal diarrhea have been reported in this population. The Academy maintains that "based on available data, the routine use of a cathartic in combination with activated charcoal is not endorsed. If a cathartic is used, it should be limited to a single dose in order to minimize adverse effects."[7] To reduce the emetic effect, consider delaying sorbitol administration until drug-induced vomiting has subsided.

Whole-bowel irrigation

Whole-bowel irrigation (WBI) involves the use of an electrolyte solution (GoLYTELY, Colyte) administered orally or by gastric tube at a rate of about 2 L/hr until the bowel is purged. Whole-bowel irrigation produces a rapid catharsis, eliminating most matter from the gastrointestinal tract within a few hours. Whole-bowel irrigation most commonly is given following ingestion of an agent that is not well adsorbed by activated charcoal, such as iron, lead, lithium, or zinc. This therapy also has been used to remove time-released drugs and other poisons with delayed absorption. Swallowed button batteries and cocaine-filled condoms also can been removed by whole-bowel irrigation.

Box **28-4**   Poisons That Respond to Hemodialysis

Acetaminophen	Ethylene glycol	Potassium
Alcohols	Isoniazid	Quinidine
Amphetamine	Meprobamate	Quinine
Antibiotics	Methanol	Salicylate
Arsenic	Paraldehyde	Strychnine
Chloral hydrate	Phenacetin	Sulfonamide
Ergotamine	Phenytoin	Theophylline

Data from Criddle L: Toxicologic emergencies. In Newberry L, editor: *Sheehy's emergency nursing: principles and practice,* ed 5, St Louis, 2003, Mosby.

Box **28-5**   Poisons That Respond to Charcoal Hemoperfusion

Digitalis
Paraquat
Phenobarbital
Tegretol
Theophylline

The Academy's position is that "there is no conclusive evidence that WBI improves the outcome of the poisoned patient ... [but] WBI may be considered for potentially toxic ingestions of sustained-release or enteric-coated drugs."[8] Do not initiate whole-bowel irrigation in patients who lack bowel sounds, have a possible bowel obstruction, or already have diarrhea.

Hemodialysis and Charcoal Hemoperfusion

Hemodialysis is indicated for certain serious poisonings associated with severe metabolic acidosis, electrolyte abnormalities, or renal failure. Peritoneal dialysis also can be used for short-term treatment. Box 28-4 lists dialyzable substances.[5]

Dialysis is *not* indicated for the following:
- For ingestion of substances that are highly protein bound
- When the agent is rarely lethal or an effective antidote exists
- If the patient is too hemodynamically unstable
- In patients with poor vascular access
- In small children

Similar to hemodialysis, charcoal hemoperfusion is an extracorporeal technique that involves filtering blood through a cartridge containing activated charcoal. However, charcoal hemoperfusion is performed infrequently, and there are only a handful of substances for which hemoperfusion is indicated (Box 28-5). Extracorporeal membrane oxygenation and liver dialysis are two other highly invasive interventions occasionally used to manage serious poisonings.

Prevention and Education

Since its passage in 1970, the Poison Prevention Act has succeeded in reducing the number of pediatric exposures and poison-related deaths. This legislation mandated child-resistant caps on toxic substances. Nonetheless, child-resistant containers are not a substitute for prevention education or aggressive poison-proofing of homes frequented by young children. Recently, denatonium benzoate (Bitrex), a taste-aversive agent, has been added to many household products to dissuade children from drinking toxic quantities. Expanding the use of this product to an even greater number of poisonous agents could decrease pediatric morbidity and mortality even further.

Abuse of alcohol and other recreational drugs has skyrocketed. Campaigns such as the ENCARE program of the Emergency Nurses Association provide injury prevention education designed to increase public awareness of the tragedies associated with alcohol and drug use. Emergency nurses are in an excellent position to teach patients and communities about proper medication use, safe storage of toxins, and the risks associated with recreational substance abuse.

SPECIFIC TOXICOLOGIC EMERGENCIES

Analgesics

The nonprescription analgesics acetaminophen, aspirin, and ibuprofen account for more calls to poison control centers than any other class of substances. These medications come in a variety of strengths, colors, sizes, and combinations, making dosing errors common in even by persons with the best of intentions. Complacency and easy availability add to the high incidence of exposures.

Acetaminophen

Acetaminophen, a metabolite of phenacetin, is consistently the leading cause of poisoning deaths in the United States. This drug is found in varying quantities in more than 200 miscellaneous remedies for pain, sleep, coughs, and colds. According to the Toxic Exposure Surveillance System, in the year 2003, acetaminophen was involved in 19% of poisoning fatalities.[9]

The toxic metabolites of acetaminophen destroy hepatocytes, resulting in hepatic necrosis and massive liver damage. Hepatotoxicity is seen following ingestion of greater than 140 mg/kg. Patients with a history of alcohol abuse or other liver disease are at increased risk for acetaminophen toxicity.

Signs and symptoms

Initial Stage (0 to 24 hours after ingestion)

- Symptoms may be mild or absent in the early phase, even in significantly toxic individuals.
- Gastrointestinal irritation (nausea, vomiting, anorexia)
- Lethargy, malaise
- Diaphoresis, pallor
- In rare cases of massive poisoning (4 hour blood level greater than 800 mg/L), metabolic acidosis and coma can develop within the first 24 hours.

Dormant Stage (24-48 hours after ingestion)

- This is a relatively symptom-free stage of toxicity. Gastrointestinal distress tends to subside, and hepatic failure is not yet significant enough to produce overt findings.
- Even though the patient is asymptomatic, liver failure has begun. Tests of hepatic function—aspartate transaminase (glutamic-oxaloacetic transaminase), alanine

transaminase (glutamic-pyruvic transaminase), bilirubin, and prothrombin time—show abnormal results.
- Right upper quadrant pain may be present.

Hepatic Stage (48 to 96 hours after ingestion)
- Progressive hepatic encephalopathy develops, characterized by confusion, lethargy, and coma.
- Vomiting
- Jaundice
- Significant right upper quadrant pain
- Bleeding disorders
- Hypoglycemia
- Transient elevation of liver enzymes
- Renal damage

Therapeutic interventions
- Provide basic and advanced supportive care as indicated.
- Obtain baseline liver enzymes, prothrombin time, blood urea nitrogen, and blood glucose levels.
- Consider gastric lavage if the ingestion was recent and the dose was greater than 7.5 g (greater than 140 mg/kg in a child).
- Administer activated charcoal.
- Consult your regional poison control center
- Draw a quantitative acetaminophen level 4 hours from the time of (acute) ingestion and plot the results on a Rumack-Matthew nomogram. Serum levels drawn before 4 hours have no clinical value.
- If the patient's plasma level falls within the toxic range of the nomogram, administer the antidote *N*-acetylcysteine (Mucomyst).[10]
  - For best results, initiate therapy within 10 hours of acetaminophen ingestion. However, *N*-acetylcysteine is still effective when started up to 24 hours after poisoning.
  - For the *N*-acetylcysteine loading dose, give 140 mg/kg orally (5% solution) mixed in a carbonated soft drink, orange juice, or grapefruit juice to mask the unpleasant taste. *N*-acetylcysteine also can be given via a gastric tube.
  - For the *N*-acetylcysteine maintenance dose, give 70 mg/kg orally every 4 hours for a total of 17 doses.
  - Typically, treatment is not considered complete until all 17 doses have been given, but alternate dosing regimens occasionally are used, particularly in pediatric patients.
  - If the patient is vomiting, give metoclopramide (Reglan). Insert a gastric tube and instill *N*-acetylcysteine in slowly. If any dose is vomited within 1 hour of administration, the dose should be repeated.
- Intravenously administered *N*-acetylcysteine has been used off label in many medical centers for years. Intravenous administration is now approved by the Food and Drug Administration. Loading and maintenance doses are the same as those used for orally administered *N*-acetylcysteine. Generally, only 12 doses are given.
- Liver dialysis and liver transplant have been used in the management of severe acetaminophen toxicity.

Salicylates

With the emergence of other over-the-counter analgesics, the number of salicylate poisonings has decreased over the last 2 decades. Nonetheless, according to the AAPCC, there are more than 20,000 cases annually. An estimated 61% of these cases are treated in health care facilities.[9] Aspirin (and other salicylates) interfere with a variety of organ systems. The half-life of aspirin is long, and the generally accepted toxic dose is 150 mg/kg. Salicylates stimulate the respiratory center, producing respiratory alkalosis, along with a compensatory renal loss of bicarbonate. These agents also interfere with lipid and carbohydrate metabolism, creating a concurrent metabolic acidosis. This combination of respiratory alkalosis and metabolic acidosis is the hallmark of salicylate toxicity.

Signs and symptoms

Mild to Moderate Toxicity (150 to 300 mg/kg)

- Tachypnea, hypernea
- Nausea, vomiting, abdominal pain
- Diaphoresis, fever, dehydration
- Tachycardia
- Tinnitus
- Hypoglycemia, electrolyte imbalances

Severe Toxicity (greater than 300 mg/kg)

- Altered mental status, seizures
- Noncardiogenic pulmonary edema
- Hemorrhagic gastritis
- Coagulation abnormalities

Therapeutic interventions

- Provide basic and advanced supportive care as indicated.
- Tracheal intubation may be necessary.
- Gastric emptying still can be effective several hours following ingestion if the patient consumed enteric-coated pills.
- Activated charcoal has a high affinity for aspirin. Multidose charcoal may be effective.
- Repeat salicylate level measurements every 6 to 12 hours.
- Alkalize the urine by adding sodium bicarbonate to IV fluids (e.g., three ampules of sodium bicarbonate added to 1 L of 5% dextrose in water and infused at 200 mL/hr).
- Correct fluid and electrolyte imbalances (these may be profound).
- Provide conventional treatment for hypoglycemia, seizures, and pulmonary edema.
- Hyperthermia usually subsides with rehydration and external cooling.
- Hemodialysis is indicated in cases of severe poisoning and in patients with renal failure. Hemodialysis can correct fluid and electrolyte disturbances and remove salicylates from the blood.

Nonsteroidal antiinflammatory drugs

Since introduction of nonsteroidal antiinflammatory drugs (NSAIDs) for nonprescription use in 1984, their use has skyrocketed. In addition to over-the-counter sales, an estimated 35 to 70 million NSAID prescriptions are written annually. Fortunately, the toxicity of these agents is low, and only 38 deaths were reported between 1997 and 2000.[11] Ibuprofen (Motrin, Advil), the most popular NSAID, has a short half-life and is absorbed and eliminated rapidly. Acute ingestion of less than 100 mg/kg is regarded as nontoxic. Ingestions of more than 300 mg/kg are considered severe. Ibuprofen has a high safety profile compared with the incidence of death associated with acetaminophen and aspirin.

Signs and symptoms
- Drowsiness, lethargy, seizures (particularly in children who ingest more than 400 mg/kg)
- Gastrointestinal irritation
- Hypotension, bradycardia
- Renal failure, hepatotoxicity
- Apnea
- Metabolic acidosis

Therapeutic interventions
- Provide basic and advanced supportive care as indicated.
- Monitor the cardiac rhythm continuously in patients with significant overdoses.
- Serum NSAID levels are not clinically useful.
- Consider gastric lavage if the ingestion was recent and involved a large dose.
- Administer activated charcoal.
- Institute seizure precautions.

Common Prescription Medications

Calcium channel blockers

Patients with toxic levels of calcium channel blockers, primarily verapamil (Calan, Isoptin) and diltiazem (Cardizem, Dilacor), present a unique and problematic profile. Because of the sustained-release nature of many of these agents, onset of toxicity may be late, characterized by waxing and waning deterioration. Death frequently occurs more than 24 hours after the overdose.[12] Symptoms are rapid in their progression and are resistant to conventional therapies.

As implied by their name, calcium channel blockers prevent the influx of calcium through the slow calcium channels in cardiac and vascular smooth muscle. They prolong the refractory period and depress impulses conduction, thereby reducing heart rate. Drugs in this class produce a variety of negative chronotropic, dromotropic, and inotropic effects. Calcium channel blockers are metabolized by the liver and are extensively protein-bound and therefore not dialyzable.

Signs and symptoms
- Hypotension
- Cardiac disturbances, especially conduction abnormalities, atrioventricular blocks, and bradycardia
- Confusion, altered mental status, syncope, seizures, coma
- Nausea, vomiting
- Dysrhythmias, congestive heart failure
- Hyperglycemia, lactic acidosis

Therapeutic interventions
- Provide basic and advanced supportive care as indicated.
- Administer crystalloids such as normal saline (0.9%) or lactated Ringer's solution.
- Monitoring cardiac rhythm continuously. Obtain a 12-lead electrocardiogram.
- Quantitative drug levels are of little value in the management of acute toxicity.
- Consider gastric lavage if ingestion was recent.
- Administer activated charcoal.
- Whole-bowel irrigation can be used for significant ingestion of sustained-release products.
- Institute cardiac pacing as needed for atrioventricular blocks and bradycardia.

- Several drugs are used to manage calcium channel blocker overdose.[10] Treat patients symptomatically.
  - *Calcium:* Increases the concentration gradient in the serum, thereby reducing intracellular calcium flow. This treatment is effective in small or therapeutic overdoses but is relatively ineffective in massive overdoses.
  - *Atropine:* Useful for the treatment of sinoatrial node bradycardia but will not reverse bradycardia caused by atrioventricular blocks (pace the patient).
  - *Glucagon:* Glucagon is an antidote for drugs that reduce intracellular calcium. Administration may reverse myocardial depression in cases of intractable bradycardia.
  - *Catecholamines:* Treat hypotension with fluids, dopamine, or norepinephrine.
  - Some research suggests that insulin and glucose administration increases myocardial carbohydrate metabolism and contractility in calcium channel blocker overdose.
- Charcoal hemoperfusion has been used in children with calcium channel blocker toxicity.

Tricyclic antidepressants

Tricyclic antidepressants (TCAs) are the second most frequent cause of poisoning deaths in the United States, and 60% of these overdoses are intentional.[11] Onset of action is rapid and symptoms may peak as soon as 60 minutes after ingestion. TCAs are highly protein bound and lipid soluble. This results in falsely low serum levels, poor hemodialyzability, and a long elimination half-life. The three pharmacologic features responsible for the toxic manifestations most commonly observed in tricyclic antidepressant overdose are the following:

- *Cardiotoxicity:* Decreased cardiac conduction results. (This is the most clinically significant effect.)
- *Adrenergic compromise:* Alpha-adrenergic stimulation is blocked, and catecholamines are depleted.
- *Anticholinergic activity:* Although prominent, anticholinergic symptoms have little impact on morbidity and mortality.

Signs and symptoms

- Anticholinergic effects (Box 28-6)
- Nausea, vomiting
- Tachydysrhythmias, prolonged P-R interval, QRS complex widening, heart blocks, asystole
- Hypotension
- Syncope, seizures, coma (Central nervous system deterioration can progress quickly.)

Box **28-6** **The Anticholinergic Toxidrome: Common Signs and Symptoms**

Peripheral Anticholinergic Effects	Central Nervous System Effects
Blurred vision	Anxiety
Decreased bowel motility	Confusion
Dilated pupils	Delirium
Dry mouth	Disorientation
Dry skin	Hallucinations
Fever	Impaired recent memory
Flushed skin	Incoherent speech
Increased heart rate	Paranoia
Reduced secretions	Purposeless movements
Urinary retention	

Therapeutic interventions

- Provide basic and advanced supportive care as indicated.
- Serum tricyclic antidepressant levels are not clinically useful in overdose situations.[10]
- Institute gastric lavage. Tracheal intubation is usually advisable before lavage because of the rapid onset of toxic symptoms.
- Consider giving multiple doses of activated charcoal (first check for the presence of an ileus).
- Administer a cathartic agent to counteract drug-induced decreased bowel motility.
- Monitor continuously for cardiac dysrhythmias; these can be severe and lethal.
- Give sodium bicarbonate by IV. Mild alkalosis reduces the incidence of dysrhythmias. Keep serum pH at 7.5.
- If dysrhythmias do not respond to sodium bicarbonate therapy alone, treat with lidocaine or phenytoin (Dilantin) by IV.
- Manage hypotension with isotonic fluids and dopamine or norepinephrine (Levophed) as needed.
- Administer diazepam (Valium) or lorazepam (Ativan) by IV for seizures.

Digoxin

Digitalis is prescribed for the treatment of congestive heart failure. Digitalis also is given to reduce ventricular response rates in certain supraventricular tachycardias. Digitalis works by slowing atrioventricular nodal conduction and augmenting contractility (positive inotropic effect). The concurrent use of other cardiac drugs and diuretics or the presence of hypokalemia can increase the incidence of mild toxicity in patients receiving therapeutic doses. Following acute ingestion, symptoms can peak in as little as 30 minutes or up to 12 hours later. Almost 3000 toxic exposures were reported to the AAPCC in 2001. Of these, 652 patients suffered moderate or major morbidity and 13 died.[13]

Signs and symptoms

Box 28-7 summarizes the signs and symptoms of digitalis toxicity.

Therapeutic interventions

- Provide basic and advanced supportive care as indicated.
- Discontinue all digoxin-containing preparations and diuretics.

Box **28-7** **Signs and Symptoms of Digitalis Toxicity**

Mild Toxicity	Severe Toxicity
Anorexia	Blurred vision
Bradycardia	Delirium
Confusion	Diarrhea
Headache	Disorientation
Malaise	Hallucinations
Nausea and vomiting	Sinoatrial or atrioventricular block
Premature ventricular contractions	Ventricular fibrillation
Visual disturbances	Ventricular tachycardia

- Obtain a quantitative serum digoxin level immediately and 6 hours after acute ingestion. Further digoxin levels are of no value.
- Administer activated charcoal.
- Correct electrolyte imbalances, hypoglycemia, and hypovolemia.
- Give atropine or use cardiac pacing for bradycardia.
- Administer digoxin immune Fab (Digibind), the digitalis antidote.[13]

Indications

- Severe dysrhythmias unresponsive to treatment
- Large ingestions in previously healthy individuals (adults, 10 mg; children, 4 mg)
- Digoxin levels in excess of 10 ng/mL
- Hyperkalemia (>5.5 mEq/L)

Precautions

- Digibind has an excellent safety profile, but allergic reactions are possible.
- Check for precipitous drops in potassium levels.
- Monitor for new onset dysrhythmias and symptoms of congestive heart failure in patients who have been taking digoxin therapeutically.

Benzodiazepines

Benzodiazepines are administered for anxiety, sedation, seizures, and muscle relaxation. Commonly prescribed agents in this class are diazepam (Valium), alprazolam (Xanax), triazolam (Halcion), lorazepam (Ativan), temazepam (Restoril), clorazepate (Tranxene), chlordiazepoxide (Librium), midazolam (Versed), and flurazepam (Dalmane). Designed to depress the CNS, these drugs also can cause hypotension and respiratory suppression in overdose quantities. Fortunately, mortality related to these substances is low. Death usually involves coingestion of another CNS depressant such as ethanol.

Signs and symptoms

- Drunken behavior without the odor of alcohol, slurred speech, impaired memory, or coma
- Respiratory depression
- Dilated pupils
- Weak and rapid pulse

Therapeutic interventions

- Provide basic and advanced supportive care as indicated.
- Monitor closely for respiratory and CNS depression.
- Administer dextrose 50%, thiamine, and naloxone by IV to rule out other causes of CNS depression.
- Do not induce emesis because of CNS depression.
- Consider gastric lavage if the amount ingested was large or was combined with other medicines.
- Give activated charcoal.
- With supportive care (possibly including mechanical ventilation), benzodiazepine overdoses generally self-resolve.
- Administer flumazenil (Romazicon), a specific antidote for benzodiazepine reversal.[10]

Indications
- Acute benzodiazepine toxicity with profound sedation, respiratory depression, or coma

Precautions
- Do not give flumazenil to patients who have also ingested a tricyclic antidepressant, cocaine, or other seizure-inducing agent.
- Do not give flumazenil to chronic benzodiazepine users. This can precipitate seizures.
- Watch for resedation 30 to 60 minutes after flumazenil administration.

Environmental Poisons

In the course of a day we all come into contact with a variety of substances with potentially toxic effects. In the home, plants, personal care products, and cleaning agents are responsible for the largest number of poison control center calls. The Occupational Safety and Health Administration (OSHA) places strict safeguards on the labeling, handling, disposal, and use of toxic substances in the workplace. Yet even with stringent guidelines, occupational exposures occur regularly.

Carbon monoxide

Carbon monoxide is emitted in the process of combustion. All fossil fuels (e.g., coal, gasoline, and natural gas) emit carbon monoxide as they burn. Carbon monoxide released from wood and other materials in house fires is the principal cause of death from smoke inhalation. Improperly vented hot water heaters, stoves, furnaces, and automobiles are also sources of carbon monoxide.

Tissue hypoxia and direct cellular toxicity are responsible for the clinical manifestations of carbon monoxide poisoning. When inhaled, carbon monoxide binds to hemoglobin molecules, forming carboxyhemoglobin (COHgb or COHb) and displacing oxygen. When carbon monoxide ties up hemoglobin binding sites, oxygen cannot attach and oxygen delivery to the tissues is severely limited. Additionally, carbon monoxide causes the oxyhemoglobin dissociation curve to shift to the left, further reducing tissue oxygen availability. On room air the half-life of COHgb is about 5 hours. The organs with the greatest sensitivity to hypoxia—the CNS and the cardiovascular system—are affected most. Children and persons with cardiac and pulmonary disorders are at greatest risk. Fetal COHgb levels rise more slowly than maternal levels but remain elevated for a longer period of time.

Signs and symptoms
Mild (COHgb Level 10% to 20%)
- Nausea, vomiting
- Mild, throbbing headache
- Malaise, flulike symptoms
- Carbon monoxide toxicity should be considered in purported outbreaks of food poisoning.

Moderate (COHgb Level 20% to 30%)
- Symptoms associated with mild toxicity increase
- Dyspnea with minimal exertion
- Exacerbation of underlying coronary artery disease
- Dizziness, confusion, agitation

Severe (COHgb Level 30% to 50%)

- Seizures, coma
- Respiratory failure
- Dysrhythmias, hypotension

Therapeutic interventions

- Remove the patient from the contaminated area.
- Give 100% oxygen by tight-fitting face mask or positive pressure; significantly reduces half-life.
- Provide basic and advanced supportive care as indicated.
- Begin continuous cardiac monitoring.
- Caution: Pulse oximeter readings will be elevated falsely. Instead, draw and follow measured arterial oxygen saturation levels.
- Draw a COHgb level (venous or arterial blood). However, COHgb levels are only a guide and may not correlate with the severity of poisoning, particularly in cases of chronic exposure.
- Infuse isotonic crystalloids for hypotension. Add a vasopressor if needed.
- Give benzodiazepines by IV for seizures.
- Treat myocardial ischemia in the standard manner.
- Consider early hyperbaric oxygen therapy for any patient with moderate or severe symptoms. Hyperbaric oxygen therapy can reduce the half-life of carbon monoxide 4 to 5 times more rapidly than normobaric oxygen.
- Indications for hyperbaric oxygen therapy include COHgb levels greater than 25%, altered mental status, pregnancy, and exacerbation of symptoms in patients with cardiac or pulmonary disease.

Cyanide

Cyanide poisonings occur as a result of occupational exposures, suicidal or homicidal ingestions, and smoke inhalation (from plastics fumes). Many "herbal" remedies contain cyanide, and hospitalized patients on continuous nitroprusside infusions also can experience cyanide toxicity after several days of therapy.

Signs and symptoms

- Tachycardia, bradycardia, asystole
- Hypotension, cardiovascular collapse
- Headache, drowsiness, seizures, coma
- Tachypnea, hyperpnea, apnea

Therapeutic interventions

- Remove the patient from the source of the exposure.
- Give 100% oxygen by tight-fitting face mask or positive pressure.
- Provide basic and advanced supportive care as indicated.
- Begin continuous cardiac monitoring.
- Administer benzodiazepines for seizure activity.
- For ingestions, gastric lavage and activated charcoal are recommended.
- For topical exposures, irrigate the area with copious amounts of water.
- In patients with serious clinical symptoms, administer cyanide antidotes as soon as possible:
  - One ampule of amyl nitrate by inhalation
  - 10 mL of 3% sodium nitrate by IV
  - 50 mL of 25% sodium thiosulfate by IV
  - Health care providers must be protected from contact with cyanide–laced vomitus or contact with any cyanide (topical exposure).

Food Poisoning

Bacterial contamination

Bacterial contamination is the most common cause of food poisoning. A majority of cases result from improper food handling and failure to maintain food at an appropriate temperature. Because of the self-limiting nature of this illness, the incidence is probably much greater than the 7 million cases reported to the AAPCC annually. About 325,000 persons require hospitalization and 5000 die each year from complications of bacterial food poisoning.[11]

The most common causative organisms are *Staphylococcus aureus*, *Salmonella*, *Escherichia coli*, *Clostridium perfringens*, *Campylobacter jejuni*, and *Bacillus cereus* (Table 28-3). Of these, *E. coli* has gained the most notoriety following several cases of severe illness and death related to contaminated, undercooked beef products.

A high index of suspicion and a careful history of a patient's recent travel experiences and eating habits may help to diagnose food poisonings of a nonbacterial nature.

Table 28-3   Differential Diagnosis of Bacterial Causes for Diarrhea and Food Poisoning

Bacterial Diarrhea	Pathogenesis	Symptoms					
		Fever	Diarrhea	Dysentery*	Abdominal Pain	Vomiting	Incubation Period
Clostridium perfringens	Enterotoxin	−	+[†]	+	++	±[†]	8-24 hr
Escherichia coli	Enterotoxin	−	±	±	±	0[§]	24-72 hr
Salmonella	Bacteria (endotoxin)	+	+	±	±	±	8-48 hr
Shigella	Bacteria (endotoxin)	±	+	+	+	±	24-72 hr
Staphylococci	Enterotoxin	−	+	0	+	+	2-6 hr
Streptococci	Bacteria	+	±	−	−	−	24-72 hr
Vibrio cholerae	Enterotoxin	±	+	0	±	±	24-72 hr
Clostridium botulinum	Neurotoxin	−	−	−	±	±	12-36 hr
Bacillus cereus							
Type I	Enterotoxin	−	±	−	+	++	1-6 hr
Type II	Enterotoxin	−	++	−	+	±	10-12 hr
Campylobacter jejuni	Enterotoxin	+	+	−	+	+	1-7 days

Data from Grady GF, Keusch GT: Pathogenesis of bacterial diarrheas, *N Engl J Med* 285:831-841, 1971.
* Dysentery means diarrhea with blood and mucus.
[†] +, Occurs regularly.
[‡] ±, May or may not occur.
[§] 0, Does not occur.

Signs and symptoms

- Nausea, vomiting, abdominal cramping, diarrhea (may be watery or contain mucus or blood)
- Fever or hypothermia
- Headache
- Dehydration
- Hemolytic uremic syndrome (seen in severe *E. coli* poisonings)

Therapeutic interventions

- Encourage oral fluid intake if the patient can tolerate it.
- Begin IV hydration for patients with symptoms of dehydration.
- Collect and send stool cultures.
- Initiate antibiotic therapy for suspected shigella or streptococcal infections. Also start antibiotics on immunocompromised patients.

Effect of Heat	Age-Group	Transmission Pattern	Extraintestinal Symptoms	Culture
Thermostable organism Thermolabile organism	Adults	Poultry, heat-processed meats (stews)	Volume depletion	Food, stool, vomitus
Thermostable toxin; capsular-thermolabile toxin	All	Contact	Volume depletion	Stool
Thermolabile organism	All	Prepared foods, poultry, egg products, pet turtles and chicks	Headache, bacteremia	Food, stool, blood
Thermolabile organism; thermolabile toxin	All	Institutions	Seizures, meningismus	Food, stool
Thermostable toxin	All	Prepared food (salami, varied salads), fowl, pastry	Volume depletion	Food, stool
Thermolabile organism	All	Proteinaceous foods	Influenza-like pharyngitis	Food, stool, blood
Thermolabile toxin	All	Water, food	Hypokalemic nephropathy	Stool
Thermolabile spore; thermolabile toxin	All	Diverse canned foods	Dysphagia descending paralysis	Serum, stool, vomitus for toxin
Thermolabile toxin	All	Fried rice	Limited	Food, stool
Thermolabile toxin	All	Meats, vegetables	Volume depletion	Food, stool
Thermolabile toxin	All	Poultry, meats, dairy produce	Limited	Food, stool, blood

- Administer an antiemetic agent.
- Replace electrolytes as needed.

Prevention and education
- Wash hands well before handling food or eating.
- Wash all utensils and cutting surfaces between food preparation sessions.
- Wash all fresh fruits and vegetables.
- Thoroughly cook all meat and poultry.
- Use warmers to keep unrefrigerated foods at a temperature of 140° F (during prolonged serving periods).
- Check the expiration dates on all food products.
- Refrigerate dairy products and other susceptible foods at 40° F (or less).

Botulism

Botulism is a paralytic illness that results from neurotoxins produced by the organism *Clostridium botulinum*. Botulism is rare but typically occurs in sporadic outbreaks within a family or other group. This condition can result from toxin ingestion or from wound contamination. The most common cause of botulism is poorly processed or spoiled home-canned vegetables, especially nonacid items such as green beans. When questioned, patients may mention a history of eating food from a can or jar with a bulging lid (a result of expanding gases released as the organisms grow). Clinical findings generally develop 8 to 36 hours following ingestion of contaminated food but may be delayed for as long as 4 days.[13]

Signs and symptoms
- Presenting signs and symptoms are often vague.
- Lethargy, weakness
- Constipation
- Headache
- Normal or subnormal temperature
- Dry, sore throat, hoarseness, inability to swallow, impaired speech
- Visual disturbances (diplopia), limited eye movement, dilated pupils
- Decreased deep tendon reflexes, descending paralysis

Therapeutic interventions
- Provide basic and advanced supportive care as indicated.
- ABCs
- Patients frequently require a tracheostomy and long-term ventilatory assistance.
- Gastric emptying is only of benefit immediately following ingestion of food *known* to contain botulinum toxin.
- Asymptomatic individuals who were probably exposed should be hospitalized, closely observed, and treated with antitoxin as soon as symptoms appear.
- Admit symptomatic patients to an intensive care unit.
- Draw and send blood to determine the specific toxin serotype. The type determines the specific antitoxin to be used for treatment.
- Specific mono-, bi-, and trivalent horse serum antitoxins are available from the Centers for Disease Control and Prevention. These agents stop disease progression but do not reverse existing problems.

Metal Poisonings

Iron

Toxic levels of iron are most commonly a result of iron supplement ingestion. Treatment is complicated by the fact that there is no physiologic mechanism for iron excretion. Normal serum iron levels range from 50 to 175 mcg/100 mL. Ingestion of greater than 20 mL/kg is thought to be toxic; ingestion of 300 mg/kg is considered lethal.[10]

Signs and symptoms

Initial Stage (within 2 hours of ingestion)

- Nausea, vomiting, abdominal pain
- Hematemesis, bloody stools
- Hyperglycemia

Second Stage (2-48 hours postingestion)

- Resolution of gastrointestinal disturbances
- Dehydration may be the only symptom present

Third Stage (48-96 hours)

- Metabolic acidosis
- Coagulopathy
- Hemorrhage and shock
- Hepatic and renal failure
- Hypoglycemia

Therapeutic interventions

- Provide basic and advanced supportive care as indicated.
- Induced emesis is preferred over gastric lavage in children because most adult-strength pills (e.g., prenatal vitamins) are large and will not fit through a pediatric lavage tube.
- Activated charcoal does *not* bind well with iron.
- Obtain abdominal radiographs. Some types of iron tablets are radiopaque on abdominal films. Chewable vitamins containing iron are usually not visible.
- Initiate whole-bowel irrigation if there is radiographic evidence of iron tablets past the pylorus or if iron remains in the stomach after other attempts at decontamination.
- Draw and send a serum iron level 4 to 6 hours after ingestion.
- Consider chelation therapy with deferoxamine (Desferal) 15 mg/kg per hour by continuous infusion.

Indications

- Symptomatic patients
- Ingestion of greater than 20 mg/kg of elemental iron
- Serum iron levels greater than 350 mcg/100 mL
- Deferoxamine administration turns the urine a pink "vin rosé" color.

End point

- Continue deferoxamine infusion until urine color normalizes.[5]
- Emergency surgery may be performed for the removal of iron bezoars from the gastrointestinal tract. Bezoars can cause necrosis, gut perforation, and massive intraabdominal hemorrhage.

- Although rarely indicated, some patients have required exchange transfusions for massively toxic levels.

Lead

An estimated 5 million tons of lead are contained in paint in homes throughout the United States. Up to 70% of houses built before 1960 have some surfaces covered with a lead-based paint. Although leaded paint is the most visible and publicized source of lead toxicity, it is certainly not the only one. The incidence of pediatric lead poisoning peaks during summer months.

Lead poisoning does not produce a classic toxidrome that facilitates easy diagnosis. Symptoms of toxicity in children range from subtle behavioral changes to acute encephalopathy and death. Lead is compartmentalized into three main areas: bones, soft tissues (including the brain), and the blood. Organic lead is assimilated rapidly by the CNS and can produce a host of neuropsychiatric manifestations. Excretion occurs slowly through urine, feces, and sweat.

Signs and symptoms
Gastrointestinal
- "Viral" symptoms
- Anorexia, nausea, vomiting, abdominal pain, colic
- Changes in bowel habits

Neuropsychiatric
- Motor coordination difficulties
- Delayed reaction times
- Changes in behavior, headache, encephalopathy
- Attention disorders, impaired cognitive skills, mental retardation

Miscellaneous
- Microcytic anemia
- Renal dysfunction (proximal tubular acidosis)
- Porphyrins in the urine
- Radiographic long bone changes (radiodense) are seen in children

Routes of entry
Oral
- Ingestion of paint chips; eating off of glazed pottery; "herbal" medicines (especially Mexican American, Indian, and Chinese folk medicines); dust particles from lead-filled homes or renovations; water contaminated by lead piping

Inhalation
- Sniffing of leaded gasoline products; exposure to fumes or dust particles during building renovations; occupational exposure

Drugs of abuse
- Homemade alcoholic beverages (especially moonshine and wine) from still pipes and lead salts. Samples of heroin, cocaine, and methamphetamine have been reported to contain as much as 60% lead by weight

Therapeutic interventions

Acute Ingestion

- Perform whole-bowel irrigation and administer cathartics for acute ingestion of lead glazes or lead products.
- Obtain abdominal radiographs (if indicated).

Chronic Exposure

- Check a serum lead level (acceptable levels less than or equal to 10 mcg/dL).
- Obtain a baseline CBC to determine whether the patient has developed a microcytic hypochromic anemia.
- Obtain radiographs of the abdomen, wrists, and knees in children with chronic exposures.
- Send an erythrocyte protoporphyrin level.
- Begin chelation therapy for symptomatic children and any patient with a level greater than 45 mcg/dL.
  - Dimercaprol (BAL, British anti-Lewisite) and calcium disodium edetate (Ca^{++} EDTA, EDTA) are administered parenterally and require hospitalization.
  - Succimer (2,3 dimercaptosuccinic acid) is approved for oral chelation therapy. The dose is 30 mg/kg for 7 days.

Poisonous Plants

According to the AAPCC, plants are the fourth most common reason for poison center notification. Children under the age of 6 are involved in 70% to 80% of all plant-related exposures.[9] Most poisonings are unintentional, and 98% of exposures result in no toxicity or only minor toxicity.[9] Dermatitis and gastrointestinal irritation are the most common side effects reported. Rarely do plant-related exposures require treatment. However, a small number of highly poisonous plants exist. Unfortunately, few antidotes to these toxins exist. Refer to Table 28-4 for information on specific poisonings.

Mushrooms

Mushroom species range from delectable to lethal. Typically, wild mushrooms ingestions are nontoxic. Only eight mushroom fatalities, resulting from more than 100,000 exposures, have been reported to the AAPCC in the last 10 years. Most fatalities involved adult mushroom hunters who failed to identify the fungi properly before consuming large quantities. Other tragic cases involve individuals seeking hallucinogenic mushrooms, who mistakenly select a toxic variety.

Signs and symptoms

- Mushroom poisoning may mimic food poisoning.
- Symptoms that develop within 2 hours of ingestion are unlikely to be fatal (gastrointestinal symptoms).
- Symptoms that develop after 6 hours suggest hepatotoxicity.
- Signs of liver failure
- CNS disturbances (vertigo, seizures, incoordination)
- Hepatorenal syndrome

Therapeutic interventions

- Provide basic and advanced supportive care as indicated.
- If the mushroom is not available, obtain a detailed description of its appearance. Occasionally, consultation with a mycologist can be helpful.

Table 28-4   Poisonous Plants and Their Treatment

Plant Name	Plant Family	Symptoms	Treatment
Castor bean	*Ricinus communis*	Gastroenteritis: may be severe and hemmorrhagic Delirium Seizures Coma Death	Whole-bowel irrigation Rapid and complete gut decontamination Observe for 8-12 hours Monitor fluids, glucose, and electrolytes
Foxglove	*Digitalis purpurea*	Nausea, vomiting Diarrhea Abdominal pain Confusion	Monitor fluids, glucose, and electrolytes May require insulin, glucose, or bicarbonate
Oleander	*Nerium oleander*	Cardiac dysrhythmias	Whole-bowel irrigation If symptomatic, treat with digoxin immune Fab (Digibind) Hemodialysis
Jequirity bean	*Abrus precatorius*	Delayed gastroenteritis: may be severe and hemorrhagic Delirium Seizure Coma Death	Whole-bowel irrigation Observe for 8-12 hours Monitor fluids, glucose, and electrolytes
Poison hemlock	*Conium maculatum*	Oral burning and dryness Tremors, weakness Diaphoresis Mydriasis Seizures *Rarely:* Paralysis Rhabdomyolysis Renal failure Bradycardia Coma Death	Whole-bowel irrigation Activated charcoal Intravenous fluid replacement Antidysrhythmics Benzodiazepines
Water hemlock	*Cicuta maculata*	Nausea, vomiting Abdominal pain Delirium Seizures Death	Whole-bowel irrigation Intravenous fluid replacement Anticonvulsants
Yew	*Taxus spp*	Nausea, vomiting *Rarely:* Seizures Cardiac dysrhythmias Coma	Whole-bowel irrigation Activated charcoal Intravenous fluid replacement Anticonvulsants Antidysrhythmics
Aloe	*Aloe barbadensis*	Abdominal pain and diarrhea within 6-12 hours of ingestion Urine may turn red	No antidote is available Intravenous fluid replacement
Azalea	*Rhododendron spp*	Salivation Lacrimation Bradycardia Hypotension Progressive paralysis	Whole-bowel irrigation Atropine for bradycardia Intravenous fluid replacement Vasopressors

Table 28-4   Poisonous Plants and Their Treatment—cont'd

Plant Name	Plant Family	Symptoms	Treatment
Cactus	Not applicable	Needles or spine embedded in the skin Pain or irritation at the site	Instruct patient to watch for wound infection
Caladium spp	Not applicable	Oral burning and irritation Oral swelling Drooling Respiratory compromise	Cold milk Ice cream Analgesics
Colchicine	Autumn crocus Meadow saffron Glory lilly	Coagulopathy Bone marrow suppression Cardiac dysrhythmias Cardiogenic shock Respiratory distress Seizure Coma Liver impairment Death	Whole-bowel irrigation Aggressive fluid resuscitation
Dumbcane	*Dieffenbachia amoena*	Oral burning and irritation Drooling Respiratory compromise	Milk Ice cream Analgesics
Fava beans	Not applicable	Gastrointestinal upset Fever Headache Jaundice	Monitor patients closely Intravenous fluid replacement
Jimson weed	*Datura* spp	Flushing Hyperthermia Dry skin and mucosa Mydriasis Hallucinations Delirium	Emesis or gastric lavage Activated charcoal Intravenous fluid replacement External cooling Physostigmine for *severe* anticholinergic symptoms: 0.5 mg for children 1.0-2.0 mg for adults
Nightshade, common or woody	*Solanum* spp	Nausea, vomiting, diarrhea Abdominal pain Delirium Hallucinations Coma	No specific treatment
Peach, apricot, pear, crab apple, and hydrangea	Not applicable	Diaphoresis Nausea, vomiting Abdominal pain	Emesis or gastric lavage Antidote therapy may be needed for cyanide toxicity
Pepper	*Capsicum* spp	Mucous membrane irritation, burning, and pain	Demulsifying agents Analgesics
Pokeweed	*Phytolacca americana*	Oral and throat burning and irritation Abdominal pain Nausea, vomiting Foamy diarrhea	Emesis or gastric lavage Activated charcoal Fluid and electrolyte replacement
Yellow sage	*Lantana camara*	Nausea, vomiting, diarrhea Weakness Coma	Emesis or gastric lavage Intravenous fluid replacement

Continued

Table 28-4   Poisonous Plants and Their Treatment—cont'd

Plant Name	Plant Family	Symptoms	Treatment
Poison ivy, oak, and sumac	Not applicable	Itching, burning, and redness leading to rash 12-48 hours after exposure	Oatmeal baths Topical steroids Ivy Block: contains bentoquatam, which binds to urushiol to prevent absorption
Holly	*Ilex* spp	Nausea, vomiting, diarrhea	Emesis or gastric lavage Intravenous fluid replacement
Poinsettia	*Euphorbia pulcherrima*	Local irritation to skin, mouth, or conjunctiva	Comfort measures
Mistletoe	*Phoradendron flavescens*	Nausea, vomiting, diarrhea	Emesis or gastric lavage Fluid and electrolyte replacement

- If a sample of the mushroom is available, save it in a *paper* bag and place it in a refrigerator.
- The type of mushroom and symptom severity determine interventions.
- Consider inducing emesis if ingestion was recent.
- Administer activated charcoal and a cathartic.
- Save all emesis and stools in the refrigerator (do not freeze) for possible microscopic study and analysis.
- Observe the patient for seizures and hypotension.
- Give analgesics, sedatives, antispasmodics, and antiemetics as indicated.

Pesticides

Organophosphates and carbamates are two related classes of insecticides that are commonly available. Both can cause serious poisonings. Patients with a toxic exposure to either of these agents have similar clinical presentations, but the duration of carbamate symptoms is usually shorter. Organophosphates and carbamates bind acetylcholinesterase, allowing accumulation of acetylcholine at the neuroreceptor sites. This produces a cholinergic crisis. Pesticides are readily absorbed by oral, dermal, and inhalation routes of exposure.[10]

Signs and symptoms

Table 28-5 summarizes the signs of pesticide toxicity.

Therapeutic interventions

- Decontaminate the patient to reduce further absorption and prevent secondary exposure of health care providers.
- Provide basic and advanced supportive care as indicated.
- Treat hypotension with fluids and vasopressors. (Resolving bradycardia will improve blood pressure.)
- Administer antidotes.
  - *Atropine:* This drug may need to be given for up to 24 hours. Massive quantities may be required. Continue to give atropine until secretions are minimal and bradycardia has resolved.

Table 28-5   Clinical Effects of Pesticide Poisoning (Acetylcholine Excess)

Tissue or Organ	Effect
Muscarinic Effects	
Sweat glands	Sweating
Pupils	Pupillary constriction
Lacrimal glands	Lacrimation
Salivary glands	Excessive salivation
Bronchial tree	Wheezing
Gastrointestinal	Cramps, vomiting, diarrhea, tenesmus
Cardiovascular	Bradycardia, fall in blood pressure
Ciliary bodies	Blurred vision
Bladder	Urinary incontinence
Nicotinic Effects	
Striated muscle	Fasciculations, cramps, weakness, twitching paralysis, respiratory embarrassment, cyanosis, arrest
Sympathetic ganglia	Tachycardia, elevated blood pressure
Central nervous system	Anxiety, restlessness, ataxia, convulsions, insomnia, coma, absent reflexes, Cheyne-Stokes respirations, respiratory and circulatory depression

- *Pralidoxime chloride (Protopam):* This antidote is administered as a loading dose followed by a continuous IV infusion in cases of severe organophosphate poisoning; effects are often dramatic.

Prevention and education

- Nonleather gloves, protective clothing, and eye shields should be used when handling pesticides.
- Use pesticides only in well-ventilated areas and spray or spread downwind.
- Read the product label before use.

Petroleum Distillates

Kerosene, lighter fluid, mineral oil, furniture polish, turpentine, gasoline, and many insecticides contain petroleum distillates. Complications usually occur as a result of aspiration or other pulmonary problems. Hydrocarbon aspiration produces transient CNS depression or excitation. Like pesticides, the skin, gut, and lungs readily absorb petroleum products.

Signs and symptoms

- Respiratory difficulty (aspiration of petroleum distillates can initiate a massive pulmonary inflammatory response)
- Infiltrates on chest radiographs
- Abnormal arterial blood gases
- Dysrhythmias

Table 28-6   Alcohols

Formulations and Uses

	Use	Approx. conc.
	1. Methanol: Gas line antifreeze	95
	Windshield washer fluid	35-95
	Antifreeze	Varied
	Industrial solvents (e.g., paint and varnish remover, shellac)	
	Sterno	
	Dry gas	
	2. Ethanol/Isopropanol	(proof/2 = % ETOH)
	Ethanol: Beverages	
	(A) Beer	4-6
	(B) Wine	10-20
	(C) Spirits	20-50
	Rubbing alcohol	70
	Aftershaves/colognes	40-60
	Mouthwashes	Up to 75
	Medicinal preparations	Varied
	Isopropanol: Rubbing alcohol	70
	Pine disinfectants	5-30
	Solvents	Varied
	3. Ethylene glycol: car radiator antifreeze	95
	Note: Longer-chain glycols (i.e., propylene glycol and polyethylene glycol) are relatively nontoxic orally.	

Comparison of toxicity

Methanol

"Highly toxic"

By history, death has been reported after 15 mL 40% methylhydroxide; blindness reported after 4 mL.

Ex: 1.5 mL of 100% methanol in a 10-kg child produces a potential level of 20 mg%; one gulp (2-8 mL) can produce levels of 26-105 mg%.

Blood levels

All are potentially toxic depending on the time of ingestion and presence of signs and symptoms.

Ethanol/Isopropanol

Isopropanol is approximately twice as intoxicating as ethanol at equivalent blood levels. (Severe toxicity with blood levels >150 mg%)

Ethanol (blood levels)

50-100 mg% = mild toxicity

100-300 mg% = moderate toxicity

>300 mg% = severe toxicity, but 1 ml/kg of pure ethanol will result in a blood level of approximately 100 mg% at 2 hours postingestion.

Ethylene Glycol

"Highly toxic"

Ex: 3 mL of 100% ethylene glycol in a 10-kg child produces a potential level of 50 mg%; one gulp (2-8 mL) can produce levels of 34-135 mg%.

Blood levels

All are potentially toxic depending on the time of ingestion and presence of signs and symptoms.

Presentation and onset of symptoms	Toxicity delayed: Usual latent period is 12-24 hr (may be delayed during concurrent ethanol ingestion). Gastritis and hangover-like effect are followed by visual disturbances and an anion gap metabolic acidosis. Anion gap = *Na minus (HCO$_3$ + Cl). Normal = 12 ± 4. Mnemonic for an anion gap metabolic acidosis is M-U-D-P-I-L-E-S: Methanol, Uremia, Diabetic ketoacidosis, Paraldehyde; phenformin, Iron, isoniazid, Lactic acidosis, Ethylene glycol, ethanol ketoacidosis, Salicylates, sympathomimetics	Rapid onset of intoxication (30-60 min). Gastritis possible from high concentrations	**Phase I (½-12 hr)** CNS ethanol-like inebriation (no odor), Anion gap metabolic acidosis, Calcium oxaluria. **Phase II (2-36 hr)** Tachypnea, tachycardia. **Phase III (2-3 days)** Renal failure
Toxicology	Metabolized by the liver via alcohol dehydrogenase to formaldehyde and then quickly to formic acid. These two metabolites, rather than the methanol, cause the visual and metabolic changes.	*Ethanol:* Direct-acting CNS (reticular activating system) depressant. *Isopropanol:* Direct-acting CNS depressant. Causes local gastritis. The metabolite acetone acts to prolong CNS effects. Produces a ketosis without an acidosis.	Neurologic symptoms. Caused by parent compound. Renal toxicity results from formation of oxalic acid metabolite.
Referral to medical facility	All suicide gestures. All symptomatic patients. All but minute amounts of dilute concentrations	All suicide gestures. Symptomatic patients with calculated ethanol level >100 mg%	All suicide gestures. All symptomatic patients. All but minute amounts of dilute concentration

Continued

Table 28-6   Alcohols—cont'd

Hospital management		
(1) ABCs (2) Gut decontamination (time dependent) (3) Laboratory tests, diagnostic Blood methanol Electrolytes ABCs Calculate anion gap Blood ethanol Fundoscopic examination of the eye (4) Ethanol therapy: (A) Loading dose followed by maintenance dose (Ethanol has 20 times the affinity for alcohol dehydrogenase compared with methanol.) Indications (B) (+) Blood methanol level OR (C) Symptomatic patient and strong suspicion Load 7.6-10 mL/kg IV of 10% ethanol in D_5W over 30 min to achieve blood ethanol level of 100 to 130 mg%. Oral route is acceptable. Maintenance 14 mL/kg/hr of 10% ethanol IV.	(1) ABCs (2) Gut decontamination (time dependent) (3) Laboratory tests, diagnostic Ethanol/isopropanol/acetone levels Blood and urine ketones Electrolytes Glucose Calculate anion gap (4) Supportive care	(1) ABCs (2) Gut decontamination (time dependent) (3) Laboratory tests Ethylene glycol (if possible) Electrolytes: including calcium ABG ABGs Calculate anion gap Electrocardiogram Urine analysis for oxalate or hippurate crystals Some brands of antifreeze may be fluorescent under Woods' lamp. (4) Ethanol therapy: loading dose followed by maintenance (same indications and dosing as in methanol management) (5) Hemodialysis (6) Possibly thiamine and pyridoxine (7) Fomepizole (Antizol) antidote therapy. This is a newer alternative to ethanol therapy. (A) Loading dose (adult or pediatric) is 15 mg/kg. (B) Maintenance dose (adult or pediatric) is 10 mg/kg every 12 hours until ethylene glycol level is less than 20 mg/dL. (C) Dilute dose in 100 mL of NS or D_5W and infuse IV over 30 minutes.

Requirements increase in chronic alcoholics and during hemodialysis Treat until level of methanol is zero.

(5) Hemodialysis

(6) Folinic or folic acid

(7) Fomepizole (Antizol) antidote therapy. This is a newer alternative to ethanol therapy.

(A) Loading dose (adult or pediatric) is 15 mg/kg.

(B) Maintenance dose (adult or pediatric) is 10 mg/kg every 12 hours until methanol level is less than 20 mg/dL.

(C) Dilute dose in 100 mL of NS or D_5W and infuse IV over 30 min.

All patients in hospital

Physician consultant   All patients with unstable vital signs (or acidosis-unrelated)   All patients in hospital

Suspect MEOH or ethylene glycol.

Modified from New York City Poison Center: *Syllabus*, 1993.

ETOH, Ethyl alcohol; *CNS*, central nervous system; *ABC*, airway, breathing, and circulation; *IV*, intravenous; *D5W*, 5% dextrose in water; *NS*, normal saline; *ABG*, arterial blood gas; *MEOH*, methyl alcohol.

Table 28-7 Antidotes

Exposure/Condition	Antidote	Comments
Black widow spider	Antivenin	*Latrodectus mactans* venom neutralizer; give 1-2 vials IV over 1 hour.
Rattlesnake	Antivenin	Crotalidae polyvalent venom neutralizer; give 5-20+ vials IV.
Carbamates	Atropine, pralidoxime	Very large quantities of atropine may be required.
Organophosphates		Give a pralidoxime loading dose followed by a continuous infusion.
Neuroleptic drugs (haloperidol, phenothiazines, thioxanthenes) and metoclopramide	Benztropine (Cogentin)	Reverses drug-induced dystonias through competitive inhibition of muscarinic receptors and blockade of dopamine reuptake.
Botulism	Botulinum antitoxin	Contact the CDC to obtain antitoxin. Draw 10 mL of serum for determination of the specific toxin serotype before treatment is started.
Calcium channel blockers	Calcium chloride (drug of choice unless the patient is acidotic)	Large amounts may be required. Keep serum Ca++ <11 mg/dL.
Hydrofluoric acid burns	Calcium gluconate	2.5% calcium gluconate gel for dermal exposure 10% calcium gluconate infiltrated locally around hydrofluoric acid burns (or can be given as an intraarterial infusion into the affected limb).
Hyperkalemia Hypermagnesemia	Calcium gluconate by IV	Administer slowly.
Lead Cadmium	Calcium disodium edetate (Ca++ EDTA, EDTA)	Precautions: Ensure adequate fluid volume, monitor urine output; avoid rapid IV infusion. Not effective for mercury, gold, or arsenic poisoning.
Cyanide Hydrogen sulfide	Cyanide kit	Follow the instructions in the kit. Oxygen and methemoglobin levels need to be monitored closely. Do not use methylene blue if excessive methemoglobinemia occurs. For hydrogen sulfide poisoning, *do not* use sodium thiosulfate. Use the nitrites only.
Iron	Deferoxamine mesylate (Desferal)	Deferoxamine forms ferrioxamine complexes that are excreted. This red complex is water-soluble and is excreted readily by the kidneys. Vin rosé–colored urine indicates the presence of iron in the urine.
Cocaine	Diazepam	
Digitalis Oleander Foxglove	Digoxin immune Fab (Digibind)	Antigen-binding fragments bind with digoxin.
Arsenic Lead encephalopathy Gold Mercury	Dimercaprol (BAL, British anti-Lewisite)	Heavy metals inhibit sulfhydryl-containing enzymes; the resulting chelated mercaptide product is less toxic and more easily excreted from the body than the heavy metals.
Phenothiazines	Diphenhydramine (Benadryl)	Diphenhydramine reverses drug-induced extrapyramidal effects.
Lead	DMSA (dimercaptosuccinic acid)	DMSA is an oral chelating agent indicated for the treatment of lead poisoning in children with lead levels >45 mg/dL.

Table 28-7   Antidotes—cont'd

Poison	*Antidote*	*Comments*
Arsenic Lead Mercury Bismuth	D-penicillamine	Contraindicated in penicillin-allergic patients.
Methanol Ethylene glycol	Ethanol or fomepizole (Antizol) by IV	Reduces the formation of toxic metabolites by competing for alcohol dehydrogenase. Monitor blood glucose levels. Adjust dosage if dialysis is performed.
Benzodiazepines	Flumazenil	Use cautiously in persons with unknown drug ingestions. Seizures can occur with reversal of benzodiazepine effects in chronic users, especially with tricyclic antidepressant or cocaine coingestions.
Beta-blockers	Glucagon	Bypasses beta-adrenergic blockade by activating non-beta receptors; increases cardiac contractility.
Aniline Nitrites Local anesthetics	Methylene blue	Methylene blue is a reducing agent that converts methemoglobin to hemoglobin.
Sulfonylureas (oral hypoglycemic agents)	Octreotide	Stimulates release of insulin from the beta islet cells of the pancreas. Use for overdoses refractory to glucose administration.
Acetaminophen	N-Acetylcysteine (Mucomyst)	N-Acetylcysteine is a glutathione substitute that prevents the formation of toxic intermediary metabolites. Best when given within 8 hours of ingestion but can be given up to 24 hours after ingestion.
Opioids Ethanol-induced coma Clonidine Propoxyphene Diphenoxylate	Naloxone (Narcan), Nalmefene (Revex)	Opioid antagonists used to reverse central nervous system and respiratory depressant effects.
Carbon monoxide	Oxygen, hyperbaric oxygen	Administer 100% oxygen by tight-fitting mask or positive pressure to reduce the half-life of carbon monoxide. Consider hyperbaric oxygen.
Anticholinergics *(rarely)* Tricyclic antidepressants *(last resort only)*	Physostigmine	Inhibits the destructive action of acetylcholinesterase. Should *not* be used routinely because of its potential for serious adverse effects.
Warfarin Long-acting anticoagulants	Phytonadione (vitamin K)	Reverses the inhibitory action of warfarin on blood clotting factors II, VII, IX, and X.
Heparin	Protamine sulfate	Protamine reacts with heparin to form a stable salt, resulting in neutralization of anticoagulant activity of heparin.
Tricyclic antidepressants	Sodium bicarbonate	Aside from gastric decontamination, sodium bicarbonate is the most useful single intervention for the management of overdose.

IV, Intravenous; *CDC,* Centers for Disease Control and Prevention.

Therapeutic interventions

- Decontaminate the patient to reduce further absorption and prevent secondary exposure of health care personnel.
- Provide basic and advanced supportive care as indicated.
- Give oxygen. Tracheal intubation may be required.
- Gastric emptying is not indicated unless the patient has a history of a large ingestion of hydrocarbons known to produce renal, liver, or CNS toxicity (e.g., halogenated hydrocarbons, petroleum, or petroleum distillates with additives).
- Monitor arterial blood gases in patients with respiratory symptoms (coughing, choking, dyspnea).
- Obtain a chest film. (Changes should be diagnostic within 6 hours of exposure.)

Alcohols

Each of the alcohols—ethanol, isopropanol, methanol, and ethylene glycol—is associated with varying degrees of toxicity. Table 28-6 compares alcohol types, their toxicity, and their management. For more information on the complications of ethanol abuse, see Chapter 29.

Substances of Abuse

For information on commonly abused substances and recreational poisoning, refer to Chapter 49.

CURRENTLY AVAILABLE ANTIDOTES

An antidote is a physiologic antagonist that reverses the signs or symptoms of poisoning. Table 28-7 is a brief guide to poisons and their antidotes.[5,10,11,13] New drugs are added and old ones are deleted regularly from this list. For current information and help with patient management, contact the experts at your regional poison control center.

References

1. Watson WA et al: 2002 annual report of the American Association of Poison Control Centers Toxic Exposure Surveillance System, *Am J Emerg Med* 21(5):353-421, 2003.
2. Krenzelok EP, McGuigan M, Lheur P: Position statement: ipecac syrup, American Academy of Clinical Toxicology; European Association of Poisons Centres and Clinical Toxicologists, *J Toxicol Clin Toxicol* 35(7):699-709, 1997 (see comment).
3. Vale JA: Position statement: gastric lavage, American Academy of Clinical Toxicology; European Association of Poisons Centres and Clinical Toxicologists, *J Toxicol Clin Toxicol* 35(7):711-719, 1997 (see comment).
4. Chyka PA, Seger D: Position statement: single-dose activated charcoal, American Academy of Clinical Toxicology; European Association of Poisons Centres and Clinical Toxicologists, *J Toxicol Clin Toxicol* 35(7):721-741, 1997 (see comment).
5. Criddle L: Toxicologic emergencies. In Newberry L, editor: *Sheehy's emergency nursing: principles and practice*, ed 5, St Louis, 2003, Mosby.
6. Anonymous: Position statement and practice guidelines on the use of multi-dose activated charcoal in the treatment of acute poisoning, American Academy of Clinical Toxicology; European Association of Poisons Centres and Clinical Toxicologists, *J Toxicol Clin Toxicol* 37(6):731-751, 1999 (see comment).

7. Barceloux D, McGuigan M, Hartigan-Go K: Position statement: cathartics, American Academy of Clinical Toxicology; European Association of Poisons Centres and Clinical Toxicologists, *J Toxicol Clin Toxicol* 35(7):743-752, 1997.
8. Tenenbein M: Position statement: whole bowel irrigation, American Academy of Clinical Toxicology; European Association of Poisons Centres and Clinical Toxicologists, *J Toxicol Clin Toxicol* 35(7): 753-762, 1997 (see comment).
9. Watson A et al: 2003 annual report of the American Association of Poison Control Centers Toxic Exposure Surveillance System, *Toxicology* 22(5):335.
10. Dart R et al, editors: *The 5 minute toxicology consult,* Philadelphia, 2000, Lippincott Williams & Wilkins.
11. Tintinalli J, Gabor D, Stapczynski J: *Emergency medicine: a comprehensive study guide,* ed 6, New York, 2004, McGraw-Hill.
12. Litovitz TL et al: 1996 annual report of the American Association of Poison Control Centers Toxic Exposure Surveillance System, *Am J Emerg Med* 15(5):447-500, 1997.
13. Schaider J et al, editors: *Rosen and Barkin's 5-minute emergency medicine consult,* ed 2, Philadelphia, 2003, Lippincott Williams & Wilkins.

29

Environmental Emergencies

Nancy J. Denke, RN, MSN, FNP-C, CCRN

SNAKEBITES

Of the more than 3000 species of snakes, 375 of these, from five different families, are venomous. The five toxic snake families are the following:
- *Crotalidae (pit vipers):* Copperheads, rattlesnakes, cottonmouths, and water moccasins
- *Elapidae:* Coral snakes, Cobras, mambas
- *Viperidae (true vipers):* Puff adders
- *Hydrophidae:* Sea snakes
- *Colubridae:* Boomslangs

Pit vipers (Crotalidae) are responsible for most envenomations in the United States. Although the American Association of Poison Control Centers reports an average of 6000 snakebites annually (about 2000 from venomous snakes), the incidence of lethal envenomation in the United States is only 5 to 10 per year.[1] The majority of bites occur when handling, teasing, or playing with snakes, and 40% of persons bitten have a blood alcohol level of greater than 0.1%. Snake venoms contain varying combinations of neurotoxic, cardiotoxic, and hemolytic proteins designed to immobilize the prey, stop the heart, and begin the digestive process. Venom is manufactured in the salivary glands and is injected through the hollow fangs of the snake. Most bites occur to the hands or legs.[2]

Signs and Symptoms

The clinical effects of snakebite range from mild local reactions to life-threatening, systemic toxicities. In fact, 25% of all pit viper bites are "dry"; no envenomation occurs.[1] The extent of the reaction depends on the following:
- The species and size of the snake
- The location and depth of the bite
- The number of bites

- The amount of venom injected
- The age of the snake: Young snakes do not release a consistent amount of venom with each bite.
- The age and size of the patient: Small children receive a proportionally greater venom dose.
- Individual sensitivity to venom
- The number of previous venom exposures: Prior envenomations increase the potential for allergic reactions.
- The concentration of microorganisms in the mouth of the snake
- The patient's general physical condition (e.g., history of diabetes, cardiovascular disease, or renal failure)

Initial reactions

Patients bitten by pit vipers describe a burning pain at the injection site, followed by an odd (metallic or rubber) taste in the mouth. This may be accompanied by oral and facial numbness and tingling. These symptoms occur about 30 to 60 minutes after the bite.

Local reactions

Signs and symptoms of a local reaction to a snakebite include the following:
- Fang marks (usually two)
- Edema (occurs within 5 minutes, can last 36 hours, and may be severe)
- Pain at the site (usually correlates with the extent of edema)
- Petechiae, ecchymosis
- Loss of limb function
- Tissue necrosis (16 to 36 hours after injury)

Systemic reactions

Signs and symptoms of a systemic reaction to a snakebite include the following:
- Abnormal vital signs: Tachycardia, tachypnea. Blood pressure may be elevated initially. Hypotension occurs with intravascular volume depletion and cardiovascular collapse.
- Dyspnea
- Nausea, vomiting
- Diaphoresis
- Syncope
- Constricted pupils (unilateral or bilateral), ptosis, diplopia
- Muscle twitching: Mouth, face, and the affected extremity (approximately 1 hour after the bite)
- Paresthesias: Numbness and tingling orally and at the wound site
- Salivation
- Difficulty speaking, confusion
- Bleeding disorders manifested by ecchymosis, hematemesis, hemoptysis, hematuria, epistaxis, melena

Severe systemic reactions

Signs and symptoms of a severe systemic reaction to a snakebite include the following:
- Pulmonary edema
- Seizures

- Severe coagulopathies and hemorrhage
- Renal failure
- Paralysis
- Hypovolemic shock

Therapeutic Interventions

Therapeutic interventions for snakebites include the following:
- Provide basic and advanced supportive care as indicated. Monitor for airway edema and respiratory distress.
- Remove potentially constricting clothing or jewelry.
- Immobilize the involved area at or below the level of the heart.[3]
- Send blood for a complete blood count (CBC), type and crossmatch, electrolytes, and coagulation studies (prothrombin time [international normalized ratio], activated partial thromboplastin time, fibrinogen, D-dimer).
- No clinical trials support the use of traditional interventions such as ice, tourniquets, constricting bands, electrotherapy, or wound suction.
- Cleanse the wound and provide tetanus prophylaxis as indicated.
- Give analgesics for pain.
- Symptomatic patients may require central and arterial pressure line placement.
- Begin antivenin therapy in patients with progressive deterioration. Antivenins are associated with significant complications and should not be given to patients with mild or resolving symptoms.
  - Antivenins are specific to the type of snake involved. Most U.S. emergency departments (EDs) have access to crotalid (pit viper) antivenin. Contact your poison control center for information on how to obtain antivenin for exotic snake species.
  - Ideally, antivenin administration is initiated within 4 hours of exposure but may be effective for up to 24 hours.
  - Because antivenin is made from animal serum, its use is associated with potentially life-threatening allergic reactions. Watch for signs of an antigen-antibody response and have medications readily available (epinephrine, antihistamines, histamine$_1$ and histamine$_2$ blockers).
  - CroFab (crotalid antivenin) is given initially in large doses (5 to 20 vials). The half-life of CroFab is shorter than the half-life of snake venom. Therefore antivenin usually is readministered 6, 12, and 18 hours after envenomation.
  - Read package inserts carefully for antivenin mixing and infusion information.[3-5]

SPIDER (ARACHNID) BITES

Most spider bites involve local reactions such as itching, swelling, redness, and stinging pain. Venoms from some species can induce systemic reactions as well. Several varieties of toxic spiders live in the United States. Black widow and brown recluse spiders cause systemic reactions and anaphylaxis, making them responsible for the greatest number of U.S. ED visits.

Black Widow (Latrodectus mactans)

Black widow spiders (or simply "widow" spiders) inhabit dark, secluded, damp, cool places such as barns and woodpiles. They can be found in all U.S. states with the exception of Alaska. Only the female is dangerous to human beings. These distinctive spiders can be identified by their shiny black bodies and red, hourglass-shaped abdominal markings. Black widow venom is neurotoxic. Patients experience an immediate pinprick sensation at the time of the bite, followed by a dull, numb pain (within 30 minutes). Systemic symptoms develop within the first hour. Symptoms peak in 2 to 3 hours and subside after 2 to 3 days. The pain may become intense and generalized.[1] Reactions vary from minor to severe and must be treated accordingly.

Signs and symptoms

Signs and symptoms of black widow spider envenomation include the following:
- Two tiny red fang marks at the point of venom entry surrounded by a papule (The presence of multiple bite marks usually excludes spider envenomation; arachnids rarely bite more than once.)
- Nausea, vomiting
- Paresthesias
- Headache
- Weakness, syncope
- Muscle spasm
- Chest, back, and abdominal pain
- Hypertension
- Elevated temperature
- Respiratory distress
- Seizures
- Shock

Therapeutic interventions

Therapeutic interventions for black widow spider envenomation include the following:
- Provide basic and advanced supportive care as indicated.
- Apply ice to the area to slow the action of the neurotoxin and control swelling.
- Check tetanus immunization status; vaccinate as needed.
- Treat the patient symptomatically. Symptoms usually resolve within 48 hours if the patient receives aggressive supportive care.
- Control pain and muscle spasms with liberal doses of opioids, benzodiazepines, and muscle relaxants.
- Calcium gluconate, traditionally used for muscle spasms, has been shown to be of no benefit.
- *Latrodectus* antivenin administration can shorten the course of illness significantly. Read the package insert carefully before administration.[6]

Brown Recluse (*Loxosceles reclusa*)

Brown recluse spiders are indigenous to the southeastern, south central, and southwestern United States. These small brown spiders inhabit dark, undisturbed areas such as basements, garages, boxes, and closets and are most active at night. *Loxosceles reclusa* can be identified by its light brown color and dark brown, fiddle-shaped mark on the cephalothorax. Brown recluse venom is cytotoxic and hemolytic.

Signs and symptoms

Signs and symptoms of brown recluse spider envenomation depend on the severity of the reaction.

Local reactions
- Mild stinging may occur at the time of the bite, but the initial event often goes unnoticed.
- A bluish ring, with local edema, appears around the bite site. This is accompanied by bleb formation.
- Erythema, edema, blistering, and pain develop over the first 2 to 8 hours.
- Local ischemia progresses to tissue necrosis on the third or fourth day.
- An area of eschar forms over the next several days or weeks; full healing may take months.

Systemic reactions (24 to 72 hours after the bite)
- Fever, chills
- Weakness, general malaise
- Nausea, vomiting
- Arthralgias, joint pain
- Petechiae

Severe systemic reactions
Rarely, patients develop profound systemic symptoms (particularly children):
- Seizures, coma
- Coagulopathies, hemolysis
- Renal failure
- Cardiopulmonary arrest

Therapeutic interventions

Therapeutic interventions for brown recluse spider envenomation include the following:
- Provide basic and advanced supportive care as indicated.
- Cleanse the wound.
- No specific antidote is available for brown recluse envenomation.
- Over the years, many therapies—including antihistamines, antibiotics, steroids, hyperbaric oxygen, electrical shock, and surgical excision—have been advocated. None of these has been demonstrated to be effective.[6]
- Dapsone inhibits the progression of crater lesions but must be used cautiously because of the risk of blood dyscrasias. The dose is 50 mg twice daily for 10 days.
- Systemic reactions are treated symptomatically. In acutely ill individuals, obtain blood for CBC, electrolytes, renal function, and coagulation studies.
- Local reactions eventually may require skin grafting.

Scorpion Stings

Scorpions are found throughout the world, particularly in warm climates, but none of the highly toxic species are indigenous to the United States. However, because of their size, scorpions can travel easily anywhere in the world as stowaways in cargo. Although there are many species of scorpions in the United States, only the venom of *Centruroides exilicauda* (the bark scorpion) is potent enough to cause systemic toxicity in human beings. This arthropod is found in California, Arizona, Texas, and Mexico. The incidence of scorpion stings increases in the cool evening and night hours when the animals are active. The neurotoxic venom is stored in the tail of the scorpion and is injected through a stinger as a defensive response. The stings of most scorpions are painful but harmless to human beings and require no specific care.

Signs and symptoms

Signs and symptoms of envenomation by *C. exilicauda* include the following:
- *Pain and numbness:* Immediate onset in the affected area that usually resolves in a few hours.
- *Respiratory:* Wheezing, stridor, tachypnea
- *Cardiovascular:* Tachycardia, palpitations, hypertension
- *Neurologic:* Anxiety, profuse salivation, visual disturbances, malaise, muscle spasms, hyperesthesias, ataxic gait, agitation or drowsiness, speech disturbances, dysphagia, seizures
- *Other symptoms:* Nausea, vomiting, trismus, incontinence, itching, edema, discoloration of the bite site, anaphylaxis

Therapeutic interventions

Therapeutic interventions for envenomation by *C. exilicauda* include the following:
- Provide basic and advanced supportive care as indicated.
- Treat the patient symptomatically.
- Administer mild analgesia to relieve pain. Narcotics may increase the toxic effects of the venom.
- Immobilize the affected area.
- Provide tetanus prophylaxis.
- Scorpion antivenin is available on an extremely limited basis (and is not approved by the Food and Drug Administration). Its use is associated with major allergic complications, and efficacy has not been established.
- Patients with severe envenomation may exhibit complicated neuromuscular and autonomic symptoms.
- Consult your regional poison control center for patient management advice.[1]

BEE, WASP, HORNET, AND FIRE ANT (HYMENOPTERA) STINGS

Bees, wasps, hornets, yellow jackets, and fire ants fall into the order of insects known as Hymenoptera. Stings from these animals can produce mild local reactions, moderate systemic symptoms, anaphylaxis, or life-threatening toxicity (e.g., from Africanized "killer" bees). Fire ants have a painful sting that forms a wheal, which eventually expands into a large vesicle. The area reddens and a pustule forms. Pustule reabsorption is later followed by crusting and scar formation.

Reactions to hymenopteran envenomation can occur immediately or up to 48 hours after the sting. The effect of stings is cumulative; the more stings, the greater the reaction. The honeybee is the only insect in this order that does not sting repeatedly. Venom composition varies among species, each producing different degrees of cytotoxic, hemolytic, allergenic, or vasoactive effects. Toxic reactions—involving multiple stings by highly potent insects—are unusual in the United States. Most severe hymenopteran-related illnesses are due to allergic reactions.

Signs and Symptoms

Signs and symptoms of stings by hymenopterans include the following:

Mild Local Reactions

- A burning sensation at the time of the sting
- Local swelling, warmth, and wheal formation
- Localized itching (pruritus)

Severe Local Reaction

- Regional edema

Systemic Reactions

- *Respiratory:* Laryngeal edema, stridor, bronchospasm, wheezing
- *Cardiovascular:* Hypotension, anaphylactic shock
- *Dermatologic:* Urticaria, pruritus, and local, regional, or generalized edema

Therapeutic Interventions

Therapeutic interventions for hymenopteran stings include the following:

Mild Reactions

- If a bee stinger is still present in the wound, use a dull object to scrape the stinger in the direction opposite the angle of penetration. Do not grasp or pull stingers from the skin; this can squeeze the attached sac and inject more venom.
- Apply ice to decrease the swelling. Elevate the involved area when possible.
- Cleanse the sting site with soap and water.
- Administer oral antihistamines (consider using one with a nondrowsy formula) and nonsteroidal antiinflammatory analgesics.

Severe Reactions

- Provide basic and advanced supportive care as indicated.
- Treat anaphylactic reactions in the standard manner. See Chapter 22.

Prevention

Because most hymenopteran emergencies are related to an allergic response, patient teaching is an important component of care. To prevent future stings and serious reactions, advise patients to do the following:
- Avoid wearing bright colors or perfumes while outdoors.
- Wear shoes when walking outside.
- Consider purchasing an anaphylaxis prevention kit (EpiPen).
- Wear a MedicAlert bracelet or some other type of allergy notification.
- Consider desensitization therapy (allergy shots). This is an option for certain patients, and the efficacy rate has been reported to be as high as 95%.

TICK-BORNE ILLNESSES

Ticks are vectors for a number of illnesses. With strong jaws and a cementlike adhesive, ticks attach to human beings and other mammals, engorge themselves on blood, and transmit disease through their saliva. In addition to spreading infection, certain ticks contain a neuro-toxin that can induce tick paralysis. This disease is characterized by a descending paralysis that resembles Guillain-Barré syndrome. Paralysis quickly resolves when the tick is removed.

Rocky Mountain Spotted Fever

Rocky Mountain spotted fever is caused by the organism *Rickettsia rickettsii,* transmitted through tick bites. This disease can be difficult to diagnose in the early stages because of its relatively long incubation period (5 to 10 days) and symptoms that resemble several other diseases. Nonetheless, without appropriate treatment, Rocky Mountain spotted fever can be fatal. Complications include renal failure and shock. More than 90% of patients with Rocky Mountain spotted fever are infected between April and September. North Carolina and Oklahoma (not states in the Rockies) have the highest infection rates. Two thirds of cases occur in children under the age of 15 years; the peak incidence is 5 to 9 years. Individuals with frequent exposure to dogs that roam in wooded or high grass areas are at increased risk for tick bites. The Rocky Mountain spotted fever incubation period is 2 to 14 days. The classic triad of symptoms involves fever, rash, and a history of tick exposure.[1]

Signs and symptoms

Signs and symptoms of Rocky Mountain spotted fever include the following:

Initial symptoms

- Tick(s) may still be attached to the patient's body.
- Fever (sudden onset), chills
- Anorexia, severe headache, myalgias
- Dermal manifestations: Small, flat, pink, nonpruritic spots (macules) on the palms, wrists, forearms, soles, and ankles during the first 10 days. Initially, the spots blanch when pressure is applied. They eventually become raised bumps.

Later signs and symptoms

- Maculopapular rash: The characteristic red, spotted (petechial) rash of Rocky Mountain spotted fever is seen 2 to 5 days after symptoms onset. The rash typically spreads in a centripetal fashion to cover most of the body, including the palms, soles, and face.
- Abdominal pain, distention, diarrhea
- Joint pain
- Decreased level of consciousness

Therapeutic interventions

Therapeutic interventions for Rocky Mountain spotted fever include the following:
- Remove the tick. Grasp the tick with forceps as close to the skin surface as possible, pull upward with steady, even pressure, being sure to retrieve the entire body and head. Do not twist or jerk the tick; this can cause mouthparts to break off and remain in the skin. Do not squeeze, crush, or puncture the body of the tick. Do not apply a hot match to the tick; burns may occur. Other methods, such as the use of petroleum jelly or alcohol to kill the tick have been recommended. Ticks must be removed to relieve the symptoms.
- Care for the bite site. After removing the tick, thoroughly wash the site with soap and water.
- Perform laboratory tests. Complete blood count, electrolytes, and liver function studies are indicated for symptomatic patients. Rocky Mountain spotted fever can cause thrombocytopenia, hyponatremia, or elevated liver enzymes.

- Send a blood sample for indirect immunofluorescence assay. This serologic test is the preferred reference standard of the Centers for Disease Control and Prevention for Rocky Mountain spotted fever.
- Administer antibiotics. Doxycycline is the drug of choice for 14 to 21 days.

Prevention

Measures to prevent tick bites and possible infection include the following:
- Tuck pants into socks in tick-prone areas to prevent insects from crawling inside the pant legs.
- Apply repellants to discourage tick attachment.
- Conduct a body check for ticks after visiting infested areas.
- Check children for ticks (especially in the hair) when returning from potentially tick-infested sites.

Lyme Disease

Ticks are the vectors for the organism *(Borrelia burgdorferi)* that causes Lyme disease. This spirochete, transmitted to human beings by the bite of infected deer ticks, causes more than 16,000 infections in the United States each year. Because of its vague viral symptomatology, Lyme disease often is misdiagnosed. The incubation period from the time of the bite to the onset of rash and other symptoms is typically 7 to 14 days.[7]

Signs and symptoms

Signs and symptoms of Lyme disease include the following:

Initial Stage (1 Week After Exposure)

- Fatigue, malaise, lethargy (flulike symptoms)
- Fever, headache
- Myalgias, stiff neck
- Joint aches (arthralgias)
- Target, bull's-eye rash formation (erythema migrans): This distinctive annular lesion, with bright red borders and a fading center, is present in only 25% of cases. The rash usually disappears without treatment.

Second Stage (4 Weeks After Exposure)

- Bell's palsy (common)
- Memory loss
- Meningitis
- Hepatitis
- Paresthesias
- Skin lesions
- Monoarticular arthritis
- Syncope, atrioventricular blocks
- Coagulopathies

Third Stage (6 Months after Exposure)

- Recurrent joint pain
- Arthritis, predominantly in the large joints

Therapeutic interventions

Therapeutic interventions for Lyme disease include the following:
- Manage headache, fever, joint pain, and myalgias with nonsteroidal antiinflammatory drugs.
- Institute antibiotic treatment.
  - *Early disease:* Orally administered doxycycline or amoxicillin are generally effective. Cefuroxime axetil or erythromycin can be used for persons who cannot take penicillin or tetracycline.
  - *Late disease:* Intravenously administered ceftriaxone or penicillin may be required for 4 weeks or more, depending on disease severity (particularly in patients with neurologic manifestations).

COLD-INDUCED INJURIES

Chilblains

Chilblains, also known as pernio, are localized areas of itching, painful redness, and recurrent edema on exposed areas such as the earlobes, fingers, and toes. Chilblains are a mild form of frostbite that develop in cool, damp climates when temperatures are above freezing. Symptoms (usually numbness and tingling) are generally self-limiting. Treatment involves placing the patient in a warm location and covering the affected area.

Immersion Foot

Immersion foot, or "trench foot," occurs when the feet are wet and subjected to cold temperatures for prolonged periods inside a nonbreathing boot or shoe. This condition is typically seen in foot soldiers and hunters. Initially, the foot appears pale and wrinkled. Tissue sloughing can develop if the condition is allowed to persist.[3]

Therapeutic interventions

Therapeutic interventions for immersion foot are as follows:
- Warm the affected foot in tepid water.
- Change into dry socks and shoes.

Frostbite

Frostbite is a traumatic condition that results when ice crystals form in the cells and extracellular spaces. The enlarging crystals disrupt metabolic processes, suspend cellular enzymatic activities, and damage delicate cell membranes. As histamine is released, capillary permeability increases, causing red cell aggregation and microvascular occlusion similar to that seen in burn injuries. Once the cells are frozen, damage is irreversible. Further exposure or trauma worsens the injury. Protecting the tissues surrounding frostbitten areas helps prevent additional tissue loss. The full extent of injury will not be apparent for several days.

Frostbite can be accompanied by hypothermia. Depending on the extent of hypothermia, treatment of this condition may take precedence over frostbite interventions.

Superficial frostbite

Superficial frostbite usually involves the fingertips, ears, nose, cheeks, or toes.

Signs and symptoms
- Local burning, numbness, tingling
- Whitish, waxy skin color
- After the skin thaws, the area will sting and feel hot. Depending on the length of exposure, large blisters may develop.

Therapeutic interventions
- Soak the affected area in warm (40° to 43.3° C or 104° to 110° F) water. Do *not* rub injured tissues.
- Elevate the area.
- Keep the patient warm. (Avoid heavy blankets or materials that may cause friction or weight on the affected area)
- Give analgesics; rewarming can be painful.
- Provide topical care for areas of open wounds.
- Ensure tetanus prophylaxis.

Deep frostbite

Deep frostbite produces local vascular and tissue changes resulting in cellular injury and death. Deep frostbite can involve muscle, fat, bones, and tendons as well as skin.

Several factors influence the probability of sustaining frostbite:
- Ambient temperature
- Windchill factor (Figure 29-1)

Estimated wind speed (in mph)	Actual Thermometer Reading (°F)											
	50	40	30	20	10	0	−10	−20	−30	−40	−50	−60
	EQUIVALENT CHILL TEMPERATURE (°F)											
CALM	50	40	30	20	10	0	−10	−20	−30	−40	−50	−60
5	48	37	27	16	6	−5	−15	−26	−36	−47	−57	−68
10	40	28	16	4	−9	−24	−33	−46	−58	−70	−83	−95
15	36	22	9	−5	−18	−32	−45	−58	−72	−85	−99	−112
20	32	18	4	−10	−25	−39	−53	−67	−82	−96	−110	−124
25	30	16	0	−15	−29	−44	−59	−74	−88	−104	−118	−133
30	28	13	−2	−18	−33	−48	−63	−79	−94	−109	−125	−140
35	27	11	−4	−21	−35	−51	−67	−82	−98	−113	−129	−145
40	26	10	−6	−21	−37	−53	−69	−85	−100	−116	−132	−148
(Wind speeds greater than 40 mph have little additional effect)	LITTLE DANGER in <5 hr with dry skin Maximum danger of false sense of security				INCREASING DANGER Danger from freezing of exposed flesh within one minute				GREAT DANGER Flesh may freeze within 30 seconds			
	Trenchfoot and immersion foot may occur at any point on this chart.											

Figure 29-1. Cooling power of wind on exposed flesh expressed as an equivalent temperature.

- Duration of exposure
- Contact with moisture or metal objects
- Type and number of layers of clothing
  Other factors that may contribute to an individual's predisposition to frostbite include the following:
- Dark skin pigmentation
- Lack of acclimatization
- Previous frostbite injury
- Poor peripheral vascular status
- Anxiety, exhaustion
- Frail body type
- Alcoholism, homelessness

Signs and symptoms

- Slight burning pain, followed by a feeling of warmth and then numbness as the area freezes
- Whitish or yellow-white discoloration of the skin, followed by a waxy appearance
- Swelling and intense burning accompanying thawing
- Blisters (usually appear in 1 to 7 days)
- Edema of the entire extremity that may persist for months
- Severe discoloration and gangrene are late findings.

Therapeutic interventions
Prehospital (or Wilderness)

- Prevent further heat loss:
  - Remove the patient's wet clothing.
  - Cover the patient with dry blankets or sheets.
  - Give warm, noncaffeinated liquids if the patient is conscious and has an intact gag reflex.
- Protect the injured part from further damage.
- Do not use ice or snow and friction to massage the frozen extremity. This outmoded intervention promotes further tissue damage.
- Do not thaw areas if they are likely to be refrozen before definitive care.

In the Emergency Department

- Immerse the frostbitten part in warm water (40° to 43.3° C or 104° to 110° F). Maintain the water at a constant temperature.
- Administer warm liquids by mouth if the patient is alert and has an intact gag reflex.
- Cover the patient with warm blankets; be careful not to place pressure on frostbitten areas.
- Administer narcotic analgesics (rewarming is painful).
- Once thawed, protect and immobilize the extremity with splints and bulky sterile dressings (avoid pressure).
- Consider tetanus prophylaxis and antibiotic administration.
- Escharotomy is indicated for severe vascular compromise.
- Amputation is not an emergency procedure. If necessary, amputation will be performed days or weeks after injury.

Prevention

- Dress properly for the climate; wear layers of loose-fitting clothing.
- When outdoors in cold areas, eat a diet high in carbohydrates and fats.
- Do not smoke or drink alcoholic or caffeinated beverages.
- Prevent bare skin contact with metal objects.
- Keep skin and clothing dry.
- Avoid exhaustion.
- Protect previously frostbitten parts from reexposure.

Hypothermia

Hypothermia is defined as a core body temperature of less than 35° C (95° F). Severe hypothermia occurs at a core temperature of 32.2° C (90° F). The American Heart Association has established 30°C (86° F) as the temperature for initiation of aggressive internal warming.[8] Below this temperature, profound physiologic derangements take place. Death usually results when core temperature falls below 25.6° C (78° F).

Pathophysiology of hypothermia

Most of the metabolic and enzymatic processes of the body are temperature dependent. Hypothermia slows cellular activity. Respirations decrease, carbon dioxide is retained, and hypoxia and acidosis ensue. Because of diminished glucose supplies, patients quickly can become hypoglycemic. Central nervous system changes—the most obvious early symptoms—include decreased level of consciousness, apathy, tiredness, and incoordination.

Furthermore, as core temperature begins to fall, the cells of the heart become sensitive and prone to dysrhythmias. Osborne, or J, waves develop on the electrocardiogram. Also known as a hypothermic hump, J waves are rounded bumps that appear at the junction of the QRS complex and the ST segment when body temperature is less than 32° C. Sudden movement of the hypothermic patient can trigger ventricular fibrillation.[3] The following groups of persons are especially prone to hypothermia:

- Neonates, because of limited body fat and an inability to shiver or seek warmth
- Elderly persons, because of medications, loss of body fat, and cardiovascular changes associated with aging
- Alcoholics and the homeless, because of poor nutrition and environmental exposure

Mild hypothermia

Signs and symptoms

- Fatigue, apathy, altered mental status
- Slow gait, muscle incoordination
- Hypotension
- Cardiac dysrhythmias

Therapeutic interventions

Therapeutic interventions for the patient who is still shivering, alert, and oriented include the following:

- Place the individual in a warm bath (40° to 43.3° C or 104° to 110° F).
- Apply a convective air warmer (e.g., Bair-Hugger), warmed blankets, and warm, humidified oxygen.
- Administer warm, sugary fluids by mouth to provide heat and calories.

Moderate and severe hypothermia

Signs and symptoms

Table 29-1 gives clinical manifestations of moderate and severe hypothermia.

Therapeutic interventions

- Provide basic and advanced supportive care as indicated.
- Avoid endotracheal intubation. Ventilate the patient with a bag-valve-mask device to prevent excessive stimulation and ventricular fibrillation.
- Chest compressions are not recommended in (pulseless) patients who still have an electrical rhythm.
- Ventricular fibrillation will not respond to the conventional advanced cardiac life support interventions unless the patient is rewarmed. Limit defibrillation to three shocks (along with intravenously administered medications) until the core temperature reaches 28° C (86° F).
- Replace volume. Rewarming causes peripheral vasodilation, and hypotension can occur as a result of this relative hypovolemia.
- Core rewarming of the severely hypothermic patient is essential to prevent rewarming shock. Rewarming shock occurs when the periphery is warmed faster than the core. This causes the lactic acid accumulated in cold extremities to be shunted rapidly to the heart, where it can induce fibrillation.
- Core rewarming can be achieved by several different means. Techniques vary from minimally to highly invasive. A combination of methods is generally preferred.
  - *Warm, humidified oxygen (40° to 45° C):* This technique is particularly effective for pediatrics patients.
  - *Warmed intravenous solutions (40° to 42° C):* Warmed fluids will not significantly raise core temperature but can help prevent further heat loss.
  - *Warmed gastric lavage:* This technique is fast and easy but not as effective as peritoneal lavage because of the smaller surface area of the stomach. Patients are at risk for ventricular fibrillation when the lavage tube is inserted.
  - *Peritoneal lavage:* Warmed normal saline or lactated Ringer's lactate solutions are used to irrigate the peritoneal cavity. Instill fluids through a cannula and remove them by suction. This procedure can raise the core temperature 6° C (10.8° F) per hour.
  - *Pleural/mediastinal irrigation:* Used in severe hypothermia in patients without cardiac activity. Instill warmed saline through chest tubes or pour it directly into the mediastinum through a thoracotomy incision.

Table **29-1**   **Clinical Manifestations of Hypothermia**

Body Temperature (C° [F°])	*Clinical Findings*
35.6-37.2 (96-99)	Shivering; loss of manual coordination
32.8-35 (91-95)	Violent shivering; slurred speech; amnesia
30-32.2 (86-90)	Shivering decreases but is replaced by muscular rigidity; cyanosis
<30 (<86)	Patients this cold can develop rewarming shock; atrial fibrillation
27.2-29.4 (81-85)	Patients become irrational and stuporous; pulse and respirations decrease
25.6-26.7 (78-80)	Coma; erratic heartbeat
<27.2 (<81)	Ventricular fibrillation can occur
<25.6 (<78)	Cardiopulmonary arrest

- *Hemodialysis or heart-lung bypass machine:* Although impractical in most emergency settings, these extracorporeal rewarming procedures may be performed if equipment and skilled personnel are available.
- *Bedside blood rewarming:* The Level 1 fluid infuser (a device routinely available in most trauma centers) can serve as an extracorporal blood rewarmer. Large-bore (dialysis-type) catheters are inserted into the femoral vein and artery and then are attached to a special tubing set (not the standard Level 1 tubing). Essentially, the patient becomes the "IV bag." Blood is pumped from the patient, through the warmer, and then back into the patient. This procedure has the advantages of being relatively easy, fast, safe, inexpensive, and effective.[9]
- Correct electrolyte disturbances.
- Give medications judiciously. Hypothermic patients metabolize drugs poorly and may receive a large bolus once rewarmed.

HEAT-INDUCED ILLNESSES

A variety of heat-related illnesses can occur and range in severity from mildly annoying to life threatening. These illnesses include prickly heat, heat cramps, heat tetany, heat exhaustion, and heat stroke.

Heat Cramps

Heat cramps are caused by sweat-induced electrolyte depletion during intense physical activity in hot weather. Patients are generally in good health but have not replaced lost fluids and electrolytes adequately.

Signs and symptoms

Signs and symptoms of heat cramps include the following:
- Cramps, particularly in the shoulders, lower extremities, and abdominal wall muscles
- Weakness
- Thirst
- Nausea
- Tachycardia
- Profuse diaphoresis
- Pale, cool, moist skin

Therapeutic Interventions

Therapeutic interventions for heat cramps include the following:
- Replace sodium chloride orally or intravenously, depending on the patient's clinical status. Commercially prepared balanced electrolyte drinks (e.g., Gatorade, POWERade, or any sports drink) work well for oral electrolyte replacement.
- Move the patient to a cool location.
- Encourage rest. Following an episode of heat cramps, patients should not return to the hot environment for 1 to 2 days.

Heat Exhaustion

Heat exhaustion occurs from a combination of prolonged periods of fluid loss (from perspiration, diarrhea, or diuretic use) and exposure to warm ambient temperatures without adequate fluid *and* electrolyte replacement. This condition is particularly common in the very young and the very old. Symptoms generally have a rapid onset. Untreated heat exhaustion can progress to heat stroke.

Signs and symptoms

Signs and symptoms of heat exhaustion include the following:
- Thirst
- Anorexia, nausea, vomiting
- Anxiety, general malaise
- Muscle cramps
- Sweating: May be profuse, but small children and the elderly have limited sweat capabilities
- Core body temperature can be normal or elevated (37° to 40° C) (98.6° to 105° F).
- Headache
- Dehydration, orthostatic hypotension
- Tachycardia
- Muscle incoordination
- Syncope

Therapeutic interventions

Therapeutic interventions for heat exhaustion include the following:
- Provide basic and advanced supportive care as indicated.
- Encourage rest.
- Place the patient in a cool environment.
- Administer fluids and electrolytes intravenously.

Heat Stroke

Exercise-induced heat stroke results from strenuous physical activity in a hot environment when a person is unable to dissipate body heat effectively. Non–exercise-induced heat stroke occurs in individuals who are vulnerable to high environmental temperatures, particularly small children and the elderly. Heat stroke also can be precipitated by medications that affect heat production (thyroid preparations, sympathomimetics), decrease thirst (haloperidol), or limit diaphoresis (antihistamines, anticholinergics, phenothiazines, and propranolol). As the body temperature rises to 41° C (105.8° F) central nervous system, cardiac, and cellular functions are affected. For every 1° C (1.8° F) rise in temperature, the metabolic rate increases by approximately 13% (Table 29-2). Such tremendous metabolic demands cannot be sustained indefinitely, and death follows if body temperature is not lowered.[3]

Table 29-2   Body Temperature and Metabolism

If Body Temperature Rises to C° (F°)	Metabolism Increases by (%)
38 (100.4)	13
39 (102.2)	26
40 (104)	39
41 (105.8)	52
42 (107.6)	Insufficient oxygen to meet cellular needs

Signs and symptoms

Signs and symptoms of heat stroke include the following:
- Rapid symptom onset
- Hyperthermia: Core temperature is greater than 41° C (105.8° F).
- Nausea, vomiting, diarrhea
- Classically, the skin is hot and dry, but perspiration is often present in the early stages, particularly in young, healthy individuals (e.g., athletes).
- Tachycardia, tachypnea
- Decreased level of consciousness, abnormal posturing, seizures
- Dilated, unresponsive pupils
- Hypotension, decreased urinary output
- Coagulopathies

Therapeutic interventions

Heat stroke is a true medical emergency. Provide the following interventions:
- Provide basic and advanced supportive care as indicated.
- Cool the patient as rapidly as possible:
- Remove clothing.
  - Spritz and fan the patient. This involves repeatedly spraying patients with a fine mist and blowing a fan over the skin. This technique minimizes shivering and promotes evaporative cooling.
  - Place ice packs in the groin and axilla.
  - Iced peritoneal lavage and cardiopulmonary bypass have been used in refractory cases.
- Rehydrate patients with room temperature intravenous fluids.
- Monitor electrolytes and clotting factors.
- Check urine for the presence of myoglobin (indicates rhabdomyolysis).
- Other supportive measures include the following:
  - Control shivering with chlorpromazine (Thorazine). Shivering causes the body temperature to rise.
  - Prepare for inpatient admission.

LIGHTNING INJURIES

Each year, 150 to 300 lightning-related fatalities occur in the United States, making this the third most common cause of death from isolated environmental injuries. Most lightening strikes occur between May and September.[10,11]

Signs and Symptoms

Signs and symptoms of injury from lightning include the following:
- Cold, pulseless extremities (indicates vasomotor instability)
- Confusion, amnesia, paralysis, and loss of consciousness (caused by the direct passage of current through the brain)
- Temporary hearing loss, possible tympanic membrane rupture
- Hypotension: May be related to intraabdominal hemorrhage, pelvis fracture, or extremity fracture
- Fixed and dilated pupils (generally transient)
- Cardiac dysrhythmias (caused by the direct passage of current through the heart)
- Burn wounds: Look for entrance and exit sites.

Therapeutic Interventions

Therapeutic interventions for injury from lightning include the following:
- Provide basic and advanced supportive care as indicated.
- Institute continuous cardiac monitoring and obtain a 12-lead electrocardiogram.
- Collect and send laboratory studies based on symptom severity: CBC, electrolytes, troponin I, creatinine phosphokinase, urinalysis, blood urea nitrogen, and creatinine.
- Watch for evidence of rhabdomyolysis (dark urine, elevated creatinine phosphokinase). Lightening-strike patients are at high risk for this syndrome.
- Perform radiographic studies of injured areas.
- Observe for the development of compartment syndrome.
- Clean and dress burn wounds.

DIVING EMERGENCIES

Scuba divers are exposed to atmospheric pressures far greater than those on land. Such hyperbaric conditions produce an array of medical problems unique to the underwater diving environment. At sea level the pressure exerted on the body is 1 atmosphere. At a water depth of 33 feet, pressure on the body is 2 atmospheres (Table 29-3).[12]

Dive Depth and Gas Volumes

According to Boyle's law, gas volume is related inversely to pressure at a constant temperature. In other words, as pressure increases (i.e., descent), gas volume decreases, and vice versa (Table 29-4).

Table **29-3** Underwater Pressures

Water Depth (Feet)	Pressure (Atmospheres)
Sea level	1
33	2
66	3
100	4
133	5
166	6
200	7
300	10
400	13
500	16

Data from Dickey LS: Barotrauma. In Rosen P, Barkin RM, editors: *Emergency medicine concepts and clinical practice*, St Louis, 1997, Mosby.

Table **29-4** The Effect of Water Depth on Gas Volume

Depth	Gas Volume (mL)
Sea level	2000
33	1000
100	500
233	250

When a diver inhales air from a scuba tank, the amount inspired remains the same regardless of submersion depth. However, with ascent, gas in the pulmonary system expands. If the diver fails to exhale on the way up, the volume of air in the lungs will increase as atmospheric pressure decreases. As this gas expands, it stretches the lungs and rupture can occur, resulting in pneumothorax and air embolism.

Air Embolism

Air embolism is a serious condition in which high-pressure air is forced into the circulatory system, causing an air embolism. Exhaling during a slow, controlled ascent is the best way to prevent air emboli. Rapid ascent and breath holding put the diver at risk. Symptoms appear within seconds or minutes of surfacing. Prompt therapy is crucial.

Signs and symptoms

Signs and symptoms of air embolism include the following:

Respiratory
- Chest tightness
- Shortness of breath
- Pink, frothy sputum
- Pneumothorax symptoms (simple or tension)

Neurologic (Caused by Air in the Cerebral Circulation)
- Vertigo (loss of a visual point of reference)
- Unilateral or bilateral limb paresthesias, sensory loss, or paralysis
- Confusion, loss of consciousness
- Seizures

Therapeutic interventions

Therapeutic interventions for air embolism include the following:
- Provide basic and advanced supportive care as indicated.
- Administer 100% oxygen.
- If tension pneumothorax is present, perform needle decompression.
- Placing the patient into a head-down Trendelenburg position used to be considered standard in emergency department management to prevent cerebral gas embolization. Recent research suggests this practice should be abandoned. Trendelenburg position actually increases intracranial pressure and exacerbates injury to the blood-brain barrier.
- Arrange for urgent recompression and controlled decompression in a hyperbaric chamber.
- If the patient must be flown to a hyperbaric chamber, pressurize the aircraft cabin to 1 atmosphere. Transport in nonpressurized aircraft (e.g., helicopters) should be done at an altitude of no more than 1000 feet, if at all possible.[13]

Nitrogen Narcosis

Air is composed of 79% nitrogen. When air is breathed under pressure (i.e., scuba diving) nitrogen is dissolved slowly in the blood. Dissolved nitrogen produces neurodepressant symptoms similar to those of alcohol intoxication. The deeper one dives, the greater the degree of nitrogen narcosis (Table 29-5). "Martini's law" estimates that every 50 feet of descent is roughly equivalent to the effects of one martini.

Table **29-5**   **Effects of Nitrogen by Depth (at 1 Hour)**

Depth (Feet)	Effects
125-150	Narcosis begins
150-200	Drowsiness; decreased mental function
200-250	Decreased strength; impaired coordination
300	Mental function and movement deteriorate
350-400	Unconsciousness; death

Therapeutic intervention consists of gradual ascent to shallow water with decompression stops along the way to allow nitrogen reabsorption.

Decompression Sickness

If a diver is at depth long enough for nitrogen to be dissolved but then ascends rapidly, there is insufficient time for the dissolved nitrogen to reabsorb. Nitrogen bubbles form in the blood and tissues, producing decompression sickness, also known as dysbarism, the bends, caisson disease, and diver's paralysis. Dive depth and duration influence the probability of decompression sickness. Dysbarism has been reported to occur at depths less than 33 feet (1 atmosphere).

Exercise (such as swimming toward the surface) stimulates more rapid release of nitrogen bubbles from solution, an effect similar to shaking an unopened bottle of a carbonated beverage. Clinical manifestations of the bends are related to nitrogen bubbles in the joints, pulmonary system, central nervous system, and skin. Decompression sickness should be considered in any patient complaining of joint soreness 24 to 48 hours after a dive, particularly those who have traveled by air (a hypobaric environment) since diving.[3]

Signs and symptoms

Signs and symptoms of decompression sickness include the following:
- Shortness of breath, crepitus (subcutaneous air), cough
- Petechial rash, itching
- Headache
- Visual loss, diplopia
- Fatigue, dizziness, unconsciousness, seizures
- Paresthesias, paralysis
- Joint soreness, progressive pain

Factors that increase symptom severity

The following factors may increase severity of symptoms:
- Extreme water temperatures
- Heavy work while diving
- Poor physical conditioning
- Increased age
- Alcohol consumption before diving
- Obesity (large amounts of nitrogen can be stored in adipose tissue)
- Preexisting peripheral vascular disease
- Fatigue

Therapeutic interventions

Therapeutic interventions for decompression sickness include the following:
- Provide basic and advanced supportive care as indicated.
- Administer 100% oxygen by nonrebreather mask. This aids nitrogen elimination.
- Fluid resuscitation: Patients are often mildly hypovolemic. Rehydration assists with gas removal and dissolution of nitrogen. Maintain a urinary output of 1 to 2 mL/hr.
- Arrange for urgent recompression in a hyperbaric chamber (except for patients who exhibit only cutaneous symptoms).
- Provide analgesics for pain relief. Because of the respiratory depressant effect of narcotics, avoid using these drugs.
- Consider aspirin (325 mg) administration for its antiplatelet effects.
- Treat nausea and vomiting.
- Consider administering a helium-oxygen combination (Heliox) to increase bubble shrinkage.

Special Notes

The Divers Alert Network is based out of Duke University Medical Center. Experts are available 24 hours a day for telephone consultation related to any diving emergency. These specialists can help facilitate transfer to a hyperbaric oxygen recompression chamber. Call 1-919-684-8111.

Alternatively, contact the U.S. Navy Experimental Diving Unit in Washington, D.C., (202-433-2790) 24 hours a day, 7 days a week. The duty officer can provide the name, location, and telephone number of the nearest recompression chamber. A useful reference book is the *Directory of Worldwide Decompression Chambers,* which is available from the Superintendent of Diving, U.S. Navy, Naval Ships Systems Command, National Center Building #3, Washington, DC 20360.

References

1. Tintinalli J, Gabor D, Stapczynski J: *Emergency medicine: a comprehensive study guide,* ed 6, New York, 2004, McGraw-Hill.
2. Juckett G: Snakebite. In Rakel RE, editor: *Saunders manual of medical practice,* ed 2, New York, 2000, Saunders.
3. Schaider J et al, editors: *Rosen and Barkin's 5-minute emergency medicine consult,* ed 2, Philadelphia, 2003, Lippincott Williams & Wilkins.
4. Auerbach PA: *Wilderness medicine: management of wilderness and environmental emergencies,* ed 4, St. Louis, 2001, Mosby.
5. Dart RC, McNally J: Efficacy, safety, and use of snake antivenoms in the United States, *Ann Emerg Med* 37(2):181-188, 2001.
6. Dart R et al, editors: *The 5 minute toxicology consult,* Philadelphia, 2000, Lippincott Williams & Wilkins.
7. Rahn DW: Natural history of Lyme disease. In Rahn DW, Evans J, editors: *Lyme disease,* Philadelphia, 1998, American College of Physicians.
8. Hazinski MF, Cummins RO, Field JM, editors: *2000 Handbook of emergency cardiovascular care for healthcare providers,* Dallas, 2000, American Heart Association.
9. Janczyk RJ et al: High-flow venovenous rewarming for the correction of hypothermia in a canine model of hypovolemic shock, *J Trauma* 53(4):639-645, 2002.
10. Fahmy FS et al: Lightning: the multisystem group injuries, *J Trauma* 46(5):937-940, 1999.
11. Jain S, Bandi V: Electrical and lightning injuries, *Crit Care Clin* 15(2):319-331, 1999.
12. Dickey LS: Barotrauma. In Rosen P, Barkin RM, editors: *Emergency medicine concepts and clinical practice,* St Louis, 1997, Mosby.
13. Holleran R: *Air and surface patient transport principles and practice,* St Louis, 2003, Mosby.

30

Genitourinary Emergencies

Louise LeBlanc, RN, BScN, ENC(c)

This chapter describes several acute genitourinary conditions encountered in the emergency department. For information on genitourinary trauma, see Chapter 38.

PROBLEMS OF THE URINARY TRACT

Pyelonephritis

Pyelonephritis is an inflammation of the kidneys that involves the tubules, glomeruli, and renal pelvis. The usual cause is a bacterial infection.

Signs and symptoms

- Severe flank or back pain at the costovertebral angle
- Tenderness over the affected flank
- Fever, chills
- Nausea, vomiting
- Urinary frequency and urgency
- Dysuria, nocturia
- Pyuria, hematuria, bacteriurea

Diagnostic aids

- Urinalysis
- Urine cultures
- Blood cultures do not contribute to diagnosis or management.
- A complete blood count will show leukocytosis but is otherwise noncontributory.[1]

Therapeutic interventions

- Encourage fluid intake to maintain brisk diuresis.
- Encourage bed rest as needed.
- Administer broad-spectrum antibiotics. Patients with severe disease, immunosuppression, pregnancy, abscesses, gram-negative septicemia, age extremes, or significant comorbidities require hospital admission and parenterally administered antibiotics. Most other patients can take antibiotics orally on an outpatient basis.

Perinephric Abscess

Patients with a perinephric abscess generally have a history of a recent skin infection (within the past month), a long-standing urinary tract infection, or pyelonephritis.

Signs and symptoms

- Fever (may be high or low grade)
- Exquisite tenderness over the flank
- A palpable mass in the flank area
- New-onset spinal scoliosis (concave on the affected side)

Diagnostic aids

- On chest radiograph, the diaphragm is elevated on the affected side and the psoas shadow is decreased.
- Ultrasound
- Computed tomography to identify the abscess(es)

Therapeutic interventions

- Incision and drainage
- Antibiotics

Renal Carbuncle

A renal carbuncle is a cortical abscess in the periphery of the kidney usually caused by *Staphylococcus aureus*.

Signs and symptoms

- Severe flank tenderness or pain
- Fever, chills
- Normal urinalysis

Therapeutic interventions

- Incision and drainage
- Antibiotic therapy
- Relapse is common if the carbuncle is incompletely treated.

Renal Calculi

The pain of renal colic typically radiates from the flank to the ipsilateral lower quadrant, the groin, and (occasionally) to the leg. This pain results from ureteral distention caused by the passage of a renal stone (calculus, kidney stone) or blood clots. The size of the stone or clot does not necessarily relate to pain severity.

Signs and symptoms

- Restlessness
- Sudden onset of severe, colicky, radiating, flank pain
- Urinary urgency, frequency, dysuria
- Nausea, vomiting
- Diaphoresis
- Low-grade fever
- Hematuria
- History of renal calculi, presence of an ileal conduit, or hypercalcemia

Diagnostic aids

- Strain the urine for calculi.
- Obtain a urine sample and perform a rapid dipstick test for blood.
- Abdominal radiographs and ultrasound may reveal calculi but are not sensitive.
- Helical computed tomography has replaced intravenous pyelogram as the diagnostic test of choice. Accuracy is 97%.[1]

Therapeutic interventions

- To help flush out stones, initiate an isotonic, intravenous crystalloid infusion. Give 1 L over the first 30 to 60 minutes and then decrease the rate to 200 to 500 mL/hr.
- Provide analgesics. Ketorolac (Toradol) is currently the drug of choice in treating patients who present with pain related to renal colic. Morphine or meperidine (Demerol) also may be given.
- Administer an antiemetic such as ondansetron (Zofran) or promethazine (Phenergan) if the patient is nauseated or vomiting.
- For ongoing care, patients may require hospital admission, pharmacologic stone dissolution, extracorporeal shock wave lithotripsy, laser lithotripsy, or surgical intervention.[2]

Urinary Retention

Urinary retention is the inability to completely empty the bladder of urine. The problem may be acute or chronic. A variety of conditions can cause urinary retention, including urethral strictures, an enlarged prostate, blood clots, renal stones, neurogenic bladder, multiple sclerosis, congenital stenosis, foreign bodies, bladder stones, and hysteria. Urinary retention is also a side effect of parasympatholytic agents and certain other drugs. Rapid drainage avoids stretch injury to the bladder.

Signs and symptoms

- Lower abdominal discomfort
- Bladder distention (A mass is palpable just above symphysis pubis.)
- An ultrasonic bladder scan can confirm urine retention quickly.

Therapeutic interventions

- Insert an indwelling urinary catheter for immediate relief.
- Investigate the cause and treat as indicated.
- Consider urologic consultation.

Hematuria

Hematuria is a symptom of nephrologic and urologic diseases. Blood may appear in the urine as a result of trauma, renal calculi, anticoagulant use, blood dyscrasias, ruptured scrotal varices, ruptured cysts, renal or bladder tumors, or recent urologic manipulation. Bleeding at the start of urination suggests a problem in the region of the anterior urethra. If blood is visualized at the end of the urinary stream, suspect bleeding from the posterior urethra. If bleeding is noted throughout urination, the most likely cause is a bladder or upper urinary tract source.

Do not to assume that all red-colored urine indicates hematuria. Urine may be tinted by the ingestion of food colorings, certain medications, or beets. In females, determine whether the bleeding is actually vaginal.

Diagnostic aids

- Carefully obtain a patient history.
- Collect a urine specimen for dipstick testing and urinalysis. In menstruating females, it may be necessary to obtain the sample via a catheter.
- If significant blood loss is suspected or signs of infection are present, check a complete blood count.

Therapeutic interventions

Interventions depend on the cause of the bleeding.

Oliguria/Anuria

Oliguria is defined as the excretion of less than 500 mL of urine per day. Anuria is the complete absence of urine. A patient with one of these conditions may complain of being unable to void, yet little or no urine is returned on catheterization. Oliguria and anuria can be caused by fluid and electrolyte imbalances, urinary tract obstructions, acute tubular necrosis, tumors, trauma, or accidental laceration of a ureter during abdominal surgery.

Signs and symptoms

- Patients (or their caregivers) complain of a significantly diminished urine output or an inability to void.
- Weakness
- Signs of dehydration or fluid overload

Therapeutic interventions

- Perform intravenous pyelogram or helical computed tomography scan (preferred) to rule out obstruction.
- Treatment is specific to the cause.
- Obtain urologic consultation if indicated.

Acute Cystitis

Acute cystitis is an infection of the bladder that results from bacterial migration from the urethra. Females are more likely to have this condition because their urethras are shorter. Males may contract acute cystitis following acute prostatitis.

Signs and symptoms

- Urinary urgency, frequency, nocturia
- Normal temperature or low-grade fever
- Suprapubic pain
- Hematuria
- Prostate tenderness
- Urinary retention in males

Diagnostic aids

- Blood, leukocyte esterase, and nitrates are readily evident on a rapid urine dipstick.
- Urinalysis is only necessary in complicated cases.

Therapeutic interventions

- Stable, uncomplicated patients can be seen in the emergency department and discharged with a prescription for oral antibiotics.
- Individuals with urosepsis, fulminant pyelonephritis, or septic shock require hospital admission.
- Begin antibiotic therapy. Fluoroquinolones (ciprofloxacin [Cipro]) and trimethoprim/sulfamethoxazole (Septra, Bactrim) are the first-line drugs of choice.[1]
- Phenazopyridine (Pyridium) is a urinary analgesic that reduces dysuria pain and bladder spasms. This drug can be prescribed or purchased over the counter. Warn patients that phenazopyridine will turn their urine bright orange.
- Encourage patients to increase fluid intake to promote bacterial excretion.

GENITOURINARY PROBLEMS UNIQUE TO MALES

Penile/Scrotal Edema

Penile or scrotal edema is frequently present in men with congestive heart failure or recent abdominal surgery in which the pelvic lymph nodes were affected. Although patients may be alarmed, this is not a medical emergency. Care is focused on identifying the cause and referring the patient for ongoing management.

Signs and symptoms

- Diffuse edema of the penis and scrotum
- Possible history of recent pelvic lymphadenectomy

Therapeutic interventions

- Treat the congestive heart failure or other underlying cause.
- Elevating the penis and scrotum on a towel or taping the penis to the abdomen may reduce edema temporarily.

Hematospermia

Hematospermia is an uncommon condition in which blood is present in semen. Anxiety may bring patients to the emergency department, but the condition is generally self-limiting and is rarely significant. Potentially serious causes of hematospermia include bleeding disorders, infections, tumors, or ureteral strictures. Patients with these conditions almost always have other significant findings.[1]

Signs and symptoms

- Blood in the semen

Therapeutic interventions

- Provide reassurance.
- Refer the patient for urologic consultation if indicated.

Hydrocele

A hydrocele results from an imbalance between the production and resorption of fluid within the space between the tunica vaginalis and the tunica albuginea. Although a hydrocele may occur within the spermatic cord, it most often is seen surrounding the testes. This disorder is generally unilateral but can be bilateral.

Signs and symptoms

- Progressive, painless swelling on the involved side of the scrotum
- Presence of a large scrotal mass

Diagnostic aids

- The scrotal mass transilluminates when a bright light is held against the skin.
- Ultrasound will identify fluid in the scrotum.

Therapeutic interventions

- No emergency interventions are indicated.
- Otherwise healthy patients can be discharge with a urologist referral.
- Drainage and sclerotherapy or surgical repair can be performed on an outpatient basis for cosmesis and discomfort.[1]

Priapism

Priapism is a prolonged, painful erection that is not relieved by ejaculation. Physiologic causes include spinal cord injury, tumors, sickle cell disease, or other hematologic disorders. Pharmacologic agents injected into the corpus cavernosum for the treatment of impotence (e.g., papaverine, phentolamine, or prostaglandin E_1) also can elicit priapism. Oral erectile stimulants such as sildenafil (Viagra) occasionally have been implicated. Priapism is considered a urologic emergency.[3]

Signs and symptoms

- Persistent and painful erection

Therapeutic interventions

- Provide analgesia and sedation.
- Manage any underlying conditions.
- Obtain urgent urologic consultation.
- An urologist may perform a needle aspiration to remove trapped blood.
- Epinephrine, phenylephrine, pseudoephedrine, or terbutaline can be injected into the penis to help reverse engorgement.

Acute Prostatitis

Acute prostatitis is an inflammation of the prostate gland, most commonly the result of a bacterial infection. Prostatitis usually is accompanied by acute cystitis.

Signs and symptoms

- Prostate tenderness
- Lower abdominal and perineal pain
- Elevated temperature
- Possible urinary retention, irritative bladder symptoms
- Positive urine culture, positive urethral culture
- Hematospermia, hematuria

Diagnostic aids

- Obtain urine for urinalysis and cultures.
- Prostate examination may reveal a firm or boggy prostate that is exquisitely tender.

Therapeutic interventions

- Provide nonsteroidal antiinflammatory drugs for pain management.
- Initiate antibiotic therapy. Trimethoprim/sulfamethoxazole (Bactrim, Septra) or doxycycline are the drugs of choice for bacterial infection. Give acyclovir for herpes proctitis.[4]
- Encourage patients to increase their fluid intake to aid bacterial elimination.

Acute Epididymitis

Acute epididymitis is an infection of the epididymis. It may result from cystoscopic examination, prostate surgery, or bladder catheterization. However, acute epididymitis most commonly is contracted by sexual contact. *Chlamydia trachomatis* and *Neisseria gonorrhoeae* are the two organisms responsible for the majority of epididymitis cases. This disorder is rare in prepubertal boys. Epididymitis in elderly men often follows urologic manipulation.

Signs and symptoms

- Gradual onset of mild to moderate testicular or scrotal pain that is usually unilateral
- Progressive scrotal swelling
- Dysuria
- Ureteral discharge
- Scrotal warmth, tenderness, and erythema
- Elevated temperature, sepsis (in severe cases)

Table **30-1**　Epididymitis vs. Torsion

	Acute Epididymitis	*Testicular Torsion*
Onset	Gradual	Sudden Pain often begins during physical activity but can occur during sleep as well.
Pain character	Mild to moderate testicular or scrotal pain that is usually unilateral	Severe, unilateral scrotal pain and tenderness followed by scrotal swelling and erythema
Cause	Infectious (usually *Chlamydia trachomatis* and *Neisseria gonorrhoeae*)	Congenital abnormality
Common age group	Postpubertal (sexually active) males	Most common in boys between the ages of 12 and 18 years (but can occur at any age)
Ureteral discharge	Yes	No
Scrotal elevation	May decrease pain	Often causes intense pain
Treatment	Antibiotics	Surgery

Diagnostic aids

- Scrotal ultrasound to differentiate epididymitis from testicular torsion (Table 30-1)
- Urethral smear for Gram stain and culture
- Urine culture

Therapeutic interventions

- Scrotal elevation may decrease pain.
- Initiate antibiotic therapy based on the suspected organisms:
- Gonococcal or chlamydia infection: Ceftriaxone (intramuscularly × 1) plus doxycycline orally
- Enteric organisms: Ciprofloxacin, ofloxacin, or amoxicillin
- Encourage patients to increase oral fluid intake.[3]

Testicular Torsion

Testicular torsion is the twisting of a testicle or the spermatic cord within the tunica vaginalis, causing strangulation of the blood supply to the testis. This condition is seen most commonly in children and adolescents. The majority of patients with testicular torsion have a congenital abnormality of the genitalia. The anomaly is generally bilateral, placing both testicles at risk. Eighty-five percent of cases of testicular torsion occur in boys between the ages of 12 and 18 years. Infants are also susceptible. Torsion is rare after the age of 30. This is an emergent condition. Failure to correct torsion of the testicle results in ischemia and necrosis.[5]

Signs and symptoms

- Sudden onset of severe, unilateral scrotal pain and tenderness followed by scrotal swelling and erythema
- Pain often begins during physical activity but can occur during sleep as well.
- Nausea, vomiting

- Tense scrotal mass (The epididymis cannot be palpated.)
- A high-riding testicle may be present
- Intense pain when the testicle is elevated

Diagnostic aids

- Doppler ultrasonography
- Scintillation scan

Therapeutic interventions

- Obtain urgent urologic consultation.
- Immediate surgical exploration is routinely the treatment of choice.
- Bedside detorsion may be attempted. Most testes twist medially. To correct torsion, manually rotate the affected testis laterally. Relief of pain indicates successful detorsion.[3]

Testicular Tumor

Testicular tumors are most common in the 20- to 30-year-old age-group. These patients come to the emergency department complaining of a scrotal mass with or without pain.

Signs and symptoms

- Scrotal swelling
- A testicular mass that is firm and nontender

Diagnostic aids

- Scrotal ultrasound
- Transillumination

Therapeutic interventions

Obtain urological consultation for surgical intervention.

SEXUALLY TRANSMITTED DISEASES

Patients frequently seek emergency department care for sexually transmitted diseases (STDs). Although initial diagnosis and interventions are important, follow-up care and sexual partner treatment are also essential. Several of the more common STDs are discussed in this section. Refer to Table 30-2 for a quick reference.

Urethritis

Patients with urethritis usually have a chief complaint of urethral discharge. Most cases of urethritis are related to sexual activity, and *N. gonorrhoeae, C. trachomatis,* and *Ureaplasma urealyticum* are the most frequently involved organisms. *Chlamydia trachomatis* is implicated in about 50% of cases.[6]

Table **30-2**   **Sexually Transmitted Diseases**

Description and Risks	Symptoms	Complications and Treatments
Scabies		
Caused by tiny insects that burrow under the skin and produce irritation *Mode of spread:* Close skin-to-skin contact Shared personal items	Intense itching at night Small red bumps and rash develop 4-6 weeks after contact. Lesions occur anywhere on the skin except the head and neck.	*Complications:* Aesthetic *Treatment:* Treat all infected partners and roommates at the same time. Personal clothing and linens should be washed, dry-cleaned, or sealed in plastic and placed in a freezer for 3 days. *Cure:* Yes, topical lotions or sprays
Acquired Immunodeficiency Syndrome (AIDS)		
Caused by the human immunodeficiency virus (HIV), which invades the immune system *Mode of spread:* Contact with infected blood, semen, or vaginal fluids Unprotected anal sex Unprotected vaginal sex Unprotected oral sex Injection of tainted blood Injection by needle sharing Sharing objects contaminated with body fluids Maternal-fetal transfer	HIV stage (1½-14 years) Flulike symptoms may occur early or late from the time of exposure. Most patients look and feel well for years, but carriers are infectious. Skin and lung infections are common as the disease advances. A positive HIV antibody test indicates infection. 25% of infants born to HIV-positive mothers will be infected.	*Complications:* HIV progresses to AIDS (over 2-5 years). The immune system is destroyed. Fatal illnesses develop (pneumonia, cancer, dementia, wasting). *Treatment:* Yes, early treatment is best *Cure:* No
Chlamydia		
A bacterial infection of the genitals, anus, and throat *Mode of spread:* Contact with infected semen and vaginal fluids Unprotected vaginal sex Unprotected anal sex Unprotected oral sex (uncommon)	Most women show *no* symptoms. Some have slight vaginal discharge, dysuria, pain during sex, or frequent urination. Most men show symptoms: penile itching, discharge, mild dysuria, infection of the anus or throat.	*Complications:* Women: Infertility, infected cervix, pelvic pain, pelvic inflammatory disease, ectopic pregnancy, arthritis Infants: Pneumonia, blindness Men: Infertility, arthritis, eye infections, urinary tract infections *Treatment:* Yes, antibiotics *Cure:* Yes
Genital Herpes		
Caused by a virus; ulcerating blisters occur on the genitals or in the anal region; may be spread to the mouth	Fatigue, fever Painful blisters that itch, redden, form into groups, and ulcerate	*Complications:* The virus hides on nerve endings and can recur at any time.

Table 30-2   Sexually Transmitted Diseases—cont'd

Description and Risks	Symptoms	Complications and Treatments
Mode of spread: Unprotected vaginal sex Unprotected anal sex Unprotected oral sex Close, intimate contact	Ulcers crust and may heal with scarring.	*Treatment:* Yes, antivirals *Cure:* No

Genital Warts

Caused by a virus; warts occur on or in the genitals and anus *Mode of spread:* Unprotected vaginal sex Unprotected anal sex Unprotected oral sex (uncommon)	Soft, moist, pink growths on the penis, around the anus, and on or in the female genitalia May form a stalk and look like a cauliflower	*Complications:* The presence of warts may indicate cancer or other immunosuppressive conditions. Bladder cancers Invasive cervical cancer Infected women need yearly Pap smear. May be passed to a fetus *Treatment:* Yes, cauterization, surgery, and drugs *Cure:* No

Gonorrhea

A bacterial infection that commonly infects the genitals, anus, and throat *Mode of spread:* By infected semen and vaginal fluids Unprotected vaginal sex Unprotected anal sex Unprotected oral sex	Most women show *no* symptoms or some vaginal discharge, pain on urination, or urinary frequency. Men usually notice a thick yellow-green discharge from the penis, dysuria, and penile pain. Rectal infection causes pain, bleeding, and discharge. Throat pain occurs if the pharynx is infected.	*Complications:* Women: Sterility, pelvic inflammatory disease Men: Sterility, swollen testes, urinary tract infections Men and women develop cardiac, neurologic, hepatic, and arthritic symptoms. *Treatment:* Yes, antibiotics *Cure:* Yes, although some strains are resistant

Hepatitis B

Caused by a virus that invades the liver *Mode of spread:* Blood transfusion (rare) Injected drugs (sharing needles) Unprotected vaginal sex Unprotected anal sex Unprotected oral sex Maternal blood to fetus Sharing items with blood (e.g., razors, toothbrushes, instruments)	A sudden flulike illness with fatigue, nausea, vomiting, anorexia, fever Dark urine; jaundice 10% of carriers can spread this disease.	*Complications:* Hepatic failure Liver cancer Death *Treatment:* Yes, rest *Cure:* No, but prophylactic vaccination is available

Continued

Table 30-2   **Sexually Transmitted Diseases—cont'd**

Description and Risks	Symptoms	Complications and Treatments
Syphilis		
Caused by bacteria that develops in stages over several years; highly contagious; affects the skin and any other organs *Mode of spread:* Contact with infected blood, semen, vaginal fluids, or pus Mother to newborn Close, intimate contact Unprotected vaginal sex Unprotected anal sex Unprotected oral sex Kissing Blood injection (needle sharing)	Early syphilis: Painless sores, swollen glands, skin rashes Sores inside the vagina or anus may go unnoticed. Late syphilis: Rash, new sores, flulike symptoms, swollen glands, brain infection	*Complications:* Skin, bone, heart, brain disease Dementia Blindness, if untreated *Treatment:* Yes, antibiotics (Sexual contacts must be examined and treated.) *Cure:* Yes, with treatment
Trichomoniasis		
Caused by *Trichomonas vaginalis*; Highly contagious Mode of spread: Contact with infected semen or vaginal secretions Unprotected sexual contact	May be asymptomatic Erythema of external genitalia, vaginal discharge, foul-smelling urethritis (males)	Complications: Pregnancy: Increased risk of delivering preterm or low-birth weight infant. Treatment: Yes: Antibiotics Cure: Yes

Compiled from University of Manitoba: Student affairs guide: STD chart. http://www.umanitoba.ca/student/handbook/chart.html. Accessed July 6, 2000; and Levine WC, Workowski KA: Sexually transmitted diseases treatment guidelines, *MMWR* 51(RR06):1-80, 2002.

Signs and symptoms

- Dysuria
- Urethral discharge
- Urinary frequency
- The first portion of the urinary stream is cloudy.[1]

Diagnostic aids

- Urinalysis
- Ureteral culture

Therapeutic interventions

- Begin antibiotic therapy for the treatment of gonorrhea and chlamydia (see the following discussions).
- Encourage the patient to have sexual partners treated.
- Refer the patient for follow-up care and STD education.

Chancroid

Chancroid infections produce an area of ulceration on the penis, anus, cervix, vagina, vulva, or perineum. Caused by the organism *Haemophilus ducreyi*, this STD occurs more frequently in patients with concomitant infection with human immunodeficiency virus.

Signs and symptoms

- One or more genital lesions
- A painful inguinal adenopathy develops 3 to 14 days after exposure

Diagnostic aids

- Perform Gram stain. A culture of the lesion will be positive for *H. ducreyi*.
- Polymerase chain reaction assays are diagnostic but are not readily available.[1]

Therapeutic interventions

- Check for the presence of other STDs.
- Initiate antibiotic therapy: Ceftriaxone, azithromycin, or ciprofloxacin. (Ciprofloxacin is contraindicated during pregnancy or lactation.)
- Encourage the patient to have sexual partners treated.
- Refer the patient for follow-up care and STD education.

Gonorrhea

Gonorrhea is an STD caused by *N. gonorrhoeae*. Coexisting chlamydial infections are common. Symptoms may be limited to genital pain and discharge, but numerous organs and tissues can be infected. Look for signs of gonococcal cervicitis, proctitis, pelvic inflammatory disease, prostatitis, pharyngitis, conjunctivitis, salpingitis, and epididymitis. Disseminated disease can lead to endocarditis or meningitis.

Signs and symptoms

- Dysuria
- Yellow-white, thick discharge (vaginal, rectal, urethral) 7 to 10 days after exposure
- Positive gonococcus culture

Diagnostic aids

- Gram-negative diplococci are present on Gram stain.
- Positive gonococcus cultures require antibiotic sensitivity testing to identify resistant stains.
- Consider serologic testing for concomitant syphilis infection.

Therapeutic interventions

- Treat uncomplicated genital infections with an initial antibiotic dose (e.g., ceftriaxone, cefixime, ofloxacin, and ciprofloxacin).
- Recommended antibiotic therapy in complicated cases (e.g., acute illness, pregnancy, or comorbid conditions) varies.
- Encourage the patient to have sexual partners treated.
- Refer the patient for follow-up care and STD education.

Chlamydial Infections

Chlamydial infections are the most prevalent STD. The *C. trachomatis* organism commonly coexists with gonorrhea. Patients treated for one infection also should be treated for the other. All recommended antibiotic regimens address both bacteria. Chlamydial infections occur in the rectum, urethra, and cervix.

Signs and symptoms

- Same as for gonorrhea
- Positive *C. trachomatis* culture

Therapeutic interventions

- One-time antibiotic dose (azithromycin) or 7-day antibiotic dose (doxycycline).

Genital Herpes Simplex Virus Infections

Genital herpes is a recurrent, incurable infection caused by the herpes simplex virus (HSV). Two serotypes of HSV have been identified: HSV-1 and HSV-2. Most cases of genital herpes are caused by HSV-2. This virus lives on the nerve root and can be reactivated at any time. Patients with HSV-2 have an average of 3 to 4 recurrences per year. The initial incubation period is 2 to 12 days. Symptoms peak in 8 to 10 days, and lesions typically heal in 3 weeks. The virus can be reactivated by events such as local trauma, emotional stress, fever, sunlight, cold, heat, menstruation, and infection.[1]

Signs and symptoms

- Local manifestations
- Groups of vesicles on an erythematous base that ulcerate, crust over, and then (eventually) heal
- Vesicles form on the vulva, vagina, cervix, perineum, buttocks, penile shaft, and glans.
- Pain and itching at the site of the lesions
- Systemic manifestations
- Fever, headache, malaise, photophobia, anorexia, myalgias, lymphadenopathy
- Patients with a primary HSV-2 infection tend to have a more severe course. Subsequent episodes may include the same symptoms, but severity is generally milder.

Therapeutic interventions

- Acyclovir is the drug of choice for the first clinical episode, recurrences, and early suppressive therapy.
- Encourage the patient to have sexual partners treated.
- Refer the patient for follow-up care and STD education.

Syphilis

Syphilis is a systemic STD caused by the spirochete *Treponema pallidum*. Sometimes referred to as "the great mimicker," syphilis resembles numerous other disease states. This slowly evolving infection can be present for decades (latent syphilis) but eventually affects virtually every body system. Symptoms occur in stages.

Signs and symptoms

First stage (early syphilis)

Signs and symptoms of primary syphilis include the following:

- Painless ulcerations or pustules (chancres) appear on the genitals several weeks after exposure
- Lesions culture positive for *Treponema pallidum*

Second stage

This stage resolves spontaneously in 1 to 2 months. Signs and symptoms include the following:
- General malaise, lethargy
- Lymphadenopathy
- Anorexia, nausea
- Fever
- Rash
- Headache
- Alopecia
- Bone and joint pain
- White sores in mouth

Third stage (tertiary or late syphilis)

The third stage of syphilis may take up to 20 years to develop. Signs and symptoms include the following:
- Soft, rubbery tumors attack all areas of the body, including the central nervous system, heart, and skeleton.
- Disease may be transmitted to fetuses, causing congenital syphilis.

Diagnostic aids

- Blood and skin (lesion) tests
- Lumbar puncture and cerebral spinal fluid testing for tertiary syphilis

Therapeutic interventions

- Intramuscularly administered penicillin G benzathine is the drug of choice for treatment in most syphilis cases.
- Encourage the patient to have sexual partners treated.
- Refer the patient for follow-up care and STD education.

EMERGENCIES IN DIALYSIS PATIENTS

Because of the chronic and serious nature of their condition, dialysis patients make frequent emergency department visits with a variety of complaints ranging from loss of access to lethal hyperkalemia and fluid overload. Some of the problems unique to this population are addressed briefly in this section.

Clotted Access

Hemodialysis patients have one of two basic types of vascular access systems. A fistula (e.g., a Cimino-Brescia fistula) is a surgically created connection between an artery and a vein. The fistula can be constructed from the patient's own vessels or from synthetic graft materials. Fistulas are contained completely under the skin. The most common fistula site is the forearm. A patent fistula will have a strong, palpable bruit. The second type of access consists of a subclavian or femoral catheter, the distal end of which is external to the patient. Catheters can be inserted for short-term use, or a tunneled catheter may be placed surgically for long-term access. Regardless of the type, all vascular access devices are subject to clotting. Most dialysis center personnel do *not* want emergency department providers accessing or manipulating these devices. Declotting is rarely an emergency procedure. Catheters and fistulas can be declotted with a fibrinolytic agent (alteplase, recombinant tissue plasminogen activator) or reopened by angioplasty or angiographic clot removal. Consultation with the patient's nephrologist is indicated.[2,4]

Bleeding

A number of conditions predispose hemodialysis patients to bleeding disorders. Uremia suppresses platelet function, dialysis causes hemolysis, renal failure limits erythropoietin production, and patients are heparinized during dialysis. Additionally, catheters and fistulas provide opportunities for significant hemorrhage.

Fistula Infection

Fistula infections generally are accompanied by signs of systemic infection. Blood cultures should be drawn and antibiotics administered in a timely manner. Synthetic grafts are more vulnerable to infection than are fistulas made from native vessels. Failure to control infection aggressively can lead to loss of the fistula.

Pulmonary Embolus

Hemodialysis patients with an arterial-venous access system can develop clots in their catheter or fistula. These thrombi are prone to detach and embolize to the lungs. Consider the possibility of pulmonary embolism in any hemodialysis patient who has a complaint of acute onset shortness of breath.

References

1. Tintinalli J, Gabor D, Stapczynski J: *Emergency medicine: a comprehensive study guide,* ed 6, New York, 2004, McGraw-Hill.
2. Schaider J et al, editors: *Rosen and Barkin's 5-minute emergency medicine consult,* ed 2, Philadelphia, 2003, Lippincott Williams & Wilkins.
3. Marx J, Hockenberger R, Walls R, editors: *Rosen's emergency medicine: concepts and clinical practice,* ed 5, St Louis, 2002, Mosby.
4. Lok CE, Oliver MJ: Overcoming barriers to arteriovenous fistula creation and use, *Semin Dial* 16(3): 189-196, 2003.
5. Tanago EA, McAninch JW: Disorders of the testis, scrotum, & spermatic cord. In *Smith's general urology,* ed 15, New York, 2000, McGraw-Hill.
6. Levine WC, Workowski KA: Sexually transmitted diseases treatment guidelines, *MMWR* 51(RR-6): 1-80, 2002.

31

Infectious Diseases

Patricia M. Campbell, RN, MSN, CCRN, ANP-CS

Persons with infectious diseases commonly are seen and diagnosed in the emergency department, and nurses are frequently the first health care providers to encounter these patients. Familiarity with contagious conditions, an ability to recognize their signs and symptoms, and rapid implementation of isolation precautions will limit the spread of communicable illnesses. This chapter outlines common infectious diseases, categorized according to their mode of transmission. Also addressed are some unusual conditions related to emerging pathogens or potential epidemics such as severe acute respiratory syndrome (SARS), monkey pox, and West Nile virus. Patients with these illnesses will present for emergency care with signs and symptoms similar to those of common infectious diseases but may pose a grave threat to the hospital and greater community. Weaponized diseases (e.g., smallpox and anthrax) are covered in Chapter 13. See Table 31-1 for information regarding disease incubation periods.

ISOLATION PRECAUTIONS

The five primary routes of transmission are contact, droplet, airborne, common vehicle (food-borne or waterborne), and vector-borne. The Centers for Disease Control and Prevention have established isolation precautions to prevent the spread of infection in health care establishments. Isolation precautions are divided into two general categories: standard precautions and transmission-based precautions.[1]

Standard Precautions

Standard precautions are designed to reduce the risk of transmitting pathogens regardless of a patient's diagnosis or potential risk for infectious disease. Standard precautions apply to

Table 31-1   Incubation Periods of Specific Diseases

Disease	Duration of Incubation
Acquired immunodeficiency syndrome	More than 3 years
Bacillary dysentery (shigella)	1 to 7 days; average 4 days
Botulism (food poisoning)	Fewer than 24 hours for food containing the toxin
Chickenpox (varicella)	14 to 16 days
Common cold	1 to 3 days
Diarrhea, viral	3 to 5 days
Diphtheria	2 to 6 days
Encephalitis	5 to 15 days; range of 4 to 21 days; varies as to the type
Hepatitis	
Infectious (virus A)	15 to 50 days
Serum (virus B)	2 to 6 months
Herpes simplex (type 1 causes the majority of cold sores) (cold sore, fever blister)	2 to 12 days; average 4 days
Herpes zoster (shingles)	4 to 24 days; average 4 days
Infectious mononucleosis (glandular fever)	Children, less than 14 days; adults, 33 to 49 days; average of 4 to 14 days
Influenza (*Haemophilus*)	24 to 72 hours
Lyme disease	3 to 33 days; average 1 week
Malaria	Varies with particular species; 12 to 14 days or as long as 30 days; some strains from 8 to 10 months
Meningitis (bacterial)	2 to 7 days
Mumps (parotiditis)	14 to 28 days
Pertussis (whooping cough)	5 to 21 days
Plague (*Yersinia pestis*)	
Bubonic	2 to 6 days
Pneumonic	2 to 4 days
Pneumococcal pneumonia (bacterial)	1 to 3 days
Poliomyelitis (infantile paralysis)	7 to 14 days
Rabies (hydrophobia)	Dogs, 3 to 8 weeks; human beings, 10 days to 2 years with an average of 2 to 6 weeks
Rocky Mountain spotted fever (tick fever)	2 to 12 days; may be as long as 14 days; average of 7 days
Rubella (German measles)	14 to 21 days, usually 18 days after exposure
Salmonella	7 to 72 hours
Scarlet fever (scarlatina)	24 hours to 10 days, but first clinical signs generally appear between 2 to 5 days
Smallpox (variola)	7 to 16 days; average of 12 days
Syphilis	3 weeks (primary); 6 to 20 weeks (secondary); 3 to 12 months (latent); more than 4 years (tertiary)
Tetanus	3 to 21 days; average of 10 days
Tuberculosis	Variable
Typhoid fever	10 to 14 days; may be as short as 7 days or as long as 21 days
Viral pneumonia (atypical pneumonia)	Varies widely, depending on specific virus; may be from a few days to a week or longer

blood, nonintact skin, mucous membranes, and all body fluids (except sweat). Standard precautions formerly were referred to as universal precautions. Standard precautions include the following:

- *Hand washing:* With soap, water, and friction after touching any contaminated surface and after glove removal. Waterless hand cleansers are also acceptable.
- *Gloves:* To be worn for all patient contacts
- *Gowns:* Worn when body fluid contact is possible

Box **31-1** **Health Care Precautions Against Infectious Diseases**

Standard Precautions

Hand washing

Gloves

Gown/mask/eye protection/face shields: Wear as needed to prevent exposure via the skin and mucous membranes.

Patient care equipment/bed linens: Handle, clean, and discard appropriately to avoid pathogen transmission.

Sharps precautions: Prevent needlesticks and other penetrating injuries.

Transmission-Based Precautions

Use standard precautions *plus* the precautions listed below.

Airborne Precautions

Private patient room with negative air pressure and a closed door.

Respiratory protection for all persons with patient contact (N-95 respirator mask).

Limit patient transport; mask the patient when travel is essential.

Droplet Precautions

Private room.

Wear mask when working within 3 feet of the patient and as needed to prevent exposure via the mucous membranes.

Limit patient transport; mask the patient when travel is essential.

Contact Precautions

Private room.

Don gloves when entering the room. Change gloves after each contact with infectious materials or wounds. Remove gloves before exiting the room.

Wear gown when entering the room if contact with infected surfaces, patient, or items is anticipated. Wear gown if the patient has diarrhea, is incontinent, or has wounds with drainage that are not contained by a dressing. Remove the gown before leaving the room.

Limit patient transport. For essential transport, take precautions to minimize the risk of transmission.

Limit all equipment to single-patient use.

From Garner JS, Hospital Infection Control Practices Advisory Committee: Recommendations for isolation precautions in hospitals. In *Guideline for isolation precautions in hospitals,* Atlanta, 1997, Public Health Service, US Department of Health and Human Services, Centers for Disease Control and Prevention.

- *Masks/eye protection/face shields:* Worn to protect mucous membranes from exposure to body fluids in situations when splashing or other contact is possible (e.g., rescue breathing, tracheal intubation, suctioning, and wound irrigation)

Transmission-Based Precautions

Additional precautions are used to prevent the spread of infectious diseases that have specific modes of transmission. See Box 31-1 for the requirements of each category.

BLOOD-BORNE INFECTIONS

Blood-borne pathogens cause diseases that spread from person to person through direct contact with infected blood or other body fluids.

Acquired Immunodeficiency Syndrome

Acquired immunodeficiency syndrome (AIDS), type 1 (HIV-1) and type 2 (HIV-2), have spread worldwide. Both variants of the human immunodeficiency virus (HIV) have the same modes of transmission and associated complications. However, they differ in their rate of disease progression, duration of infectiousness, and geographic distribution. The United States currently has few HIV-2 cases.[2] By affecting T cell and B cell immunity, the virus compromises the immune system. AIDS is a chronic, progressive, incurable disease. Opportunistic infections are the usual cause of death. Human immunodeficiency virus immunization research is ongoing, but no vaccine is currently available.

High-risk groups

- Intravenous (IV) drug users
- Persons sexually active without protection, those with multiple sexual partners, and those engaged in homosexual or bisexual activities
- Blood transfusion recipients (includes all blood products and clotting factors)
- Hemodialysis patients
- Health care workers

Transmission

- Blood, semen, vaginal secretions, breast milk, and other body fluids
- Maternal-fetal viral transfer
- Needle sharing
- Sexual intercourse, oral sex
- Tattoos and body piercings with contaminated needles or ink

Signs and symptoms

- Chronic infections
- Cough
- Disseminated cytomegalovirus
- Disseminated herpes zoster
- Encephalopathies
- Fatigue, arthralgias
- Fever
- Fungal infections
- Headache, aseptic meningitis
- Secondary complications such as Kaposi's sarcoma, non-Hodgkin's lymphomas, primary lymphomas of the brain, recurrent pneumonia, *Pneumocystis carinii* pneumonia, and toxoplasmosis
- Tuberculosis
- Unexplained weight loss, diarrhea

Diagnostic studies

- Multiple types of HIV tests are available, including rapid, point-of-care detection systems. Refer tested patients for follow-up and counseling.
- Complete blood count (CBC), electrolytes, cultures (blood, sputum, wounds, viral load studies), immune studies (CD4)
- Chest radiograph
- Other tests as indicated by patient presentation

Therapeutic interventions

- Antiviral medications (e.g., nonnucleoside reverse transcriptase inhibitors, nucleoside/nucleotide reverse transcriptase inhibitors)
- Counseling, referral services
- Fluid, electrolyte, and nutritional support
- Fusion inhibitors
- Protease inhibitors
- Symptomatic support
- Treatment for opportunistic infections

Prevention

- Avoid high-risk behaviors, including tattoos and body piercing.
- Use protective barriers during sexual encounters.
- Ensure sharps protection.
- Follow standard precautions.

Discharge instructions

Provide information regarding the following:
- Counseling services
- HIV prevention measures
- HIV support groups
- Medical follow-up
- Nutritional support

Hepatitis B

Hepatitis B virus (HBV) is a chronic, progressive disease of the liver that can cause cirrhosis, liver cancer, hepatic failure, and death. A small percentage of patients recover from the disease; most develop chronic hepatitis.

Transmission

- HBV is transmitted through contact with blood or other body fluids from an infected person (see Acquired Immunodeficiency Syndrome).
- Blood transfusions
- Body piercing, tattooing
- Hemodialysis
- Needle sharing
- Unprotected sex, especially with multiple partners

Signs and symptoms

- Abdominal pain
- Anorexia, nausea, vomiting
- Fatigue
- Jaundice, dark urine
- Joint pain
- Clay-colored stools

Diagnostic studies

- Serum hepatitis panel (screen for types A, B, C, D)
- CBC and platelets
- Prothrombin time (international normalized ratio), activated partial thromboplastin time
- Electrolytes, complete metabolic panel
- Liver enzymes, amylase, lipase, ammonia level

Therapeutic interventions

- Provide fluids, electrolytes, and nutrition.
- Observe for bleeding disorders.
- Administer approved medications: Interferon-alpha, pegylated interferon (Pegasys), adefovir dipivoxil (Hepsera), lamivudine (Epivir)

Prevention

- Use standard precautions.
- Obtain HBV vaccination. Routine vaccinations are given between birth and 18 years of age (Figures 31-1 to 31-3).
- Avoid high-risk behaviors, including tattoos and body piercing.

Discharge instructions

- Receive medical follow-up for ongoing care.
- Avoid alcohol.
- Do not donate organs, blood, or other tissue.
- Do not share personal items (e.g., toothbrush and razors).
- Use protective barriers during sexual encounters.

Hepatitis C

The hepatitis C (HCV) virus attacks the liver and progressively causes severe hepatic disease that culminates in liver failure, cancer, and death. Patients may be asymptomatic for up to 20 years and can be unaware of the disease until signs of liver failure occur. Hepatitis C infection is the most common reason for liver transplant in the United States.

Transmission

- Needle sharing (past or present) accounts for two thirds of all HCV cases in the United States.
- Accidental needlesticks and other sharps-related injuries
- Blood transfusion or organ transplant before 1992
- Body piercing or tattooing with contaminated needles or ink
- Clotting factor infusion before 1987 (hemophiliacs)
- Hemodialysis
- History of liver disease
- Intranasal cocaine use
- Sexual transmission is unlikely unless blood exposure occurs.

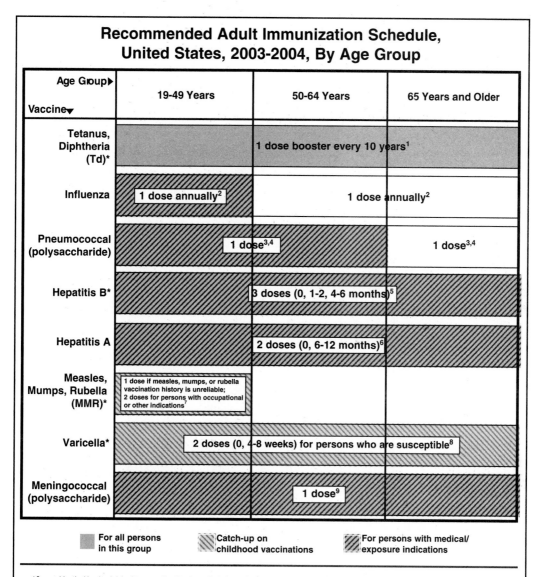

Figure 31-1. Recommended Adult Immunization Schedule, United States, 2003-2004 (by age). (Reprinted with permission from the Centers for Disease Control and Prevention.)

Recommended Adult Immunization Schedule, United States, 2003-2004, By Medical Conditions

Medical Conditions ▼ Vaccine ▶	Tetanus-Diphtheria (Td)*,1	Influenza2	Pneumo-coccal (polysacch-aride)3,4	Hepatitis B*,5	Hepatitis A6	Measles, Mumps, Rubella (MMR)*,7	Varicella*,8
Pregnancy		A					
Diabetes, heart disease, chronic pulmonary disease, chronic liver disease, including chronic alcoholism		B	C		D		
Congenital Immunodeficiency, leukemia, lymphoma, generalized malignancy, therapy with alkylating agents, antimetabolites, radiation or large amounts of corticosteroids			E				F
Renal failure/end stage renal disease, recipients of hemodialysis or clotting factor concentrates			E	G			
Asplenia including elective splenectomy and terminal complement component deficiencies		H	E,I,J				
HIV infection			E,K			L	

See Special Notes for Medical Conditions below also see Footnotes for Recommended Adult Immunization Schedule, by Age Group and Medical Conditions, United States, 2003-2004 on back cover.

■ For all persons in this group   ▨ Catch-up on childhood vaccinations   ▨ For persons with medical/exposure indications   ■ Contraindicated

Special Notes for Medical Conditions

A. For women without chronic diseases/conditions, vaccinate if pregnancy will be at 2nd or 3nd trimester during influenza season. For women with chronic diseases/conditions, vaccinate at any time during the pregnancy.

B. Although chronic liver disease and alcoholism are not indicator conditions for influenza vaccination, give 1 dose annually if the patient is age 50 years or older has other indications for influenza vaccine, or if the patient requests vaccination.

C. Asthma is an indicator condition for influenza but not for pneumococcal vaccination.

D. For all persons with chronic liver disease.

E. For persons < 65 years, revaccinate once after 5 years or more have elapsed since initial vaccination.

F. Persons with impaired humoral immunity but intact cellular immunity may be vaccinated. *MMWR*1999;48 (RR-06):1-5.

G. Hemodialysis patients: Use special formulation of vaccine (40 mcg/mL) or two 1.0 mL 20 mcg doses given at one site. Vaccinate early in the course of renal disease. Assess antibody titers to hep B surface antigen (anti-HBs) levels annually. Administer additional doses if anti-HBs levels decline to <10 milliinternational units (mIU)/ mL.

H. There are no data specifically on risk of severe or complicated influenza infections among persons with asplenia. However, influenza is a risk factor for secondary bacterial infections that may cause severe disease in asplenics.

I. Administer meningococcal vaccine and consider Hib vaccine.

J. Elective splenectomy: vaccinate at least 2 weeks before surgery.

K. Vaccinate as close to diagnosis as possible when CD4 cell counts are highest.

L. Withhold MMR or other measles containing vaccines from HIV-infected persons with evidence of severe immunosuppression. *MMWR* 1998;47 (RR-8):21-22; *MMWR* 2002;51 (RR-02):22-24.

Figure 31-2. Recommended Immunizations for Adults With Medical Conditions, United States, 2003-2004. (Reprinted with permission from the Centers for Disease Control and Prevention.)

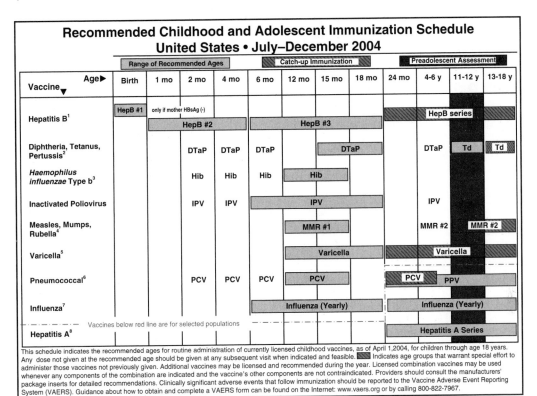

Figure 31-3. Recommended Childhood and Adolescence Immunization Schedule—United States, 2004 (Reprinted with permission from the Centers for Disease Control and Prevention.)

Signs and symptoms

- Abdominal pain
- Anorexia, nausea
- Fatigue
- Jaundice, dark urine
- Clay-colored stools

Diagnostic studies

- Liver biopsy
- Hepatitis panel (screen for types A, B, C, D)
- Hepatitis C virus RNA polymerase chain reaction becomes positive 2 to 4 weeks after exposure.

Therapeutic interventions

- Interferon
- Ribavirin

Prevention

- Follow standard precautions.
- Avoid high-risk behaviors (see Acquired Immunodeficiency Syndrome and Hepatitis B).

Discharge instructions

- Same as for HBV

Hepatitis D

Hepatitis D virus (HDV) is a defective RNA virus that requires the presence of the HBV for duplication and survival. All patients who have HDV will also have HBV. Superinfection with HDV in a patient with HBV increases the incidence of cirrhosis. See Table 31-2 for a summary of hepatitis types.

Transmission

- Same as for HBV
- Perinatal transmission is less common.

Signs and symptoms

- Same as for HBV

Diagnostic studies

- Same as for HBV

Therapeutic interventions

- Same as for HBV

Prevention

- Same as for HBV

AIRBORNE INFECTIONS

Airborne pathogens are transmitted by exposure to respiratory droplets, aerosols, and secretions. A number of common bacterial and viral pathogens are distributed by this route.

Epiglottitis

See Chapter 19.

Influenza

Influenza viruses are endemic throughout the world, including the United States. Disease prevalence is greatest in winter and early spring. Influenza A and B are the most common flu viruses. Influenza is a respiratory pathogen; there is no "stomach flu."

Transmission

- Readily spread from person to person by respiratory droplets

Table 31-2   Types of Hepatitis

Type	Transmission	High Risk for Infection	Signs and Symptoms	Long-Term Complications	Treatment	Prevention
Hepatitis A	Food-borne/ waterborne Enteric	Household contacts Sexual contacts Endemic areas Travelers Homosexual contacts Drug users	Jaundice, abdominal pain, fatigue, anorexia, nausea, vomiting, fever	No chronic infection 15% may have a relapse of symptoms within 1 year.	Supportive treatment	HAV vaccine: series of two injections (>2 years old) Good sanitation and personal hygiene
Hepatitis B	Blood-borne	Unprotected sex Multiple partners Intravenous (IV) drug users Needlestick/sharp exposure Maternal transfer at birth Persons with HCV or HIV Household contacts of infected persons	Jaundice, abdominal pain, fatigue, anorexia, nausea, vomiting, dark urine, joint pain	Chronic infection 90% of infants are infected at birth if the mother is HBV-positive. 30% of children are infected by age 1-5. 6% infected >5 years Mortality is 15%-25% in patients with chronic infection.	Antiviral medications: adefovir dipivoxil, interferon-alpha, lamivudine Pregnant women cannot take these drugs. Avoid alcohol.	HBV vaccination for all ages: series of three injections Avoid IV drug use. Avoid unprotected sex. Use latex condoms. Avoid tattoos/ piercings. Avoid sharing personal items that may be contaminated with blood. If pregnant, get tested. Infants of infected mothers should receive (hepatitis B immune globulin) within 12 hours of birth.

Continued

Table 31-2   Types of Hepatitis—cont'd

Type	Transmission	Risk factors	Symptoms	Treatment	Prevention
					HBV-positive persons should never donate blood, organs, or tissues.
Hepatitis C	Blood-borne	IV drug users Recipients of clotting factors before 1987 Hemodialysis patients Recipients of blood/organs before 1992 Infants of infected mothers Health care workers Multiple sexual partners/infected partner	May be asymptomatic for years, then symptoms are the same as HBV	Interferon and ribavirin for treatment of chronic HCV. Avoid alcohol.	No vaccine for HCV. Avoid IV drug use. Do not share personal items that may be contaminated with blood. Get vaccinated for HBV and HAV. Use latex condoms. HCV-infected persons should never donate blood, organs, or tissues.
Hepatitis D	Blood-borne	Same as HBV Requires coinfection with HBV	Same as HBV	Same as HBV	Prevent HBV infection.
Hepatitis E	Foodborne/waterborne Enteric	Same as HAV	Same as HAV Rare in the United States	Same as HAV	No vaccine Good sanitation/personal hygiene Avoid contaminated/endemic areas.

National Center for Infectious Diseases: *Viral hepatitis fact sheets*, Atlanta, 2004, Centers for Disease Control and Prevention.
HAV, Hepatitis A virus; *HBV*, hepatitis B virus; *HCV*, hepatitis C virus; *HIV*, human immunodeficiency virus.

Signs and symptoms

- Abrupt onset of high fever: 38° to 40° C (100° to 104° F)
- Anorexia
- Conjunctivitis, coryza, pharyngitis, nasal discharge
- Dry cough[3]
- General body aches, myalgias
- Headache
- Malaise, lassitude

Diagnostic studies

- Diagnosis usually is made clinically based on presenting complaints.
- A CBC and complete metabolic panel are indicated for patients with significant compromise.
- Nasopharyngeal swabs or aspirate can confirm the diagnosis.

Therapeutic interventions

- Adequate hydration and nutrition
- Antiviral medications
- Influenza A: Amantadine (Symmetrel), rimantadine (Flumadine)
- Influenza A and B: Zanamivir (Relenza), oseltamivir (Tamiflu) for treatment and prophylaxis

Prevention

- Use standard precautions; use droplet precautions for *Haemophilus influenzae* type B.
- Annual influenza vaccinations are recommended for persons at risk, including those who are immunosuppressed, over the age of 50 years, health care workers, chronic care facility residents, women in the second or third trimester of pregnancy, and anyone with chronic disease.

Discharge instructions

- Increase fluid intake, and ensure adequate nutrition and rest.
- Take antiviral drugs as instructed.
- Use acetaminophen or ibuprofen for fever and pain.
- Seek medical care for persistent symptoms or dehydration.

Pneumonia

See Chapter 20.

Tuberculosis

Tuberculosis is a respiratory disease caused by *Mycobacterium tuberculosis*. Not long ago, tuberculosis was largely considered a disease of the past for developed countries. However, in recent years the incidence of tuberculosis has risen dramatically, complicated by the emergence of drug-resistant strains. Tuberculosis is endemic among the poor, those living in overcrowded situations (jails, homeless shelters), and recent U.S. immigrants. Elderly and immunosuppressed patients are at particularly high risk for activation of latent tuberculosis.

Tuberculosis is classified as active (infectious) or latent (inactive). Even though individuals may skin test positive, those with latent tuberculosis infection are asymptomatic and non-contagious. These carriers can develop tuberculosis at any time later in life if the disease is not eliminated with medications. Patients with active tuberculosis require aggressive drug treatment and respiratory precautions.

Transmission

Tuberculosis is transmitted by respiratory droplets. The concentration of organisms in the sputum, cough severity and frequency, and the extent of the disease determine a patient's infectivity. Tuberculosis is known primarily as a pulmonary disease, but the bacilli can be transported throughout the body, resulting in a disseminated infection. Other tissues that can become infected include the heart, lymph nodes, bones, kidneys, urinary tract, meninges, eyes, gastrointestinal system, adrenal glands, and the skin.

Signs and symptoms

Initial infection with tuberculosis is usually asymptomatic. In healthy individuals the disease moves rapidly into the latent phase. Symptoms begin once the tuberculosis is activated, possibly decades after exposure:
- Cough that persists for more than 2 weeks
- Hemoptysis
- Night sweats, fever, chills
- Unexplained weight loss, fatigue

Diagnostic studies

- Sputum for acid-fast organisms, culture, and sensitivity
- CBC, complete metabolic panel
- Chest radiographs
- Acutely ill individuals and those with nonpulmonary disease require further studies.

Therapeutic interventions

- Treat acutely ill patients symptomatically.
- Antituberculosis drug therapy regimens are long-term (at least 6 months) and include multiple drugs such as isoniazid (INH), rifampin, pyrazinamide, ethambutol, and streptomycin.

Prevention

- Standard and airborne precautions
- Compliance with a medication regimen prevents the conversion of latent tuberculosis to active (and contagious) tuberculosis.
- Teach patients with active tuberculosis to contain their respiratory secretions. Specific precautions include covering the mouth and nose with a tissue when coughing, sneezing, or laughing.
- Dispose of contaminated articles in a sealed bag.
- Do not go to work or school until medically cleared.
- Avoid close contact with others. Sleep in a bedroom away from family members.
- Air out the patient's room each day; tuberculosis spores can exist for years in small closed spaces with stagnant air.

Discharge instructions

Provide information regarding the following:
- Medical follow-up
- Medication compliance (Continue all drugs until the prescribed regimen is complete.)
- Nutrition and hydration
- Preventative measures
- When to seek medical care (fever, hemoptysis, medication reactions)

Chickenpox (Varicella Zoster)

Chickenpox is a highly contagious disease caused by the varicella zoster virus. Before the advent of routine immunization, chickenpox was a common childhood illness. Most U.S. adults have developed immunity through childhood exposure. In children, varicella zoster is generally a mild illness, although secondary bacterial infections can occur. However, adults who contract the disease often experience severe complications such as varicella pneumonitis. Chickenpox mortality in adults is 15 times greater than in children. In addition to the initial illness, anyone who has contracted varicella zoster still may have the virus dormant in sensory nerve ganglia. Reactivation of the virus produces shingles (see Herpes Zoster [Shingles]).

Transmission

Varicella zoster virus usually is spread by respiratory droplets. Contagion is possible (although much less common) through secondary contact with the live virus in skin lesions. Individuals are infectious for 48 hours before the rash appears and remain contagious until all skin lesions have crusted over and no new lesions have formed.[3]

Signs and symptoms

- Fever
- Headache, anorexia
- Lymphadenopathy
- Malaise
- Pruritus
- Purulent vesicular rash that initially forms on the trunk and face and then becomes generalized
- Urticaria

Diagnostic studies

- CBC, metabolic panel
- Chest radiographs if respiratory involvement occurs

Therapeutic interventions

- Respiratory and contact isolation
- Symptomatic care: Rest, oral fluid intake
- Medications
  - Antiviral agents: Acyclovir (Zovirax), foscarnet (Foscavir) (not generally necessary in uncomplicated cases)
  - Antihistamines: Diphenhydramine for pruritic symptoms
  - Antipyretics/analgesics: Acetaminophen, ibuprofen

- Administer varicella-zoster immune globulin for pregnant patients. This drug also can be used for prophylaxis in nonimmune pregnant patients with chickenpox exposure.
- Antibiotics if a secondary bacterial infection occurs

Prevention

- Follow standard, contact, and airborne precautions.
- The varicella vaccine is a live virus. One dose is recommended for all children at 12 to 18 months of age. (Immunosuppression is a contraindication to immunization.)
- Children and adults who have not been vaccinated and have never had chickenpox should be immunized as well.

Discharge instructions

Provide information regarding the following:
- Medications
- Nutrition, hydration
- Rest and symptomatic treatment
- Skin care: Do not scratch lesions; this may cause a secondary bacterial infection.
- When to seek medical care: Cough, red/purulent lesions, persistent vomiting, persistently high fever, or secondary infection.

Monkeypox

Monkeypox, caused by the monkeypox virus, is a disease that originated in Africa. Although it is in the same family as smallpox (variola) and cowpox, symptoms are usually milder. This pathogen is currently rare in the United States.

Transmission

Monkeypox is transmitted by direct contact with infected animal blood, body fluids, or lesions. Human-to-human transmission occurs via respiratory droplets and prolonged close contact. Touching contaminated surfaces, linens, and clothing also can spread the virus. *Monkeypox is a reportable disease. Contact the National Notifiable Diseases Surveillance System at the Centers for Disease Control and Prevention, 404-639-3311.*

Signs and symptoms

- Incubation of about 12 days
- Headache, backache, myalgias, exhaustion
- Fever, swollen lymph nodes
- A papular rash usually first appears on the face. Lesions progress through several stages but finally crust over and fall off.
- The illness lasts 2 to 4 weeks.

Diagnostic studies

- CBC, metabolic panel

Therapeutic interventions

- Acetaminophen or ibuprofen for fever and aches
- Oral or intravenous hydration

- Supportive care
- Treatment of secondary infections

Prevention

- Standard, contact, and airborne precautions
- Smallpox vaccination appears to provide immunity to monkeypox. Clinicians caring for monkeypox patients should be immunized against smallpox. Postexposure vaccination is effective up to 14 days after contact and may prevent the disease or lessen its severity.[4]

Discharge instructions

- Increase fluid intake, and ensure adequate nutrition and rest.
- Use acetaminophen for fever and aches.
- Provide topical care for rash.
- Wash all linens and clothes in very hot water; separate them from other household laundry.

Measles

The two types of measles are rubeola and rubella (or German measles). These once-common childhood illnesses have largely disappeared from developed nations as a result of aggressive immunization campaigns. Vaccination is highly effective. However, cases still are seen occasionally in persons who escaped immunization, such as the elderly, immigrants, and individuals with religious objections to vaccination.

Transmission

Measles is a highly contagious disease that is transmitted via nasal secretions, either directly to another individual or via respiratory droplets. The incubation period for rubeola is 8 to 12 days; for rubella it is 14 to 21 days. These viruses can be transmitted 5 days after initial exposure and up to 5 days after the rash has appeared. Both types of measles have fairly similar symptoms. Fetuses exposed to rubella during the first trimester are at risk for abnormalities including heart defects, mental retardation, deafness, and stunted growth.

Signs and symptoms

- Conjunctivitis, eyelid edema, photophobia
- Dry cough, coryza
- Fever
- Joint pain (rubella)
- Rash
- Koplik's spots (These lesions are diagnostic for measles. They are small, red specks with a blue-white center. These spots are found on the buccal mucosa, especially near the molars. Koplik's spots appear 2 days before the rash and disappear within 48 hours of rash onset.)
- Malaise, irritability
- Tender, enlarged lymph nodes (rubella)

Diagnostic studies

- Diagnosis is made based on clinical findings.
- Leukopenia may be present.

- Viral cultures and antibody testing are possible but are generally impractical and rarely contribute to patient management.
- Chest radiograph may be necessary for suspected pneumonitis.

Therapeutic interventions

- Antipyretics for fever
- Diphenhydramine for itching
- Supportive care, hydration, nutrition
- Symptomatic treatment of patients with oxygen, IV fluids, and analgesics

Prevention

- Follow standard and airborne precautions.
- Refer to Figures 31-1 to 31-3.

Discharge instructions

- Increase fluid intake, and ensure adequate nutrition and rest.
- Use antipyretics for fever.
- Use diphenhydramine for pruritus.
- Seek medical care for respiratory, cardiac, or neurologic complications.

Mumps

The mumps virus is a paramyxovirus most frequently seen in the spring months. This virus causes glandular enlargement, primarily of the parotid gland. Complications include orchitis, in which the testicles become swollen and painful. Twenty percent to 50% of postpubertal males with mumps develop orchitis. Other complications include pancreatitis, aseptic meningitis, oophoritis, and central nervous system involvement.

Transmission

Viral transmission is via respiratory droplets and saliva. Patients are most contagious 1 to 2 days before the appearance of parotitis and remain infectious for up to 5 days after the onset of glandular enlargement.[3]

Signs and symptoms

- *Parotitis:* Swelling is bilateral in two thirds of cases.
- *Fever:* 37.8° to 39.4° C (100° to 103° F)
- *Nonspecific symptoms of upper respiratory tract infection:* malaise, anorexia, and headache

Diagnostic studies

- Diagnosis usually is based on clinical findings. Further studies are noncontributory in uncomplicated cases.
- The virus can be isolated from throat swabs, secretions, cerebral spinal fluid, or urine.
- An immunofluorescence assay indicates viral antigens in oropharyngeal cells.

- An enzyme-linked immunosorbent assay (ELISA) for rapid detection can be performed with unclear cases.
- Leukocytosis with a left shift may be present in severely ill patients.
- Amylase level may be elevated (pancreatitis).

Therapeutic interventions

- Analgesics, antipyretics
- Orally administered steroids if orchitis is severe
- Scrotal support or ice packs to reduce discomfort
- Supportive care

Prevention

- Follow standard and droplet precautions.
- Refer to Figures 31-1 to 31-3.

Discharge instructions

- Increase fluid intake, and ensure adequate nutrition and rest.
- Seek medical care for complications such as orchitis.
- Take antipyretics and analgesics as needed.
- Maintain respiratory isolation.

Pertussis (Whooping Cough)

Pertussis is a highly contagious respiratory disease caused by the gram-negative organism *Bordetella pertussis*. These bacteria attach to the respiratory tract and produce toxins that limit a patient's ability to clear secretions. This predisposes patients to a secondary pneumonia. Pertussis remains a major health issue in countries where vaccination is not routine. Occasional cases have been reported in unimmunized individuals in the United States.

Transmission

Bordetella pertussis is transmitted through respiratory droplets or contact with airborne respiratory secretions. There have been rare cases of transmission via contaminated surfaces and clothing. The pertussis incubation period is usually 7 to 10 days but may be as long as 4 to 42 days. Children are infected more frequently than are adults and tend to have a more severe disease course.

Signs and symptoms

- *Stage I (catarrhal stage):* Approximately 1-week duration with coryza, sneezing, low-grade fever, and occasional cough that progressively becomes worse
- *Stage II (paroxysmal stage):* 1 to 6 weeks in duration. One to 2 weeks after onset, the cough worsens. Patients experience unremitting paroxysmal bursts of coughing that end with a high-pitched "whoop." Cyanosis may be present during the coughing episode. Coughing fits happen more frequently at night.
- *Stage III (convalescent stage):* Gradual recovery as the cough becomes less severe and frequent. Superinfections can occur because of trapped secretions.

Diagnostic studies

- Diagnosis of uncomplicated cases is based on clinical findings.
- Collect posterior nasopharyngeal cultures (not throat cultures) for isolation of *B. pertussis*. Use a Dacron (not cotton) swab and place it directly on the medium. This organism is difficult to isolate. Culturing is easiest in the catarrhal stage, before antibiotic use.
- Other diagnostic studies have been used but vary in reliability and availability.

Therapeutic interventions

- Respiratory isolation
- Supplemental oxygen as needed to maintain saturation
- Intravenous fluid administration if the patient is unable to tolerate liquids orally
- Suction as needed to keep the airway clear
- Antibiotics: Clarithromycin or erythromycin

Prevention

- Follow standard and droplet precautions.
- Obtain pertussis vaccination.
- Household contacts should be treated with antibiotics regardless of vaccination status.

Discharge instructions

- Persons younger than 1 year, those with severe disease, and patients with complications usually are admitted to the hospital under respiratory isolation.
- *Pertussis is a reportable disease. Contact the National Notifiable Diseases Surveillance System.*

Diphtheria

Diphtheria is an infection of the mucous membranes caused by the pathogen *Corynebacterium diphtheriae*. The bacteria is uncommon in the United States because most persons are vaccinated in childhood. Diphtheria still is seen in unimmunized immigrants, particularly those living in overcrowded situations.

Transmission

Diphtheria is spread by respiratory droplets. The incubation period is 1 to 8 days.

Signs and symptoms

- Low-grade fever
- Sore throat
- A thick, gray, membranous covering forms on the tonsils and pharynx. The covering may extend over the larynx, causing airway obstruction.
- Complications include systemic diseases such as myocarditis and peripheral neuritis.

Diagnostic studies

Swab the throat for culture, sensitivity, and Gram stain.

Therapeutic interventions

- Diphtheria antitoxin: The dose depends on the extent of the disease.
- Erythromycin 20 to 25 mg/kg every 12 hours for 7 to 14 days.[5]
- Membrane removal will cause bleeding.

Prevention

- Standard and droplet precautions
- Diptheria vaccination

Discharge instructions

Patients with severe disease require hospital admission for airway and ventilatory management.

Severe Acute Respiratory Syndrome

Severe acute respiratory syndrome (SARS) was first identified in China in the winter of 2003. The SARS virus is a member of the coronavirus family, similar to the common cold. This emerging disease originally was transmitted from animals to the human population. Human transmission is now typically face to face. *Severe acute respiratory syndrome is a disease warranting quarantine and must be reported to the Centers for Disease Control and Prevention and local health authorities.*

Transmission

The SARS virus is largely transmitted via respiratory droplets and surface contact, but the possibility of respiratory transmission has not been ruled out. Live viruses also can be found in urine and feces. The incubation period is 2 to 10 days.

Signs and symptoms

- Fever: temperature greater than 38° C (100.4° F)
- Signs of respiratory illness (cough, dyspnea, labored respirations, hypoxia)
- Severe illness: Radiographic signs of pneumonia, severe respiratory distress, respiratory failure
- History of travel to an endemic area or exposure to persons who have traveled. Check the Centers for Disease Control and Prevention Web site *(www.cdc.gov)* for current disease information.

Diagnostic studies

- CBC, complete metabolic panel, cultures (sputum, urine, stool, blood)
- Chest radiographs
- Tests specific for SARS
  - Enzyme immunoassay
  - Indirect fluorescent antibody
  - Reverse transcription polymerase chain reaction test for serum, stool, and nasal secretions

Therapeutic interventions

- Supportive care, hydration, nutrition
- Respiratory support, supplemental oxygen as needed
- Antiviral medications

Prevention

- Standard, airborne, droplet, and contact precautions
- Avoid travel to high-risk areas.
- Avoid exposure to infected individuals.

Discharge instructions

- Severe disease: Patients require hospital admission.
- Mild cases: Patients must be isolated at home with standard, airborne, droplet, and contact precautions for any household members.
- Teach patients about isolation and quarantine measures.

WATER-BORNE AND FOOD-BORNE INFECTIONS

Many pathogens are transmitted via contaminated food and water supplies. These infections commonly accompany foreign travel but readily occur in the United States as well because of inadequate sanitation and poor food preparation or storage practices.

Hepatitis A

The hepatitis A virus (HAV) infects the liver. The virus is prevalent in areas with poor hygiene and sanitation or crowded living conditions. Hepatitis A is a self-limited illness that usually does not cause chronic liver disease. Infection with HAV provides immunity. The incubation period is 2 to 6 weeks.

Transmission

HAV is spread via the fecal-oral route from contaminated food, water, or objects:
- High-risk individuals:
  - Household contacts with infected individuals
  - Persons living in, or traveling to, an area in which HAV is endemic

Signs and symptoms

- Anorexia, nausea, abdominal pain, diarrhea
- Fatigue
- Jaundice
- Low-grade fever

Diagnostic studies

- Serum HAV antibodies
- Stool cultures that are positive for the virus

Therapeutic interventions

- Provide symptomatic care.
- Maintain fluid and electrolyte balance.

Prevention

- HAV vaccination is recommended for the following:
  - Persons age 2 years or older
  - High-risk individuals
  - Health care workers
  - Travelers to endemic areas
- Immune globulin prevents infection if given before, or within 2 weeks, of exposure.
- Wash hands with soap, water, and friction after using the toilet and before eating or food preparation.

Discharge instructions

- Provide information regarding HAV transmission, prevention, and treatment.
- Increase fluid intake, and ensure adequate nutrition and rest.

Hepatitis E

Hepatitis E virus (HEV), a single-stranded RNA virus, is responsible for most of the non-A, non-B enterically transmitted hepatitis. This organism causes an inflammatory liver disease similar to HAV. The course of the disease is self-limiting. Most patients recover, although mortality rates are higher in pregnant women. No evidence indicates chronic disease.

Transmission

- HEV is excreted in the stool.
- Transmission is by the fecal-oral route.
- The incubation period is 15 to 60 days.

Signs and symptoms

- Abdominal pain, nausea, vomiting
- Fever, malaise
- Jaundice, dark urine, hepatomegaly
- Clay-colored stools

Diagnostic studies

- Same as for hepatitis A

Therapeutic interventions

- Same as for hepatitis A

Prevention

- Same as for hepatitis A

Traveler's Diarrhea

This generic illness is caused by a wide variety of organisms including salmonella, toxigenic *Escherichia coli,* campylobacter, shigella, and *Giardia.* High-risk individuals have a history of foreign travel or immunosuppression. Also at risk are persons on recent antibiotic, antacid, or antimotility medication therapy. Traveler's diarrhea is inconvenient, but usually self-limiting, and requires only supportive care.

Transmission

- Any contaminated food or water
- Salmonella often is transmitted in contaminated eggs and chicken.

Signs and symptoms

- Bloody stools (shigella, *E. coli,* salmonella, amebic dysentery)
- Fever (salmonella)
- Nausea, vomiting, abdominal cramps, diarrhea

Diagnostic studies

- Stool and blood cultures
- CBC, complete metabolic panel

Therapeutic interventions

- Maintain hydration.
- If the patient is immunosuppressed or has severe illness, treat with antibiotics:
  - *Mild cases:* Ciprofloxacin (Cipro) 750 mg, one oral dose
  - *Severe cases:* Ciprofloxacin 500 mg orally twice daily for 3 to 7 days or azithromycin (Zithromax) 1 g × 1 then 500 mg orally for 6 days
- Antidiarrheals: Loperamide (Imodium). Do not use this drug in the presence of bloody stools.
- Use antiemetics as needed.

Prevention

- Follow standard and contact precautions.
- Avoid contaminated food and drink.
- Wash all food preparation surfaces well, especially after working with raw chicken or eggs.
- Thoroughly cook all food.
- Wash hands and cooking utensils with soap and water.

Discharge instructions

Instruct patients to do the following:
- Maintain hydration.
- Take medications to control nausea and vomiting as needed.
- Seek medical care for dehydration and persistent nausea, vomiting, or diarrhea.
- Schedule medical follow-up for culture results and reevaluation.

Botulism

See Chapter 28.

Typhoid Fever

Typhoid, or enteric, fever is caused by the organism *Salmonella typhi*. This disease is contracted by ingestion of contaminated food, water, or milk. In the United States, typhoid fever is most common in recent immigrants from underdeveloped countries but can occur in travelers. The average incubation period is 10 days.[6]

Transmission

- Contaminated food, water, milk

Signs and symptoms

- Altered level of consciousness
- Headache, malaise, anorexia
- High fever and chills for 2 to 3 weeks
- Relative bradycardia (bradycardia in the presence of fever)
- "Rose spots"—erythematous macules on the upper abdomen

Diagnostic studies

- Diagnosis generally is based on patient history and clinical findings.
- Blood and stool cultures
- CBC, metabolic panel, urinalysis

Therapeutic interventions

- Administer fluoroquinolones (e.g., oral ciprofloxacin [Cipro] 500 mg twice a day for 10 days).
- Administer azithromycin (Zithromax) 1 g orally and then 500 mg daily for 6 days.
- If the patient has mild disease, typhoid fever can be managed on an outpatient basis.
- For severe disease, admit patients to the hospital.

Prevention

- Food and water precautions during travel
- Hygienic food preparation and storage
- Typhoid fever vaccination before travel

Discharge instructions

Instruct patients to do the following:
- Replace fluid losses with electrolyte drinks.
- Maintain adequate nutrition.
- Take antibiotics as directed and complete the entire course.
- Seek medical care for dehydration or persistent fever, nausea, vomiting, and diarrhea.
- Arrange for medical follow-up for continued care and reevaluation.

VECTOR-BORNE INFECTIONS

Vector-borne diseases involve pathogens are that are spread by contact with an infected animal or insect host.

West Nile Virus

West Nile virus, a mosquito-transmitted flavivirus, is quickly spreading across the United States. This organism has an incubation period of 3 to 14 days.[7]

Transmission

- Virus generally is transmitted by the bite of infected mosquitoes.
- There have been instances of West Nile virus transmission through blood transfusion, organ transplantation, breast-feeding, and percutaneous injury (laboratory worker needlestick).[4]

Signs and symptoms

- Anorexia, nausea, vomiting
- Encephalitis or neurologic disorders can develop in severe cases.
- Eye pain
- Lymphadenopathy
- Malaise, headache
- Myalgias
- Rash: Maculopapular or morbilliform on the neck, trunk, arms, and legs

Diagnostic studies

- Lumbar puncture with cultures
- Immunoglobulin M antibody in the serum and cerebral spinal fluid
- CBC, complete metabolic panel, urinalysis

Therapeutic interventions

- Severe disease requires hospitalization.
- Supportive care includes hydration, respiratory assistance, and prevention and treatment of secondary infections.

Prevention

Avoid mosquitoes. Use an insect repellant that contains DEET (*N,N*-diethyl-*m*-toluamide); wear long sleeves, long pants, and light colors. Avoid outdoor activities at dawn and dusk when mosquitoes are most active.

Discharge instructions

Seek medical care for persistent headache, vomiting, fever, or worsening symptoms.

Rocky Mountain Spotted Fever

See Chapter 19.

Rabies

See Chapter 12.

DERMAL INFECTIONS

Scabies

Scabies is a contagious skin infection caused by the mite *Sarcoptes scabiei.*

Transmission

Scabies is transmitted by direct, close, skin-to-skin contact with an infected person, bedding, or clothing.

Signs and symptoms

Patients have a red, intensely pruritic rash with burrow channels obvious under the skin. Infestation can occur anywhere on the body but is most common in the webbing between the fingers and toes or in skinfolds over joints. Scratch marks are often present.

Diagnostic studies

- Diagnosis usually is made clinically based on patient history and rash characteristics.
- Skin scrapings can be done to look for mites or eggs.

Therapeutic interventions

Topical treatment includes lindane 1% lotion (Kwell) or permethrin 5% dermal cream (Lyclear). Use according to directions.

Prevention

- Follow standard and contact precautions.
- Wash all linens and clothing in very hot water to prevent insect spread.
- Avoid contact with infected individuals.

Discharge instructions

Instruct patients to do the following:
- Institute preventive measures.
- Take medications as directed.
  - Insecticidal cream or lotions
  - Antipruritics
- Avoid scratching to prevent secondary infection.
- Seek medical care for fever, increased rash, or signs of secondary infection.

Ringworm

Ringworm, tinea corporis, is a nonemergent, superficial fungal infection of the skin. There are several varieties of tinea (capitis, cruris, pedis), each named for the body region infected. Tinea corporis generally is limited to the arms, legs, and trunk.

Transmission

Ringworm is transmitted through contact with an infected person or animal. Pets are often the vectors for this organism.[3]

Signs and symptoms

- Sharply marginated anular lesions with raised margins and central clearing.

Diagnostic studies

- Diagnosis usually is made by clinical examination.
- If potassium hydroxide–stained skin scrapings are examined under a microscope, hyphae or yeast buds are seen.

Therapeutic interventions

- Antifungal creams generally eradicate the infections.
- In cases of severe infestation, systemic antifungal agents can be used.

Prevention

- Follow standard and contact precautions.
- Follow good skin hygiene.
- Limit contact with infected pets.

Discharge instructions

Instruct patients to do the following:
- Maintain good skin hygiene.
- Use medications as prescribed.
- Have pets treated.
- Seek medical care for signs of increased infection or secondary bacterial infection.

Eye, Ear, Nose, and Throat Infections

See Chapter 33.

Genitourinary Infections

See Chapter 30.

MISCELLANEOUS INFECTIOUS CONDITIONS

Herpes Zoster (Shingles)

Herpes zoster, commonly known as "shingles," is caused by the reactivation of dormant varicella zoster viruses (see Chickenpox [Varicella Zoster]). Lesions occur along the path of nerve dermatomes, which explains their unilateral distribution (lesions do not cross the midline). Shingles can occur anytime after initial varicella infection and may recur repeatedly over a lifetime.

Transmission

Vesicles contain live virus and can be contagious to unvaccinated or susceptible hosts.

Signs and symptoms

- Severe, localized, unilateral pain
- Within 48 hours of pain onset, vesicular lesions erupt along nerve dermatomes.

Diagnostic studies

- The diagnosis of shingles is made clinically.
- Viral cultures can be obtained, but they rarely contribute to diagnosis or management.

Therapeutic interventions

- Antiviral medications
- Cover lesions to minimize viral transmission
- Supportive care and comfort measures

Prevention

- Varicella zoster vaccination
- Standard, airborne, and contact precautions around persons with active chickenpox

Discharge instructions

- Ensure hydration and rest.
- Take analgesics for pain.
- Take antiviral medications as directed.

Meningitis

Meningitis is an acute inflammation of the meninges in the brain and spinal cord. Its cause can be viral or bacterial. Viral (aseptic) meningitis is usually a mild, self-limited condition that resolves spontaneously with basic symptomatic care. Bacterial meningitis is more severe and can cause serious complications if not appropriately treated. Common causative agents for bacterial meningitis are *Streptococcus pneumoniae*, *H. influenza*, and *Neisseria meningitidis*.

Transmission

- Bacterial meningitis: Via respiratory droplets and secretions
- Viral meningitis: Not usually contagious

Signs and symptoms

- Headache, fever, malaise
- Irritability, restlessness, altered level of consciousness can occur in severe cases
- Nausea, vomiting
- Petechial rash: Characteristic of *N. meningitidis* (meningococcal meningitis)
- Stiff neck, photophobia

Diagnostic studies

- Lumbar puncture for cerebrospinal fluid analysis and culture
- CBC, complete metabolic panel
- Blood cultures

Therapeutic interventions

- Viral meningitis: Supportive care, nutrition, hydration, rest, analgesics, antipyretics
- Bacterial meningitis: Urgent antibiotic therapy targeted at suspected organisms
  - These patients can be extremely ill and progress to septic shock within hours of initial symptoms.
  - Treat septic shock. See Chapter 22.
  - Place in isolation

Prevention

- Follow standard and droplet precautions.
- Close contacts of patients with bacterial meningitis should receive antibiotic prophylaxis.
- Vaccines are available for *N. meningitidis* and *H. influenza* (Hib vaccine). Although immunization against *H. influenzae* is effective, *N. meningitidis* vaccination only confers immunity against certain pathogen serotypes.

Discharge instructions

- Bacterial meningitis: Admit or transfer to an intensive care unit as soon as possible.
- Viral
  - Provide supportive care, nutrition, hydration, and rest.
  - Provide analgesics for pain.
  - Provide antipyretics for fever.
  - Seek medical care for increased fever, uncontrolled vomiting, rash, worsening symptoms.

Mononucleosis

Mononucleosis is a mildly contagious, self-limiting disease caused by the Epstein-Barr herpesvirus. Mononucleosis commonly affects adolescents and young adults and is usually mild. Older persons who contract the disease have more severe symptoms.

Transmission

Mononucleosis is transmitted through saliva and (less commonly) through blood transfusion.

Signs and symptoms

- Fatigue (may be profound)
- Fever
- Hepatomegaly, splenomegaly (Splenic rupture can occur.)
- Sore throat, cervical lymphadenopathy

Diagnostic studies

- Mono-spot laboratory test
- CBC

Therapeutic interventions

- Supportive care: Fluids, analgesics, antipyretics

Prevention

- Follow standard precautions.
- Avoid close contact with infected individuals.

Discharge instructions

- Increase fluid intake, and ensure adequate nutrition and rest.
- Take analgesics and antipyretics.
- Avoid contact sports or other activities that may cause abdominal trauma (because of splenomegaly and hepatomegaly).

Tetanus

Clostridium tetani, the organism responsible for tetanus, is prevalent in the soil worldwide. This disease occurs in unimmunized persons who have sustained a laceration, abrasion, burn, or puncture with exposure to the soil. In the wound, this anaerobic, spore-forming pathogen germinates and produces toxins. These toxins block the release of inhibitory neurotransmitters in the presynaptic terminals, causing persistent muscle contraction.

Transmission

Transmission occurs when soil contaminated with *C. tetani* enters an open wound. The incubation period is 2 days to 3 weeks.[3] However, spores can lie dormant in tissue for years.

Signs and symptoms

- Autonomic dysfunction
- Contraction of facial muscles (Contraction of back muscles results in arching of the back.)
- Dysphagia
- Increased masseter muscle tone (trismus or "lockjaw")
- Neck, shoulder, and back pain and stiffness
- Possible fever
- Violent muscle spasms

Diagnostic studies

- Diagnosis is made from clinical examination and history.
- Wound cultures are unreliable.
- *Clostridium tetani* titers can be obtained but are not generally useful.

Therapeutic interventions

- Provide basic and advanced supportive care as indicated.
- Provide airway management. Patients are at risk for laryngeal spasm. Tracheal intubation can be complicated by trismus and neck rigidity.
- Administer fluids intravenously.
- Administer penicillin G potassium (1.2 million units IV every 6 hours for 10 days) to eliminate live bacteria.

- Adminster human tetanus immune globulin 3000 to 6000 units intramuscularly to neutralize circulating toxins. This drug has no effect on toxins that are already bound to the central nervous system.
- Adminster Diazepam (Valium) for muscle spasms.
- Neuromuscular blockade may be required for severe muscular contractions.
- Surgical wound debridement usually is performed several hours after administration of human tetanus immune globulin.
- Adminster tetanus/diphtheria vaccine.[3]

Prevention

- Avoid injuries in soil-contaminated areas. Clean wounds quickly and thoroughly. Never close puncture wounds.
- Obtain tetanus/diphtheria vaccine: initial immunization series and then 1 booster dose every 10 years.

Discharge instructions

Admit or transfer the patient to an intensive care unit.

References

1. Garner JS, Hospital Infection Control Practices Advisory Committee: Recommendations for isolation precautions in hospitals. In *Guideline for isolation precautions in hospitals.* Atlanta, 1997, Public Health Service, US Department of Health and Human Services, Centers for Disease Control and Prevention.
2. Centers for Disease Control and Prevention: Division of HIV/AIDS Prevention, October 1998, Atlanta, 1998, Public Health Service, US Department of Health and Human Services, Centers for Disease Control and Prevention. Retrieved from http://www.cdc.gov/hiv/partners/AHP/progressfacts.htm.
3. Schaider J et al, editors: *Rosen and Barkin's 5-minute emergency medicine consult,* ed 2, Philadelphia, 2003, Lippincott Williams & Wilkins.
4. Centers for Disease Control and Prevention: *Smallpox vaccine and monkeypox,* Atlanta, 2003, The Centers.
5. Gilbert DN, Moellering RC, Sande MA: *The Sanford guide to antimicrobial therapy 2003,* ed 33, Hyde Park, Vt, 2003, Antimicrobial Therapy.
6. Tintinalli J, Gabor D, Stapczynski J: *Emergency medicine: a comprehensive study guide,* ed 6, New York, 2004, McGraw-Hill.
7. Koll B: West Nile virus infection: are you prepared? *Consultant* 43(9):1144-1149, 2003.

32

Allergies and Hypersensitivity

Faye P. Everson, RN, CEN, EMT-B

An allergy is an abnormal, exaggerated immune response to substances such as foods, plants, animals, or other materials. These reactions range from minor inconveniences to life-threatening problems. This chapter reviews the types, clinical manifestations, and treatment of allergic responses and hypersensitivity reactions.

DEFINITIONS

The following definitions are important to understanding allergic responses:

Antigen: Any substance that causes antibody formation. Antigens are introduced into the body by absorption, ingestion, inhalation, or injection. Drugs, venoms, foods, inhaled pollens, and latex are common antigens.

Antibody: A protective protein substance developed by the body in response to exposure to a specific antigen. Normally, antibodies are neutralized by binding to their target antigen and do not cause any further reactions.

Allergen: A substance that can produce an immune hypersensitivity reaction.

Allergic reactions: An abnormal, increased physiologic response to an antigen *after* previous sensitization to the same antigen.

Anaphylaxis: An intense antigen-antibody reaction to an allergen to which the body has been previously exposed.

IMMUNE RESPONSE

Cells involved in the immune response include the following:

Leukocytes: The blood component of the immune response.

Monocytes: These cells initiate antibody production by capturing, processing (phagocytosis), and presenting antigens to the lymphocytes.

Lymphocytes: The two categories of lymphocytes are the following:

- *T cells:* These cells defend against viruses, tumors, and fungi by recognizing and attaching to antigens. They produce cells with identical antigen receptors. Some T cells destroy invading pathogens, whereas others become memory cells, ready to respond to subsequent exposures.
- *B cells:* B cells produce antibodies (immunoglobulins). They contain antigen-specific receptors, retain memory, and enhance the work of the phagocytic cells.[1]

IMMUNOGLOBINS

Immunoglobulins are molecules produced by B cells in response to an antigen exposure. The five immunoglobulin (Ig) types are the following:

- *IgA:* These antibodies combine with proteins in the mucosa to protect the body surface from microorganisms. This is the second largest class of immunoglobulins.
- *IgD:* The function of these immunoglobulins remains unknown.
- *IgE:* Immediate hypersensitivity reactions are a result of class E immunoglobulins.
- *IgG:* These are the antibodies primarily responsible for fighting bacterial and viral infections. Immunoglobulin G is the largest class of immunoglobulins and the only type that crosses the placenta, conferring passive immunity to the fetus.
- *IgM:* Immunoglobulin M is the dominant antibody in ABO incompatibilities (transfusion reactions).

TYPES OF ALLERGIC RESPONSE

Four types of allergic reactions occur in response to antigen exposure (Table 32-1).

Type I: Immediate Hypersensitivity Reactions

Immediate hypersensitivity responses are IgE-mediated reactions. Type I hypersensitivities (anaphylaxis) can range in severity from mild (allergic rhinitis or hay fever) to life threatening (anaphylactic shock).[1] Immediate hypersensitivities are the most important type of allergic reactions seen in emergency departments. They are responsible for 400 to 800 deaths each year in the United States. Hypersensitivities can form to any protein, but certain substances commonly are associated with antibody development.

Common antigens

- Drugs and biologic agents
  - Analgesics: aspirin, nonsteroidal antiinflammatory drugs, opiates
  - Anesthetics
  - Antibiotics
  - Chemotherapeutic agents
  - Insulins
  - Vaccines
- Foods
  - Chocolate
  - Eggs

Table 32-1   Types of Hypersensitivity Reactions

	Type I: Anaphylactic Reactions	Type II: Cytotoxic Reactions	Type III: Immune Complex–Mediated Reactions	Type IV: Delayed Hypersensitivity Reactions
Antigen	Exogenous pollen, food, drugs, dust	Cell surface of red blood cell Basement membrane	Extracellular, fungal, viral, bacterial	Intracellular or extracellular
Antibody involved	IgE	IgG IgM	IgG IgM	None
Complement involved	No	Yes	Yes	No
Mediators of injury	Histamine SRS-A	Complement lysis Neutrophils	Neutrophils Complement lysis	Cytokines T cytotoxic cells Monocytes/macrophages Lysosomal enzymes
Examples	Allergic rhinitis Asthma	Transfusion reaction Goodpasture's syndrome	Serum sickness Systemic lupus erythematosus Rheumatoid arthritis	Contact dermatitis Tumor rejection Transplant rejection
Skin test	Wheal and flare	None	Erythema and edema in 3 to 8 hours	Erythema and edema in 24 to 48 hours (e.g., tuberculin test)

From Lewis S et al, editors: *Medical-surgical nursing assessment and management of clinical problems*, ed 6, St Louis, 2004, Mosby.
Ig, Immunoglobulin; *SRS-A,* slow-reacting substance of anaphylaxis.

- Food additives (monosodium glutamate)
- Milk
- Nuts and seeds (including soy and cottonseed)
- Shellfish, fish
- Strawberries
- Wheat
- Bites and stings
  - Animal venom (See Chapter 19.)
  - Insects: Hymenoptera (bees, wasps, fire ants, hornets, yellow jackets)

Pathophysiology

Immediate hypersensitivity responses require previous exposure to the offending antigen. The initial exposure stimulates the immune system to produce IgE. Immunoglobulin E stays in the mast cells until another exposure occurs. With each subsequent contact, mast cells are destroyed, histamines and other chemical mediators are released, and a cascade of complex chemical processes occurs. The clinical manifestations of an anaphylactic reaction depend on whether the mediators remain local or become systemic.[1] Responses vary widely and include the following signs and symptoms:

- Respiratory
  - Bronchospasm, complete airway obstruction
  - Coughing
  - Sneezing
  - Throat tightness, voice changes, stridor
  - Wheezes, dyspnea
- Cardiovascular
  - Dysrhythmias: Tachycardia, bradycardia, ventricular fibrillation, asystole
  - Hypotension, vascular collapse, shock
- Cutaneous
  - Angioedema: Swelling of the face, tongue, and airway
  - Cyanosis (a late finding that is due to hypoxemia)
  - Skin warmth, pruritus
  - Urticaria (hives)
  - Wheals: 1 to 6 cm in diameter with raised margins and blanched centers
- Central nervous system
  - Agitation, weakness
  - Feeling of impending doom
  - Headache
  - Syncope, seizures, coma
- Gastrointestinal
  - Nausea, vomiting, abdominal cramps, diarrhea

Management of immediate hypersensitivity reactions

Management of immediate hypersensitivity reactions includes the following (also see Anaphylactic Shock in Chapter 22):

Initial management

- Airway
  - Watch for increasing edema, voice changes, and tongue swelling.

- Provide early tracheal intubation. Angioedema can progress quickly. Do not delay interventions in patients with progressive symptoms.
  - Perform a cricothyrotomy if the upper airway is swollen closed.
- Breathing
  - Administer 100% oxygen at 10 to 15 L/min using a non-rebreather mask.
  - Assess respiratory rate, effort, chest excursion, and breath sounds.
  - Assist ventilation as needed (bag-valve-mask, mechanical ventilator).
- Circulation
  - Initiate continuous cardiac and oxygen saturation monitoring.
  - Assess heart rate, rhythm, and blood pressure. Reassess frequently.
  - Establish large bore vascular access and intravenously infuse isotonic crystalloids (normal saline or Ringer's lactate). Patients in shock are vasodilated and may require substantial amounts of fluid.
- Disability
  - Assess level of consciousness.
  - Monitor for changes: Anxiety, restlessness, and lethargy may indicate early or progressing tissue hypoxia.

Medications

- Epinephrine
  - Epinephrine (0.3 to 0.5 mL of 1:1000 dilution) subcutaneously for mild to moderate reactions (children, 0.01 mL/kg)
  - Epinephrine (0.3 to 0.5 mL of 1:10,000 dilution) intravenously for severe reactions (anaphylactic shock) (children, 0.01 mg/kg = 0.1 mL/kg)
  - May be repeated every 5 to 15 minutes (give slowly)
- Diphenhydramine (Benadryl) 25 to 50 mg slow intravenous or intramuscular administration (children, 1 to 2 mg/kg)
- Nebulized racemic epinephrine (2.25% solution in 2.5 mL normal saline) for upper airway edema
- Nebulized albuterol (Ventolin, Proventil) for bronchospasm
- Steroids
- Methylprednisolone (Solu-Medrol) 125 mg intravenous (children, 1 to 2 mg/kg)
- Hydrocortisone or prednisone may be used as well.
- Histamine$_2$ blockers (select one)
- Cimetidine (Tagamet) 300 mg intravenously
- Ranitidine (Zantac) 50 mg intravenously[2]
- Pepcid 20 mg intravenously

Type II: Cytotoxic Hypersensitivity Reactions

Cytotoxic (or cytolytic) hypersensitivity reactions involve IgG or IgM antibodies that attach to cells and cause cellular lysis. This type of response is seen most commonly in ABO transfusion reactions.[1]

Signs and Symptoms

- Anginal chest pain
- Fever
- Headache, flank pain
- Hematuria
- Nausea, vomiting
- Tachycardia, hypotension
- Urticaria

Management

1. Stop the transfusion (save the bag).
2. Maintain intravenous access.
3. Monitor vital signs.
4. Treat any life-threatening symptoms as for type I reactions.
5. Obtain urine and blood samples as directed by the institutional transfusion reaction protocol.

Type III: Immune Complex–Mediated Hypersensitivity Reactions

Immune complex–mediated hypersensitivity reactions are antigen-antibody responses in which IgG or IgM antibodies form complexes with an antigen. However, these complexes are too small to be removed effectively by phagocytes in the blood, and they are deposited in the tissues or small blood vessels. Common deposit sites are the kidneys, joints, lungs, skin, and blood vessels. In these tissues the complexes cause inflammation and destruction of the involved tissue. This damage can result in acute (e.g., serum sickness) or chronic (auto-immune) diseases such as systemic lupus erythematosus, rheumatoid arthritis, and acute glomerulonephritis.[1]

Primary serum sickness typically occurs 6 to 21 days after exposure to the inciting antigen. The development of serum sickness has been linked to many common pharmaceuticals (e.g., allopurinol, barbiturates, captopril, methyldopa, penicillins, phenytoin, procainamide, and sulfonamides). Insect venoms, vaccines, blood products, and antivenins are associated with an even higher incidence of serum sickness.[2]

Signs and Symptoms

- Clinical findings depend on the organ or system affected.
- Joints: Rheumatoid arthritis
- Kidneys: Glomerulonephritis
- Skin: Erythema multiforme, toxic epidermal necrolysis
- Vessels: Arteritis

Management

- Obtain a history of events. Is this an acute or chronic situation?
- Manage acute issues symptomatically.
- Refer patients for ongoing management of chronic autoimmune disorders.
- Discontinue any pharmaceutical agents that may be causing serum sickness.

Type IV: Delayed (or Cell-Mediated) Hypersensitivity Reactions

Delayed hypersensitivity responses, also known as cell-mediated immune reactions, involve the T cells. These responses are slow to develop and usually occur 24 to 72 hours after exposure. Instead of antibodies or complement, sensitized T lymphocytes attack antigens or release cytokines. Some of these cytokines damage local macrophages, which then release enzymes that cause tissue destruction.[1] Examples of delayed hypersensitivity reactions include the following:

- Contact dermatitis following exposure to cosmetics, adhesives, topical medications, drug additives, plant toxins (e.g., poison ivy), and latex rubber
- Graft-versus-host disease and tissue rejection in transplant patients

- Microbial hypersensitivity reactions, commonly seen after purified protein derivative (tuberculin) antigen injection

Signs and Symptoms

- Usually no reaction occurs with the first exposure.
- Any subsequent exposure can stimulate a response that includes itching, erythema, and vesicular lesion formation.

Prevention

Avoid contact with allergenic substances.

DIAGNOSTIC TESTS FOR ALLERGIES

The following are diagnostic tests for allergies:
- Assay of IgE levels
  - Radioallergosorbent test
  - Radioimmunosorbent test
  - Eosinophil levels
- Pulmonary function tests
- Skin testing
  - Scratch, prick, patch, or intradermal
- Elimination of allergenic foods from the diet to see whether the condition improves
- Perform challenge testing for food allergies

LATEX ALLERGY

Latex allergies involve an IgE-mediated response to the proteins contained in natural rubber latex. Until recent efforts to reduce exposure, latex was a component of dozens of items routinely stocked in emergency departments. These included such everyday objects as gloves, catheters, Penrose drains, tourniquets, adhesive tape, medication vial stoppers, and intravenous tubing ports. Most hospitals and medical product manufacturers have worked diligently to limit latex-containing equipment and supplies in health care facilities. Nonetheless, many items still exist. In fact, latex can be found in about 40,000 different products. Even paints commonly contain latex. One percent to 6% of the general population and 8% to 12% of health care workers are estimated to have an allergy to latex. Additionally, 54% of health care workers with latex allergies will have latex asthma.[3]

Aerosolization is the process by which latex becomes airborne. Latex molecules readily bind with substances (cornstarch, talcum powder) used to enhance glove application. These powders increase the number of latex particles in the air, thus increasing latex contact through the respiratory tract and mucosa. Even "low powder" or "nonpowdered" gloves potentially can aerosolize latex particles. Once sensitization has taken place, exposure to even small amounts of latex may stimulate a response.

Latex Exposure Prevention

Emergency nurses can take the following precautions to reduce exposure to latex:
- Screen patients for allergies at the time of emergency department arrival.
- Ask specifically about prior reactions to latex, rubber items, or any hospital product.

- Patients at particularly high risk are those with a history of multiple genitourinary procedures, spinal surgeries, or spina bifida.
- Patients sensitive to latex often have cross-reactivity to avocados, potatoes, bananas, tomatoes, chestnuts, kiwi fruit, or papaya.
- In sensitized individuals, prevent exposure to products containing latex such as the following:
  - Gloves, catheters, other tubes, vial stoppers, intravenous tubing medication ports
  - Blood pressure cuffs, tourniquets, adhesive bandages, and some airway products.
  Most manufacturers now provide nonlatex alternatives.

Types of Latex Allergies

Type IV: delayed hypersensitivity reactions (contact dermatitis)

- Rash with itching, erythema, and vesicular lesions may form.
- Typically, no symptoms occur with the first exposure.
- Reactions may be delayed up to 48 hours after contact.
- Reactions usually are not life threatening.

Type I: immediate hypersensitivity (anaphylaxis)

- Reactions can be immediate or up to 2 hours after exposure.
- Signs and symptoms range from mild to severe: sneezing, runny eyes and nose, itching, wheals (hives), vocal changes, dyspnea, chest tightness, nausea, vomiting, diarrhea, abdominal cramping, airway edema, shock, tachycardia, and death.

Treatment for Latex-Induced Asthma and Anaphylaxis

Refer to the previous section of this chapter (or Chapter 22) for specific information regarding the treatment of type I hypersensitivity reactions. Importantly, interventions for sensitized individuals need to be provided in a latex-safe environment. The treatment room must not share a ventilation system with any area in which latex products are used. An environment cannot be termed *latex-free* unless no latex has been in the area for at least 12 hours. Examine all prepackaged kits to identify latex-containing items. The U.S. Food and Drug Administration now requires package labels to state the presence or absence of latex.[3]

Inform patients about the seriousness of latex allergies; provide tips for prevention and information regarding ways to decrease exposure. Explain the need to prepare for future reactions by carrying an Epi-Pen (prepackaged injectable epinephrine), liquid diphenhydramine (Benadryl), and (possibly) steroids. Rapid recognition and management of symptoms can prevent lethal reactions.

Latex Information and Support

The following resources provide information and support for latex-related issues:
1. National Institute for Occupational Safety and Health: *Preventing allergic reactions to natural rubber latex in the workplace*, DHHS Pub #97-135, Washington, DC, 1997, US Department of Health and Human Services.
2. American Latex Allergy Association, *http://www.latexallergyresources.org*
3. Latex Allergy Links, *http://www.latexallergylinks.org*
4. MedicineNet.com

References

1. Lewis S, Kang D: Genetics and altered immune responses. In Lewis S et al, editors: *Medical-surgical nursing assessment and management of clinical problems,* vol 1, ed 6, St Louis, 2004, Mosby.
2. Schaider J et al, editors: *Rosen and Barkin's 5-minute emergency medicine consult,* ed 2, Philadelphia, 2003, Lippincott Williams & Wilkins.
3. Miller K, Weed P: The latex allergy triage or admission tool: an algorithm to identify which patients would benefit from "latex safe" precautions, *J Emerg Nurs* 24(2):1-8, 1998.

33

Facial, Ocular, ENT, and Dental Emergencies

Anne Marie E. Lewis, RN, BSN, BA, MA, CEN

Medical problems of the face, eyes, ears, nose, throat, and mouth involve a myriad of conditions including infectious and inflammatory processes, foreign bodies, embolic or thrombotic events, and hemorrhage. Regardless of the chief complaint, the first priority for these patients is assessment and management of their airway, breathing, and circulatory status. The focus of this chapter is medical processes; refer to Chapter 40 for discussion of trauma to the head and face.

FACIAL EMERGENCIES

Bell's Palsy

Bell's palsy is a unilateral facial paralysis caused by damage to the facial nerve (cranial nerve VII), often as a result of the herpes simplex virus. Symptoms can take weeks or months to resolve, and some individuals will have permanent sequelae. Before definitive diagnosis, patients must be evaluated fully to rule out acute stroke or a neoplasm affecting the facial nerve.

Signs and symptoms

- Unilateral facial paralysis with facial drooping (Figure 33-1)
- Inability to blink or close the affected eye
- Ear pain or pain near the ear, on the affected side
- Increased or decreased unilateral tear production
- Drooling
- Ipsilateral loss of taste (one side of the tongue)
- A perception that sounds are louder in the ear on the affected side
- Headache

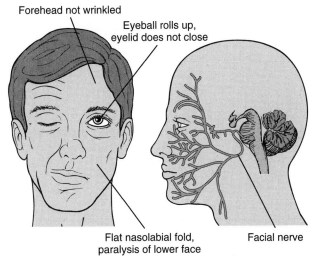

Forehead not wrinkled

Eyeball rolls up,
eyelid does not close

Flat nasolabial fold,
paralysis of lower face   Facial nerve

Figure 33-1. Bell's palsy: facial characteristics. (From Lewis SM, Heitkemper MM, Dirksen SR: *Medical-surgical nursing: assessment and management of clinical problems*, ed 6, St Louis, 2004, Mosby.

Diagnostic aids

- Clinical examination
- Computed tomography (CT) scan of the head to determine whether findings are due to stroke or some other intracranial event
- Electromyography may be performed as part of a comprehensive workup.

Therapeutic interventions

- Antiviral medications and corticosteroids may shorten the disease course.
- Administer analgesics.
- Check for corneal abrasions or ulcers and facial spasm.

Patient education and discharge instructions

- If the affected eye is dry, use artificial tears at night and an eye patch or shield.
- Consider facial massage to prevent contracture of paralyzed muscles.

Trigeminal Neuralgia (Tic Douloureux)

Trigeminal neuralgia, also referred to as tic douloureux, is a disorder of the fifth cranial nerve that usually occurs only in persons over the age of 50, predominantly in females. The right side of the face is affected more commonly than is the left. Painful episodes can last only seconds, may repeat immediately, or can continue unabated for days. Pain onset is spontaneous or initiated by simple maneuvers such as toothbrushing, chewing, speaking, or touching the face.

Signs and symptoms

- Excruciating, stabbing, electric shock–like pain
- Generally limited to one side of the face but both sides can be affected at different times
- Usually involves the lips, cheeks, jaw, eyes, forehead, scalp, and nose

Therapeutic interventions

- Administer analgesics for pain.
- Treat neurogenic pain with anticonvulsant medications such as phenytoin (Dilantin), carbamazepine (Tegretol), and gabapentin (Neurontin).

Patient education and discharge instructions

- Take medications as directed.
- Consult helpful websites for further information and tips on dealing with the pain:
  - Trigeminal Neuralgia Association at *http://www.tna-support.org*
  - American Chronic Pain Association at *http://www.theacpa.org*

Periorbital Cellulitis

Periorbital cellulitis refers to inflammation of the soft tissues surrounding the eye. Pneumococcal, staphylococcal, or streptococcal bacteria produce this condition. Infection can spread rapidly to adjacent sinuses and from there to the meninges.

Signs and symptoms

- Aching pain in and around the affected eye
- Conjunctival chemosis (swelling of the conjunctiva because of fluid accumulation)
- Diminished visual acuity
- Exophthalmos (an abnormal bulging of the eye)
- Facial and globe edema
- Fever
- Papilledema
- Paralysis of the extraocular muscles
- Vascular congestion in the eyelids

Diagnostic aids

- Clinical examination
- Culture the site of primary infection
- Complete blood count (CBC), erythrocyte sedimentation rate (ESR), and blood cultures
- CT scan
- Magnetic resonance imaging (MRI) scan

Therapeutic interventions

- Analgesics
- Bed rest and hospitalization
- Ophthalmologic consultation
- Parenterally administered broad-spectrum antibiotics
- Warm compresses to the eye

Cavernous Sinus Thrombosis

Cavernous sinus thrombosis is a potentially life-threatening infection of a blood clot in one or both of the cavernous sinuses. This condition usually follows midfacial cellulitis or a paranasal sinus infection. *Staphylococcus aureus* and *Streptococcus* are the most frequent causative organisms. Cavernous sinus thrombosis survival has improved significantly with the advent of antibiotic therapy; nonetheless, mortality remains nearly 30%.[1] Death occurs from overwhelming sepsis or neurologic infection. Patients with cavernous sinus thrombosis and periorbital cellulitis have similar clinical presentations.

Signs and symptoms

- Chemosis
- Decreased visual acuity
- Dysfunction of cranial nerves III, IV, and especially VI (Cranial nerve VI controls lateral gaze.)
- Exophthalmos
- Eyelid and periorbital edema
- Facial pain
- Fever, tachycardia, sepsis
- Headache, with nuchal rigidity
- Impaired eye movement
- Lethargy, seizures, or coma
- Proptosis (bulging eye, caused by an intraorbital space-occupying lesion)
- Ptosis (eyelid drooping)

Diagnostic aids

- Clinical examination
- Culture the site of primary infection
- CBC, ESR, and blood cultures
- CT scan
- MRI scan

Therapeutic interventions

- Parenterally administer broad-spectrum antibiotics.
- Administration of anticoagulants and steroids is controversial. Use should be based on individual patient considerations.
- Provide systemic analgesics.
- Maintain bed rest.
- Obtain ear, nose, and throat (ENT) (otolaryngology) specialist consultation.
- Admit the patient to the hospital for aggressive therapy and monitoring.

OCULAR EMERGENCIES

Assess and manage potentially life-threatening conditions before addressing eye problems. Check the visual acuity of both eyes in all patients who have an ophthalmologic complaint (Box 33-1 and Table 33-1). Visual acuity should be determined before manual eye examination because manipulation increases blurring and decreases acuity. The exception to this

Box **33-1**   How to Perform a Visual Acuity Examination

1. If the patient wears corrective lenses (i.e., glasses or contact lenses), test vision with lenses in place.
2. If the patient's corrective lenses are not available, have the patient read the chart through a pinhole poked in a piece of cardboard (or use a similar commercially available device).
3. Check each eye separately; instruct the patient to cover the other eye.
4. Eye charts come with specific instructions regarding how to conduct the examination:
   The Snellen chart is read at 20 feet. Record the lowest line the patient can read, and indicate the number of letters misread.
   Children and the illiterate may be tested with a chart that uses pictures rather than letters.
   The Rosenbaum Pocket Vision Screener is read 14 inches from the tip of the nose.

Table **33-1**   Documenting Visual Acuity

Score	Explanation
20/20	When standing 20 feet from the Snellen chart, the patient can read what the normal eye can read at 20 feet.
20/40-2	When standing 20 feet from the Snellen chart, the patient can read what the normal eye can read at 40 feet and has missed two letters.
10/200	If the patient cannot read any of the letters on the Snellen chart, have the patient stand half the distance (10 feet) and read what the patient can. Record this distance from the chart (e.g., 10/_) over the smallest line that could be read.
CF/3 feet	The patient can count fingers at a maximum distance of 3 feet.
HM/4 feet	The patient can see hand motion at a maximum distance of 4 feet.
LP/position	The patient can perceive light and determine from which direction it came.
LP/no position	The patient can perceive light but cannot determine from which direction it came.
NLP	The patient cannot perceive light.

caveat is the patient with chemical burns to the eye. In this situation, treatment must begin immediately to limit further damage. A topical anesthetic agent can be instilled before manual eye examination and may be needed before the patient can read an eye chart. Figure 33-2 illustrates key ocular structures. Remove contact lens whenever it is necessary to examine the eye, perform ocular irrigation, or patch the eye. Figure 33-3 illustrates how to remove hard and soft contact lens. Refer to Chapter 40 for discussion of corneal abrasions and other ocular injuries.

Conjunctivitis (Pink Eye)

Acute conjunctivitis is an infection of the conjunctiva (the membrane that lines the eyelids and sclera) typically caused by bacteria or a virus. Other causes include chemical irritation, allergies, and certain systemic diseases (e.g., tuberculosis or Stevens-Johnson syndrome).

Signs and symptoms

- Eyelids are "stuck together" on awakening
- Sensation of "something in my eye"

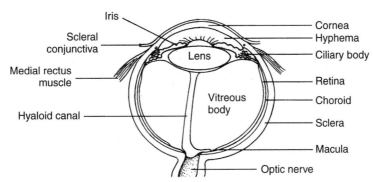

Figure 33-2. Horizontal section of left eye seen from above.

- Reddened sclera
- Purulent discharge (bacterial conjunctivitis)
- Serous discharge (allergic or viral conjunctivitis)
- Pruritus (allergic conjunctivitis)

Diagnostic aids

- Perform a clinical examination.
- Culture the discharge only if conjunctivitis is severe, chronic, and recurrent or does not respond to treatment.

Therapeutic interventions

- Apply antibiotic ophthalmic ointments for bacterial infections.
- Systemic antibiotics may be required for serious conditions.
- Cool compresses and topical vasoconstrictors can provide symptomatic relief for viral or allergic conjunctivitis.
- Administer systemic antihistamines for allergic conjunctivitis.
- Perform immediate eye irrigation for chemicals in the eye (Box 33-2 and Figure 33-4).

Patient education and discharge instructions

- Bacterial or viral conjunctivitis is highly contagious. Pay strict attention to hygiene and perform frequent hand washing.
- Stay out of swimming pools until symptoms have resolved completely.
- Sunglasses decrease photophobia.
- Avoid eye cosmetics.
- Do not wear contact lenses until the infection has resolved.
- Do not share towels, pillowcases, and cosmetics or have facial contact while infected. Change pillowcases daily.
- Persons with viral or bacterial infections who prepare food or have direct contact with others should not return to work until the infection is healed.
- Take medications as directed.

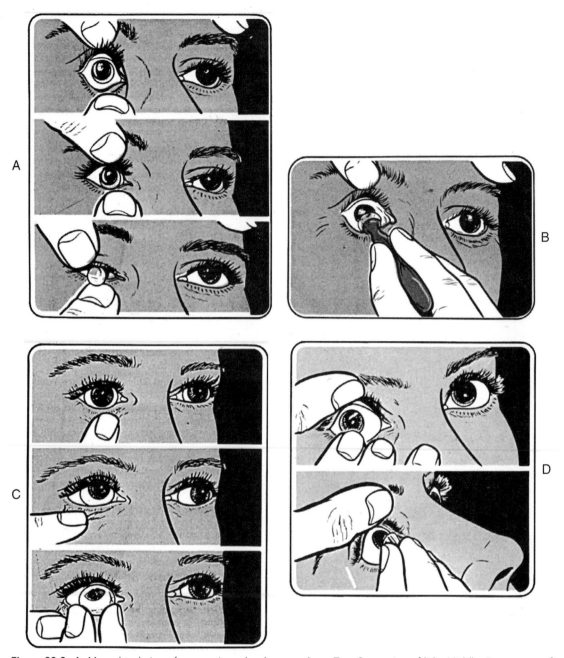

Figure 33-3. A, Manual technique for removing a hard contact lens. *Top,* Separation of lids. *Middle,* Entrapment of lens edges with lids. *Bottom,* Expulsion of lens by forcing of lower lid under inferior edge of lens. **B,** Use of a moistened suction cup to remove a hard contact lens. **C,** Removal of a hard scleral lens. *Top,* Separation of lids. *Middle,* Forcing of lower lid beneath edge of scleral lens by temporal traction on lower lid. *Bottom,* Lifting of lens off eye. **D,** Removal of soft contact lens. *Top,* Separation of lids and movement of contact onto sclera using index finger. *Bottom,* Pinching of lens between thumb and index finger. (From Grant HD, Murray RH, Bergeron JF: *Brady emergency care,* ed 5, Englewood Cliffs, NJ, 1990, Prentice-Hall. Reproduced with permission.)

Box **33-2** Eye Irrigation with the Morgan Lens

The Morgan lens (see Figure 33-4) is a concave, scleral lens composed of flexible plastic that is placed on the eye to provide continuous ocular lavage or medication instillation. The tubing is made of soft silicone and has a female adapter at the distal end.
1. Attach the Morgan lens to a syringe filled with the solution of choice (for medication installation) or to an intravenous infusion tubing set connected to a bag of normal saline or Ringer's lactate solution (for irrigation).
2. Prime the tubing and Morgan lens with fluid before insertion.
3. Explain the procedure to the patient.
4. Instill an anesthetic ophthalmic medication in the affected eye(s).
5. Ask the patient to look downward.
6. Retract the upper eyelid.
7. Grasp the lens by the tubing and its small, finlike projections.
8. Slip the superior border of the lens under the upper eyelid.
9. Have the patient look upward.
10. Retract the bottom eyelid and place the lower border of the lens beneath it.
11. Have the patient turn the head toward the affected side and place a folded towel or shampoo basin under the head. Alternatively, attach a Medi-duct device to collect irrigation solution.
12. To remove the lens, follow steps 4 through 9 in reverse order.
13. Do not allow the tubing to run dry before removing the lens. The resulting vacuum can cause a corneal abrasion when the lens is removed.
14. Dispose of the lens.
15. Use a different lens for each eye.

The Morgan Lens and Medi-duct are products of MorTan Inc., Missoula, Montana.

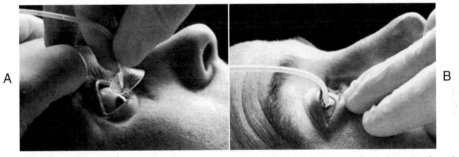

Figure 33-4. Placement of the Morgan lens for eye irrigation. **A,** Have the patient look downward, and then insert the lens under the upper lid. Have the patient look upward, and then retract the lower lid. **B,** For removal, have the patient look upward, and then retract the lower lid; hold the position and slide the lens out. (Courtesy of MorTan, Inc. Instructional chart for Morgan lens. Copyright 1996 by MorTan, Inc, Missoula, Mont.)

- Avoid any offending allergens, and apply cool compresses to the eyelids (allergic conjunctivitis).
- Follow up with a primary care provider or ophthalmologist in 2 to 3 days.

Retinal Detachment

A tear in the retina allows vitreous humor to leak between the retina and the choroid, separating these two layers. This diminishes the supply of blood and oxygen to the retina, and permanent vision loss can ensue. Retinal detachment is an ocular emergency. Detachment can occur following trauma or without a known cause. Spontaneous retinal detachment is more frequent in nearsighted individuals because myopia makes the retina thinner.

Signs and symptoms

- Flashes of light
- Shower of "floaters" (particles) or "cobwebs" in the visual field
- Sudden decrease or loss of vision
- "Veil" or "curtain" effect in the visual field
- "Wavy" visual distortion

Diagnostic aids

- Clinical examination
- Visual acuity testing
- Dilated fundus examination
- Ophthalmoscopy

Therapeutic interventions

- Immediate referral to an ophthalmologist for possible surgical repair

Central Retinal Artery Occlusion

Central retinal artery occlusion produces sudden, painless, unilateral blindness. This disorder is usually embolic and is associated with concomitant atherosclerosis and systemic hypertension. Prognosis for regaining sight is poor if the occlusion lasts longer than 90 minutes.

Therapeutic interventions

- Place the patient in a supine position to optimize circulation.
- Gentle, intermittent (5 to 15 seconds at a time) ocular massage can be performed to increase circulation and potentially dislodge the embolus.
- To decrease intraocular pressure, administer acetazolamide (Diamox) by IV and a topical beta-blocker such as timolol (Timoptic).
- Assist with anterior chamber paracentesis (performed by an ophthalmologist).
- Consider anticoagulant administration.
- Assist with injection of recombinant tissue plasminogen activator (alteplase) or urokinase into the ophthalmic or internal maxillary artery. (Some studies have found this treatment more effective than conservative management.)[2,3]
- Surgical intervention by an ophthalmologist may be necessary.
- Treatment also must be aimed at identifying and controlling the condition that precipitated arterial occlusion (e.g., hypertension or atrial fibrillation).

Patient education and discharge instructions

Follow up with a primary care provider to identify and treat the underlying disorder.

Corneal Ulcer

The most common cause of corneal ulcers is inadequately cleaned contact lenses or lenses left in place for long periods of time. Corneal foreign bodies, various eyelid defects, and eye infections also are associated with ulcer formation. An untreated corneal ulcer, infected with *Pseudomonas,* can lead to blindness within 24 to 48 hours.

Signs and symptoms

- Whitish spot on the cornea
- Pain, sensation of "something in my eye"
- Photophobia
- Profuse tearing
- Reddened eye
- Possible purulent discharge

Diagnostic aids

- Stain the eye with fluorescein, and then assess the cornea with a cobalt light.
- Perform a slit lamp examination.
- Culture any eye discharge.

Therapeutic interventions

- Administer topical or intravenous (IV) antibiotics.
- Provide analgesics.
- Obtain an immediate ophthalmologic consultation.

Patient education and discharge instructions

- Take antibiotics as directed.
- Follow up with an ophthalmologist.

Blepharitis

Anterior blepharitis is an inflammation of the lid margin at the site where the eyelashes originate. This condition usually is caused by *Staphylococcus aureus*. Blepharitis frequently is ulcerative and may become chronic.

Signs and symptoms

- Burning, or a sensation of "something in my eye"
- Eyelid edema
- Loss of eyelashes
- Photophobia
- Possible blurred vision
- Pruritus
- Pustules or ulcers may be present at the lid follicles.
- Reddened eyelid margin
- Tearing
- The eye drains and forms crusts during sleep.

Therapeutic interventions

Administer an antibiotic ophthalmic ointment (Box 33-3).

Patient education and discharge instructions

- To keep the eyelid clean and remove crusts, apply a warm compress to the lid and then wash the area thoroughly with water and baby shampoo.
- Instill topical antibiotics as directed.

Box **33-3** **How to Instill Ophthalmic Medications**

Ophthalmic Drops

1. Explain the procedure to the patient.
2. Pull the lower eyelid down.
3. Have the patient look up.
4. Instill one or two drops of solution into the cul-de-sac (the center of the lower lid).
5. Have the patient blink gently to distribute the solution.
6. Instruct the patient not to squeeze the eyelids shut tightly; this will cause the solution to leak out.

Ophthalmic Ointment

1. Explain the procedure to the patient.
2. Pull the lower eyelid down.
3. Have the patient look up.
4. Apply ointment in a 1-cm line into the inner aspect of the lower lid.
5. Have the patient blink to distribute the ointment.
6. Instruct the patient not to squeeze the eyelids shut tightly; this will expel the ointment.

Hordeolum

A hordeolum or sty is an infection of the eyelash follicle caused by *S. aureus*. This condition may occur in association with blepharitis and is usually self-limiting.

Signs and symptoms

- Small external abscess
- Pain
- Redness
- Swelling

Therapeutic interventions

- Consider systemic antibiotics; ophthalmic antibiotic ointments are ineffective.
- Administer systemic analgesics.
- Assist with abscess incision and drainage.

Patient education and discharge instructions

- Apply warm compresses 3 times a day.
- Take antibiotics, if ordered.

Chalazion

A chalazion is a (usually) sterile inflammation of the meibomian gland on the inner surface of the eyelid. Without treatment, a chalazion will resolve spontaneously in a few months.

Signs and symptoms

- Small mass beneath the lid
- Pain (infrequently)

- Reddened conjunctiva
- Swelling

Therapeutic interventions

- Administer an antibiotic ophthalmic ointment or drops if bacterial infection is suspected.
- Administer systemic analgesics as needed.
- Assist the ophthalmologist or plastic surgeon with steroid injection or incision and drainage.

Patient education and discharge instructions

- If the chalazion is being managed medically, apply warm compresses 3 to 4 times a day.
- Instill an antibiotic ointment or drops, if ordered.
- Consult an ophthalmologist if the chalazion does not resolve.

Glaucoma

Glaucoma occurs when aqueous humor cannot escape the anterior chamber. This increases intraocular pressure and compresses the optic nerve. High intraocular pressures are a risk factor for glaucoma, but even patients with normal intraocular pressures can experience vision loss from glaucoma.[4] Several types of glaucoma occur, and therapeutic interventions vary according to the cause.

Primary open-angle glaucoma is caused by an obstruction within the canal of Schlemm, which decreases drainage of aqueous fluid from the anterior chamber. This disorder develops slowly, and patients are asymptomatic except for a gradual loss of peripheral vision.

Secondary glaucoma refers to increased intraocular pressure caused by trauma, eye surgery, inflammation, diabetes, corticosteroid use, or various other conditions that interfere with aqueous humor drainage.

Angle-closure glaucoma (acute glaucoma or narrow-angle glaucoma) occurs when the opening of the canal is blocked. This condition is less common but progresses rapidly and can cause blindness within hours if it is untreated. Only angle-closure glaucoma is a medical emergency; signs, symptoms, and interventions are discussed next.

Signs and symptoms

- Acute eye pain
- Decreased peripheral vision
- Elevated intraocular pressure
- Fixed and slightly dilated pupil
- Foggy-appearing cornea
- Halos around lights
- Hard globe
- Possible nausea and vomiting
- Reddened eye
- Severe headache

Diagnostic aids

- Clinical examination
- Slit lamp examination
- Tonometry to measure intraocular pressure (Box 33-4)

Box **33-4** How to Measure Intraocular Pressure With a Tonometer

Schiøtz Method

Have the patient lie supine and loosen any tight clothing around the neck. (Tight clothing may increase intraocular pressure.)

Anesthetize the eye with an ophthalmic anesthetic agent.

Have the patient stare upward at a spot on the ceiling.

Place the sterile, previously calibrated tonometer on the globe for a few seconds. Allow the plunger to indent the surface. Be careful not to put pressure on the globe while retracting the lids.

A normal indentation tonometer reading is 12 to 20 mm Hg. (Readings commonly reach 40 to 65 mm Hg with angle-closure glaucoma.)

Applanation Method

Loosen any tight clothing around the neck. (Tight clothing may increase intraocular pressure.)

Anesthetize the eye with an ophthalmic anesthetic agent.

Apply fluorescein to the eye.

Using the slit lamp, touch the patient's eye with the tonometer attached.

Ocular tonometry also can be performed with a Tono-Pen. This device produces an immediate digital readout.

Therapeutic interventions

Therapeutic interventions for acute glaucoma focus on reducing pupil size to promote aqueous humor drainage:

- Frequently administered (every 15 minutes) miotic eye drops (e.g., pilocarpine) increase outflow.
- Administer acetazolamide (Diamox), an oral carbonic anhydrase inhibitor, to decrease the production of aqueous humor.
- Instill a topical beta-blocker (e.g., timolol 0.5%) to decrease aqueous humor production further.
- Provide systemic analgesics.
- Consider giving a prostaglandin analog such as latanoprost (Xalatan) to increase aqueous outflow.

Patient education and discharge instructions

- Follow up with an ophthalmologist for monitoring and possible surgery (e.g., iridotomy or laser trabeculoplasty) if medications are ineffective.
- Use oral and topical medications as directed.
- Watch for signs that the medication is ineffective (i.e., continued symptoms).
- Avoid activities that increase intraocular pressure such as bending with the head below the waist, coughing, straining, and lifting more than 2.3 kg (5 lb).
- Drink water in small amounts. Water consumed in large quantities may increase intraocular pressure.

Keratitis

Keratitis is an inflammation of the cornea, often caused by herpes viruses (herpes simplex type I and herpes zoster), but it may be caused by bacteria, fungi, or general ocular dryness. Trauma to the cornea, particularly from contact lenses, is also a risk factor. Untreated, keratitis can cause permanent corneal damage and blindness.

Signs and symptoms

- Blurred vision
- Pain, a sensation of "something in my eye"
- Photophobia
- Profuse tearing
- Purulent discharge (bacterial infections)
- Reddened cornea

Diagnostic aids

- Perform a clinical examination.
- Consider corneal smear and culture.

Therapeutic interventions

- Depending on the organism involved, administer oral or topical antibacterial, antiviral, or antifungal agents.
- Instill a cycloplegic (tropicamide [Mydriacyl], cyclopentolate [Cyclogyl]).
- Give analgesics.
- Assist with corneal debridement.

Patient education and discharge instructions

- Administer ophthalmic medications as directed.
- Follow up with an ophthalmologist for frequent monitoring until the infection has resolved.
- Fully disinfect contact lenses using sterile solutions. Do not wear contact lenses until symptoms resolve.
- Administer artificial tears as directed (patients with ocular dryness).
- Do not touch the eyes after touching a cold sore (patients with herpetic infections).

Uveitis

In developed countries, uveitis is the third leading cause of blindness. Uveitis results from an immune reaction that produces inflammation of the iris (iritis), the iris and the ciliary body (iridocyclitis), the choroid (choroiditis) or the choroid and retina (chorioretinitis). Without effective treatment, permanent structural eye damage occurs with subsequent visual loss. Uveitis often is associated with infections (e.g., herpes or syphilis), or it may be related to an autoimmune disorder such as systemic lupus erythematosus or rheumatoid arthritis. Although only a small percentage of persons with this condition are children, children develop *posterior* uveitis more frequently than do adults. Posterior uveitis carries a greater risk for permanent vision loss.

Signs and symptoms

- Blurred vision
- Pain
- Photophobia
- Possible constricted, nonreactive pupil
- Reddened eye
- Tearing

Treatment/interventions

Treatment is aimed at aggressive reduction of the inflammation, whether or not the patient has yet experienced visual changes.
  Administer systemic analgesics:

- Anterior uveitis (affecting the iris and/or the ciliary body)
  - Cycloplegics and mydriatics
  - Topical steroids
- Posterior uveitis (affecting the choroid and/or retina).
  - Systemic steroids

Patient education and discharge instructions

- Continue frequent doses of topical steroids, mydriatics, and cycloplegics as directed (e.g., every 30 to 60 minutes while awake).
- Follow up with an ophthalmologist within 24 hours.
- Preliminary research by the National Institutes of Health indicates that monthly IV doses of humanized anti-Tac monoclonal antibody eventually may replace traditional, long-term steroid therapy.[5]

Amaurosis Fugax (Transient Monocular Blindness)

Amaurosis fugax is a transient ischemic attack in which an embolus, thrombus, or plaque in the carotid artery decreases perfusion to the retinal circulation. This condition lasts from seconds to a few minutes without any permanent damage, but patients are at high risk for subsequent stroke or central retinal artery occlusion. This condition occurs more often in persons with sickle cell disease.

Signs and symptoms

- Painless monocular visual loss

Diagnostic aids

- Carotid ultrasound
- Magnetic resonance angiography scan

Therapeutic interventions

Amaurosis fugax usually resolves without treatment. However, anticoagulant and antiplatelet therapy may be indicated for stroke prevention.

Patient education and discharge instructions

- Follow up with a primary care provider to determine and treat the underlying cause.
- Stop smoking, decrease serum cholesterol levels, and control hypertension.
- Carotid endarterectomy or balloon angioplasty with stent placement may be needed.

Cyanoacrylate Exposure (Crazy Glue or Super Glue)

Cyanoacrylate glue containers resemble eye drop bottles or ointment tubes. Therefore it is not surprising that there have been case of patients who have inadvertently confused the tubes, inserting glue in their eyes. Contamination also can occur when persons with fresh glue on their fingers touch the eyes or lids. Cyanoacrylate dries quickly with a strong bond.

Signs and symptoms

- Pain
- Tearing
- Lids may be sealed.

Therapeutic interventions

- Immediate and copious eye irrigation with saline, lactated Ringer's solution, or warm water (if the eye can be opened at all).
- Do not attempt to pry the lids apart. They usually will loosen on their own in a few days.
- Administer systemic analgesics.

Patient education and discharge instructions

- Do not attempt to separate the lids.
- Follow up with an ophthalmologist.
- Wear safety goggles when working with cyanoacrylate.

EAR, NOSE, AND THROAT EMERGENCIES

Some medical historians believe that George Washington, the first U.S. president, died of advanced epiglottitis.[6] Although seldom fatal today, ear, nose, and throat ailments still cause discomfort and debilitation and bring many patients to emergency departments.

Otitis Externa

Acute otitis externa, or swimmer's ear, is an infection of the external auditory canal, usually caused by bacteria. Excessive moisture and trauma to the ear canal are the two most common predisposing factors.[7]

Signs and symptoms

- Severe external ear pain
- Swelling and erythema of the ear canal
- Possible periauricular cellulitis
- Discharge from the ear
- Pruritus
- Hearing loss

Therapeutic interventions

- Administer topical and/or systemic analgesics.
- Insert an ear wick and saturate the wick with a topical antibiotic solution.

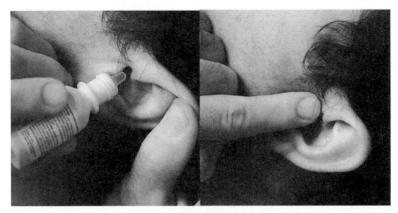

Figure 33-5. Ear drop instillation. Turn the head to the side so that the affected ear faces upward. The orifice is exposed, and the drops of medicine are directed toward the internal wall of the canal. Pull the pinna up and back in a person older than 3 years of age and down and back in a younger child. Then push the tragus against the ear canal to ensure that the drops stay in the canal. (From Potter PA, Perry AG: *Fundamentals of nursing*, ed 6, St Louis, 2004, Mosby.)

Patient education and discharge instructions

- Do not insert cotton swabs or other items in the ear.
- Administer eardrops, as directed (Figure 33-5). Warming the medication bottle between the hands before instillation decreases dizziness.
- Avoid getting water in the ear(s) until the infection has resolved.
- Swimmers should wear a tight-fitting bathing cap. Ear plugs predispose swimmers to otitis externa.[8]
- Avoid using earphones or headphones.

Otitis Media

Otitis media is an inflammation of the middle ear caused by the buildup of infected fluid behind the tympanic membrane. Complications include rupture of the tympanic membrane and acute mastoiditis.

Signs and symptoms

- Sharp middle ear pain
- A sensation of fullness in the ear
- Hearing loss
- Bulging tympanic membrane
- Fever
- Possible nausea and vomiting
- History of a recent upper respiratory infection
- Infants and children may pull on the affected ear(s).

Therapeutic interventions

- Administer decongestants.
- Administer oral antibiotics.
- Administer systemic analgesics.

Box **33-5** **How to Perform Ear Irrigation**

---

1. Consider instilling a ceruminolytic in the affected ear canal(s) before the procedure.
2. Use a large syringe (e.g., 30 mL) with a soft intravenous catheter attached (e.g., an 18-gauge butterfly catheter with the needle cut off). Trim the catheter to avoid accidental tympanic membrane perforation. Do not irrigate with a Waterpik (Water Pik Technologies, Inc., Newport Beach, Calif.); the stream is too forceful.
3. Use body temperature water. (The water may be mixed with hydrogen peroxide.) Water that is too hot or too cold causes dizziness when it contacts the tympanic membrane.
4. With the patient sitting upright, straighten the ear canal by pulling it up and back for adults, down and back for young children.
5. Fill the syringe with water, insert it into the outer portion of the ear canal, and direct the stream at the *side* of the canal. Be careful not to scratch the ear canal with the catheter.
6. If the patient feels water in the mouth or throat, *stop immediately.* This indicates tympanic membrane perforation.
7. Collect the irrigation water in a basin held under the patient's ear.
8. Repeat the procedure until all cerumen has been removed from the ear canal.

Patient education and discharge instructions

- Use medications as directed.
- Follow up with a primary care provider or ENT specialist if the infection does not resolve in several days. A myringotomy may be needed.

Cerumen Impaction

Cerumen (ear wax) is produced by the outer ear canal to repel moisture and trap debris and microorganisms. Cerumen normally moves to the canal opening where it can be washed away. Overproduction of cerumen may cause an impaction. However, impaction frequently occurs when objects inserted in the ears (e.g., cotton swabs) push cerumen deep into the inner canal where it obstructs the tympanic membrane.

Signs and symptoms

- Progressive hearing loss
- Pain or fullness in the ear
- Tinnitus

Therapeutic interventions

- Instill a ceruminolytic such as Cerumenex or liquid docusate sodium (Colace) to soften and loosen debris.
- If there is no suspicion of tympanic membrane perforation, irrigate the ear(s) with warm water (Box 33-5).

Patient education and discharge instructions

- Do not put any object in the ear.
- To prevent cerumen buildup, instill 2 to 3 drops of mineral oil in the ear. Leave it in place for 2 to 3 minutes and then gently rinse with warm water. Dry the ear after rinsing; repeat weekly.

Foreign Body in the Ear

Common foreign bodies in the ear include beans, beads, and bugs. Bleeding and tympanic membrane rupture can occur if the patient attempts to remove the object. Live insects moving in the ear also may rupture the tympanic membrane.

Therapeutic interventions

- After the object has been visualized, assist with removal.
- Do not push the object deeper into the ear canal.
- Remove foreign bodies with an ear curette (hook), rubber-tipped suction, or alligator forceps.
- Immobilize a live insect by instilling a few drops of lidocaine or mineral oil. Once the insect is immobilized, it can be removed with alligator forceps. Never wrestle with a bug inside a patient's ear canal. Alternatively, try shining a light in the affected ear. Live insects may move toward the light.
- Certain items can be irrigated out of the ear canal. Do *not* irrigate vegetable matter, soft objects, or any substance that will absorb water and expand.

Mastoiditis

The infection and inflammation of otitis media can spread from the middle ear to the porous mastoid bone. The resulting infection then may erode the mastoid and surrounding structures, leading to intracranial infection. The incidence of mastoiditis has dropped significantly since the advent of antibiotic therapy for otitis media.

Signs and symptoms

- Discharge from the ear if the tympanic membrane has ruptured
- Earache
- Fever
- Headache
- History of recent or current otitis media
- Pain and swelling in the mastoid area (behind the ear)
- Possible hearing loss
- Redness of the ear or behind the ear

Diagnostic aids

- Obtain a CT scan.
- If the patient has not yet received antibiotics, culture any discharge from the ear canal or any fluid obtained from myringotomy.

Therapeutic interventions

- Give systemic analgesics.
- Initiate IV antibiotic therapy.
- Admit the patient to the hospital.
- Consult an ENT specialist. Mastoidectomy may be required. Myringotomy is performed to treat persistent otitis media if antibiotic therapy is unsuccessful.

Labyrinthitis

Inflammation of the semicircular canals and labyrinth of the inner ear often follows acute otitis media, upper respiratory infections, and allergies. Labyrinthitis also can result from the ototoxic effects of certain medications. This distressing disorder can last for hours or weeks but is usually self-limiting.

Patients with Meniere's disease have symptoms similar to labyrinthitis, with the additional complaint of "fullness" in the affected ear(s). Meniere's disease is caused by the presence of an abnormally large amount of inner ear fluid (endolymph).

Signs and symptoms

- Difficulty standing or walking
- Dizziness
- Hearing loss
- Intense vertigo, often associated with movement of the head or body
- Nystagmus
- Possible nausea and vomiting
- Tinnitus

Diagnostic aids

- Perform a clinical examination.
- Exclude other possible causes of dizziness and ataxia (e.g., cerebellar stroke).

Therapeutic interventions

- Administer meclizine (Antivert) for vertigo.
- Give antiemetics.
- Sedate with benzodiazepines.
- Initiate antibiotic therapy if labyrinthitis is associated with a bacterial infection.
- Encourage bed rest.

Patient education and discharge instructions

- Avoid sudden changes in head or body position.
- Lie still, with the eyes closed.
- Use a cane or walker when walking is necessary.
- Do not drive or operate dangerous machinery.
- Follow up with a primary care provider if attacks increase in frequency or severity or are associated with additional neurologic symptoms.

Epistaxis (Nosebleed)

Epistaxis results from nose-picking, trauma, inhalant use, hypertension, nasal mucosal drying, infections, tumors, septal perforation, intranasal administration of drugs (e.g., cocaine), and anticoagulation or coagulopathies that predispose the patient to bleeding. Epistaxis originates in the vessels of the anterior nose or the posterior nasal chamber (Figure 33-6).

Anterior epistaxis

Anterior epistaxis is the most common type of epistaxis. Simply pinching the nostrils shut for 10 minutes is usually sufficient to control bleeding.

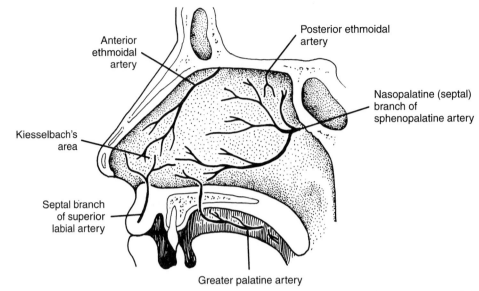

Figure 33-6. Arterial supply to nasal septum. (From Rosen P et al: *Emergency medicine: concepts and clinical practice*, ed 4, St Louis, 1998, Mosby.)

Diagnostic aids

- Patients with anterior epistaxis rarely need diagnostic studies. However, if the patient is in a high-risk category and bleeding persists, perform the following:
  - Check blood pressure to rule out a hypertensive event.
  - Draw and send coagulation studies.

Therapeutic interventions

- Have the patient sit upright and pinch the nostrils continuously for a full 10 minutes (no peeking). If mild bleeding persists, repeat for an additional 10 minutes. If the patient is still bleeding significantly, try the following:
  - Soak a cotton pledget in a vasoconstrictor and anesthetic combination (e.g., 4% cocaine solution with 0.25% phenylephrine and 4% lidocaine or epinephrine 1:10,000 solution with 4% lidocaine). Insert the pledget in the nostril for approximately 10 minutes.
  - Alternatively, use a commercially available hemostatic nasal sponge.
  - Or assist with cauterization of the bleeding site(s) with silver nitrate.
  - Or assist with firmly packing the nostril with petroleum gauze, a nasal tampon, or an anterior epistaxis balloon (Figure 33-7).

Patient education and discharge instructions

- Avoid behaviors that lead to episodes of epistaxis (e.g., nose-picking).
- Follow up with a primary care provider for management of any contributory medical problems.
- If the nasal mucosa is dry, apply a thin coat of petroleum jelly to the nostrils once or twice a day.
- If anterior packing is in place, follow up with an ENT specialist.

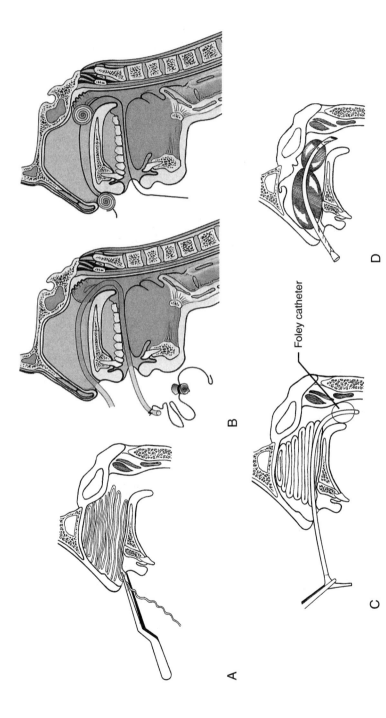

Figure 33-7. A, Anterior nasal packing. **B,** Method of placing posterior nasal pack. *Left,* Catheter is passed through the bleeding side of the nose and pulled out through the mouth with a hemostat. Strings are tied to the catheter, and the pack is pulled up behind the soft palate and into the nasopharynx. *Right,* Nasal pack in position in the posterior nasopharynx. Dental roll of the nose helps maintain correct position. **C,** Nasal packing for severe epistaxis. **D,** Anterior and posterior nasal balloon tamponade for control of anterior and posterior epistaxis. (**A** and **B** from Lewis SM, Heitkemper MM, Dirksen SR: *Medical-surgical nursing: assessment and management of clinical problems,* ed 6, St Louis, 2004, Mosby.)

Age/developmental considerations

Socks, gloves, or mittens over the hands may prevent children from unconsciously nose-picking while asleep.

Posterior epistaxis

Posterior epistaxis accounts for only 10% of all epistaxis cases but is considerably more difficult to control and can result in significant blood loss. Unlike anterior epistaxis, which is usually benign, patients with posterior bleeds often have underlying medical disorders or major facial trauma.

Diagnostic aids

- Ask about the patient's medical history and medication use.
- Monitor vital signs including oxygen saturation. Consider cardiac monitoring.

Therapeutic interventions

- Administer IV crystalloids and transfuse as necessary.
- Assist with posterior nasal packing according to the product manufacturer's directions (see Figure 33-7, *B* to *D*).
- Alternatively, insert an indwelling urinary (Foley) catheter. Box 33-6 gives directions.
- Analgesics and sedatives usually are required during posterior packing.
- Consider the need for antibiotic administration.
- Obtain ENT specialist consultation.
- Patients with posterior packs generally are admitted to the hospital while the packing is in place (commonly 3 to 5 days). Not only do these patients often have serious underlying disorders, but posterior packing can decrease oxygenation, requires ongoing analgesia and sedation, and potentially can cause airway obstruction.
- Ligation of the internal maxillary artery or of the anterior or posterior ethmoid arteries or embolization of the internal maxillary artery may be required if the bleeding is intractable.

Nasal Foreign Bodies

Foreign bodies in the nose are common in children, often discovered only after a purulent, foul-smelling discharge is noted. Unlike the child with a cold, this discharge is from a single nostril. Patients may be at risk for choking if the object is aspirated from the nose.

Therapeutic interventions

- Have the patient blow his or her nose while the unaffected nostril is pressed closed.
- Remove visible objects with a ring curette, alligator forceps, or suction.

Box 33-6 How to Insert a Foley Catheter for Posterior Epistaxis

Insert a 12- to 16-French Foley catheter into the affected nostril until the tip of the catheter is visible in the posterior pharynx.
Inflate the balloon with approximately 10 mL of saline.
Gently pull the catheter forward until the inflated balloon is lodged firmly in the posterior nasal cavity.
Secure the anterior portion of the catheter in place with an umbilical clamp.
Pack the nostril around the catheter with petrolatum or petrolatum-impregnated gauze to prevent pressure ulcers.
Consult an ear, nose, and throat specialist.

- Using a bag-valve-mask device, cover the child's mouth (only) with the mask, occlude the unaffected naris, and ventilate (squeeze the bag) firmly against a closed glottis (if the child can cooperate). This procedure can blow the object from the nose.
- Administer decongestant nose drops as needed. Pretreatment with a decongestant facilitates foreign body removal.

Esophageal Obstruction

See Chapter 24.

Epiglottitis

See Chapter 19.

Peritonsillar Abscess

A peritonsillar abscess is a collection of purulent material in the area around the tonsils. The abscess typically follows an episode of pharyngitis or tonsillitis.

Signs and symptoms

- Deviation of the uvula toward the unaffected side
- Drooling
- Dysphagia (difficulty swallowing)
- Fever
- Halitosis
- Muffled voice
- Pain in the throat, radiating to the ear
- Soft palate swollen on the affected side
- Tonsil deviation medially or anteriorly
- Trismus (tonic contraction of the jaw muscles)

Diagnostic aids

- Culture purulent drainage.
- Obtain CT scan if direct visualization is not possible.

Therapeutic interventions

- Establish an IV and infuse crystalloids for dehydration.
- Initiate IV antibiotic therapy.
- Administer IV steroids such as dexamethasone (Decadron) to decrease edema.
- Give systemic analgesics.
- Obtain ENT specialist consultation.
- Assist with needle aspiration or incision and drainage when the abscess points.

Patient education and discharge instructions

- Take antibiotics as directed.
- Assume a position of comfort.
- Call 911 for respiratory distress.

Ludwig's Angina

Ludwig's angina is bacterial cellulitis involving the floor of the mouth and neck. (This condition is unrelated to cardiac angina.) Ludwig's angina may arise from an untreated dental abscess, an abscess not responding to therapy, or trauma to the mouth. One reported case of Ludwig's angina occurred following tongue piercing.[9] Swelling may progress to the point of airway occlusion.

Signs and symptoms

- Deviation of the tongue upward and backward because of swelling under the tongue
- Difficulty breathing
- Drooling
- Fever
- Muffled voice
- Pain
- Possible toothache
- Swelling in the submandibular and sublingual spaces
- Trismus
- Children may adopt a tripod position and develop stridor.

Diagnostic aids

- Perform a clinical examination.
- Obtain soft tissue neck radiographs.
- Consider CT scan of the neck.
- Obtain a complete blood count and blood cultures.

Therapeutic interventions

- Establish an IV and infuse crystalloids for dehydration.
- Initiate IV antibiotic therapy.
- Administer IV steroids to decrease edema.
- Give systemic analgesics.
- Obtain ENT specialist consultation.
- Assist with incision and drainage.
- Facilitate tracheal intubation or cricothyrotomy as needed for airway management.
- Admit to the hospital.

DENTAL EMERGENCIES

Dental Pain

Causes of dental pain or referred pain to the teeth include the following:
- Carcinoma and radiation therapy
- Coronary artery disease (referred pain to the jaw)
- Dry socket
- Exposed root surfaces from receding gums
- Foreign bodies such as a toothbrush bristle embedded in the gums
- Fractured teeth
- Glossodynia (a burning pain in the tongue)

- Hematomas (usually related to trauma but can result from local anesthetic injection)
- Mandibular fractures
- Pericoronitis (inflammation of the gingiva around a partially erupted tooth)
- Periodontal disease in supporting tissues
- Pressure from a prosthetic device
- Teeth eruption
- Temporomandibular joint dysfunction
- Tooth decay or pulpal disease
- Trigeminal neuralgia (See Facial Emergencies.)
- Vincent's angina (also known as necrotizing ulcerative gingivitis or "trench mouth")

Dental and Periodontal Abscesses

The development of a dental abscess usually follows pulpal necrosis, caused by caries or trauma. Destruction of the periodontal ligament and alveolar bone causes periodontal abscess formation. Chronic periodontal disease or a foreign body lodged in the gingiva are common culprits.

Therapeutic interventions

- Administer analgesics.
- Most patients will be treated with antibiotics, although this practice is controversial.[10]

Patient education and discharge instructions

- Take medications as directed.
- Follow up with a dentist. Abscess incision and drainage, tooth extraction, or root canal therapy may be indicated. Table 33-2 describes specific periodontal emergencies that call for dental referral.

Table 33-2   Periodontal Emergencies Requiring Dental Referral

Type	Description
Gingivitis	Inflammation of the gums characterized by redness, swelling, and bleeding caused by plaque buildup. Usually painless. Good dental hygiene can prevent or reverse this condition.
Periodontitis (pyorrhea)	Occurs when gingivitis extends into the surrounding structures and bone is destroyed. The patient has symptoms of severe gingivitis. Radiographs are used to determine the amount of bone loss. Eventually, teeth will loosen and fall out. Antibiotics and surgery may be required.
Vincent's angina (necrotizing ulcerative gingivitis or trench mouth)	Painful bleeding, halitosis, lymphadenopathy, chills, fever, dysphagia, and malaise are present. The top of the gums (between the teeth) erodes and becomes covered with a layer of gray-colored, dead tissue that must be debrided by a dentist.
Pericoronitis	A flap of gum overlying an erupting tooth, often a wisdom tooth, under which bits of food and bacteria accumulate. Accompanied by swelling, lymphadenopathy, and trismus. Treatment involves removing the tissue over the tooth. Rinse with warm saline, take antibiotics, and follow up with a dentist for possible tooth extraction.

Bleeding After Tooth Extraction

Postoperative bleeding after tooth extraction is not usually a life-threatening condition. In rare instances the bleeding can cause airway compromise and require emergency airway management.[11]

Therapeutic interventions

- Apply moist gauze over the extraction site and have the patient bite down for 45 minutes. Placing a wet tea bag over the socket also may help; tannic acid promotes hemostasis.
- If the bleeding persists, the socket requires packing with a hemostatic dressing (e.g., oxidized cellulose, thrombin, or an absorbable gelatin sponge).
- Assist with suturing or cautery of bleeding vessels.

Patient education and discharge instructions

- To avoid dislodging the blood clot, do not suck through a straw, smoke, or spit for 1 week.
- Chew with teeth other than those near the extraction site.
- Eat soft foods and increase fluid intake.
- Avoid carbonated drinks and hot liquids.

Dry Socket (Alveolar Osteitis)

If a clot becomes dislodged following tooth extraction (usually a mandibular molar), localized inflammation can develop, filling the socket with necrotic tissue. Dry socket occurs 1 to 4 days after surgery and is accompanied by halitosis and severe pain that may radiate to the ear.

Therapeutic interventions

- Assist with a nerve block or administer an analgesic.
- Assist with socket irrigation.
- Assist with packing the socket using a material that contains lidocaine and an antiseptic.

Patient education and discharge instructions

- Take analgesics as directed.
- Follow up with an oral surgeon.

BODY PIERCING OF THE FACE, EARS, AND TONGUE

All forms of body piercing have the potential for causing serious infections, local or systemic. Unsterile piercing equipment can transmit hepatitis, tetanus, and human immunodeficiency virus.[12] In severe local infections, jewelry removal actually promotes abscess formation. Table 33-3 highlights specific complications associated with various piercings on the head. One of the challenges encountered when caring for pierced patients is removal of unique items such as captive bead rings and barbells. Figure 33-8 illustrates different types of body jewelry.

Table 33-3   **Ear, Nose, and Throat Complications Related to Body Piercing**

Location	Complications
Tongue	Hemorrhage that may require transfusion; swelling that threatens the airway (from the piercing or from infection); nerve damage; difficult orotracheal intubation; chipped teeth
Pinna	Infection and deformity of the ear cartilage
Uvula	May present an obstacle to intubation. Leave uvula jewelry in place; removal entails a significant risk of dropping jewelry down the airway.[13]

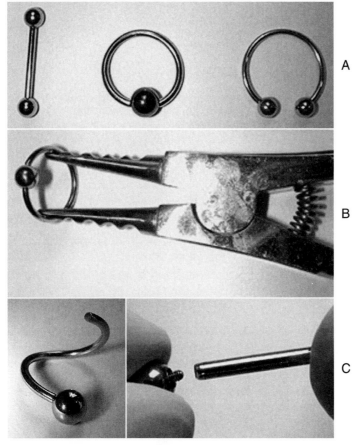

Figure 33-8. Removal of body jewelry. **A,** Barbell, bead ring, circular barbell. **B,** Ring-expanding pliers with bead ring. **C,** Bead ring removed with hemostats. Removal of internal threaded barbell. (Courtesy Association of Professional Piercers, Chamblee, Ga.)

References

1. Ebright JR, Pace MT, Niazi AF: Septic thrombosis of the cavernous sinuses, *Arch Intern Med* 161(22):2671-2676, 2001.
2. Schmidt DP, Schulte-Monting J, Schumacher M: Prognosis of central retinal artery occlusion: local intraarterial fibrinolysis versus conservative treatment, *AJNR Am J Neuroradiol* 23(8):1301-1307, 2002.
3. Padolecchia R et al: Superselective intraarterial fibrinolysis in central retinal artery occlusion, *AJNR Am J Neuroradiol* 20(4):565-567, 1999.
4. Distelhorst JS, Hughes GM: Open-angle glaucoma, *Am Fam Physician* 67(9):1937-1944, 2003.
5. National Institutes of Health: New eye disease treatment may improve patients' quality of life. http://www.nih.gov/news/pr/jun99/nei-21.htm. Accessed June 21, 1999.
6. Wallenborn WM: George Washington's terminal illness: a modern medical analysis of the last illness and death of George Washington. http://gwpaperw.virginia.edu/articles/wallenborn/. Accessed August 19, 2003.
7. Sander R: Otitis externa: a practical guide to treatment and prevention, *Am Fam Physician* 63(5): 927-936, 2001.
8. Nichols AW: Nonorthopaedic problems in the aquatic athlete, *Clin Sports Med* 18:395-411, 1999.
9. Perkins CS, Meisner J, Harrison JM: A complication of tongue piercing, *Br Dent J* 182:147-148, 1997.
10. Herrera D, Roldan S, Sanz M: The periodontal abscess: a review, *J Clin Periodontol* 27(6):377-386, 2000.
11. Moghadam HG et al: Life-threatening hemorrhage after extraction of third molars: case report and management protocol, *J Can Dent Assoc* 68(11):670-674, 2002.
12. American Dental Association: Statement on intraoral/perioral piercing. http://www.ada.org/prof/resources/positions/statement/piercing.asp. Accessed October 23, 2000.
13. Meyer D: Body piercing: old traditions creating new challenges, *J Emerg Nurs* 26(6):612-614, 2000.

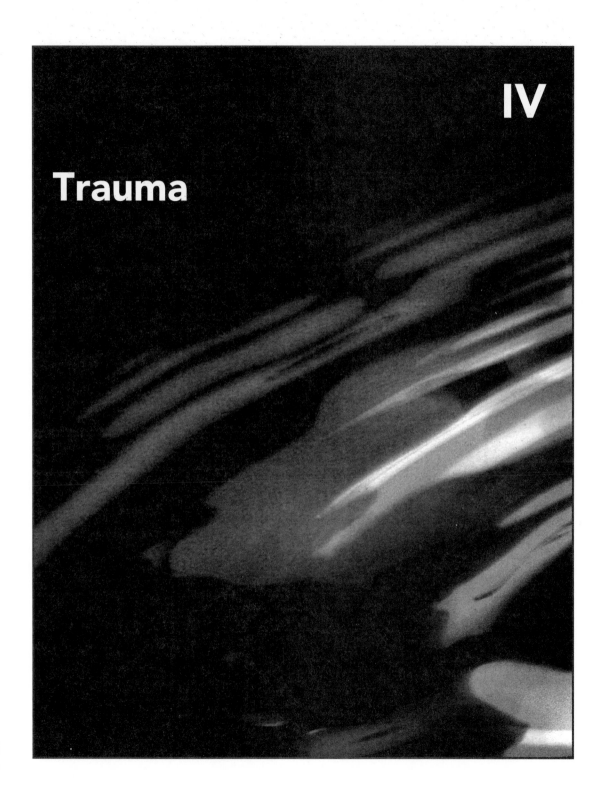

IV

Trauma

34

Assessment of the Trauma Patient

LCDR Andrew A. Galvin, APRN, BC, MSN, CEN

TRAUMA EPIDEMIOLOGY

Trauma is defined as injury that results when energy is transferred from the environment to human tissue.[1] Injuries are a major cause of disability in the United States, accounting for more than 150,000 deaths annually.[2] Trauma can be classified as *intentional* or *unintentional*. In the United States, unintentional injury is the fifth leading cause of death in all age groups and the number one killer of persons 1 to 34 years old.[3] Every emergency nurse must be prepared to care for critically injured trauma patients.

MECHANISM OF INJURY

Mechanism of injury refers to the means by which energy is transferred from the environment to the trauma patient. Energy is the agent that causes physical damage. Types of energy involved in trauma are mechanical, electrical, thermal, chemical, and radiation. Of these, injuries resulting from mechanical energy are by far the most common. Mechanical energy is transferred to patients through mechanisms such as motor vehicle collisions, falls, blunt assaults, stabbings, and gunshot wounds. Injuries caused by mechanical force can be subcategorized as blunt or penetrating. Motor vehicle crashes and falls are considered blunt trauma, whereas gunshot wounds and impalement injuries are examples of penetrating injuries.

Mass and velocity influence the amount of force an object exerts. Of the two, velocity is significantly more influential (Box 34-1). A linear association exists between mass and force, but the relationship between velocity and force is logarithmic. If the mass of an object is doubled, its force doubles as well. But in the kinetic energy equation, velocity is squared, resulting in much greater energy gains as speed (velocity) increases. This explains why a tiny bullet (very small mass) can do such tremendous damage (very high velocity).

Box **34-1** The Relationship Between Mass, Velocity, and Force

$$\text{Kinetic energy} = \frac{\text{Mass} \times \text{Velocity}^2}{2}$$

Table 34-1   Mechanisms and Patterns of Injury (Unrestrained Driver in a Multivehicle Collision)

Mechanism of Injury	Predicted (Suspected) Injury Patterns
Frontal Impact	
Spider-web or bull's-eye pattern on the windshield	Cervical spine fracture; facial trauma
Bent steering wheel	Anterior flail chest; blunt cardiac injury; pneumothorax; splenic or hepatic injury; aortic disruption
Knee imprint on the dashboard	Fractures/dislocations of the knee, femur, and hip
Lateral Impact	
Head contact on the side window	Cervical spine fracture; head injury
Door intrudes into passenger space	Lateral flail chest
	Splenic or hepatic rupture (depending on the side of impact)

Mechanical energy can affect the body through deceleration forces (most common), acceleration forces, or both. For example, an unrestrained passenger in a motor vehicle collision is subject to deceleration forces as the vehicle comes to a sudden halt. Energy is transferred to the patient through contact with the windshield, dashboard, and pavement. Not all anatomical structures decelerate at the same speed. Certain organs and tissues are more susceptible to deceleration forces. The opposite of deceleration is acceleration, a rapid increase in speed, which also can damage the tissues. An acceleration injury occurs when a pedestrian or bicyclist is struck by a moving vehicle and is thrown suddenly into motion. However, the same pedestrian also experiences deceleration injuries when landing on the roadway.

By gathering a careful history of events, clinicians often can predict injuries based on typical trauma constellations. Besides mechanism, specific injury patterns are influenced by patient age, the body area affected, and the presence or absence of safety devices designed to reduce energy transfer. Using this information, clinicians can predict the location and type of tissue damage likely to affect a particular patient.

For example, an unrestrained driver in a frontal motor vehicle collision is at risk for abdominal, thoracic, and facial injury caused by rapid deceleration against the steering wheel at the time of the crash. A patient who falls from a second-story window, landing on his feet, has a high probability of sustaining calcaneal fractures and compression fractures of the lumbar spine. Table 34-1 describes patterns of injury common to unrestrained drivers involved in a vehicle collision.

APPROACH TO THE MULTITRAUMA PATIENT

A systematic approach is essential for optimal management of the trauma patient. Urgent care priorities are (1) establish and maintain an adequate airway, (2) ensure effective ventilation, and (3) control hemorrhage. These priorities direct the course of the primary trauma survey.

Death from trauma has a trimodal pattern of distribution.[4] The first morbidity peak occurs within seconds or minutes of injury. These deaths are due to lacerations of the heart, large vessels, brain, or spinal cord. Because of the severity of such injuries, few patients are salvageable. The second death peak takes place minutes or hours after the traumatic event. Deaths in this period are generally due to intracranial hematomas or uncontrolled hemorrhage from pelvic fractures, solid organ lacerations, or multiple wounds. Care received during the first (so-called golden) hour after injury is crucial to trauma patient survival. The Trauma Nursing Core Course (Emergency Nurses Association) and Advanced Trauma Life Support (American College of Surgeons) use the primary and secondary survey approach. This approach focuses largely on preventing death and disability in the first hours after injury.[5] The third morbidity peak occurs days to weeks following trauma. Death during this period is due to sepsis, multi-organ failure, and respiratory or other complications.

Because of the complexity and severity of injury and the need for simultaneous evaluation and intervention, major trauma patients require a coordinated team effort for successful resuscitation. The team leader (or captain) oversees the course of patient resuscitation. Team composition varies from facility to facility but usually consists of at least one physician, one nurse, and ancillary care personnel.

THE PRIMARY SURVEY: A, B, C, D, AND E

Initial assessment of the trauma patient consists of a primary and secondary survey. This approach is designed to provide a consistent method of caring for individuals with multiple injuries and to keep the team focused on care priorities. Life-threatening problems related to the patient's airway, breathing, circulation, and disability status are identified, evaluated, and treated within minutes of emergency department arrival. Potentially lethal conditions—such as pneumothorax, hemothorax, pericardial tamponade, flail chest, and hemorrhage—can be detected during the primary survey. As each major problem is identified, appropriate interventions are initiated.

The primary survey involves a continuous process of assessment, intervention, and reevaluation (assess, mess, reassess). The components of the primary trauma survey are as follows:
A: Airway
B: Breathing
C: Circulation
D: Disability (neurologic deficits)
E: Exposure and environmental control

A: Airway

Assessment of the airway is always the initial step in trauma patient care. Because of the potential for cervical spine injury in this population, airway assessment is performed simultaneously with neck stabilization. Maintain the head and neck in a neutral position while placing a rigid cervical collar and immobilizing the patient on a long spineboard.

Listen for spontaneous vocalization indicating air movement across the cords. If vocalization is absent, open the patient's airway using a chin-lift or modified jaw-thrust maneuver. Examine the oropharynx. The airway may be partially or entirely obstructed by fluids (blood, saliva, emesis) or debris such as teeth, food, or foreign bodies. Intervene as appropriate (e.g., digital removal, suctioning, and repositioning) and then reassess airway patency.

A nasopharyngeal airway (nasal trumpet), oropharyngeal airway, laryngeal mask airway, tracheal tube, Combitube, or cricothyrotomy may be necessary to establish and preserve the airway. See Chapter 19 for discussion of these devices.

B: Breathing

The trauma patient's respiratory status may be compromised by ventilation or perfusion defects or as a result of a serious neurologic condition. To assess breathing, observe for spontaneous respirations and note their rate, depth, and effort. Examine the chest wall for use of accessory muscles and symmetrical rise and fall during respiration. Additionally, visually inspect the thorax. Certain traumatic injuries, such as open wounds or flail chest, may be easily observed. Auscultate breath sounds if ventilation is compromised. Breath sounds can be assessed as part of the secondary examination in patients without obvious respiratory issues. Always assume uncooperative or restless patients are hypoxic until proved otherwise.

Interventions during this phase of care include the following:

- Provide supplemental oxygen to all patients. For those with an adequate tidal volume, use a non-rebreather mask[5] with a reservoir at a flow rate of 10 to 12 L/min.
- Assist ventilations as needed. Use a bag-valve-mask device to deliver positive-pressure oxygen to patients with ineffective respirations. Obtain definitive airway control (tracheal intubation), and place the patient on a mechanical ventilator. (For information on ventilatory assistance, see Chapter 19.)
- Confirm tracheal tube placement. Once the patient is intubated, verification of correct tube placement is imperative; reverify as needed. Visualize symmetrical chest rise and fall, auscultate over the stomach and then the lung fields, confirm the presence of carbon dioxide (exhaled carbon dioxide detector), and monitor oxygen saturation per pulse oximeter.
- Treat serious thoracic injuries. Cover sucking chest wounds, relieve tension pneumothoraces, stabilize flail segments, and insert chest tubes. (See Chapter 37.)
- In addition to reassessing previously monitored parameters, ongoing evaluation of respiratory status includes measurement of oxygen saturation and arterial blood gases.

C: Circulation

Primary assessment of the trauma patient's circulatory status involves evaluation of bleeding, pulses, and perfusion.

Bleeding

Inspect for signs of significant external blood loss and apply direct pressure to the affected area. If possible, elevate hemorrhaging extremities above the level of the heart. Large amounts of blood can be lost internally. Splinting long bone and pelvic fractures can reduce ongoing orthopedic losses. (See Chapter 39.) Facilitate surgical management of internal hemorrhage.

Pulses

Pulses are palpated for presence, quality, rate, and rhythm. Peripheral pulses may be absent following direct injury, hypothermia, hypovolemia, or vasoconstriction caused by an intense sympathetic nervous system response. Palpate carotid, radial, and femoral pulses. Box 34-2 lists approximate minimal systolic blood pressures palpable in adults at various sites.

Circulation also is evaluated by apical auscultation. Listen for muffled heart tones that indicate pericardial tamponade. Begin basic and advanced life support measures for pulseless patients. (See Chapter 18.) However, patients in traumatic cardiopulmonary arrest have a dismal prognosis, especially following blunt trauma.[6,7] The position of the American College of Surgeons Committee on Trauma is that providers may cease efforts in patients with witnessed traumatic cardiopulmonary arrest who have had 15 minutes of unsuccessful

Box **34-2** **Estimating Adult Systolic Blood Pressure**

If the pulse is palpable,	Systolic blood pressure is at least
Radial	80 mm Hg
Femoral	70 mm Hg
Carotid	60 mm Hg

resuscitation attempts.[8] In the trauma patient population, always consider tension pneumothorax and cardiac tamponade as potential causes of pulselessness. These quickly reversible conditions can be managed with needle thoracentesis and pericardiocentesis, respectively. See Chapter 37 for more information about these disorders and interventions.

Skin perfusion

Several nonspecific signs (cool, clammy skin; pallor; cyanosis; or mottling) may indicate the presence of hypovolemic shock. Assess the skin for color, temperature, the presence of diaphoresis, and capillary refill. Capillary refill time is a good measure of perfusion in children but its usefulness decreases with patient age and diminishing health status. Unfortunately, all of these signs of shock are imprecise and observer-dependent.[9] In addition to the skin, signs of hypoperfusion are evident in other organs. Look for oliguria, altered level of consciousness, tachycardia, and dysrhythmias. Also assess for distended or abnormally flattened external jugular veins. See Chapter 22 for a more complete discussion of shock.

Restoring circulating blood volume as soon as possible is crucial. Insert two (or more) large-bore (14- to 16-gauge) peripheral intravenous (IV) lines. Infuse warmed IV fluids via Y (blood) tubing. Y tubing has a wider diameter than standard tubing (allowing faster flow) and will already be in place in the event of blood transfusion. Give patients a bolus with 1 to 2 L (children, 20 mL/kg) of an isotonic crystalloid solution (0.9% normal saline or Ringer's lactate).[1] Give fluids according to patient response. Remember, it takes approximately 3 mL of crystalloids to replace the intravascular volume of every 1 mL of blood lost. See Chapter 8 for a discussion of crystalloid solutions.

Several recent studies have suggested caution when providing IV fluids to the trauma patient.[9] Data indicate that in certain populations, aggressive volume replacement actually may worsen hemorrhage by overcoming hemostatic plugs formed to stop bleeding.

As a general rule, a patient that remains hemodynamically unstable after 2 to 3 L of rapidly infused crystalloids should receive blood transfusions.[10] Type-specific, crossmatched blood is ideal. However, in emergency situations, uncrossmatched O-negative blood is acceptable for transfusion in patients with any blood type. Males and females beyond childbearing may receive O-positive blood safely. See Chapter 8 for a discussion of blood products.

D: Disability

This component of the trauma survey focuses on the patient's general neurologic status. Level of consciousness can be assessed grossly and communicated using the AVPU mnemonic (Box 34-3).

Additionally, check pupillary size, shape, equality, and reactivity to light. During the primary survey, only a brief, focused, neurologic assessment is performed. If the patient is exhibiting motor posturing, or has gross pupillary dilation or asymmetry, consider mannitol infusion, maneuvers to maximize cerebral venous outflow, brief hyperventilation, or emergent

Box **34-3** AVPU Mnemonic

A, Awake
V, Responsive to verbal stimuli
P, Responsive to painful stimuli
U, Unresponsive

surgical intervention. (See Chapter 35.) Patients at risk for hypoglycemic events (e.g., known diabetic patients) should have a capillary glucose level checked. Give dextrose 50% only for documented hypoglycemia.

Any decreased level of consciousness or pupil abnormality will be investigated further during the secondary survey. Glasgow Coma Scale scores can be calculated after the secondary examination is complete.

E: Exposure and Environmental Control

Exposure

Completely and rapidly remove the patient's clothing to assess for injuries, hemorrhage, or other abnormalities. Observe the patient's overall general appearance, noting body position, guarding, or the presence of odors such as alcohol, gasoline, and urine.

Environmental control

Trauma patients must be protected from hypothermia. Hypothermia is particularly significant in this population because of its relationship with vasoconstriction and coagulopathies. Maintain or restore normothermia by drying the patient and using heat lamps, blankets, slippers, head covers, convective air warming systems (e.g., Bair Hugger [Arizant Healthcare, Eden Prairie, Minnesota]), and the administration of warmed IV fluids and warm, humidified oxygen. See Hypothermia in Chapter 29.

THE SECONDARY SURVEY

Once the primary survey is complete and issues involving the patient's airway, breathing, circulation, and disability status have been addressed, proceed to the secondary survey. This is not a final examination; it is a rapid, thorough inspection of the patient's entire body from head to toe. Unlike the primary survey, issues noted on secondary examination are not treated immediately. They are noted and then prioritized for later intervention. If at any time the patient develops an airway, breathing, or circulatory problem, return at once to the primary survey and intervene as indicated. The mnemonic used to remember the components of the secondary survey are the letters F through I.[1]

F: Full Set of Vital Signs, Five Interventions, and Facilitation of Family Presence

Full Set of Vital Signs

If a complete set of vital signs (including temperature and oxygen saturation) has not yet been obtained, it is appropriate to do so at this point. These vital signs will serve as a baseline

Box **34-4**   **Common Trauma Laboratory Tests**

Type and crossmatch or type and screen*
Complete blood count
Basic chemistry panel (electrolytes, glucose, renal function)
Urinalysis
Urine or blood human chorionic gonadotropin (females of childbearing potential)
Ethanol level
Toxicologic screens (urine, serum)
Clotting studies (prothrombin time [international normalized ratio], activated partial thromboplastin time, fibrinogen, D dimer) for patients with evidence of coagulopathy

*This is the most important laboratory test in major trauma patients.

for continued reassessment. Patients with suspected chest trauma should have apical *and* radial pulse rates documented; assess blood pressure in both arms.

Five Interventions

Interventions to consider at this juncture include the following:
- Initiate continuous cardiac monitoring.
- Place a nasogastric or orogastric tube (if indications exist and contraindications do not).
- Insert an indwelling urinary (Foley) catheter (if indications exist and contraindications do not).
- Collect and send appropriate laboratory studies (Box 34-4).
- Initiate continuous monitoring of oxygen saturation.

Facilitation of Family Presence

Facilitating family presence means granting significant individuals the opportunity to be with patients, even in life-threatening situations. Emergency care providers have mixed feelings about this practice, and family presence during resuscitation remains controversial.[11] Nonetheless, in 1993, Emergency Nurses Association members approved a resolution in support of offering families the option of being present during invasive procedures and resuscitation.[9,12] Medical facilities that permit or encourage family presence need to have a protocol describing how to provide comfort, support, and information to family members. Assignment of a health care worker (nurse, social worker, chaplain, or even a trained volunteer) to stay with the family, provide updates, explain procedures and tests, and continually evaluate the family's emotional status is essential. See Chapter 15 for more information on family presence.

G: Give Comfort Measures

The trauma victim is often in physical and psychological distress. Pharmacologic and non-pharmacologic methods of reducing pain and anxiety are available for this population. The trauma team is obliged to recognize pain and intervene as necessary. See Chapter 14.

H: History and Head-to-Toe Examination

History

If the patient is awake, alert, and cooperative, try to elicit pertinent medication, allergy, and medical history information. Family members are also a resource for this data. Important

Box **34-5**   **MIVT Mnemonic**

M,   Mechanism
I,   Injuries suspected
V,   Vital signs on scene
T,   Treatment received

prehospital information regarding the scene, mechanism of injury, assessment, and interventions should be obtained from the transporting medics. A useful tool for gathering history pertinent to trauma is the MIVT mnemonic (Box 34-5).

Head-to-Toe Examination

Items to be considered during the head-to-toe examination are addressed only briefly in this section. Refer to Chapters 35 to 42 for information on trauma to specific body regions.

Head

The head is inspected systematically and assessed for any obvious wounds, deformities, or asymmetry. Palpate the skull for depressed bony fragments, hematomas, lacerations, or tenderness. Note any areas of ecchymosis or discoloration. Ecchymosis behind the ears, over the mastoid process (battle sign) or in the periorbital region (raccoon eyes) is indicative of a basilar skull fracture.

Interventions
- Do not allow the patient to become hypotensive or hypoxic.
- Mannitol may be administered IV to decrease intracranial pressure.
- In brain-injured patients who continue to deteriorate, consider short-term hyperventilation therapy to reduce $PaCO_2$ to 30 to 35 mm Hg.
- Facilitate surgical intervention or intracranial pressure monitoring.

Face

Inspect the face for wounds and asymmetry. Note any fluid from the ears, nose, eyes, or mouth. Clear fluid from the nose or ears is assumed to be cerebrospinal fluid until proved otherwise. Reassess the pupils for symmetry, light response, and accommodation. Check gross visual acuity. Ask the patient to open and close the mouth to check for malocclusion, lacerations, loose or missing teeth, or foreign bodies.

Diagnostics
- Noncontrast computerized axial tomographic scans
- Panoramic radiographic views of the jaw

Intervention
- Wound care

Neck

While another team member provides cervical immobilization, partially remove the rigid cervical collar in order to assess the patient's neck. Palpate and inspect for obvious wounds, ecchymosis, neck vein distention, subcutaneous air, or tracheal deviation. The carotid arteries may be auscultated for bruits. Palpate for deformities, defects, or cervical vertebral tenderness before reapplying the collar. Penetrating neck trauma rarely results in vertebral injuries.[10] Nonetheless, cervical spine damage should be considered a possibility until it can be ruled out with an appropriate clinical or radiographic assessment.

Four radiographic views are needed to visualize the cervical spine fully:
1. Cross-table lateral (must visualize C1 to T1)
2. Anterior-posterior
3. Lateral
4. Open-mouth odontoid

Obtain computed tomography (CT) studies if plain films are inconclusive. Flexion/extension views are used to check for soft tissue damage and are performed much less frequently. A cervical spine cannot be cleared adequately in the presence of alcohol or drug intoxication or major distracting injuries. Conversely, the cervical spine of a low-risk, alert, oriented, non-intoxicated patient can be cleared based on clinical examinatioin alone in the absence of pain, tenderness, or neurologic findings.

Chest

Visually inspect the chest for asymmetry, deformity, penetrating trauma, or other wounds. Auscultate the heart and lungs. Palpate the chest wall for deformities, subcutaneous air, and areas of tenderness.

Diagnostics

- Obtain a portable chest radiograph if the patient cannot sit upright for posterior-anterior and lateral views.
- Record a 12-lead electrocardiogram in patients with suspected or actual blunt chest trauma.
- Consider drawing arterial blood gases if the patient has any airway distress or has been placed on a mechanical ventilator.

Abdomen

Inspect the abdomen for bruising, masses, pulsations, or penetrating objects. Observe for distention or evisceration of bowel contents. Auscultate bowel sounds in all four quadrants. Gently palpate the abdomen checking for rigidity and areas of tenderness, rebound pain, or guarding.

Diagnostics

- FAST study (focused abdominal sonography for trauma): This is a rapid, bedside, sonographic examination of four specific abdominal areas (pericardial, perihepatic, perisplenic, and pelvic) used to identify intraperitoneal fluid in patients with blunt abdominal trauma.
- Diagnostic peritoneal lavage (used less and less as the speed of CT increases)
- CT scan of the abdomen (usually performed with a contrast medium)
- Abdominal or kidneys-ureter-bladder radiographic series

Pelvis

Visually inspect the pelvis for bleeding, bruising, deformity, or penetrating trauma. In males, check for priapism; in females look for bleeding. Inspect the perineum for blood, feces, or any obvious injury. A rectal examination is performed to assess sphincter tone, identify blood, and check the position of the prostate. A high-riding prostate, blood at the urinary meatus, or the presence of a scrotal hematoma are contraindications to bladder catheterization until a retrograde urethrogram can be performed. Gently press inward (toward the midline) on the iliac crests to assess pelvic stability. Also palpate over the symphysis pubis. *Stop* if pain or motion are elicited, and obtain radiographic studies.

Extremities

Inspect all four limbs for deformity, dislocation, ecchymosis, swelling, or other wounds. Check the sensory-motor and neurovascular status of each extremity. Palpate for areas of tenderness, crepitus, and temperature abnormalities. If injuries are present, reassess distal neurovascular status regularly.

Diagnostics

- Radiographs of the affected extremity

Interventions

- Splinting
- Wound care

I: Inspect the Posterior Surfaces

While maintaining neutral spinal alignment, logroll the patient to the side. This procedure requires several team members. The team leader assesses the patient's posterior surfaces by looking for bruising, discoloration, or any open wounds. Palpate the vertebral bony prominences for deformity, movement, and pain. If a rectal examination was not performed while assessing the pelvis, it can be done at this time. This is also a good opportunity to remove any clothing or wet items left under the patient. If the spine is cleared, or the patient can lie still, remove the backboard as well (according to institutional protocol).

Diagnostics

- Spinal series (cervical, thoracic, lumbar)
- Spinal CT scan

Interventions

- Maintain spinal immobilization until the patient has been cleared.
- Consider padding or removing the board. Assess for signs of skin breakdown.

REEVALUATION/MONITORING

Once the secondary survey has been completed, prioritize and treat injuries in an appropriate and timely manner. Specific injuries identified on secondary examination now can be assessed in a detailed, focused fashion. Repair and dress open wounds as appropriate.

Multitrauma patients routinely are subjected to a variety of radiographic studies (chest, pelvis, spine). If blood specimens were not collected when IV access was established, draw and send laboratory work at this point. Box 34-4 lists commonly ordered tests. Determine whether tetanus prophylaxis is indicated. Obtain specialist consultation as needed. Prepare patients and family members for possible admission, transfer, or surgery.

As long as the trauma patient is in the emergency department, assessment is never complete. Reevaluate patients regularly to identify deterioration and injuries that were overlooked. Additionally, trauma patients may have underlying medical conditions that were not addressed during the initial resuscitation. Remediate the patient for pain (as indicated) but watch for respiratory depression. Narcotic analgesics also may mask subtle signs of neurologic deterioration. Monitor urinary output; intervene as necessary.

Glasgow Coma Scale

The Glasgow Coma Scale is a measure of the patient's level of consciousness. The scale is not a full neurologic examination. The Glasgow Coma Scale consists of a scale that corresponds with the patient's *best response* in three specific areas: eye opening, verbal responses, and motor responses (Table 7-8). The emergency nurse must remember that chemically paralyzed patients cannot be evaluated using the Glasgow Coma Scale. For information regarding the Glasgow Coma Scale, see Chapter 35.

A number of different scoring systems have been developed to predict trauma patient outcome. These scores generally are based on specific injuries, physiologic data, or a combination of the two. The Revised Trauma Score, displayed in Table 34-2, is an example of one popular scoring system. The Revised Trauma Score incorporates the Glasgow Coma Scale and certain physiologic parameters to derive a score ranging from 0 to 12. The Revised Trauma Score is easy to use and has been applied primarily in prehospital trauma triage situations.[13] The revised Trauma Score scores can predict survival, although less accurately than injury-based scoring systems.

PEDIATRIC AND GERIATRIC PATIENTS

Pediatric and geriatric patients represent special trauma victim subsets. Although the emergency nurse must consider a number of important anatomic, physiologic, developmental, and assessment differences when working with these patients, priorities of care do not change. Perform primary and secondary surveys in the same sequence. See Chapters 43 and 44 for information unique to these populations. Chapter 47 discusses nonaccidental trauma.

DOCUMENTATION

As in all aspects of health care, good documentation is essential. Because of their multiple assessments, interventions, and reassessments, recording trauma patient care in a timely fashion is crucial. Most facilities have developed a trauma flowsheet in order to achieve this goal. Assessment of the trauma patient requires a systematic, coordinated team effort to maximize resources and provide optimal patient care. Table 34-3 briefly summarizes components of the primary and secondary surveys.

Table **34-2**   **Revised Trauma Score**

Measurement	Numeric Score	Probability of Survival	
		Total Score	Percent Survivors
Systolic blood pressure (mm Hg)			
>89	4	12	99.5%
76-89	3		
50-75	2	11	96.9%
1-49	1		
0	0	10	87.9%
Respiratory rate (spontaneous inspirations per minute)*		9	76.6%
10-29	4	8	66.7%
>29	3		
6-9	2	7	63.6%
1-5	1		
0	0	6	63%
*Patient initiated breaths, *not* mechanically ventilated		5	45.5%
Glasgow Coma Scale score		3 or 4	33.3%
13-15	4		
9-12	3	2	28.6%
6-8	2		
4-5	1	1	25%
3	0	0	3.7%

Data from Emergency Nurses Association: *Trauma nursing core course,* ed 5, Des Plaines, III, 2000, The Association.

Table **34-3**   **Primary and Secondary Assessment of the Trauma Patient**

	Component	Assessment(s)	Potential Intervention(s)
A	Airway	Listen for vocalization. Patent? Obstructed? Inspect for debris, blood, vomitus, and foreign bodies.	Open the airway with a chin-lift or modified jaw-thrust maneuver. Clear the airway: suctioning and foreign body removal. Provide artificial airway: oropharyngeal or nasopharyngeal airway, tracheal intubation, or surgical airway.
B	Breathing	Observe for spontaneous respirations, chest excursion, rate and depth of respirations, and respiratory effort. Auscultate breath sounds.	Administer high-flow oxygen via a non-rebreather mask. Ventilate with positive pressure (bag-valve-mask). Assist with tracheal intubation or surgical airway placement.

Data from Emergency Nurses Association: *Trauma nursing core course,* ed 5, Des Plaines, III, 2000, The Association.
*M, Mechanism; I, injuries suspected; V, vital signs on scene; T, treatment received.

Table 34-3   Primary and Secondary Assessment of the Trauma Patient—cont'd

	Component	*Assessment(s)*	*Potential Intervention(s)*
C	Circulation	Inspect for obvious bleeding. Check skin for color, temperature, moisture, and capillary refill. Palpate central and distal pulses.	Apply direct pressure/elevation to external bleeding sites. Insert two or more large-bore intravenous catheters. Give a bolus of crystalloids or blood. Perform autotransfusion of chest blood. Apply splints to control hemorrhage. Facilitate surgical intervention for severe internal or external bleeding. Provide cardiopulmonary resuscitation/advanced cardiac life support as needed.
D	Disability	Assess neurologic status using the AVPU mnemonic. Inspect pupils for symmetry and light reactivity.	Do not allow the patient to become hypotensive or hypoxic. Maintain spinal precautions. Consider mannitol administration, measures to improve cerebral venous outflow, surgery, or a brief trial of (mild) hyperventilation.
E	Exposure and environment	Inspect the entire body.	Remove all clothing. Provide warming measures.
F	Full set of vital signs, five interventions, and family presence	Obtain baseline vital signs. Assess the patient's and family's psychosocial needs.	Initiate continuous cardiac monitoring and monitoring of oxygen saturation. Consider insertion of nasogastric or orogastric tube and urinary catheter.
G	Give comfort measures	Assess pain level.	Provide pain medications as directed. Use nonpharmacologic forms of pain relief.
H	History	If the patient is alert, gather a medical history.	Get MIVT* information from emergency medical services.
	Head-to-toe examination	Perform head-to-toe examination; inspect, auscultate, and palpate the patient from head to toe.	
I	Inspect posterior surfaces	Logroll the patient. Inspect and palpate all posterior surfaces.	

References

1. Emergency Nurses Association: *Trauma nursing core course,* ed 5, Des Plaines, Ill, 2000, The Association.
2. National Center for Injury Prevention and Control: WISQARS injury mortality reports, 1999-2002. http://webapp.cdc.gov/sasweb/ncipc/mortrate10_fy.html. Accessed August 11, 2004.
3. National Center for Injury Prevention and Control: WISQARS leading causes of death reports, 1999-2002. http://webapp.cdc.gov/sasweb/ncipc/leadcaus10.html. Accessed August 17, 2004.
4. American College of Surgeons Committee on Trauma: *Advanced trauma life support manual,* Chicago, 1997, The College.
5. Rosenblatt WH, Murphy M: The intubating laryngeal mask: use of a new ventilating-intubating device in the emergency department, *Ann Emerg Med* 33(2):234-238, 1999.
6. Pasquale MD et al: Defining "dead on arrival": impact on a level I trauma center, *J Trauma* 41: 726-730, 1996.

7. Hopson LR et al: Guidelines for withholding or termination of resuscitation in prehospital traumatic cardiopulmonary arrest: joint position statement of the National Association of EMS Physicians and the American College of Surgeons Committee on Trauma. *J Am Coll Surg* 196(1):106-112, 2003.

8. Drummond JC, Petrovitch CT: The massively bleeding patient, *Anesthesiol Clin North America* 19(4):633-649, 2001.

9. Boie ET et al: Do parents want to be present during invasive procedures performed on their children in the emergency department? A survey of 400 parents, *Ann Emerg Med* 34(1):70-74, 1999.

10. Butler KH, Clyne B: Management of the difficult airway: alternative airway techniques and adjuncts, *Emerg Med Clin North Am* 21(2):259-289, 2003.

11. Family presence at the bedside during invasive procedures and resuscitation, Emergency Nurses Association policy statement, July 2001, http://www.ena.org/about/position.

12. Kuhls DA et al: Predictors of mortality in adult trauma patients: the Physiologic Trauma Score is equivalent to the Trauma and Injury Severity Score, *J Am Coll Surg* 194(6):695-704, 2002.

13. Long JA, Klein MD: Trauma in infants in children. In Wilson RF, Walt AJ, editors: *Management of trauma: pitfalls and practice,* ed 2, Philadelphia, 1996, Lippincott Williams & Wilkins.

35

Head Trauma

Laura M. Criddle, MS, RN, CCNS, CEN, CRFN, CNRN

Brain injury is the primary cause of death in 40% to 50% of trauma patient fatalities.[1] The Centers for Disease Control and Prevention estimates that 1.5 million persons in the United States sustain a traumatic brain injury each year.[2] Of these, 50,000 persons die before reaching medical care,[3] 800,000 are seen in emergency departments or outpatient care centers,[4] and 20% are admitted to the hospital.[2] Traumatic brain injury is most common in the 15- to 44-year-old age-group,[3] and males are 3 times more likely to sustain a head injury than are females. The incidence of injury peaks during evenings, nights, and weekends and is highest among patients from low- to median-income families.[4] With more than 82,000 new patients sustaining severe brain injuries each year,[3] traumatic brain injury is also the leading cause of long-term disability in young Americans.[2] Annual expenditures for direct care of victims of head trauma exceed $4.5 billion.[1]

Common causes of traumatic brain injury are the following[3]:

- Motor vehicle crashes (50%)
- Falls (21%)
- Assaults and interpersonal violence (12%)
- Sports and recreational activities (10%)

PHYSICAL ASSESSMENT OF THE HEAD-INJURED PATIENT

Obtain an initial neurologic evaluation as soon as possible following head injury. Reevaluation should be performed frequently.

Glasgow Coma Scale

The Glasgow Coma Scale (GCS) (see Table 7-8) allows caregivers to perform a brief examination of level of consciousness in a precise, consistent manner that rapidly identifies patient improvement or deterioration. The GCS quantifies a traumatic brain injury patient's eye opening, verbal responses, and motor responses to a set of standardized stimuli. Higher scores are assigned to responses that indicate increasing degrees of arousal.[1]

Eye opening

The examiner determines the minimum stimulus that evokes opening of one or both eyes. Do not score this item if the patient cannot realistically open the eyes because of bandages or lid edema.

4 points: Spontaneous—Eyes open spontaneously without verbal or noxious stimulation.

3 points: To speech—Eyes open with verbal stimuli.

2 points: To pain—Eyes open with various forms of noxious stimuli.

1 point: None—No eye opening occurs with any type of stimulation.

Verbal response

The examiner determines the patient's best verbal response after arousal. Noxious stimuli are used if necessary. Do not score this item if the patient is dysphasic, has interfering oral injuries, or is tracheally intubated.

5 points: Oriented—Patient is aware of person, place, and time.

4 points: Confused—Answers are not appropriate to the question, but the patient demonstrates correct use of language.

3 points: Inappropriate words—Patient uses disorganized, random speech. No sustained conversation occurs.

2 points: Incomprehensible sounds—Patient moans, groans, and mumbles incomprehensibly.

1 point: None—No verbalization occurs, even to noxious stimulation.

Motor response

The examiner determines the patient's best motor response. Do not score this item if the patient is chemically paralyzed.

6 points: Obeys commands—Patient performs simple tasks on command (e.g., sticks out tongue, releases grip, wiggles toes, or holds up a specified number of fingers on request).

5 points: Localizes pain—Patient makes an organized attempt to localize and remove painful stimuli. Patient fails to obey commands but can move toward, and eventually contacts, a noxious cutaneous stimulus. (The stimulus should be maximal and applied in various locations, for example, supraorbital pressure or a trapezius pinch.)

4 points: Withdraws from pain—Patient withdraws the extremity from the source of a painful stimulus.

3 points: Abnormal flexion—(Adducts shoulder, flexes and pronates arm, flexes wrist and makes a fist) occurs spontaneously or in response to noxious stimuli.

2 points: Abnormal extension—(Adducts and internally rotates shoulders, extends forearm, flexes wrist, and makes a fist) occurs spontaneously or in response to noxious stimuli.

1 point: None—No response to noxious stimuli occurs; muscles are flaccid.

The Cranial Nerves

There are twelve pairs of cranial nerves. A description of each follows:

Olfactory (I). This nerve is responsible for olfaction, which is tested by checking the patient's ability to smell. Damage to the olfactory nerve (common in head injury) results in loss of the sense of smell (anosmia) and an ability to discern only sweet and bitter tastes.

Optic (II). The optic nerve controls vision. If the optic nerve is intact, the patient will be able to count fingers, perceive light, or blink when the eyes are threatened.

Oculomotor (III), trochlear (IV), abducens (VI). These nerves control eye movement. In addition, the oculomotor nerve regulates pupil size and accomodation. Check the patient's pupil size, shape, reactivity, and extraocular movements to assess the function of these nerves. The third cranial nerve passes through the tentorium; herniation through the tentorium puts pressure on the third nerve, causing the pupil to dilate and become fixed on the side ipsilateral to the herniation. Even a 1-mm difference in pupil size may indicate significant pressure. However, 12% to 17% of the population normally has slightly unequal pupils (anisocoria).[3]

Trigeminal (V). The trigeminal nerve controls facial sensation and mandible movement. Check for strength of mastication muscles, jaw mobility, and facial sensation.

Facial (VII). The facial nerve controls facial expression as well as taste on the anterior two thirds of the tongue. Have the patient raise the eyebrows, close the eyelids tightly to resistance, show the teeth, smile, frown, and puff out the cheeks.[5]

Acoustic (VIII). The eighth cranial nerve is responsible for hearing and balance. This nerve has two branches: the *vestibular* branch, which controls balance, and the auditory branch, which is responsible for hearing. Test the auditory branch by checking the patient's response to voice or a loud clap. In the unconscious patient, the eighth nerve can be assessed using the ice water caloric test.

Glossopharyngeal (IX), vagus (X). These nerves are evaluated together because they are closely related anatomically and functionally. The glossopharyngeal nerve controls taste on the posterior two thirds of the tongue and sensation in the pharynx and nostrils. The vagus nerve controls the soft palate, pharynx, larynx, the heart, the lungs, and the stomach. Both nerves are tested by checking gag and swallow reflexes and by assessing the patient's ability to discriminate between salty and sweet tastes.

Spinal accessory (XI). The spinal accessory nerve controls movement of the sternocleidomastoid and trapezius muscles. To assess this nerve, have the patient turn the head against resistance or shrug the shoulders. Do not test this nerve until cervical spine injury has been ruled out.

Hypoglossal (XII). The hypoglossal nerve controls tongue movement. Have the patient stick out the tongue. If the tongue is in the midline, the nerve is considered intact.

Pupillary Responses

Test pupillary reflexes using a bright, focused light:

Normal Reactions

- Pupils constrict when exposed directly to light.
- Light shined into one pupil causes the other pupil to constrict as well (consensual response).

Abnormal Reactions

- Fixed, pinpoint pupils indicate pons involvement or the use of opiates.
- A dilated, fixed pupil (unilateral) indicates (early) third cranial nerve involvement.
- Bilateral, fixed pupils indicate severe brainstem injury and possible brain death. (Pupils also may be fixed and dilated in certain reversible conditions and toxic exposures.)
- Ptosis (a drooping eyelid) indicates third cranial nerve impairment.

Reflexes

Corneal (cranial nerves V and VII)

Touch the cornea with a wisp of cotton from a swab or a drop of normal saline solution:
- Normal reaction: Eye blink
- Abnormal reaction: No response

Gag (cranial nerves IX and X)

Stimulate the back of the throat with a swab, tongue depressor, or suction catheter:
- Normal reaction: Intact gag
- Abnormal reaction: Loss of gag reflex

Deep tendon

Test deep tendon reflexes with a rubber reflex hammer. The test is scored from 0 to 4:
0 = Absent
1 = Decreased
2 = Normal
3 = Increased
4 = Hyperactive
- Normal reaction: Normal reflexes, score of 2
- Abnormal reaction: Hypoactivity or absence of reaction indicates cerebellar lesions, peripheral nerve, or anterior horn disease; hyperactivity indicates pyramidal tract lesions or psychogenic disorders. (Certain electrolyte disturbances can also alter deep tendon reflexes. See Chapter 26.)

Babinski

Check for a Babinski reflex by applying brisk cutaneous stimulation to the plantar surface of the foot:
- Normal (negative) reaction: Great toe and other toes flex (curl downward).
- Abnormal (positive) reaction: Great toe extends upward and other toes fan out toward the head. (This reaction is normal in children under age 2.) No response at all also is considered abnormal.

Posturing

Elicit posturing by verbal, tactile, or noxious stimulation:
- Abnormal flexion (Figure 35-1): Arms flex, wrists flex, and legs and feet extend. Abnormal flexion indicates a lesion above the midbrain.
- Abnormal extension (Figure 35-2): Arms extend, wrists flex, and legs and feet extend. Abnormal extension indicates brainstem herniation.

DIAGNOSTIC EXAMINATION TECHNIQUES AND DEVICES USED IN HEAD INJURY

Plain Radiography

Plain films can be obtained easily and rapidly but lack the diagnostic accuracy of computerized radiographic studies and are rarely used.

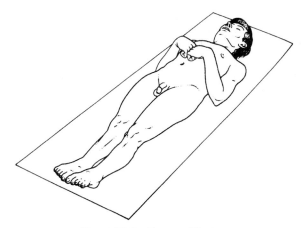

Figure 35-1. Abnormal flexion.

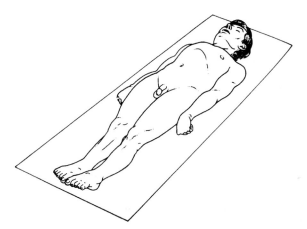

Figure 35-2. Abnormal extension.

Cross-table lateral cervical spine

About 10% of patients with significant head trauma have a concurrent spinal cord injury. Caregivers must ensure that the cervical spine is immobilized and protected until radiographic studies and clinical examination have ruled out injury.

Swimmer's view

If a cross-table lateral film cannot visualize the cervical spine adequately from C1 to T1, a "swimmer's view" should be obtained (Figure 35-3). Alternatively, obtain a computed tomography (CT) scan of the neck.

Skull

In most situations, skull radiographs offer little clinically useful information in terms of treatment intervention. In the head trauma patient, CT is usually the study of choice. However,

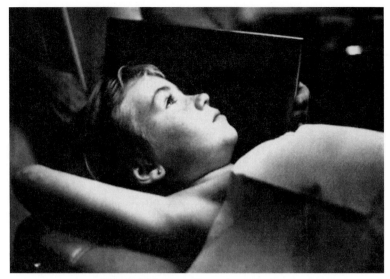

Figure 35-3. X-ray film, swimmer's view.

certain conditions—bony changes around the base of the skull, fractures, the size of the pituitary fossa, and the relationship of the cervical spine to the skull—are better seen on general skull radiographs than on CT.[6]

Computerized Axial Tomography

A noncontrast CT scan (also called a CAT scan [computerized axial tomography] or EMI scan) can detect acute bleeding accurately in about 85% of head trauma patients.[6] This test should be performed quickly in any patient with an altered level of consciousness, hemiparesis, aphasia, or other focal findings.

Magnetic Resonance Imaging

The atoms of the body broadcast signals from which images may be created. These signals can be tracked through nuclear magnetic resonance using ionizing radiation or sound waves. This noninvasive technique is an excellent method for obtaining visual images of soft tissues. Nonetheless, magnetic resonance imaging (MRI) rarely is indicated in the emergent trauma population because it is not feasible when patients are unstable, uncooperative, or otherwise unable to remain still. Magnetic resonance imaging (MRI) also is contraindicated if the patient is dependent on traction, ventilators, pumps, or other equipment that contains ferrous metals. Additionally, persons with ferrous metallic implants (pacemakers, artificial joints, implanted pumps, stents, coils, bullets) are ineligible for MRI scanning. MRI is costly and time consuming. In spite of these drawbacks, MRI can detect early changes in diffuse axonal injuries, can identify even small amounts of subarachnoid blood, and may be the test of choice if a strong suspicion of posterior fossa abnormalities exists.[6]

Angiography

Cerebral and carotid artery angiographic studies occasionally are used to diagnose the presence of traumatic cerebrovascular abnormalities such as tears or thromboses. Although traditional invasive angiography (using injected contrast media) remains the gold standard, noninvasive magnetic resonance angiography and computerized tomographic angiography are gaining in popularity and are becoming more widely available.

Intracranial Pressure Monitoring

Intracranial pressure monitoring is indicated for any patient with severe head injury (GCS ≤ 8) and for those with abnormal CT scan findings such as hematomas, contusions, edema, or severe brain swelling.[7]

Intracranial pressure monitoring systems

Intracranial pressure (ICP) is monitored most commonly using a fiberoptic transducer system inserted through a parenchymal or an intraventricular catheter. Parenchymal catheters are positioned in brain tissue. Intraventricular catheter placement (in one of the lateral ventricles) allows pressure monitoring and cerebral spinal fluid (CSF) drainage. Newer ICP monitoring systems also can measure brain temperature, brain tissue PaO_2, and certain brain chemistries.

Cerebral perfusion pressure

Normal ICP is 0 to 10 mm Hg, but an even more important number to track is cerebral perfusion pressure (CPP). Cerebral perfusion pressure is equal to the mean arterial blood pressure (MAP) minus intracranial pressure (CPP = MAP – ICP).[8] This number indicates the actual pressure of blood perfusing the brain. In head-injured adults, cerebral perfusion pressure should be maintained at greater than 70 mm Hg at all times.[7]

Clinical application

ICP monitoring is useful as a guide to osmotic diuretic administration, patient positioning, hyperventilation, sedation, analgesia, CSF drainage, and surgical intervention. ICP/CPP monitoring improves prognostic accuracy and may improve patient outcome. Nevertheless, familiarity with ICP monitoring and equipment troubleshooting is essential before use.[8]

MANAGEMENT OF PATIENTS WITH SEVERE TRAUMATIC BRAIN INJURIES

Severe head injury is defined as a GCS score of 8 or less after resuscitation. Traditionally, traumatic brain injury has been managed in a variety of ways. In 1995 the Brain Trauma Foundation, the Joint Section on Neurotrauma and Critical Care of the American Association of Neurological Surgeons, and the Congress of Neurological Surgeons developed standardized, evidence-based practice guidelines applicable to the management of all patients with severe traumatic brain injury. In 2003, pediatric guidelines were released as well. These interventions have been shown to minimize the extent and impact of secondary brain injury irrespective of the underlying pathologic condition.[9]

The interventions are as follows:

Airway

- Orally intubate patients with a GCS less than or equal to 8.
- Insert an oral gastric tube to decompress the stomach. Avoid nasogastric tubes.

Breathing

- Maintain PaO_2 greater than 100 mm Hg and oxygen saturation greater than 95%.
- Maintain eucapnia ($PaCO_2$ of 35 to 38 mm Hg).
- Avoid hyperventilation unless signs of herniation are present.
- Initiate end-tidal carbon dioxide monitoring.
- Consider neuromuscular blockade for patients who are difficult to ventilate.

Circulation

- Establish normovolemia. Keep mean arterial pressure 70 to 90 mm Hg.
- Maintain cerebral perfusion pressure greater than 70 mm Hg (an ICP catheter is required to monitor cerebral perfusion pressure).
- Restore volume as needed with isotonic fluids and blood products.
- Insert an indwelling urinary catheter. Maintain an hourly urine output of 0.5 to 1 mL/kg.
- Keep serum osmolality less than 320 mOsm.

Disability

- Perform and document serial neurologic examinations.

Facilitate Diagnosis and Neurosurgical Consultation

- Rapidly obtain appropriate diagnostic studies (e.g., CT scan).
- Monitor ICP in all patients with a GCS score of 8 or lower.
- Facilitate surgical intervention.
- Admit to a neurologic critical care unit or transfer to an appropriate facility.

Reduce Intracranial Pressure

- Provide sedation and analgesia.
- Infuse mannitol (an osmotic diuretic) 0.25 to 1 g/kg in intermittent boluses.
- Maintain the head in a neutral, midline (chin and umbilicus aligned) position.
- Keep the patient's head elevated 30 degrees, unless contraindicated by a spinal injury. (Most patients will benefit from this position, but some do better when the head rests flat.)
- Minimize external stimulation.
- Consider administration of lidocaine and sedation before suctioning.
- Consider neuromuscular blockade for increased ICP unresponsive to treatment.
- Consider ventriculostomy placement for CSF drainage.
- Consider surgical decompression (hematoma evacuation, lobectomy, craniectomy) for increased ICP unresponsive to medical management.

General Care

- Assess for and manage other injuries.
- Immobilize the spine and obtain cervical spine films.
- Perform toxicologic or alcohol screening as indicated.
- Regulate temperature to maintain normothermia.
- Treat seizures. Consider seizure prophylaxis for the first week after injury.
- Do not use IV dextrose infusions.
- Do *not* give dextrose 50% except in the presence of documented hypoglycemia.

- Do *not* give steroids.
- Consider organ donation in patients with a GCS of less than or equal to 4 who remain unresponsive to treatment.

SPECIFIC HEAD INJURY CONDITIONS

Scalp Wounds

Scalp wounds, caused by blunt or penetrating trauma, are the most frequently seen head injuries. Because of its generous vascular supply, the scalp will bleed profusely when skin integrity is breached.[10]

Signs and symptoms

- Direct observation of the wound
- Bleeding (may be profuse)

Diagnosis

- Clinical observation of the wound

Therapeutic interventions

- Apply direct or peripheral pressure to stop the bleeding. Clips or clamps may be used to control major blood loss.
- Palpate the underlying skull for fractures. Do not apply direct pressure over a depressed fracture.
- Immobilize and evaluate the cervical spine.
- Manage hypovolemia. (Small children, in particular, are prone to significant volume loss from large scalp wounds.)
- Cleanse the wound.
- Debride devitalized tissue.
- Sutures, staples, hair ties, or wound glue may be used to close the scalp.
- Keep wound margins moist with an antibiotic ointment to promote healing.
- Apply a sterile dressing or leave the wound open to air.
- Systemic antibiotics are indicated for contaminated wounds such as bites.
- Ensure appropriate tetanus prophylaxis.
- Provide aftercare instructions for wound management and head trauma.

Skull Fractures

Examine the patient's head for bumps, depressions, bruises, lacerations or other defects. The presence of a skull fracture does not necessarily indicate that intracranial injury has occurred. Skull fractures commonly are classified by type and location[1]:

Type

- Simple (linear)
- Depressed

Location

- Cranial vault
- Basilar

Simple (linear, nondisplaced) skull fractures

A simple skull fracture is a linear crack in the surface of the skull; the bone is not displaced, and the fracture itself does not require any special care. Therapeutic intervention involves observation of the patient for potential intracranial injuries. If there are no other obvious findings and a good support system (family or friends) is available, the patient may be discharged home with careful head trauma aftercare instructions.

Depressed skull fractures

A depressed skull fracture involves depression of a segment of the cranium. If the fragment is depressed below the table of the adjacent bone by more than 5 mm, surgical elevation must be performed to identify underlying brain contusions and reduce the incidence of intracranial infection.[1] If the depression overlies one of the sinuses (sagittal or lateral), there may be profuse bleeding. Because of their softer skulls, young children are more prone to depressed skull fractures than are adults.

Signs and symptoms
- Observation and palpation of the deformity
- Bleeding (either external blood loss or hematoma formation)
- Altered level of consciousness

Diagnosis
- Observation and palpation of the deformity
- CT scan

Therapeutic interventions
- Provide airway management with cervical spine protection as needed.
- Control external bleeding.
- Place sterile dressings over open wounds.
- Repair lacerations.
- Consider administration of systemic antibiotics.
- Ensure tetanus prophylaxis if an open wound is present.
- Facilitate surgical intervention to do the following:
  - Elevate the depressed segment.
  - Remove embedded fragments.
  - Debride necrotic brain tissue.
  - Evacuate hematomas.

Basilar skull fractures

A basilar skull fracture describes a fracture location, not a type. Most basilar fractures are linear. Fractures may occur in any of the three fossae of the skull base: anterior, middle, or posterior.

Signs and symptoms

General

- Headache
- Nausea and vomiting
- Altered level of consciousness

Anterior fossa fracture

- *Periorbital ecchymosis (raccoon eyes, Figure 35-4):* Bilateral periorbital ecchymosis occurs as a result of blood seeping through the fracture and pooling in the soft tissues around the eyes.[6] This finding may appear several hours after injury.
- *Rhinorrhea:* Leaking of CSF into the nasal passages

Middle Fossa Fracture

- *Battle sign:* Ecchymosis formation behind the ear in the mastoid region; usually becomes obvious 12 to 24 hours after injury (Figure 35-5)[6]
- *Hemotympanum:* Blood behind the eardrum caused by a fracture near the tympanic membrane

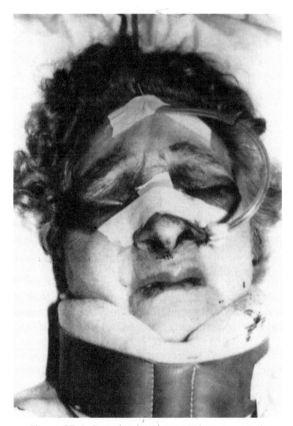

Figure 35-4. Periorbital ecchymosis (raccoon eyes).

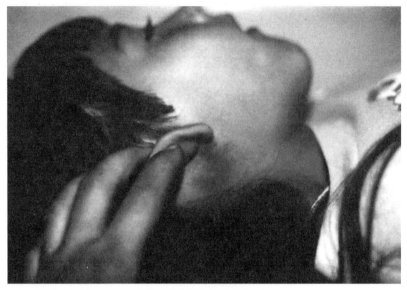

Figure 35-5. Battle sign.

- *Otorrhea:* CSF leakage from the ear canal caused by a crack in the petrous portion of the temporal bone, with an associated meningeal tear. If the tympanic membrane is intact, CSF will exit via the eustachian tube (instead of through the ear canal), and the patient may complain of a salty taste in the mouth (Box 35-1).

Posterior Fossa Fracture

- The posterior fossa is formed of thick, smooth bone that rarely is fractured. However, because of the proximity of the brainstem, even a small amount of bleeding into this fossa can put fatal pressure on the brainstem.
- MRI may provide better visualization of the posterior fossa than CT scan.

Therapeutic interventions

- Immobilize and evaluate the cervical spine.
- Do not attempt to plug CSF leaks; allow them to drain freely.
- Do not put gastric or tracheal tubes through the nose; use the oral route.
- Perform baseline and serial neurologic examinations.
- Quickly obtain a CT scan of the head to identify intracranial injury.
- Consider prophylactic antibiotic administration if a CSF leak is present (controversial).

Box **35-1** **Cerebrospinal Fluid Testing**

> To check for the presence of cerebrospinal fluid (CSF) in blood draining from the nose or ear, perform the halo test:
> Place a drop of the bloody fluid on a paper towel.
> If the substance contains CSF and blood, two distinct rings will form. Blood will pool in the center with a halo of CSF around it.
> If only blood is present, no such halo will form.
> This is also known as the "target" or "ring" sign.[4]

- Provide tetanus prophylaxis.
- Admit the patient for observation.

Diffuse Brain Injuries

Concussion

Concussion results from acceleration, deceleration, or blast injuries that cause brain movement within the bony skull. A brief interruption of the reticular activating system occurs, causing a short period of diminished consciousness. Duration of loss of consciousness is usually less than 5 minutes but by definition may be as long as 6 hours.[2] A concussion is a transient, limited process that usually requires no therapeutic intervention, although patients occasionally require months to recover fully. Concussion often accompanies other, more significant brain injuries.

Signs and symptoms

Common

- Loss or dimming of consciousness
- Flaccid paralysis (while unconscious)
- Dizziness, vertigo
- Headache
- Retrograde (posttraumatic) amnesia
- Nausea, vomiting
- Visual disturbances

Occasional

- Behavior disorders
- Hypertension or hypotension
- Apnea
- Seizures

Diagnosis

- History of a sudden loss of consciousness
- Serial neurologic examinations
- Computed tomography (CT) scan will be normal if concussion is the only injury
- MRI may show subtle changes, but is rarely clinically indicated.

Therapeutic interventions

- Immobilize and evaluate the cervical spine.
- Perform serial observations of level of consciousness.
- Administer nonnarcotic analgesics for headache.
- Admit to the hospital for observation if the following are present:
  - Level of consciousness does not quickly return to normal.
  - Vomiting is severe.
  - The skull is fractured.
- Discharge home if a family member or friend can reliably follow careful verbal and written aftercare instructions.
- Encourage the patient to obtain follow-up neuropsychiatric consultation for any postconcussive syndrome symptoms.

Postconcussive syndrome

Late sequelae of concussion may include the following[2]:
- Headache
- Syncopal episodes
- Nausea
- Loss of coordination
- Memory loss
- Numbness
- Decreased concentration
- Tinnitus (ringing in the ears)
- Decreased organizational skills
- Diplopia (double vision)
- Difficulty handling multiple tasks

Diffuse axonal injury

A diffuse axonal injury (DAI) is the most severe form of diffuse brain injury and differs from concussion in degree, rather than in type of brain injury. Tension, shearing, and compression strains—created by rotational acceleration forces—cause widespread, microscopic axonal disruption throughout the brain. Severity and outcome depend on the extent and degree of structural damage.[2] This injury is almost always associated with high-speed motor vehicle crashes.

Signs and symptoms
- Immediate and prolonged coma lasting greater than 6 hours
- Abnormal posturing
- Confusion, amnesia, and behavioral problems following coma emergence
- Possible persistent vegetative state

Diagnosis
- History of sudden loss of consciousness following head injury
- Serial neurologic examinations
- Initial CT scan: Small hemorrhagic lesions may be visible, or the CT scan may be negative if DAI is the only injury. Subsequent CT scans (days to weeks following injury) will show diffuse cerebral edema, neuronal loss, and brain shrinkage.
- MRI will show lesions more effectively than CT, particularly in the early acute phase, but this study rarely is indicated emergently.

Therapeutic interventions

See Management of Patients With Severe Traumatic Brain Injuries.

Focal Brain Injuries

Contusion

A contusion is a bruising of the surface of the brain.[3] Findings and prognosis vary extensively based on contusion size, number, and location.

Signs and symptoms
- Altered level of consciousness for more than 6 hours
- Nausea, vomiting

- Visual disturbances
- Neurologic dysfunction
- Weakness
- Ataxia
- Hemiparesis
- Confusion
- Speech problems
- Posttraumatic seizures

Diagnosis
- Clinical signs and symptoms
- CT scan
- MRI

Therapeutic interventions
- Immobilize and evaluate the cervical spine.
- Admit to the hospital for observation.
- Administer antiemetics as needed.
- See Management of Patients With Severe Traumatic Brain Injuries.
- Surgical intervention may be performed as indicated.

Intracranial bleeding

The three meningeal layers of the brain (from outer to proximal) are the dura mater, the arachnoid mater, and the pia mater. Bleeding sites in the head are named according to their location with respect to these meningeal layers (Figure 35-6). Bleeding (intracerebral hemorrhage) can occur directly into the brain tissue as well.

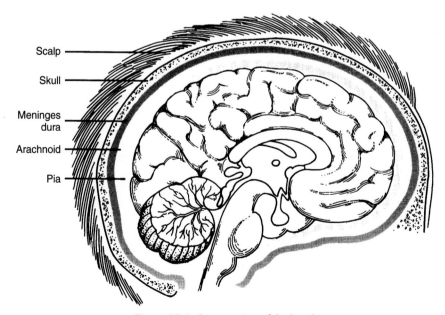

Scalp

Skull

Meninges dura

Arachnoid

Pia

Figure 35-6. Cross section of the head.

Epidural (extradural) hematomas

An epidural hematoma is a collection of blood between the skull and the dura mater. Epidural hematomas occur in only 1% to 2% of all traumatic brain injuries.[4] This bleeding is usually arterial. The most common cause is a rupture or tear of the middle meningeal artery that runs directly beneath the fractured temporal bone.[6] Venous bleeding is rare and may be manageable medically. Deterioration is generally rapid because accumulating arterial blood causes increasing pressure on the brain tissue, resulting in uncal herniation. Mortality is about 8%, the lowest of all intracranial hematomas.[4]

Signs and symptoms
- Agitation and complaint of severe headache *or*
- Sudden loss of consciousness *or*
- Progressive loss of consciousness *or*
- Short period of unconsciousness (concussion) followed by a lucid interval (as the concussion resolves) and then a subsequent deterioration of consciousness caused by accumulating pressure from the bleed
- Contralateral (opposite side) weakness or hemiparesis
- Ipsilateral (same side) dilated pupil
- Bradycardia
- Increased blood pressure
- Abnormal respiratory patterns

Diagnosis
- Emergent CT scan
- Burr holes (rarely done since the advent of ready access to CT scans and neurosurgery)
- Increased ICP

Therapeutic interventions
- See Management of Patients With Severe Traumatic Brain Injuries.
- Emergent surgical evacuation may be required.

Subdural hematoma

A subdural hematoma results from hemorrhage between the dura and the arachnoid mater in the subdural space (Figure 35-7). The cause of acute bleeding is generally severe blunt trauma, such as an acceleration/deceleration incident, in which cortical tissue is lacerated, bridging veins between the cortex and venous sinuses are torn, or a dural tear into a venous sinus occurs.[6] Subdural hematomas are much more common that epidural hematomas.[10] They are reported to occur in 10% to 20% of traumatic brain injuries[4] and have the highest mortality rate (50% to 60%).[2] Bleeding is bilateral in 15% to 20% of cases.[6] Subdural hematomas may develop rapidly (acute) or over a period of days or weeks (subacute or chronic).[3] In alcoholics and the elderly, chronic subdural bleeds may develop atraumatically or following minor injury. The most common cause of subdural hematoma in persons less than 1 year of age is child maltreatment (shaken baby syndrome). If bleeding is not surgically controlled in a timely manner, pressure from an acute expanding subdural hematoma can cause transtentorial herniation and death (Figure 35-8).

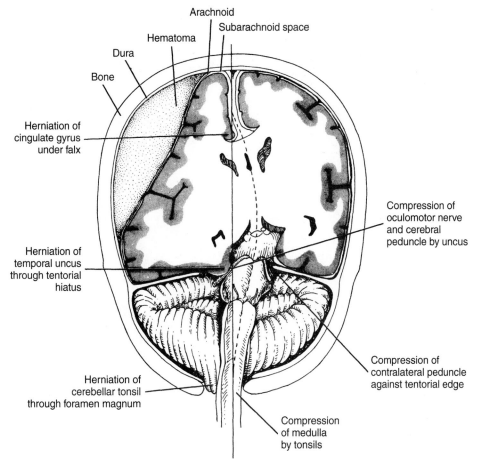

Figure 35-7. Mechanism of injury in subdural hematoma.

Signs and symptoms

Acute subdural hematoma

- Headache
- Sudden or progressive loss of consciousness
- Positive Babinski reflex
- Fixed and dilated pupil(s) (first ipsilateral and then bilateral)
- Contralateral hemiparesis
- Progression from hyperreflexia to abnormal flexion to abnormal extension to flaccidity
- Abnormal respiratory patterns (type depends on the level of involvement)
- Elevated temperature
- Increased ICP
- Nausea and/or vomiting

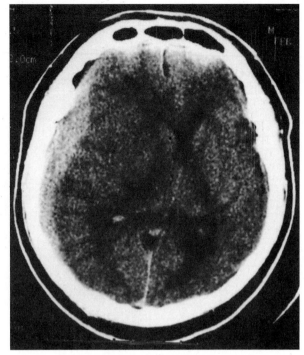

Figure 35-8. Subdural hematoma.

Subacute (24 hours to 2 weeks after injury) and chronic (2 weeks to months after injury) subdural hematoma
- Headache
- Ataxia
- Incontinence
- Increasing confusion/dementia
- Decreasing level of consciousness
- Worsening nausea and/or vomiting

Diagnosis
- Clinical findings
- Emergent CT scan. The old (isodense) blood of chronic subdural hematomas may be difficult to visualize on CT.[6]

Therapeutic interventions

Acute subdural hematoma
- See Management of Patients With Severe Traumatic Brain Injuries.

Subacute and chronic subdural hematoma
- Surgical evacuation of the clot or burr holes with gradual drainage of the hematoma to prevent recurrence[6]

Traumatic subarachnoid hemorrhage

A subarachnoid hemorrhage occurs between the arachnoid membrane and the pia mater (Figure 35-9). This can result from head injury, severe hypertension, or aneurysm or arteriovenous malformation rupture. The most common cause of subarachnoid hemorrhage is trauma.[6] However, the most devastating bleeds are generally aneurysmal. In the trauma population, subarachnoid hemorrhage is usually an incidental finding associated with other, more serious brain injuries.

Signs and symptoms
Signs of meningeal irritation such as the following:
- Headache
- Vomiting
- Photophobia
- Nuchal rigidity

Diagnosis
- Clinical signs and symptoms
- CT scan
- Blood in the CSF

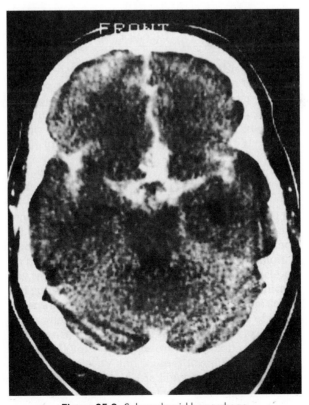

Figure 35-9. Subarachnoid hemorrhage.

Therapeutic interventions

- Because traumatic subarachnoid hemorrhage is rarely the primary brain injury, treatment focuses on associated conditions.
- Bloody CSF, which can lead to the development of obstructive hydrocephalus, may be drained through a ventriculostomy or shunt.

Intracerebral (brain) hemorrhage

Traumatic intracerebral hemorrhage (Figure 35-10) involves bleeding into brain tissue or the ventricles. Bleeding may result from penetrating wounds, diffuse brain injury, or laceration of brain tissue, particularly in the basilar area of the skull where the bony prominences of the skull tend to tear delicate brain tissue during acceleration/deceleration events. In addition to the area of hemorrhage, an even larger surrounding zone of edema and tissue ischemia forms. Overall prognosis is poor.[3]

Signs and symptoms

- Presenting signs and symptoms vary dramatically based on the size, location, and number of hemorrhagic sites and on the presence of concomitant injuries.
- Loss of consciousness

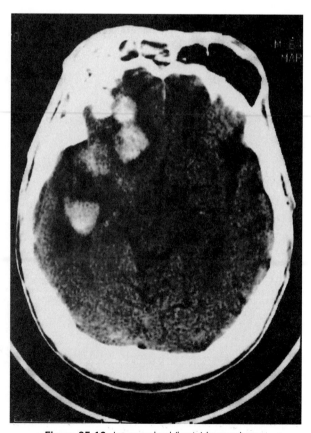

Figure 35-10. Intracerebral (brain) hemorrhage.

- Abnormal size of pupil(s)
- Abnormal respiratory patterns
- Abnormal motor function

Diagnosis
- Clinical observation
- CT scan
- Magnetic resonance imaging

Therapeutic interventions
See Management of Patients With Severe Traumatic Brain Injuries.

Penetrating injuries

Penetrating trauma to the head includes gunshot wounds, stab wounds, missile wounds, and impalement injuries. Because of the high velocity of bullets, bullet wounds have a devastating effect on extensive areas of fragile brain tissue. Objects impaled in the cranial vault commonly travel at much lower velocities. Consequently, they may or may not produce severe injury. The extent of trauma depends on the location of the wound and on the size (caliber) and velocity of the penetrating object.

Diagnosis
- Direct observation
- Skull radiography
- CT scan

Therapeutic interventions
- See Management of Patients With Severe Traumatic Brain Injuries.
- Impaled objects:
  - Do *not* attempt to remove impaled objects.
  - Stabilize impaled objects to prevent movement or dislodgment.
  - Control associated bleeding.
  - Apply a sterile dressing around the impaled object.
- Ensure tetanus prophylaxis.

SPECIAL CONSIDERATIONS

Increased Intracranial Pressure

The brain, along with its CSF and blood, are contained within a rigid skull that allows little space for expansion. When one of these components increases, the others attempt to compensate by reducing their volume, thereby maintaining a constant ICP. Such compensation is effective only for slight or gradual increases in volume. If volume increase is extensive or rapid, ICP will rise. When ICP exceeds mean arterial pressure (MAP), all blood flow to the brain ceases. Therefore management of brain-injured patients focuses heavily on avoiding or moderating increases in ICP and subsequent secondary brain trauma.[7]

Herniation

Herniation occurs whenever portions of the brain extend beyond their normal location and impinge on other areas of brain tissue. Herniation can result from an expanding hematoma, cerebral edema, or a mass (e.g., tumor or impaled object) that propels brain tissue toward the path of least resistance.

Uncal (or lateral, transtentorial) herniation

Uncal transtentorial herniation occurs when a lesion in the temporal lobe region causes the uncus (inner portion of the temporal lobe) to be pushed toward the midline and then over the edge of the tentorium.[2] Pressure builds at the tentorial notch, forcing brain tissue to the contralateral side and through the foramen magnum. This entraps the third (oculomotor) cranial nerve and the posterior cerebral artery between the herniated uncus and the edge of the tentorial notch, producing severe neurologic deficits.[2]

Early signs of transtentorial herniation

- Decreasing level of consciousness
- Ipsilateral pupil dilation
- Cheyne-Stokes respirations
- Contralateral hemiparesis
- Positive Babinski reflex
- Elevated ICP

Late signs of transtentorial herniation

- Unconsciousness
- Bilateral fixed and dilated pupils
- Central neurogenic breathing or other abnormal respiratory patterns
- Flexion or extension posturing
- Elevated ICP unresponsive to therapy
- Bradycardia

Central herniation

When ICP increases and is fairly uniformly distributed throughout the supratentorial region of the brain (e.g., cerebral edema), brain tissue begins to shift. This compresses the ventricles and forces both hemispheres of the cerebrum downward through the tentorial notch.[2]

Early signs of central herniation

- Restlessness progressing to lethargy
- Pupils: Constricted, but equal and reactive
- Cheyne-Stokes breathing with yawns and sighs
- Elevated ICP

Late signs of central herniation

- Loss of consciousness (coma) from reticular activating system impairment
- Pupils: Midpoint or dilated, and fixed
- Decreased or abnormal motor response: posturing or flaccidity
- Cheyne-Stokes, central neurogenic, or ataxic respirations
- Elevated ICP unresponsive to therapy
- Bradycardia

Diagnosis

- Clinical observation

- CT scan
- Elevated ICP

Therapeutic interventions

See Management of Patients with Severe Traumatic Brain Injuries.

Seizures After Head Trauma

Patients often develop seizures following a head trauma incident. These seizures can manifest within minutes, hours, days, or months of the incident. Early posttraumatic seizures result from direct injury to the brain or increased ICP. Late posttraumatic seizures are associated with areas of tissue scarring. Seizure activity greatly increases metabolic demands and reduces respiratory effectiveness, causing PCO_2 to rise and PO_2 to fall. This can significantly aggravate preexisting cerebral hypoxia and edema in patients who are still in the acute phase of injury.[3]

Signs and symptoms

- Loss of consciousness
- Seizure activity
  - Generalized
  - Focal
- Autonomic findings
- Bowel/bladder incontinence

Diagnosis

- Clinical observation
- History of traumatic brain injury
- Electroencephalography (intermittent or continuous) is required to diagnose seizures in the heavily sedated or chemically paralyzed patient.

Therapeutic interventions

- Airway management with spinal immobilization (if there is a history of falling).
- Provide supplemental oxygen.
- Give benzodiazepines to control seizure activity; titrate to effect.
- For ongoing seizure control, administer phenytoin (Dilantin) or fosphenytoin (Cerebyx) intravenously.
- Consider phenobarbital or deep sedation (e.g., propofol) if seizures remain uncontrolled.

References

1. Howard P: Head trauma. In Newberry L, editor: *Sheehy's emergency nursing: principles and practice,* ed 5, St Louis, 2003, Mosby.
2. McQuillan K: Traumatic brain injuries. In Whalen E, et al, editors: *Trauma nursing: from resuscitation through rehabilitation,* ed 3, Philadelphia, 2002, Mosby.
3. Hickey J: Craniocerebral trauma. In Hickey J, editor: *The clinical practice of neurological and neurosurgical nursing,* ed 5, Philadelphia, 2003, Lippincott Williams & Wilkins.
4. Blank-Reid C, Barker E: Neurotrauma: traumatic brain injury. In Barker E, editor: *Neuroscience nursing: a spectrum of care,* St Louis, 2002, Mosby.

5. Degowin R: *Degowin's diagnostic examination,* ed 7, New York, 2000, McGraw-Hill.
6. Schwartz G: Headache and facial pain. In Schwartz G, editor: *Principles and practice of emergency medicine,* ed 4, Philadelphia, 1999, Lippincott Williams & Wilkins.
7. Bullock R, Chesnut R, Clifton G: *Guidelines for the management of severe head injury,* Baltimore, 1995, The Brain Trauma Foundation.
8. Barker E: Intracranial pressure and monitoring. In Barker E, editor: *Neuroscience nursing: a spectrum of care,* ed 2, St Louis, 2002, Mosby.
9. Adelson PD: Critical pathway for the treatment of established intracranial hypertension in pediatric traumatic brain injury, *Pediatr Crit Care Med* 4(3 suppl):S65-S66, 2003.
10. Emergency Nurses' Association: Brain and craniofacial trauma. In Hoyt K, editor: *Trauma nursing core course provider manual,* ed 5, Des Plaines, Ill, 2000, The Association.

36

Spinal Cord and Neck Trauma

John Fazio, MS, RN

An estimated 8000 to 10,000 new cases of spinal cord injury occur (SCI) in the United States each year (28 to 50 per 1 million population). Motor vehicle crashes are the leading cause of SCI, responsible for about 40% of cases. Other causes include acts of violence, falls, and recreational sports. Alcohol, substance abuse, and risk-taking behaviors (e.g., extreme sports) combine to make the incidence of spinal cord injuries highest among males between the ages of 15 and 30 years.[1]

Spinal trauma can involve injury to the cord itself, the vertebral column structures (bones, ligaments, muscles), the spinal nerves, or the vascular supply. Each of these components can be damaged individually or along with other structures. Injury can result from mechanical disruption, ischemia, transection, distraction of neural elements, or an extradural process. Trauma to the cord usually is associated with fracture or dislocation of the vertebral column. However, spinal cord injury without radiographic abnormalities also can occur in the absence of vertebral disruption.[2]

MECHANISMS OF INJURY

Abnormal anatomic movements that can damage the spine and spinal cord include the following[3]:

Hyperextension: The head is bent backward and the neck is forced into an overextended position.

Hyperflexion: The head is bent forward and the neck is forced into an overflexed position.

Lateral bend: The head and neck are bent to one side, beyond normal limits.

Overrotation: The head and neck are turned beyond normal limits.

Distraction: The vertebrae are pulled out of alignment.

Compression: A force is applied from above along with a concurrent force or nongiving surface from below.

Axial loading: A force is transmitted along the length of the spinal column (e.g., blow to the top of the head, fall from a height onto the feet, or fall on the buttocks).

THE SPINAL CORD

The spinal cord is the major pathway for the interconnections between the brain and the rest of the body. The spinal cord regulates body movement, transmits nerve impulses, and controls voluntary and involuntary functions. The spinal cord begins at the base of the skull and terminates near the lower margin of the body of vertebra L1. Organized segmentally, the cord is connected to the periphery by 31 pairs of cervical, thoracic, lumbar, sacral, and coccygeal spinal nerves. These nerves are joined to the cord by an anterior (motor) and posterior (sensory) nerve root. Because of the difference in length between the shorter spinal cord and the longer spinal column, cervical and upper thoracic nerve roots attach at right angles to the spinal cord; lower nerve roots are arranged obliquely, making them more prone to disruption. Lesions of the spinal cord can be complete (no function beyond the point of damage) or incomplete. In an incomplete lesion, some degree of motor or sensory function remains intact below the level of injury.[3,4]

The openings in the vertebrae form a canal through which the spinal cord passes. The vertebrae, spinal ligaments, and the paravertebral muscles protect and support the cord. Similar to the brain, the cord is covered by three meningeal layers: the pia mater, arachnoid mater, and dura mater. Like the brain, the spinal cord also may be concussed, contused, or torn (transected). A concussed cord produces transient functional losses that resolve within minutes or hours of injury. A contused spinal cord involves a structural defect that may or may not result in permanent disability. Spinal cord transection (complete or partial) causes permanent loss of motor and/or sensory function below the level of the lesion. Acute transection above the T6 level causes neurogenic shock (see Chapter 22).[3] Table 36-1 summarizes the clinical presentation with injury at various levels.

The most immediate complication of cervical spine injury is inadequate ventilation. Cervical vertebrae 3, 4, and 5 encase the phrenic nerve. Significant injury at or above this level causes loss of diaphragm control, the primary muscle of respiration. Death quickly results from hypoventilation or apnea. Survival from such injuries is rare. Rapid prehospital care and recent advances in resuscitation have enabled more persons with quadriplegia to survive despite the dramatic nature of this type of injury.[4]

Table 36-1   Spinal Nerves and Injury

Level	Areas Innervated	Effect on Function Following Injury
C2-C4	Diaphragm, neck muscles	Respiratory arrest; flaccid paralysis; quadriplegia
C5-C6	Biceps brachii, deltoids, triceps brachii, wrist extensors	Reduced respiratory effort; total dependence; flaccid paralysis; quadriplegia
C6-T1	Latissimus dorsi, hand muscles	Reduced respiratory effort; near total dependence; splints necessary for forearms to function; quadriplegia
T2-T7	Intercostal muscles	Reduced respiratory effort; partial dependence; paraplegia
T6-L1	Abdominal muscles	Reduced respiratory effort; partial independence; paraplegia
T12-L2	Quadratus lumborum	Partial independence; paraplegia
L1-L5	Leg muscles	
L4-L5	Tibialis anterior	Complete independence; walk with foot braces; mild paraplegia
S1	Bowel and bladder	

From Moore G, Mattox K, Feliciano D, editors: *Trauma manual,* ed 4, New York, 2003, McGraw-Hill.

Complete Cord Lesions

Because the spinal cord is a small and delicate structure, most traumatic events produce complete cord injuries. Literal transections (in which the cord is cut in two) are unusual; functional transection is the norm. The hallmark of a complete lesion is paraplegia or quadriplegia (also called tetraplegia), manifested by an absence of all motor, sensory, and reflex function below the level of injury. Pathological reflexes, such as Hoffmann's sign (abnormal flexion reflex of thumb caused by flicking the distal interphalageal joint of the index, middle, or ring finger) and Babinski reflex (extension of the great toe), may be noted hours to days following the injury. Priapism, loss of the bulbocavernous reflex, and lax rectal tone signal urinary retention and fecal incontinence. Watch for the development of neurogenic shock, characterized by bradycardia (relative or absolute), hypotension, and peripheral vasodilation (Chapter 22).

Incomplete Cord Lesions[2-4]

Central cord syndrome

The leading cause of central cord syndrome is cervical hyperextension. This injury typically occurs in the elderly following a fall. Central cord syndrome produces greater motor weakness in the upper extremities than in the lower. Sensory loss varies, dysesthesias (e.g., burning sensation in hands or arms) are common, and bowel and bladder function is maintained.

Anterior cord syndrome

Hyperflexion is the usual mechanism of injury for anterior cord syndrome. Hyperflexion can cause occlusion of the anterior spinal artery, herniation of the nucleus pulposus (ruptured disk), or transection of the anterior portion of the cord. Depending on the extent of injury, patients experience variable degrees of motor function loss while retaining the senses of position, proprioception, and vibration. Anterior cord syndrome has the worst prognosis of all the cord syndromes.

Brown-Séquard syndrome

Hemisection of the cord in the anterior-posterior plane is known as Brown-Séquard syndrome. This rare injury is associated with penetrating trauma, such as gunshot or stab wounds. The hallmark of this syndrome is ipsilateral (same side) loss of motor function and proprioception, with a contralateral (opposite side) inability to sense pain and temperature. Individuals with Brown-Séquard syndrome have feeling on one half of their body but can only move the side without sensation.

Cauda equina syndrome (root injuries)

Cauda equina syndrome involves injury to the lumbosacral nerve roots. This condition is characterized by varying degrees of motor and sensory loss in the lower limbs. Patients with cauda equina syndrome experience problems with bowel and bladder control.

Posterior cord syndrome

This unusual syndrome may be related to spinal hyperextension but more commonly is associated with certain disease states such as syphilis. Below the level of injury, vibratory and light touch sensations are decreased. Proprioception is affected, and these patients demonstrate a positive Romberg's sign (abnormal swaying when the eyes are closed).

THE VERTEBRAE

Although additional vertebrae are not uncommon, the human body generally has 7 cervical, 12 thoracic, and 5 lumbar vertebrae. In addition, the sacrum is composed of 5 fused vertebrae with 1 or 2 coccygeal segments attached (Figure 36-1). Depending on the mechanism of injury, the vertebrae may be subluxated, dislocated, fractured, or compressed.

Two special types of cervical spine injuries are Jefferson's fractures and hangman's fractures. A Jefferson's ("burst") fracture involves the arch of the first cervical vertebra (atlas, C1). As serious as this injury is, no neurologic deficits may occur initially. A hangman's fracture is a bilateral arch fracture of the second cervical vertebra (axis, C2). Patients with either of these unstable injuries require traction and surgical fixation.[4]

General Assessment

Before performing an assessment, stabilize the patient's spine to ensure minimal movement. Spinal immobilization must be maintained throughout the evaluation process to decrease the potential for further harm.

Assessment measures include the following:
- Check airway patency. Inspect for a hematoma in the posterior pharyngeal area.
- Assess respiratory rate, rhythm, and depth. Can the patient cough? Take a deep breath? Patients without abdominal muscle innervation (injuries at or above T2) may appear to breathe well initially but tend to decompensate over time. Watch for progressive respiratory deterioration.
- Measure blood pressure and pulse. Check skin signs (color, temperature, diaphoresis).
- Evaluate the patient's level of consciousness.
- Identify associated injuries, especially of the head, chest, abdomen, and pelvis.[2]

Signs and Symptoms of Spine and Spinal Cord Injury

Signs and symptoms of spine and spinal cord injury include the following:
- Ecchymosis, edema, pain, tenderness, guarding, crepitus, or step-off deformities over the spine and paraspinal area
- Weakness, paralysis, or any decreased motor activity distal to the level of the injury: Test and document motor strength and level of function (Figure 36-2).
- Numbness, tingling, or loss of sensation (touch, pain, temperature, position): Assess and document the level of sensation. Use a pen to mark the level on the patient's skin (Figure 36-3).
- Sympathetic nervous system disruption (associated with injuries above T6): This injury produces vasodilation below the level of the injury because of an inability to vasoconstrict.
- Hypotension in the absence of hypovolemia (neurogenic shock)
- Priapism
- Loss of the bulbocavernous reflex: Place a finger in the patient's rectum, and then compress the glans or the clitoris or tug on an indwelling urinary (Foley) catheter. Normally, the anal sphincter will contract. If this reflex is initially absent but reappears within 24 hours, it is highly unlikely that significant neurologic function will ever return.
- Loss of rectal tone
- Loss of the "anal wink": The anal sphincter normally contracts when a pinprick is applied in proximity.
- Cough tenderness (coughing induces neck pain)
- Feelings of an "electric shock" or "hot water" running down the patient's back

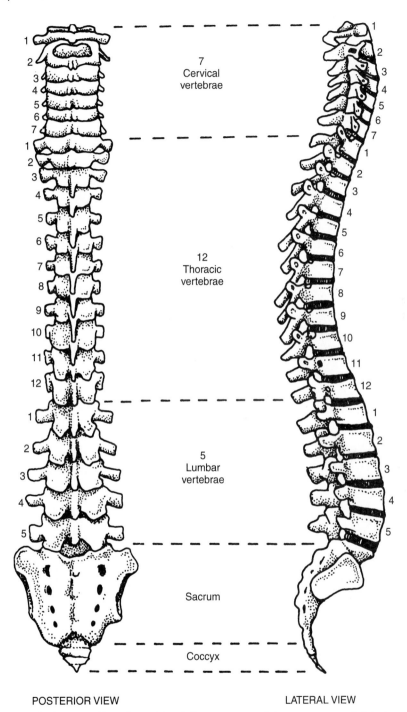

POSTERIOR VIEW   LATERAL VIEW

Figure 36-1. Vertebral column. (From Rosen P et al: *Emergency medicine: concepts and clinical practice,* ed 2, St Louis, 1988, Mosby.)

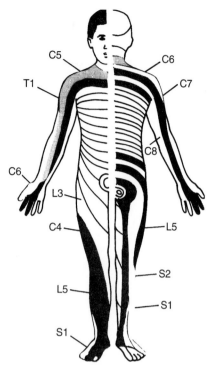

C = Cervical   T = Thoracic   L = Lumbar   S = Sacral

Figure 36-2. Nerve roots and the muscles they innervate.

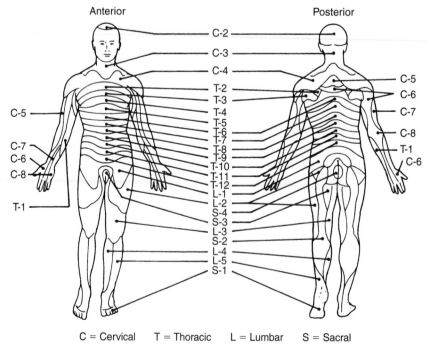

C = Cervical   T = Thoracic   L = Lumbar   S = Sacral

Figure 36-3. Dermatome chart demonstrating sensory and motor levels.

- Mouth breathing: The patient laps air because of loss of diaphragmatic control.
- "Cock Robin" appearance of the head and neck: Cranial rotation, slight flexion, head tilting contralateral to the direction of rotation) can indicate C1-C2 injury.
- Arms folded across the chest or up by the head (the "don't shoot" position) can indicate a C5-C6 injury.

Diagnosis

Diagnosis of spine and spinal cord injuries is made through careful clinical assessment and imaging studies. To clear the cervical spine, a minimum of three radiographic views are necessary: cross-table lateral, anteroposterior, and odontoid. Good visualization of all seven cervical vertebrae and T1 is essential. The arms, particularly those of muscular patients, may need to be pulled downward while shooting the film. This causes the shoulders to drop and facilitates visualization of the lower cervical spine and T1. Ensure adequate neck immobilization during this procedure. If T1 cannot be visualized on a lateral view, obtain a swimmer's view (shot upwards, through the axilla).[3]

If a high probability of injury exists, obtain a computed tomography scan of the neck or flexion-extension views to check for soft tissue injuries that can compromise vertebral column alignment. Even when cervical spine radiographs are read as negative, it is important for the patient who has a concomitant head injury or is intoxicated to remain in a collar until flexion/extension views can be done or the patient can be cleared clinically.

Plain radiographs can identify subluxations, fractures, dislocations, and narrowing of the paravertebral spaces. Assess the films for the following:
- Anterior-posterior column alignment
- Anterior-posterior diameter of the spinal canal
- Presence of bone fragments or bony displacement
- Presence of linear fractures or comminuted fractures
- Soft tissue edema at or below C3 (may indicate the presence of a retropharyngeal hematoma)
- Vertebral inclination: An angle that is greater than 11 degrees (or exceeds one fourth of the vertebral body) is considered unstable.

Obtain radiographic images of the thoracic and lumbar spinal regions in unconscious patients and those with clinical findings suggestive of injury. Magnetic resonance imaging is particularly suited for viewing compression injuries, extradural spinal hematomas, tumors, abscesses, spinal cord hemorrhage, contusions, and edema.[2]

Measures to Prevent Further Injuries

Observe the following measures to prevent further spinal injuries:
- Align and stabilize the cervical, thoracic, and lumbar spine.
- Ensure that sufficient personnel are available whenever the patient must be moved. Carefully maintain alignment during repositioning.

Therapeutic Interventions

Therapeutic interventions for spinal injury include the following:
- Support the patient's airway, breathing, and circulation while stabilizing the cervical, thoracic, and lumbar spine.
- Check for airway patency. The airway is always at risk because of edema associated with cervical cord injuries. Ninety-six percent of persons with neck fractures can be safely intubated orally.[5]

- Provide supplemental oxygen, monitor saturation, and assist ventilation as needed.
- Initiate two large-bore intravenous lines, and infuse isotonic crystalloids. Once the patient is hemodynamically stable, run fluids at a keep-open rate.
- Monitor circulation closely and provide ongoing assessment for neurogenic shock.
- Insert an indwelling urinary catheter and monitor hourly output.
- Place an orogastric or nasogastric tube.
- Facilitate early neurosurgical consultation.
- Consider placement of tongs or a halo ring and cervical traction (Figure 36-4). Ensure that traction weights hang freely at all times.
- Consider surgical intervention.
- Consider implementing a high-dose steroid infusion to minimize the secondary effects of acute spinal cord injury (Table 36-2). Despite its popularity, this practice has little scientific support and is associated with serious complications. Steroids are *not* indicated in penetrating spinal trauma.[6]
- Pad pressure points and remove patients from backboards as soon as possible.
- Administer tetanus prophylaxis and antibiotics as appropriate.
- Admit or transfer the patient to a facility with neurosurgical and rehabilitation capabilities.
- Provide hopeful but honest information and psychological support.

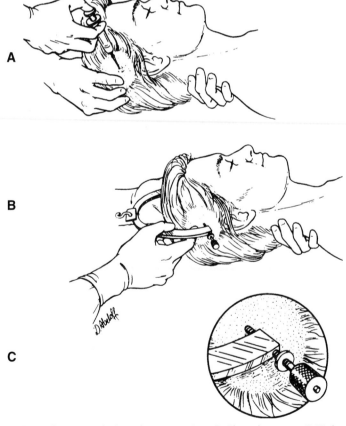

Figure 36-4. Tong placement. **A,** Anesthetize pin sites. **B,** Place the tongs. **C,** Tighten the pins.

Table 36-2 Methylprednisolone Administration for Spinal Cord Injury

Time from Injury	Bolus Dose (Over 15 Min)*	Infusion Dose (Start 45 Min After the Bolus)
<3 hours	30 mg/kg	5.4 mg/kg/hr for 23 hours
3-8 hours	30 mg/kg	5.4 mg/kg/hr for 47 hours

From Moore G, Mattox K, Feliciano D, editors: *Trauma manual*, ed 4, New York, 2003, McGraw-Hill.
*Followed by 45-minute infusion of normal saline solution.

Cervical Spine Stabilization

Spinal stabilization should be considered simultaneously with airway management as the first priority of care in any patient whose mechanism of injury suggests the possibility of cervical trauma. The responsibility to "do no further harm" cannot be overemphasized. Extreme caution and a high index of suspicion are required when handling all trauma patients until spinal injury has been ruled out.[4]

Equipment used to stabilize the neck varies with the situation, and many commercial devices are available (Figure 36-5). However, in the absence of specialized equipment, everyday materials are adequate for achieving stabilization.

Equipment list

- Semirigid cervical collar
- Kendrick extrication device
- Short spine board with straps
- Long spine board with straps
- Lightweight head supports
- Blankets and towels for padding
- 2-inch wide adhesive tape

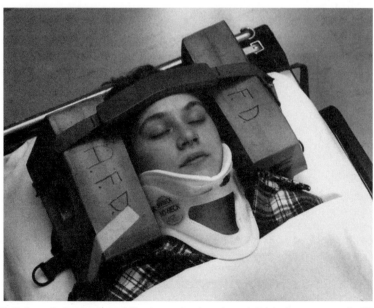

Figure 36-5. Full cervical spine immobilization, using long board, C-blocks, straps, and stiff-neck collar.

Procedure

1. To alleviate anxiety, reduce movement, and elicit cooperation, talk to the patient and keep them informed of each step.
2. Assess the airway. Open the airway with a jaw-thrust or chin-lift maneuver; do not hyperextend the neck. If tracheal intubation is necessary but not possible without hyperextension, consider nasotracheal or digital intubation or cricothyrotomy.
3. Gently apply manual immobilization by placing the hands on either side of the patient's head, stabilizing the head and neck in a neutral, vertical position. In children this is defined as the "sniffing" position. Do not cover the ears of a conscious patient.
4. Once stabilization is applied, it must be maintained manually until immobilization devices are in place.
5. Evaluate the cervical spine. Observe and palpate each spinous process; note deformity, crepitus, pain, and instability.
6. Check motor and sensory status.
7. Gently remove the patient's clothing (if possible). At a minimum, remove any sharp or bulky items that may cause soft tissue pressure injury (e.g., keys in the pocket). Liberally pad bony prominences.
8. Use padding or commercial devices to obtain neutral spinal alignment:
   - *Adults:* Pad behind the head and neck, making a 1- to 1½-inch thick towel "pillow."
   - *Small children:* Pad under the shoulders and upper body (1½ to 2 inches) to overcome the large occiput.
9. Remove earrings and necklaces that will interfere with neck radiographs.
10. Place an appropriately sized semirigid cervical collar.
11. Have team members gently logroll the patient onto a long board while the team leader continues manual head and neck stabilization.
12. Secure the patient to the board with the following:
    - Straps across the patient's chest, hip, and legs. Snugly attach the straps to the board but do not restrict chest wall or abdominal excursion.
    - Secure the patient's head to the spine board using lightweight head blocks and 2-inch wide tape applied just above the eyebrows; this tape must be firmly secured to both sides of the spine board.
13. When the patient is fully immobilized, release manual stabilization.
14. Reassess the patient's motor and sensory status.
15. Be prepared to turn the entire board if the patient begins to vomit; have suction readily available.
16. If a short spine board or other extrication device was used, place the patient on a long board or scoop stretcher before further movement.[5]
17. Remove the spine board as soon as possible to reduce the risk of skin breakdown.

Helmet Removal

Many styles of helmets are available to provide head protection for a variety of sports, including motorcycling, bicycling, kayaking, ice hockey, football, auto racing, skating, rock climbing, and horseback riding. Modern helmets are fit tightly so careful removal is imperative to prevent further cervical spine damage. Helmets should be removed initially only if they compromise airway management. Otherwise, leave helmets in place until the spine has been assessed and measures can be taken to ensure safe removal. Figure 36-6 shows the steps involved in this procedure. Cast saws can be used for helmet removal as well.

A new product called Hats Off (Motorcycle UK Limited, Kent, England) is a simple and ingenious means of helmet removal. It involves an inflatable bladder that can be placed in

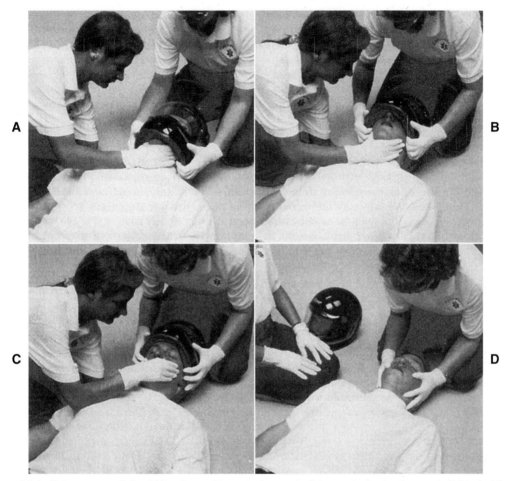

Figure 36-6. Helmet removal should be done with manual control of the cervical spine by one individual while the other person spreads the helmet laterally and removes it. **A,** Rescuer 1 immobilizes the helmet and head in an in-line position. Rescuer 2 grasps the patient's mandible by placing the thumb at the angle of the mandible on one side and two fingers at the angle on the other side. Rescuer 2 places the other hand under the neck at the base of the skull, producing in-line immobilization of the patient's head. **B,** Rescuer 1 carefully spreads the sides of the helmet away from the patient's head and ears. **C,** The helmet then is rotated toward the rescuer to clear the nose and removed from the patient's head in a straight line. **D,** After removal of the helmet, Rescuer 1 applies in-line immobilization. A rigid cervical collar is applied. (From Sanders MJ: *Mosby's paramedic textbook,* St Louis, 1994, Mosby.)

the crown of any standard sports helmet. When emergency removal is required, the bladder is inflated by hand and the helmet slowly lifts itself off the top of the head. The Hats Off device is gaining in popularity. Look for a Hats Off sticker on a helmet before pulling or cutting. Available in Europe, but not yet in the United States, is the Hats Off 1st Response Kit, which consists of an insertion tool that allows an airbag to be slid inside to the top of a helmet not previously equipped with the Hats Off device.

SOFT TISSUE INJURIES OF THE NECK

Fractured Larynx

The most common cause of a fractured larynx is blunt trauma resulting from sudden deceleration against a steering wheel, an assault (e.g., punch or karate chop), or a "clothesline" injury in which the patient's neck hits a rope or wire stretched between two fixed points.[7]

Signs and symptoms

- Hoarse voice or any vocal changes
- Cough with hemoptysis
- Difficulty breathing, respiratory distress
- Subcutaneous emphysema of the neck, face, or upper chest

Diagnosis

- History and clinical observation
- Ecchymosis or abrasions on the anterior neck
- Progressive inspiratory stridor
- Displacement of neck landmarks

Therapeutic interventions

- High-flow oxygen therapy
- Position of comfort
- Careful tracheal intubation (may require bronchoscopy)
- Emergency cricothyrotomy or tracheostomy (See Chapter 19.)
- Administration of broad-spectrum antibiotics

Penetrating Neck Wounds

Penetrating objects, such as bullets and knife blades, can cause significant damage to the important tissues of the neck. The extent of injury depends on the type of penetrating object, the force of the object, and the location and angle of penetration. For clinical purposes, the neck is divided into three anatomic zones[1,7]:

Zone 1: Extends from the thoracic inlet to the level of the cricoid cartilage. Structures at greatest risk are the following:

- Great vessels (subclavian, brachiocephalic, and jugular veins; carotid arteries; aortic arch)
- Trachea
- Esophagus
- Upper lung tissue
- Cervical spine, cervical cord, and nerve roots

Zone 2: Extends from the cricoid cartilage to the angle of the mandible. Structures at greatest risk are the following:

- Vessels: Carotid and vertebral arteries; jugular veins
- Pharynx, larynx
- Trachea
- Esophagus
- Cervical spine and cervical cord

Zone 3: Extends from the angle of the mandible to the base of the skull. Structures at greatest risk are the following:

- Salivary and parotid glands
- Carotid arteries and jugular veins

- Trachea
- Esophagus
- Cervical spine
- Cranial nerves IX to XII

Signs and symptoms

- Obvious penetrating wounds
- Airway obstruction or stridor
- Hemorrhage
- Signs of hypovolemia, hemothorax, or shock
- Presence of a large or expanding hematoma
- Subcutaneous air

Diagnosis

- Clinical observation
- Arteriography
- Exploratory surgery

Therapeutic interventions

- Airway management: Consider surgical airway interventions.
- Breathing: Ensure adequate oxygenation.
- Circulation: Control bleeding and replace volume.
- Prepare patient for surgery if indicated.[7]

References

1. Moore E, Mattox K, Feliciano D, editors: *Trauma manual,* ed 4, New York, 2003, McGraw-Hill.
2. Marion D, Przybylski G: Injury to the vertebrae and spinal cord. In Mattox K, Feliciano D, Moore E, editors: *Trauma,* ed 4, New York, 2000, McGraw-Hill.
3. Hockberger R, Kirshenbaum K: Spine. In Marx J, Hockenberger R, Walls R, editors: *Rosen's emergency medicine: concepts and clinical practice,* ed 5, St Louis, 2002, Mosby.
4. Russo-McCourt T: Spinal cord injuries. In McQuillan K et al, editors: *Trauma nursing: from resuscitation through rehabilitation,* ed 3, Philadelphia, 2002, WB Saunders.
5. Emergency Nurses Association: *Trauma nursing core course,* ed 5, Des Plaines, Ill, 2000, The Association.
6. Walker J, Criddle LM: Methylprednisolone in acute spinal cord injury: fact or fantasy? *J Emerg Nurs* 27(4):401-403, 2001.
7. Newton K: Neck. In Marx J, Hockenberger R, Walls R, editors: *Rosen's emergency medicine: concepts and clinical practice,* ed 5, St Louis, 2002, Mosby.

37

Chest Trauma

Christopher Schmidt, APRN, BC, MSN, CEN, ENP, CDR, NC, USN

In the United States, thoracic injuries are the second most common cause of trauma mortality, accounting for about 16,000 lives lost each year, or 25% of all trauma deaths.[1-3] Many potentially lethal thoracic conditions can be reversed if assessment and lifesaving interventions are performed in a timely manner.

THORACIC CAVITY ANATOMY

The thoracic cavity extends from the first rib, located beneath the clavicles, to the diaphragm (Figure 37-1). The diaphragm is a constantly moving structure, the location of which varies from the fourth intercostal space (full exhalation) to the tenth (deep inhalation) throughout the respiratory cycle (Figure 37-2). Therefore injuries sustained in this area must always be considered potential insults to the chest *and* the abdominal cavity. Penetrating trauma just below the right nipple easily can involve the lungs, the liver, or both structures.

The thoracic cavity contains the lower airway (the right and left main stem bronchi and the lungs), and heart, great vessels, and the esophagus. Twelve pairs of ribs enclose the chest cavity, providing support and organ protection. Breathing is a mechanical process that relies on thoracic cavity expansion and relaxation. Normally, the ribs and the diaphragm move in harmony, but traumatic injury inhibits this process.

When inspiration occurs, the diaphragm drops down and the intercostal muscles pull the ribs upward, increasing negative pressure within the thoracic cavity. Accessory muscles of respiration, including abdominal wall, pectoralis, and sternocleidomastoid muscles, assist this process. The lungs respond to the negative pressure by filling with air. Because of their elasticity, any loss of negative pressure results in lung collapse.

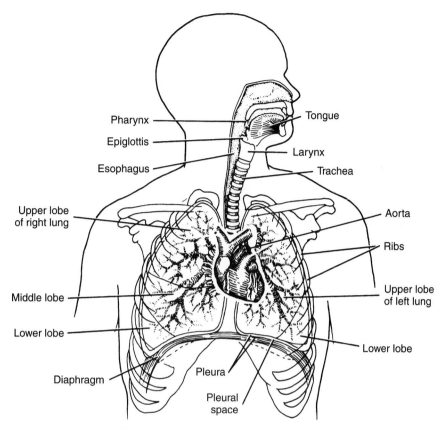

Figure 37-1. Anatomy of the thoracic cavity.

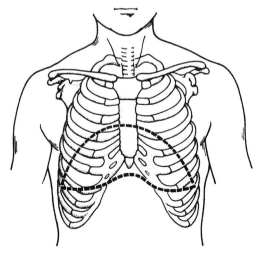

Figure 37-2. Level of diaphragm on inspiration (*upper dashed line*) and expiration (*lower dashed line*).

The phrenic nerve innervates the diaphragm to initiate breathing. Irritation of this nerve by blood or other substances can cause hiccups or referred pain to the shoulder (Kehr's sign). Intercostal veins, arteries, and nerves run along the inferior border of each rib. These structures must be carefully avoided during procedures such as needle thoracostomy or chest tube insertion. The angle of Louis on the sternum is the most constant landmark on the anterior chest wall, where it commonly serves as a reference point. The second intercostal space, a site used for needle thoracostomy, is located just below and lateral to the angle of Louis. Because hypoxia, compromised circulation, and pulmonary or vascular obstruction are frequent complications of thoracic trauma, all chest injuries must be assumed to be serious until proved otherwise.[2]

PRIORITIES IN THE TREATMENT OF PATIENTS WITH CHEST INJURIES

Regardless of the mechanism of injury, priorities in the management of patients with thoracic trauma remain the same. The following sections discuss assessment and interventions to consider. Treatment is based on the actual problems identified.[4]

Airway
Assessment

Is the airway patent or compromised?

Intervention

Clear obstructions: Vomitus, teeth, tongue blood, secretions, foreign bodies.

Breathing
Assessment

- Respiratory effort: Rate, depth, breathing patterns, use of accessory muscles
- Paradoxical or asymmetric chest movement *(flail chest)*
- Wounds *(open pneumothorax)*
- Hyperexpansion *(tension pneumothorax)*
- Subcutaneous air *(tracheal or bronchial tears)*
- Breath sounds
  - Unequal *(endotracheal tube misplacement, pneumothorax, hemothorax, lung injury, foreign body obstruction)*
  - Adventitious: Wheezing, stridor, crackles
  - Bowel sounds in the chest *(ruptured diaphragm)*
- Oxygen saturation: Pulse oximetry (oxygen saturation [SpO_2])
- Ventilation: End-tidal carbon dioxide monitoring

Interventions

- Administer supplemental oxygen via a nonrebreather mask or tracheal tube.
- Assist ventilations: Bag-valve-mask, mechanical ventilator.
- Cover open wounds *(open pneumothorax)*.
- Perform needle thoracostomy *(tension pneumothorax)*.
- Insert chest tubes *(pneumothorax, hemothorax)*.
- Draw arterial blood gas samples.

Circulation

Assessment

- Pulses: Present, absent, weak, strong, fast, slow
- Skin signs: Color, temperature, moisture, capillary refill
- Cardiac rhythm
- Heart sounds: Clear, muffled, murmur, S_3 or S_4
- Blood pressure and pulses in both upper extremities *(aortic disruption)*

Interventions

- Insert two (or more) large-bore (14- to 16-gauge) intravenous (IV) catheters.
- Infuse warmed, isotonic crystalloid solutions: lactated Ringer's solution or normal saline.
- Transfuse blood components as needed: Packed red blood cells, other blood products, autotransfused chest blood.
- Perform pericardiocentesis *(cardiac tamponade)*.
- Perform closed chest compressions *(traumatic arrest)*.
- Perform emergency thoracotomy and internal cardiac compressions *(penetrating traumatic arrest)*.

Disability

Assessment

- Level of consciousness
- Complaints: Pain, dyspnea, numbness
- Obvious neck trauma
- Gross motor or sensory function

Interventions

- Initiate or maintain spinal immobilization.
- Obtain spinal radiographs.

Miscellaneous

Assessment

- Mechanism of injury and prehospital events
- Medical history
- Chest entrance or exit wounds
- Major injuries to other body sites

Interventions

- Obtain chest radiographs.
- Perform a 12-lead electrocardiogram.
- Insert an indwelling urinary (Foley) catheter and monitor output.
- Place an orogastric or nasogastric tube for stomach decompression.
- Facilitate surgical intervention.

BONY THORAX FRACTURES

Rib fractures are the most prevalent thoracic injuries. Fractures commonly result from a direct blow to the chest but also can be caused by penetrating objects such as a fence post or a bullet. Iatrogenic rib fractures occur as a consequence of chest compression or abdominal thrusts. Ribs generally fracture at angle junctures, their weakest point. The most frequently fractured ribs are ribs three through nine.[3] Always consider the possibility of serious injury to underlying structures if a first rib fracture, multiple rib fractures, or a flail chest is present. Trauma to the first rib routinely is associated with clavicular fractures and, occasionally, disruption of the scapula. Fractures of the first, second, and third ribs carry a 15% to 30% mortality, given their proximity to the subclavian vessels, aorta, and tracheobronchial tree. Blunt force on the lower ribs can cause them to penetrate vascular abdominal organs, producing serious bleeding. Injured right lower ribs may impale the liver, whereas those on the left potentially can rupture the spleen.[5]

Uncomplicated Rib Fractures

Signs and symptoms

- Pain that increases with inspiration (bone spicules irritate the parietal pleura)
- Point tenderness (the patient can identify the site of pain precisely)
- Splinting of the chest muscles (to reduce chest wall movement)
- Ecchymosis or abrasions at the site of injury
- A palpable deformity (step-off defect) if the fracture is displaced
- Bony crepitus (palpable bone motion) at the fracture site
- Subcutaneous emphysema (if there is associated lung or tracheobronchial injury)

Diagnostic aids

- Chest radiographs
- Rib series radiographs
- Computed tomography (CT) scan of the chest to evaluate soft tissue injuries

Therapeutic interventions

Simple Fractures

- Rest
- Intermittently applied ice for the first 24 hours to decrease swelling and then heat to promote blood flow and healing
- Systemic analgesics or regional anesthesia

Displaced Fractures or Any Rib Fractures in the Elderly

- Hospital admission
- Regional anesthesia for severe pain
- Local infiltration
- Intercostal nerve blocks
- Epidural analgesia
- Incentive spirometry
- Close monitoring of respiratory status

Age/developmental considerations

- Elderly patients and those with preexisting comorbidities may lack the pulmonary reserves necessary to compensate when the ribs are fractured. This population requires careful monitoring for signs of respiratory deterioration.[6]
- The ribs of small children are cartilaginous, generally bending instead of cracking. Consider maltreatment in any child who has an unexplained rib fracture or multiple fractures.

Complications

- Atelectasis and pneumonia caused by pain-induced hypoventilation
- Lacerated organs or great vessels, internal hemorrhage
- Pneumothorax, hemothorax[5]

Patient education and discharge instructions

- Pain will occur with breathing, coughing, and laughing. Perform deep breathing exercises or incentive spirometry to prevent atelectasis and pneumonia.
- Use narcotic analgesics as prescribed.
- Healing normally occurs in 3 to 6 weeks.
- Avoid rib binders, belts, or other devices that may restrict respiratory effort and promote atelectasis.

Flail Chest

Flail chest, a life-threatening condition, is present in 30% of patients with extensive thoracic trauma. A flail occurs when two or more adjacent ribs are fractured in two or more places, or when the sternum is detached. The flail segment loses continuity with the remainder of the chest wall and responds to intrathoracic pressure changes in a paradoxical manner. Paradoxical motion refers to movement of the flail segment in the direction opposite that of the intact chest wall. Instead of expanding outward with the rest of the thorax, the flail segment is drawn inward on inspiration (Figure 37-3, *A*). Conversely, as negative pressure decreases with exhalation, the flail segment is pushed outward (Figure 37-3, *B*). Extreme force is required to create a flail chest. Therefore presence of this injury indicates a high potential for serious associated trauma.

Signs and symptoms

- Pain, bony crepitus
- Respiratory distress (dyspnea, tachypnea, respiratory failure)
- Subcutaneous air (associated pulmonary or tracheobronchial injuries are common)
- Hemothorax, pneumothorax
- Paradoxical motion of the chest wall
  - Because of muscle spasms and chest wall splinting, paradoxical motion is not always evident.
  - To visualize paradoxical motion best, crouch down at the foot of the patient's gurney and observe both sides of the chest simultaneously.

Diagnostic aids

- Clinical observation
- Chest radiographs

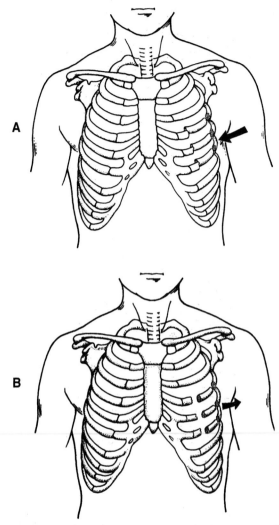

Figure 37-3. Flail chest. **A,** When the diaphragm is drawn down and respiratory effort is made, the flail segment pulls inward. **B,** When the diaphragm rises and exhalation occurs, the flail segment moves outward.

- Chest CT scan
- Continuous SpO_2 and end-tidal carbon dioxide monitoring
- Arterial blood gases

Therapeutic interventions

- Most patients with a flail chest will require the following:
  - Supplemental oxygen
  - Tracheal intubation
  - Mechanical ventilation with positive end-expiratory pressure to splint the flail from the inside[3]

- Avoid outmoded treatments such as placing sandbags on the flail segment.
- Insert chest tubes for pneumothorax or hemothorax.
- Manage pain: Systemically effective narcotics, intercostal nerve blocks, epidural analgesia.
- Once hypovolemia is corrected, administer IV crystalloids judiciously (because of underlying pulmonary contusions).
- Consider arterial catheter placement for frequent arterial blood gases.
- Consider pulmonary artery catheter insertion to guide fluid replacement.
- Admit to an intensive care unit for close observation and pulmonary management.
- Facilitate surgical intervention: Internal fixation of the flail segment sometimes is indicated.

Complications

- Hypoxia, pulmonary contusions, atelectasis, pneumonia

Sternal Fractures

It takes a great deal of force to fracture the sternum. A fractured sternum is rarely an isolated injury, so patients should be assessed carefully for concomitant thoracic or multisystem trauma. The most common cause of fractured sternum is high-speed impact against a steering wheel. Sternal fractures also may be a complication of cardiopulmonary resuscitation, particularly in the elderly. A totally detached sternum is considered a flail segment and is treated accordingly.

Signs and symptoms

- Chest pain, especially on inspiration
- Bruising, soft tissue swelling
- Dysrhythmias, electrocardiographic changes
  - Premature ventricular contractions, atrial fibrillation, right bundle branch block, and ST segment elevation

Diagnostic aids

- Palpation of the fracture
- Chest radiographs
- Continuous cardiac monitoring; 12-lead electrocardiogram
- CT scan of the chest

Therapeutic interventions

- Close observation and monitoring
- Analgesia
- Dysrhythmia management
- Possible surgery for sternal fixation
- Hospital admission

Complications

- Blunt cardiac injury
- Mediastinal hematoma[5]

Clavicular Fractures

The clavicles are frequently and easily fractured. Clavicular fractures can result from almost any blunt force and are typically seen in athletic injuries from a lateral blow or a fall on an outstretched hand. These fractures are the most common of all pediatric fractures and generally are not considered serious. Clavicular fractures are usually closed injuries and are categorized as type I to III based on the location of the break: distal, middle, or medial. Medial fractures (near the sternum) are less common and often are associated with other trauma (e.g., first rib fractures, sternal fractures, and great vessel injuries).[6]

Signs and symptoms

- Pain (especially on palpation)
- Palpable step-off defect

Diagnostic aids

- Carefully assess pulses in the arm on the side of injury to identify possible subclavian or internal jugular vessel injuries.
- Check neurologic status in the arm on the side of injury. Damage to the brachial plexus can occur.
- Obtain a chest radiograph.
- Consider an angiogram to rule out vascular injury.

Therapeutic interventions

- Ice packs to the affected area
- Figure-of-eight shoulder splint (controversial)
- Analgesia: Nonsteroidal antiinflammatory drugs or narcotics
- Closed reduction of displaced fractures
- Open reduction of open fractures

Complications

- Extensive bleeding if the fractured bone lacerates the subclavian artery or vein
- Nerve injury

Patient education and discharge instructions

- Pain may persist for days following the fracture; use ice, rest, splint, and analgesics.
- Contact an orthopedist for follow-up.

PNEUMOTHORAX AND HEMOTHORAX

Simple (Closed) Pneumothorax

A simple, or closed, pneumothorax occurs when a leak in the lungs, bronchi, or lower trachea allows air to enter the pleural space (Figure 37-4). This causes a loss of negative pressure and partial or total lung collapse. In the trauma patient, closed pneumothorax is associated with puncture of the lung by a rib or compression of the chest against a closed glottis (similar to blowing up and popping a paper bag). Less commonly, pneumothorax is a consequence of

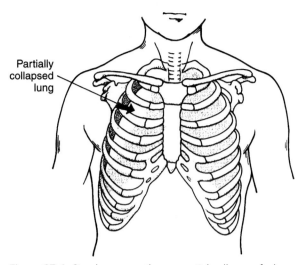

Figure 37-4. Simple pneumothorax; partial collapse of a lung.

barotrauma following a high-energy shock wave or explosion.[5,7-8] Atraumatic spontaneous pneumothoraces are produced by a ruptured bleb or cyst (see Chapter 20).

Signs and symptoms

- History of blunt chest trauma or blast injury
- Sudden onset of sharp, pleuritic chest pain
- Diminished breath sounds on the affected side
- Dyspnea
- Tachypnea
- Asymmetric chest wall movement
- Hamman's sign (a crunching sound heard with each heartbeat, caused by accumulation of air in the mediastinum

Diagnostic aids

- Clinical observation
- Chest radiographs (loss of pulmonary vascular markings on the affected side)

Therapeutic interventions

- Closely observe and monitor the patient.
- Provide oxygen as needed to maintain saturation.
- Keep the patient in the semi-Fowler position.
- Very small pneumothoraces, without ventilatory compromise, may not require chest tube insertion. However, unlike patients with a spontaneous pneumothorax, trauma patients are at risk for associated injuries and generally require at least short-term monitoring and supplemental oxygen.
- Small pneumothorax: Consider needle thoracostomy (placement of a large-bore needle through the anterior chest wall in the second intercostal space at the midclavicular line) with attachment to a one-way (flutter, Heimlich) valve (Box 37-1).

Box **37-1** **Needle Thoracostomy Procedure**

A severely symptomatic patient warrants immediate therapeutic intervention. Do not wait for a chest radiograph to confirm tension pneumothorax.

Gather the equipment:

14- to 16-gauge intravenous catheter

30- to 60-mL syringe with a Luer-Lok tip

Three-way stopcock (optional)

Skin preparation solution (e.g., povidone-iodine)

Identify the correct insertion site (second intercostal space, midclavicular line, on the affected side).

Prepare the skin.

Attach the catheter to the syringe (this procedure also can be performed without a syringe attached).

Insert the catheter at a 90-degree angle into the second intercostal space in the midclavicular line. Insert the catheter just over the top of the rib to avoid the vein, artery, and nerve that lie just below each inferior rib border.

A hissing sound should be audible as the needle enters the pleural cavity. The syringe will fill easily. The accumulated pressure actually can blow the plunger from the syringe.

Remove the needle from the catheter and attach the catheter to a three-way stopcock, a flutter (Heimlich) valve, or short tubing and a syringe filled with saline.

Secure the catheter until a chest tube is placed.

Continue to provide supplemental oxygen and ventilate as needed.

Continuously observe the patient for signs of air reaccumulation. Open the stopcock to release air as needed.

Prepare for immediate chest tube insertion.

Once the chest tube is in place, the intravenous catheter can be removed from the chest.

- Moderate or large pneumothoraces and those with associated hemothorax require chest tube insertion (refer to Boxes 37-2, p. 663 and 37-3, p. 664).

Complications

- Hypoxia
- Tension pneumothorax
- Hemothorax

Patient education and discharge instructions

A follow-up chest radiograph is required to verify reinflation.

Tension Pneumothorax

Tension pneumothorax occurs when air enters the pleural space during inspiration and becomes trapped, causing air accumulation within the thoracic cavity. This not only collapses the affected lung, reducing oxygenation and ventilation, but also is detrimental to hemodynamic function. As the affected half of the pleural cavity inflates, the heart and great vessels are shifted to the opposite side where they are compressed, producing an effect similar to pericardial tamponade. Tension pneumothorax may occur as the result of a penetrating injury (open pneumothorax), as a consequence of blunt trauma (closed pneumothorax), or as a complication of mechanical ventilation. Tension pneumothorax (Figures 37-5 and 37-6) is a life-threatening condition requiring emergent intervention.[5,7-8] Frequently, patients with a small pneumothorax will develop signs of tension pneumothorax shortly after the initiation of positive-pressure ventilation (bag-valve-mask/endotracheal tube or mechanical ventilator).

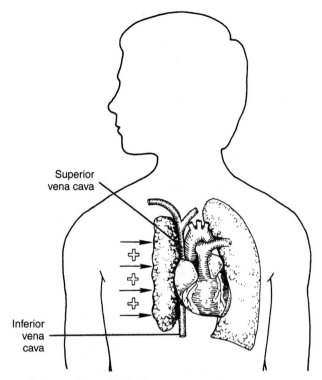

Superior
vena cava

Inferior
vena
cava

Figure 37-5. Tension pneumothorax.

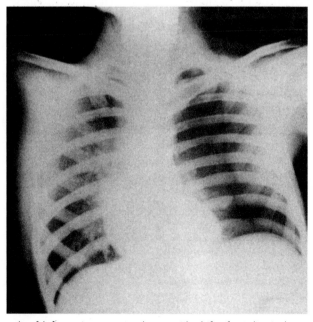

Figure 37-6. Radiograph of left tension pneumothorax with shift of mediastinal structures to right. (From Rosen P, Barkin RM, Hockberger RS et al: *Emergency medicine: concepts and clinical practice*, ed 4, St. Louis, 1999, Mosby.

Signs and symptoms

- Tachycardia
- Restlessness
- Severe respiratory distress
- Jugular vein distention caused by cardiac compression
- Deviated trachea, away from the affected side
- Mediastinal shift, away from the affected side
- Cyanosis caused by poor oxygenation
- Hypotension caused by low cardiac output
- Hyperresonance on percussion
- Hyperexpansion of the affected side
- Distant heart sounds

Diagnostic aids

- Clinical observation
- Chest radiographs
- *Never wait for a radiograph if a patient demonstrates clinical signs of tension pneumothorax.*

Therapeutic interventions

- Immediate needle thoracostomy (see Box 37-1)
- Other emergent and supportive care as indicated

Open Pneumothorax

An open pneumothorax is a chest wall defect that allows ambient air to enter the thoracic cavity. This causes loss of negative pressure in the pleural space, collapsing the lung. Penetrating injuries, such as stab wounds or high-velocity missiles, can produce an open pneumothorax. If the hole in the chest wall is open, air passes into the pleural space and back out again with each inspiration and exhalation. However, if a one-way flap develops, air in the chest accumulates with each breath and pressure builds until a tension pneumothorax has formed.[1] An open pneumothorax sometimes is referred to as a "sucking" chest wound. The sucking sound is produced when the patient takes a spontaneous breath (negative pressure) and "sucks" air though the chest wall defect. However, once the patient is intubated and given positive-pressure breaths (bag-valve-endotracheal tube or mechanical ventilator), the wound will be bubbling, *not* sucking.

Signs and symptoms

- Dyspnea
- Chest pain
- Chest wound (may be small, such as from an ice pick)
- Sucking sound (negative-pressure ventilation)
- Bubbling from the wound (positive-pressure ventilation)
- Possible signs of tension pneumothorax

Diagnostic aids

- Clinical findings

Therapeutic interventions

- Support the patient's airway, breathing, and circulation.
- Deliver oxygen under positive pressure.
- Cover the wound with an occlusive dressing. This helps reestablish negative pressure in the pleural space, allowing the lung to reexpand. *Observe closely for the development of a tension pneumothorax. If tension develops, remove the occlusive dressing and allow the air to escape.*
- Prepare for immediate chest tube placement.

Chest tube placement (tube thoracostomy)

Chest tubes are placed to facilitate the removal of air, blood, or other fluid (pus, lymph, or effusion fluid) from the intrathoracic cavity. Chest tubes must have some means of preventing air from entering the pleural space. This typically is done with a water seal system, but a one-way (e.g., Heimlich) valve also may be used for cases of simple pneumothorax. Chest tube systems that are attached to a water seal and a collection chamber frequently are attached to suction as well. Suction facilitates evacuation of the pleural cavity and is usually standard practice when tubes are placed. A chest tube insertion site is selected based on whether its purpose is to remove air, fluid, or both. Box 37-2 lists equipment and supplies for chest tube insertion, and Box 37-3 summarizes chest tube insertion steps.

Indications

- Hemothorax
- Pneumothorax
- Empyema
- Chylothorax

Box **37-2**   **Chest Tube Insertion: Equipment and Supplies**

Chest tubes
  Adult: 36 to 40 French
  Pediatric: 16 to 32 French
Povidone-iodine or other skin preparation solution
Preparation sponges
Sterile drapes
6- to 10-mL syringe for lidocaine
18-gauge needle (to draw up lidocaine)
25-gauge needle (to administer lidocaine)
1% lidocaine
Sterile surgical gloves
Scalpel and blade (for skin incision)
Two large, curved Kelly clamps (to hold the chest tube)
Chest drainage collection device (e.g., Pleuravac or Atrium)
Sterile water to fill the chest drainage device (some models)
Tubing to attach the collection device for suction
Silk suture to secure the chest tube to the skin
Needle holder (to pull the suture)
Occlusive dressing material (e.g., Xeroform or petrolatum-impregnated gauze)
Razor if chest hair removal is required (so the tape will stick)
Benzoin (so the tape will stick)
Dry, sterile dressing (to absorb insertion site drainage)
Wide adhesive tape (to tape the dressing to the chest and to tape all tubing connections to prevent accidental disconnection)

Box **37**-3   Chest Tube Insertion: Procedure

Monitor the patient closely throughout the procedure.
Identify the appropriate chest tube placement site:
  Pneumothorax: second intercostal space, midclavicular line
  Hemothorax: fourth or fifth intercostal space, slightly anterior to midaxillary line
Prepare and drape the site.
Infiltrate the skin and rib periosteum with lidocaine.
Using a scalpel and blade, make a 2- to 3-cm transverse incision through the skin.
With a Kelly clamp, bluntly dissect and spread through the subcutaneous tissue over the superior edge
  of the rib.
Puncture the tip of the Kelly clamp (carefully) through the pleura. (Air will rush from the puncture site
  if a pneumothorax is present).
Explore the intrathoracic area with a sterile, gloved index finger to free adhesions or clots.
Place one half of a Kelly clamp tip through the perforation on the distal end of the chest tube (making
  the tip of the tube firm).
Advance the distal tip of the tube into the intrathoracic cavity; ensure that it is inserted beyond the
  most proximal fenestration.
Attach the chest tube to a closed chest drainage system. (Many brands and models require that water
  be added.)
Confirm that suction equipment is in working order and attach it to the closed chest drainage
  system.
Note the amount of initial drainage and any subsequent drainage by marking directly on the collection
  chamber.
Once the tube is in place, secure it to the skin with silk suture.
Apply an occlusive dressing (e.g., Vaseline gauze) to seal the hole and prevent air leaks. Some
  practitioners choose to suture the hole first.
Apply benzoin to the skin surrounding the chest tube.
Secure the dressing and the chest tube with adhesive tape.
Obtain a chest radiograph to verify tube placement.

Hemothorax

A hemothorax is a collection of blood within the intrathoracic space. Hemothorax generally occurs when a lung or vessel (intercostal or internal mammary) is lacerated as the result of blunt or penetrating trauma. Because hemothorax can precipitate hemorrhagic shock, patients must be monitored closely. (See Chapter 22.)

Hemothorax often is seen along with simple or tension pneumothorax (Figure 37-7). Radiographic findings suggestive of hemothorax may not be visualized directly on an anterior-posterior chest film until 200 to 300 mL of blood has accumulated in the pleural space. More than 1500 mL of blood in the intrathoracic cavity is considered massive hemothorax.[5,8,9]

Signs and symptoms

- Similar to signs of simple or tension pneumothorax
- Clinical signs of hemorrhagic shock: Cool clammy skin, decreased capillary refill, hypotension, tachycardia, tachypnea, restlessness, anxiety, agitation, confusion, or unconsciousness
- Dullness to percussion on the affected side
- Diminished breath sounds on the affected side

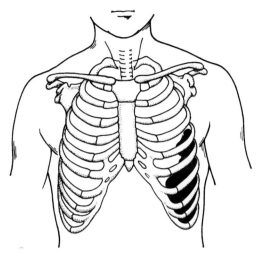

Figure 37-7. Hemothorax. (From Sheehy SB et al: *Manual of clinical trauma care: the first hour,* ed 3, St. Louis, 1999, Mosby.

Diagnostic aids

- Clinical observation
- Chest radiographs: Look for the presence of an air-fluid level in the affected lung field and a blunted costophrenic angle.

Therapeutic interventions

- Support the patient's airway, breathing, and circulation.
- Replace volume loss with IV crystalloids and blood products.
- Assist with chest tube placement; attach to suction.
- Consider autotransfusion.
- Evaluate for concurrent injuries (abdominal, cardiac, head).
- Emergent thoracotomy or surgery is indicated if the initial chest drainage is as follows:
  - Greater than 1500 mL
  - Greater than or equal to 1000 mL, followed by at least 200 mL/hr for the next 4 hours[9]

Complications

- Hypovolemia
- Hypoxia

Autotransfusion of chest blood

Chest blood autotransfusion involves collection of blood that is drained via a chest tube, filtered, and then returned to the patient. This process requires the use of a special chest drainage collection chamber. This procedure has a number of advantages.

Autotransfused blood

- Is immediately available
- Is warm (not chilled)
- Contains all clotting factors except fibrinogen

- Is fresh
- Carries no infectious disease risk
- Is perfectly cross-matched
- Is relatively inexpensive
- Does not require two professionals to check and hang

Indications

- Major hemothorax
- Myocardial rupture
- Great vessel rupture
- Nonavailability of banked blood
- A history of transfusion reactions
- Refusal of homologous blood for religious or personal reasons

Contraindications

- Chest wounds greater than 4 hours old
- Patients with preexisting impairment of kidney or liver function
- Chest blood contaminated by the following:
  - Outside sources
  - Abdominal or intestinal contents
  - Cancer cells[5,8]

LUNG INJURIES

Pulmonary Contusion

Pulmonary contusions typically occur with other severe blunt chest injuries, high-velocity missile wounds, or significant barotrauma from an explosion. Pulmonary contusion causes blood to extravasate into the lung parenchyma. As a result, the affected tissues are deprived of oxygen, becoming ischemic and edematous. Occasionally, pulmonary contusion can be so severe it causes tracheal obstruction. Like all bruises, pulmonary contusions may be slow to blossom, at times taking many hours to develop fully.[2] For this reason, pulmonary contusions more commonly become apparent during a patient's stay in the intensive care unit rather than during initial resuscitation. Diagnosis usually is made based on mechanism of injury and clinical findings.

Signs and symptoms

- Progressive deterioration of oxygenation and ventilation status
- Dyspnea
- Ineffective cough
- Restlessness and agitation
- Presence of other severe chest injuries
- Hemoptysis (occasionally)

Diagnostic aids

- Clinical observation
- SpO_2 monitoring
- Chest radiographs
- Arterial blood gases

Therapeutic interventions

- Administer high-flow oxygen (humidified if possible).
- Perform tracheal intubation and ventilatory support for deterioration.
- Consider independent lung ventilation. A special dual-lumen tracheal tube attaches to two ventilators to inflate each lung selectively.
- Conservatively use fluids during resuscitation (once hypovolemia is corrected) to minimize water in the lung.
- Peform aggressive pulmonary toilet.
- Consider use of diuretics.
- Consider use of steroids.
- Implement pain control.

Complications

- Respiratory failure
- Pneumonia
- Hypoxia

Lung Parenchyma Laceration

Lacerations of the lung parenchyma most commonly are caused by penetrating trauma or jagged rib fractures. They are usually self-limiting and rarely need surgical intervention. Severe pulmonary lacerations require thoracotomy to arrest bleeding and repair associated bronchial and vascular tears.

Signs and symptoms

- Hemothorax, pneumothorax
- Hemoptysis
- Subcutaneous emphysema

Diagnostic aids

- Clinical observation
- Chest radiographs (showing hemothorax, pneumothorax, or subcutaneous emphysema)
- Deteriorating SpO_2 and arterial blood gases

Therapeutic interventions

- Supplemental oxygen
- Chest tube placement for hemothorax or pneumothorax
- Ventilatory support as needed
- Surgical repair for severe lacerations

Tracheobronchial Tree Injury

Injury to the tracheobronchial tree involves tears of the trachea or main stem bronchus, most commonly near the carina. This injury can be caused by blunt or penetrating forces. Mortality from such tears is as high as 50% in the first hour following trauma.[2] Alternatively, signs and symptoms of a small leak can be subtle and slowly progressive and may not appear for up to 5 days following the initial event. Concomitant injuries, including cervical or thoracic fractures, must be suspected if the patient sustained a direct blow or penetrating injury to the neck. (See Chapter 36.)

Signs and symptoms

- Airway obstruction, sudden or progressive
- Respiratory distress or failure
- Hemoptysis (can be massive)
- Mediastinal and subcutaneous emphysema (can be extensive)
- Possible tension pneumothorax
- Atelectasis
- Prolonged air leak in chest drainage device

Diagnostic aids

- Clinical findings
- If the disruption is below the carina, chest radiographs will demonstrate mediastinal air.
- Bronchoscopy

Therapeutic interventions

- Airway protection
- High-flow oxygen
- Chest tubes, mediastinal tube
- Semi-Fowler's position
- Surgical repair

CARDIAC AND GREAT VESSEL INJURIES

Blunt Cardiac Injury

Blunt cardiac injury, formerly called myocardial contusion, occurs more frequently than is diagnosed. Although most incidents are mild, severe cases sometimes are overlooked because of other, more obvious problems. The possibility of blunt cardiac injury should be considered in any patient with a history of blunt chest trauma involving significant acceleration/deceleration force. At particular risk are persons involved in motor vehicle collisions in which the steering wheel was bent. Blunt cardiac injury also can be induced by chest compressions during cardiopulmonary resuscitation.[5,8]

Signs and symptoms

- Chest pain that ranges from mild to severe
- Chest wall contusions, ecchymosis
- Dysrhythmias and other electrocardiogram changes:
  - Usually apparent within the first hour but can be delayed up to 24 hours
  - Premature ventricular contractions, atrial fibrillation, right bundle branch block, or ST segment elevation
- Tachycardia
- Hypotension
- Dyspnea

Diagnostic aids

- High index of suspicion
- Elevated ST segments in leads V_1, V_2, and V_3
- Echocardiography
- Elevated cardiac isoenzymes and troponin levels

Therapeutic interventions

- Therapeutic interventions for blunt cardiac injury are similar to those for acute myocardial infarction *without thrombolysis.*
- Supplemental oxygen administration
- Semi-Fowler's position (complete bed rest)
- Analgesia
- Dysrhythmia management
- Admission to a monitored intensive care unit bed for at least 48 hours

Complications

- Myocardial injury
- Pericardial effusion
- Coronary vessel rupture
- Cardiogenic shock[5,8]

Penetrating Cardiac Injuries

Penetrating cardiac injuries are associated with a very high mortality rate. If the patient survives the prehospital phase of care and arrives at the emergency department with vital signs, immediate thoracotomy and surgical repair are indicated.[10] Penetrating cardiac injuries most frequently result from direct stab or gunshot wounds.

Signs and symptoms

Myocardial Disruption

- Severe hypotension
- Elevated central venous pressure
- Distended jugular veins
- Decreased electrocardiogram voltage
- Muffled heart sounds
- Hemothorax, pneumothorax

Aortic or Mitral Valve Disruption

- Severe chest pain
- Severe dyspnea
- Hemoptysis
- Loud "roaring" murmur
- Signs of severe heart failure and pulmonary edema

Diagnostic aids

- Clinical signs of a penetrating wound
- Chest radiographs

Therapeutic interventions

- Support the patient's airway, breathing, and circulation.
- Establish IV access and infuse crystalloids and blood.
- Prepare for emergency thoracotomy.
- Facilitate immediate surgical intervention to repair a rupture or replace a valve.
- Infuse inotropic agents to improve myocardial contractility.

Complications

- Myocardial infarction
- Heart failure
- Cardiogenic shock
- Coronary artery aneurysm
- Valve rupture
- Ventricular aneurysm

Pericardial Tamponade

Pericardial tamponade is a condition in which the heart is compressed by an accumulation of fluid in the pericardial space, resulting in abnormalities of cardiac function. When fluid accumulated rapidly, as little as 100 to 150 mL of fluid in the pericardial sac can be fatal. Gunshots and stab wounds, causing laceration of the myocardium or coronary vessels, are the most common causes, but severe blunt trauma also can be the source of traumatic pericardial tamponade.

As the volume of blood in the inelastic sac rises, the chambers of the heart are compressed. atrial and ventricular filling are impeded, and stroke volume drops dramatically. Consequently, cardiac output, systolic pressure, and pulse pressures are reduced. Poor forward flow creates a backup in the vena cava, increasing central venous pressure. Oxygen delivery to all vital organs is compromised. In an attempt to compensate, the sympathetic nervous system increases vasoconstriction, cardiac contractility, and heart rate. However, the compensatory responses of the body can be quickly overwhelmed, and cardiogenic shock ensues (see Chapter 22).

Pericardial tamponade is a life-threatening emergency that demands immediate intervention. Always consider the possibility of tamponade when there is unexplained pump failure that is no response to volume replacement. Because many clinical findings are similar, pericardial tamponade often is confused with tension pneumothorax.

Signs and symptoms

- Early symptoms: fullness in the head, neck, and abdomen
- Nausea, chest pain
- Tachycardia, dyspnea
- Pulsus paradoxus (drop in systolic blood pressure greater than 10 mm Hg during inspiration)
- Beck's triad
  - Hypotension
  - Distended jugular veins (may not be evident in patients with concomitant hypovolemia)
  - Muffled or distant heart sounds
- Cyanosis
- Altered mental status
- Hamman's crunch

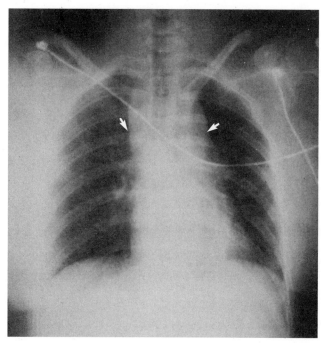

Figure 37-8. Widened mediastinum: Collection of blood or fluid within the mediastinal space denoted by greater opacity.

- Low-voltage QRS complex
- Electrical alternans (P wave, QRS complex, and ST segment amplitude changes with alternating beats). This finding is rare in patients with traumatic tamponade.[5,6]

Diagnostic aids

- Clinical observation
- Bedside ultrasound/echocardiography
- Chest radiographs (widened mediastinum; Figure 37-8)
- Pericardiocentesis
- Electrocardiogram

Therapeutic interventions

- Support the patient's airway, breathing, and circulation.
- Run isotonic IV fluids wide open to (temporarily) increase cardiac filling pressures.
- Prepare for pericardiocentesis to decompress the heart temporarily in unstable patients.
- Facilitate immediate surgical intervention for relief and repair.[6]

Aortic Disruption

Tears of the aorta usually occur following deceleration injuries (e.g., motor vehicle collisions or fall from a height). The majority of aortic disruptions occur at points of attachment, particularly the ligamentum arteriosum and aortic root. Other sites of disruption include the aortic arch, the ascending aorta, the distal descending aorta, and the diaphragm.[5,8]

Patients who sustain significant aortic tears rarely survive the injury. On-scene mortality has been reported as high as 90%. Of the patients still alive on emergency department arrival, 30% perish within 6 hours, and another 20% die within 24 hours if emergent care is delayed.[8] Death from aortic disruption usually results from pericardial tamponade or massive exsanguination. Patients generally exhibit signs of multisystem injury, but in some cases, there is no obvious external trauma.

Signs and symptoms

- Hypovolemic shock
- Pericardial tamponade
- Chest wall ecchymosis
- First or second rib fracture
- Sternal fracture
- Scapula or multiple rib fractures
- Loud murmur auscultated at the left parascapular region
- Blood pressure is higher in the upper extremities than in the lower (this may be impossible to assess in moribund patients).
- Right tracheal deviation
- Paraplegia
- Traumatic cardiac arrest

Diagnostic aids

- Chest radiographs
  - Widened mediastinum
  - Obliteration of the aortic knob
  - Presence of a pleural cap
  - Hemothorax
  - Esophageal deviation (gastric tube deviates to the right)
  - Elevated right main stem bronchus and a low left main stem bronchus
- Thoracic aortogram
- Chest CT scan
- Transesophageal echocardiogram

Therapeutic interventions

- Support the patient's airway, breathing, and circulation.
- Establish IVs and infuse crystalloids.
- Transfuse blood as needed.
- Provide medications: Beta-blockers or sodium nitroprusside lower blood pressure and decrease vessel wall shearing forces (for patients who are not hypotensive or hypovolemic).
- Prepare for urgent surgical repair.

Complications

- Hypovolemic shock
- Exsanguination

Table **37-1**   **Survival Following Emergency Thoracotomy**

Mechanism of Injury	Survival Rate
Penetrating trauma (stab wound)	16.8%
Penetrating trauma (gunshot wound)	4.3%
Blunt trauma	1.4%

From Rhee PM et al: Survival after emergency department thoracotomy: review of published data from the past 25 years, *J Am Coll Surg* 190(3):288-298, 2000.

Emergent Thoracotomy

An emergent thoracotomy (also called an ERT, emergency room thoracotomy) is a potentially lifesaving procedure in which the chest is opened rapidly and the vessels, lungs, or myocardium are patched, plugged, or clamped just enough to arrest hemorrhage, restore circulatory function, and move the patient to the operating room. Emergent thoracotomies are performed in moribund individuals to relieve acute cardiac tamponade, facilitate internal cardiac compressions, deliver electricity directly to the myocardium (internal defibrillation), treat massive air embolism, and cross-clamp the aorta (to shift blood to vital organs including the coronary vessels).[11]

Nationally, the overall survival rate following emergent thoracotomy is only 7.5%.[12] The mechanism and location of injury significantly influence outcome (Table 37-1). Emergent thoracotomy generally is limited to the left side of the chest, but a clamshell thoracotomy may be performed (opening the entire chest from axilla to axilla) when trauma on the right side also is suspected. Holes in the myocardium, vessels, or lungs can be plugged temporarily with sutures, staples, Teflon pledgets, clamps, a finger, or the balloon of a Foley catheter.

Because of the poor prognosis and high costs associated with emergent thoracotomy, criteria such as mechanism of injury (blunt vs. penetrating), prehospital vital signs (present or absent), cardiac rhythm (pulseless electrical activity or asystole), and neurologic status should be considered carefully before making a decision in favor of thoracotomy. Figure 37-9 is an example of one such decision algorithm. Box 37-4 lists equipment and supplies required for an emergent thoracotomy.

The role of the nurse during emergent thoracotomy includes the following:
- Support the patient's airway, breathing, and circulation.
- Continue fluid resuscitation.
- Perform cardiac compressions.
- Assist with the thoracotomy procedure.
- Provide postresuscitation monitoring during transit to the operating room.

MISCELLANEOUS THORACIC INJURIES

Ruptured Esophagus

A ruptured esophagus is a rare event that can occur following penetrating injury or a severe blow to the epigastric region. When the cause is blunt trauma, the tear is generally just above the diaphragm, but esophageal rupture also must be considered whenever there is evidence of a first or second rib fracture, cervical fracture, or laryngotracheal tears.

Signs and symptoms

- Sudden onset of severe chest pain or upper abdominal pain following trauma
- Clinical findings similar to those of pneumothorax

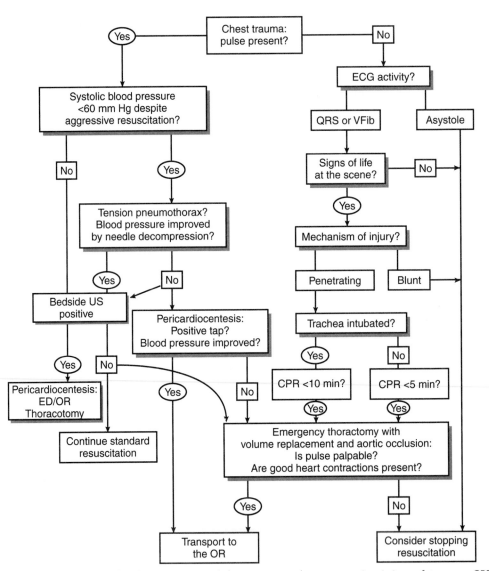

Figure 37-9. Algorithm for determining need for emergent thoracotomy in victims of trauma. *CPR*, Cardiopulmonary resuscitation; *ECG*, electrocardiogram; *ED*, emergency department; *OR*, operating room; *US*, ultrasound; *VFib*, ventricular fibrillation. (From Roberts JR, Hedges JR, editors: *Clinical procedures in emergency medicine*, ed 4, Philadelphia, 2004, WB Saunders.)

Box **37-4** **Equipment Required for Emergent Thoracotomy**

(Commonly prepackaged as a surgical tray)
#3 Bard-Parker knife handle
#10 and #11 blades
5½-inch Metzenbaum scissors, curved
Bailey rib contractor
6-inch tissue forceps
10-inch DeBakey tangential vessel clamp
Towel clamps
Gauze sponges
8¾-inch Mayo scissors (curved)
6¾-inch Mayo scissors (curved)
10½-inch Masson needle holder
Finochietto retractor (rib spreaders)
10-inch tissue forceps
Yankauer suction
Towels

- Pain on swallowing
- Mediastinitis
- Subcutaneous emphysema
- Mediastinal crunch sound (Hamman's sign) from air in the mediastinum
- Elevated temperature
- Tachypnea
- Dyspnea
- Pneumothorax, hemothorax
- Pleural effusion
- Gastric contents or bile in the chest tube drainage
- Shock

Diagnostic aids

- Clinical observation
- Upper gastrointestinal series
- Esophagoscopy
- Esophagography
- Flexible endoscopy

Therapeutic interventions

- Support the patient's airway, breathing, and circulation.
- Establish IV access and infuse crystalloids.
- Facilitate surgical intervention.

Complications

- Subcutaneous emphysema
- Mediastinitis
- Empyema
- Tracheal-esophageal fistula development

Diaphragmatic Rupture

In the setting of acute trauma, diaphragmatic rupture can be a life-threatening injury. Diaphragmatic tears (almost always on the left side) allow abdominal contents (stomach, bowel) enter through the diaphragm into the thoracic cavity.[2] This significantly interferes with ventilation. Diaphragmatic injury should be suspected in any patient who sustains a blow to the abdomen below the level of the nipples or experiences a sudden increase in intraabdominal pressure (e.g., lap belt injuries). A ruptured diaphragm generally is associated with other significant trauma and often is diagnosed after the initial resuscitation period as the abdominal contents continue to move upward into the chest.

Signs and symptoms

- Bowel sounds in the thoracic cavity
- Chest pain referred to the shoulder (Kehr's sign)
- Severe dyspnea
- Decreased breath sounds
- Undigested food or fecal matter in the chest tube drainage

Diagnostic aids

- Chest radiographs demonstrate the following:
  - An elevated left hemidiaphragm
  - Bowel herniation into the thoracic cavity
  - A nasogastric tube coiled in the chest
  - Absence of the costophrenic angle on the side opposite the injury[1]
- A gastrointestinal series shows stomach and/or intestines in the thoracic cavity.

Therapeutic interventions

- Support the patient's airway, breathing, and circulation.
- Place a gastric tube to decompress the stomach.
- Facilitate surgical repair.

References

1. American College of Surgeons Committee on Trauma: *Advanced trauma life support manual,* ed 2, Chicago, 1998, The College.
2. Lawrence P: *Essentials of general surgery,* ed 3, Baltimore, 1998, Williams & Wilkins.
3. Sherwood S, Hartsock R: Thoracic injuries. In McQuillan K et al, editors: *Trauma nursing: from resuscitation through rehabilitation,* ed 3, Philadelphia, 2002, WB Saunders.
4. Emergency Nurses Association: *Trauma nursing core course,* ed 5, Des Plaines, Ill, 2000, The Association.
5. Marx J, Hockenberger R, Walls R, editors: *Rosen's emergency medicine: concepts and clinical practice,* ed 5, St Louis, 2002, Mosby.
6. Schaider J et al, editors: *Rosen and Barkin's 5-minute emergency medicine consult,* ed 2, Philadelphia, 2003, Lippincott Williams & Wilkins.
7. Holmes H: *Atlas of pathophysiology,* Philadelphia, 2002, Springhouse.
8. Ferrera PC et al: *Trauma management: an emergency medicine approach,* St Louis, 2001, Mosby.
9. Sheehy SB et al: *Manual of clinical trauma care: the first hour,* ed 3, St Louis, 1999, Mosby.
10. Cavatorta F, Campisi S, Fiorini F: Fatal pericardial tamponade by a guide wire during jugular catheter insertion, *Nephron* 79(3):352, 1998.

11.   Bartlett RL: Resuscitative thoracotomy. In Roberts JR, Hedges JR, editors: *Clinical procedures in emergency medicine,* ed 2, Philadelphia, 1998, WB Saunders.
12.   Rhee PM et al: Survival after emergency department thoracotomy: review of published data from the past 25 years, *J Am Coll Surg* 190(3):288-298, 2000.

38

Abdominal Trauma

Dennis B. MacDougall, RN, MS, ACNPBC, CEN

Thirteen percent to 15% of traumatic deaths are a direct result of injury to abdominal structures, making this the third leading cause of trauma-related mortality.[1] Knowing the mechanism of injury, conducting a diligent physical examination, maintaining a high degree of suspicion, and performing serial evaluations are essential for reducing the morbidity and mortality related to abdominal trauma. The two mechanisms of injury most commonly associated with abdominal trauma are blunt and penetrating; each of these forces produces distinctive patterns of organ damage.

BLUNT TRAUMA

Blunt abdominal trauma results when force is applied to the abdominal wall without creating an open wound. The abdominal viscera and other structures are injured by direct blows, compression, or deceleration. In the United States, motor vehicle collisions are the number one cause of blunt abdominal trauma, responsible for 50% to 75% of significant injuries.[2,3] Other mechanisms of blunt abdominal trauma are contact sports, falls, and physical abuse.[4]

Because the spleen, liver, and kidneys are solid organs and more likely to rupture in response to blunt force, they are the intraabdominal structures most frequently injured. Although seat belts save lives, they nonetheless are associated with their own constellation of injuries, including visceral rupture, organ compression, orthopedic fractures, and abdominal vessel tears.

PENETRATING TRAUMA

In the United States, the leading cause of penetrating abdominal trauma is interpersonal violence, particularly in urban settings. Penetrating trauma results when an object such as a bullet, knife blade, or projectile fragment pierces the belly wall, entering the abdominal cavity. Stab wounds most commonly produce intestinal injury, but a surprising number of stabs do not actually penetrate the peritoneal cavity. Thus they are associated with a low mortality rate (1% to 2%) and may not even require surgery. However, 96% to 98% of abdominal gunshot wounds involve significant damage to intraabdominal organs and vessels, necessitating emergent operative intervention.[3,5]

GENERAL CONSIDERATIONS

Although penetrating injuries may be restricted to the abdomen, blunt abdominal trauma is rarely an isolated event. Head and chest trauma and other life-threatening injuries routinely complicate assessment. Hemorrhage is the usual proximate cause of death.

When assessing patients, the emergency nurse should pay particular attention to those who cannot provide information reliably, such as individuals who are unconscious, intoxicated, or very young and persons with spinal cord injuries. Importantly, the absence of clinical findings does not rule out the presence of abdominal injury, especially in pregnant patients and those with neurologic deficits. Frequent reassessment and serial diagnostic studies are essential.[3] Box 38-1 lists general signs and symptoms of abdominal trauma, and Box 38-2 briefly summarizes findings associated with hemorrhagic shock. Refer to Chapter 22 for more details.

MANAGEMENT OF THE PATIENT WITH ABDOMINAL TRAUMA

A basic knowledge of injury mechanism, location, and prevalence guides initial care of the abdominal trauma patient. Immediate determination of specific structures that have been injured is not essential; the most important management decision is whether the patient

---

Box **38-1** **Signs and Symptoms of Abdominal Trauma**

Bruises or abrasions	Masses
Bruits	Open wounds
Decreased or absent bowel sounds	Pain, rebound tenderness
Distention or rigidity	Pelvic instability
Guarding	Rectal bleeding or tenderness
High-riding prostate	Testicular pain or swelling

Box **38-2** **Signs of Hypovolemic Shock**

Cool, clammy skin	Poor capillary refill
Decreased level of consciousness	Tachycardia
Hypotension	Tachypnea
Narrowed pulse pressure	

requires immediate surgery. With this in mind, care is focused on basic stabilization, frequent reassessment, and diagnostic testing.[1]

Airway

Assessment

Ensure that the patient has a patent airway.

Intervention

Clear the airway and use adjuncts as indicated.

Breathing

Assessment

- Evaluate respiratory rate, depth, effectiveness, and work of breathing. Consider the possibility of concurrent thoracic injury (see Chapter 37).

Interventions

- Administer supplemental oxygen via a non-rebreather mask or tracheal tube.
- Assist ventilations as needed with a bag-valve-mask or mechanical ventilator.

Circulation

Assessment

- Assess circulatory status: Pulses, skin signs, and blood pressure. Patients with abdominal injuries can lose tremendous amounts of blood.

Interventions

- Insert two (or more) large-bore (14- to 16-gauge) intravenous catheters.
- Infuse warmed, isotonic crystalloid solutions: lactated Ringer's solution or normal saline.
- Transfuse blood components as needed: Packed red blood cells or other blood products.
- Because of the potential for fluid boluses to displace newly formed clots, the role of fluid resuscitation in the patient with abdominal trauma is controversial. A judicious approach to volume replacement is recommended. Administer fluids based on clinical status and test results.[6,7]
- Consider central line (subclavian or jugular) placement in unstable patients for infusion of large fluid volumes and central venous pressure monitoring.

Miscellaneous

Assessment

- Identify the mechanism of injury and prehospital events (e.g., crash speed, restraint use, fall height, type and size of weapon, time since the injury, and estimated external blood loss).

- Determine medical history.
- Inspect the anterior and posterior abdomen to identify all wounds.
- Check for major injuries to other body sites.

Interventions

- Place an orogastric or nasogastric tube for stomach decompression.
- Insert an indwelling urinary (Foley) catheter and monitor output.
- Cover open abdominal wounds with sterile saline dressings. Do not allow exposed viscera to dry.
- Facilitate diagnostic studies and surgical intervention.

SPECIFIC ORGAN INJURIES

Spleen

The spleen is the organ most frequently injured in blunt abdominal trauma; splenic injuries occur in nearly 40% of patients with major abdominal damage. The spleen is a dense, highly vascular, encapsulated organ with a blood flow of approximately 200 ml/min. Thus rupture can cause significant hemorrhage. Trauma to the spleen (located behind ribs 9, 10, and 11) should be suspected following any blow to the left upper quadrant of the abdomen. Clinical findings suggestive of injury are left upper quadrant tenderness, pain referred to the left shoulder (Kehr's sign), peritoneal irritation, and hypotension. A diagnosis of splenic injury is made by abdominal ultrasound or computed tomography (CT) scan. Hemodynamically stable individuals often can be managed nonsurgically. Admit these patients for close observation, serial hematocrit tests, and repeated CT scans. Surgery is avoided if possible because splenic preservation helps maintain immune function.[3] To significantly reduce the incidence of future pneumococcal sepsis following splenectomy, patients should receive a Pneumovax vaccination before discharge.

Liver

The liver is the largest solid organ in the body. The liver is injured in about 19% of blunt or penetrating abdominal trauma cases. This structure is damaged readily because of its anterior location, large size, denseness, and relatively unprotected status. In addition, the liver is highly vascular, with a blood flow of approximately 400 to 100 ml/min, making it a major source of potential. Be particularly suspicious of hepatic injuries whenever trauma involves the upper central abdomen or ribs 8 to 12 on the right.[3] Box 38-3 lists clinical manifestations of liver trauma. Definitive diagnosis of hepatic injuries is made by CT scan and in surgery. Large stellate lacerations must be repaired operatively, whereas small lacerations are generally self-healing.

Box **38-3**   **Clinical Manifestations of Liver Trauma**

Abdominal wall muscle spasm and rigidity
Hypoactive or absent bowel sounds
Involuntary guarding
Rebound tenderness
Right upper quadrant pain
Signs of hypovolemic shock

Stomach

The stomach is a hollow and fairly mobile organ. Therefore the stomach rarely is wounded in blunt abdominal trauma. However, the stomach often is injured by penetrating objects. To check for stomach damage, insert a nasogastric tube and examine the aspirate for blood. A plain abdominal radiograph will demonstrate free air, indicative of gastric or intestinal injury. Computed tomography scanning can provide a definitive diagnosis. Surgical repair is required.

Pancreas

The pancreas is a solid organ that is normally well protected by the stomach and the liver. A direct blow to the epigastric region, such as a kick by a horse or a fall against bicycle handle-bars, is the most common cause of blunt trauma to the pancreas. Because the pancreas is located in the retroperitoneum, damage will not be evident on peritoneal lavage and can be difficult to visualize even on CT scan. Posttraumatic pancreatitis, the major concern follow-ing pancreatic injury, often has a delayed onset. Symptoms include epigastric pain, nausea, vomiting, abdominal distention, and altered vital signs. Draw serial serum amylase levels in patients at risk for pancreatic trauma.

Kidneys

The kidneys are retroperitoneal organs located in the flank area. In response to injury, these bean-shaped structures may be contused or lacerated (fractured). Box 38-4 lists signs of renal trauma. Diagnosis is made by urinalysis (hematuria) and intravenous pyelogram or CT scan. Contusions, a generally self-limiting condition, are treated with bed rest, observation, and increased fluid intake. Renal lacerations are associated with hemorrhage and urine extra-vasation. Serious parenchymal, ureteral, or vascular damage requires surgical repair or nephrectomy.[3]

Ureters

Because of their hollow and flexible nature, the ureters are injured infrequently in blunt abdominal trauma. However, they may be disrupted by penetrating objects. Diagnosis is made by intravenous pyelogram. If disruption is present, surgical reanastomosis is indicated.

Bladder

Two common mechanisms of blunt cystic trauma occur. As a hollow organ the bladder may rupture in response to a direct blow (like a water balloon) or a bony fragment from a pelvic fracture can puncture it. All patients with pelvic fractures are at risk for concurrent bladder trauma. Clinical findings of bladder injury include lower pelvic pain, distention, and an inability to void. Consider cystic trauma in patients with an indwelling urinary catheter, who have had several liters of fluid, appear to be volume resuscitated, and yet fail to produce urine.

Box **38-4 Clinical Manifestations of Renal Trauma**

Ecchymosis over the flank (Grey Turner's sign)
Flank or abdominal tenderness
Palpable mass
Hematuria, frank or microscopic (>50 red blood cells per high-power field)

Bladder rupture is diagnosed readily by cystogram (sensitivity is nearly 100%). Lacerations or rupture require surgical repair; suprapubic catheter placement may be necessary.[8,9]

Urethra

Because of the external location of the urethra in males, disruptions are considerably more common in males than in females. Typically, trauma results from a straddle injury, such as impact with the crossbar on a bicycle or motorcycle. Also look for urethral trauma in any patient with a pelvic fracture. Box 38-5 lists signs and symptoms of urologic injuries. Initial diagnosis is made by the presence of blood at the urinary meatus, sometimes associated with a high-riding prostate on rectal examination. The presence of these findings mandates a retrograde urethrogram. Obtain urologic consultation if disruption is detected.

Intestines

The intestines, both large and small, fill the majority of the abdominal cavity. These organs are injured routinely in blunt and penetrating trauma because of their size, anterior position, points of fixation, and vascularity. The small bowel is the most frequently injured hollow organ.[1] Box 38-6 lists clinical manifestations of intestinal trauma. Although abdominal radiographs, peritoneal lavage, and CT scans are used to identify injury, definitive diagnosis typically is made by exploratory laparotomy. Additionally, small tears provide a diagnostic challenge, often requiring serial examinations to diagnose. Intestinal disruptions must be repaired surgically to control hemorrhage, return bowel function, and cleanse the abdominal cavity of spilled bowel contents. These wounds are prone to severe infections.

Diaphragm

The diaphragm is the primary muscle of respiration; any tears or herniated abdominal contents can cause severe respiratory compromise. Clinical findings of a ruptured diaphragm

---

Box **38-5**   **Clinical Manifestations of Urologic Injuries**

Abdominal wall rigidity, spasm, or guarding
Blood at the urethral meatus
Displaced prostate gland
Hematuria, frank or microscopic (>50 red blood cells per high-power field)
Pelvic or suprapubic pain
Rebound tenderness
Scrotal swelling

Box **38-6**   **Clinical Manifestations of Intestinal Trauma**

Abdominal rigidity, spasm, or guarding
Hypoactive or absent bowel sounds
Obvious evisceration
Positive diagnostic peritoneal lavage results
Rebound tenderness
Rectal blood (positive Hemoccult test)

include bowel sounds in the chest (almost always on the left side), progressive respiratory distress, a gastric tube visible in the thorax on chest films, or the presence of food or fecal material in chest tube drainage.[10] Surgical repair is required.

Major Abdominal Vessels

The aorta, inferior vena cava, and hepatic and mesenteric veins are just some of the major blood vessels in the abdomen. When disrupted, serious hemorrhage and death will occur if bleeding is not controlled rapidly. The abdomen is a large and highly distensible structure that can easily accommodate the entire blood volume of the body. Vessel injuries can be identified by diagnostic peritoneal lavage (DPL), CT scan, and angiography. If significant vascular disruption is present, immediate surgery or embolization is indicated.

DIAGNOSIS

Although signs of penetrating injury are usually obvious, diagnosing blunt abdominal trauma may be difficult. Often a thorough history of the mechanism of injury will be the most important clue to the presence of trauma. Potential and actual injuries must be prioritized to ensure that those that threaten life or limb are addressed first (see Chapter 34). Use of a systematic approach to the patient with potential abdominal trauma is important. Figure 38-1 is an example of a diagnostic algorithm for abdominal trauma.

Patients most likely to require emergent surgery are those with involuntary guarding, abdominal expansion, hemodynamic instability, penetrating trauma, or gastrointestinal bleeding (Box 38-7). The following section describes some commonly used tools for assessment of the patient with abdominal trauma.

Focused Abdominal Sonography for Trauma

A focused abdominal sonography for trauma (FAST) examination is a rapid, bedside, ultrasound of four specific abdominal areas (pericardial, perihepatic, perisplenic, and pelvic; Figure 38-2). This test is used to identify intraperitoneal fluid in patients with blunt abdominal trauma. The FAST is extremely sensitive and can detect fluid volumes of less than 100 mL. Additionally, the test is noninvasive, can be done concurrently with resuscitation, and takes less than 5 minutes. Unfortunately, FAST cannot assess the retroperitoneal or colorectal areas adequately, nor is it very sensitive for evaluating solid organ and visceral damage.[11] Indications for FAST include the following:
- Evidence of blunt or penetrating abdominal trauma
- Any patient with a mechanism highly suspicious for blunt injury

Abdominal Computed Tomography

Today's CT scanners are a fast and accurate way to evaluate a large number of intraabdominal injuries. These scans have a high sensitivity for detecting solid organ lesions, vascular injuries, and intraperitoneal hemorrhage.[6] Additionally, with the current trend toward nonoperative management of abdominal trauma, serial CT scans offer an excellent way to perform ongoing evaluation of intraabdominal structures.[2,3,12]

Indications for abdominal CT include the following:
- Persons with obvious abdominal injuries or suggestive physical findings
- Hemodynamically stable patients whose FAST examination revealed intraperitoneal fluid
- Patients with a mechanism of injury highly suspicious for intraabdominal trauma

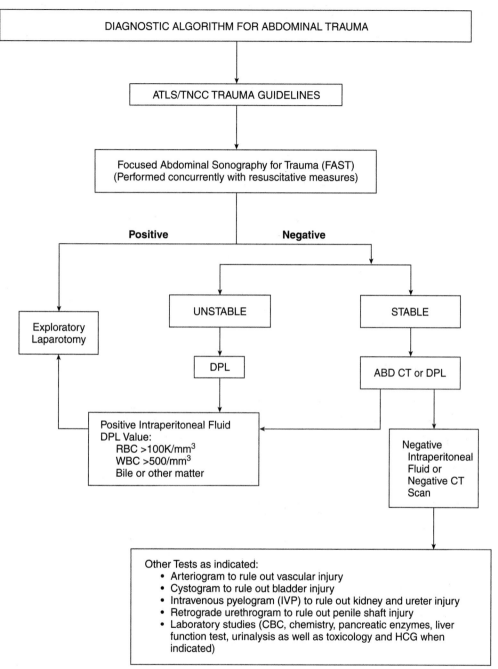

Figure 38-1. Diagnostic algorithm for abdominal trauma. *ABD,* Abdominal; *ATLS/TNCC,* Advanced Trauma Life Support/Trauma Nursing Core Course; *CBC,* complete blood count; *CT,* computed tomography; *DPL,* diagnostic peritoneal lavage; *HCG,* human chorionic gonadotropin; *RBC,* red blood cell; *WBC,* white blood cell. (Written by DB MacDougall, RN, MS, ACNP-C, CEN. Courtesy of Emergency Nurses Association.)

Diagnostic Peritoneal Lavage

Diagnostic peritoneal lavage (DPL) is an abdominal injury assessment technique that has been used sporatically over the years (Box 38-8). Once common practice, DPL was replaced largely by the advent of routine CT scanning. However, this procedure lately has regained popularity in some trauma centers, and it retains a place in the assessment of patients with blunt abdominal trauma. DPL is *not* indicated in penetrating injury; these wounds require surgical exploration. Indications for DPL include the following:

Box 38-7 Indications for Exploratory Laparotomy

Abdominal mass
Continuing drop in hemoglobin or hematocrit level
Evidence of peritonitis
Free air in the abdomen
Increasing abdominal tenderness, girth, or rigidity
Peritoneal perforation
Positive diagnostic peritoneal lavage results
Retroperitoneal fluid
Unexplained hemorrhagic shock

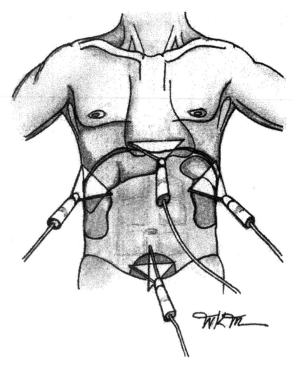

Figure 38-2. The FAST examination consists of ultrasound views of four sites: pericardial, perihepatic (right upper quadrant), perisplenic (left upper quadrant), and pelvic. (Courtesy William Mallon, MD.)

Box **38-8** **Diagnostic Peritoneal Lavage Procedure**

Equipment

Gather supplies based on institutional policy and available equipment.

Patient Preparation

- Explain the procedure to the conscious patient and provide instructions regarding how to cooperate.
- Empty the bladder by inserting an indwelling urinary (Foley) catheter.
- Empty the stomach with a nasogastric or orogastric tube attached to suction.

Procedure

1. Prepare the anterior abdominal wall with a surgical solution such as 1% povidone-iodine (Betadine) and drape the belly with sterile towels.
2. Inject lidocaine 1% with epinephrine to form a subcutaneous wheal 2 to 3 cm above or below the umbilicus.
3. Make a 2-cm or larger incision through the skin and subcutaneous adipose tissue. Ensure *absolute* hemostasis; even a small amount of wound blood can produce a false-positive lavage reading.
4. Engage the trocar into the linea alba at a 30- to 45-degree angle. (Instruct the patient to tense the abdomen if possible.) Apply rotary motion and pressure until the peritoneum is perforated or place the trocar through a surgical incision.
5. Direct the trocar tip toward the caudad pelvis and slide the catheter 15 to 20 cm into the peritoneal cavity.
6. Attach a 20-mL syringe to the catheter and aspirate. If aspiration yields 20 mL of blood, the tap is immediately considered positive and the procedure is terminated. If little or no blood is obtained, attach an intravenous line to the catheter and infuse 1000 mL of warmed Ringer's lactate over 15 minutes. Manually manipulate the abdomen to permit the solution to mix with abdominal cavity fluids.
7. Place the empty intravenous bag on the floor to siphon off the infused fluid.
8. When the majority of the fluid is returned, remove the catheter.
9. Close the skin with 4-0 nylon suture.
10. Dress the incision site with a small sterile dressing.

From Lynn-McHale DJ, Carison KK: Performing percutaneous peritoneal lavage. In American Association of Critical Care Nurses: *AACN procedure manual for critical care*, ed 4, Philadelphia, 2001, WB Saunders.

- Rapid assessment of the multitrauma patient who requires immediate surgery for severe head or chest injuries in whom abdominal trauma has not yet been ruled out. A DPL can be performed quickly in the operating room while other interventions are in progress.
- Evidence of blunt trauma to the abdomen in hemodynamically unstable patients, *when no CT scan is immediately available.*
- Hemodynamically stable patients in whom it is impossible to elicit reliable signs of blunt abdominal trauma *and no CT scan is available.* This would include patients who are unconcious or intoxicated or who have spinal cord injuries.

Contraindications

Contraindications to DPL include the following:
- Diagnostic peritoneal lavage is unnecessary for the patient going directly to the operating room for exploratory laparotomy (e.g., penetrating trauma).
- This procedure is not recommended for children.

- The only absolute contraindication to DPL is a distended bladder. The bladder must be emptied (Foley catheter) and the stomach decompressed (gastric tube and suction) before DPL.
- Relative contraindications to DPL mandate that the location of the incision be changed, but the procedure still can be performed. Relative contraindications include the following:
  - A gravid uterus
  - An abdominal wall hematoma
  - Abdominal scars from previous surgery

Analysis of Contents from Diagnostic Peritoneal Lavage

A quick, bedside analysis of DPL contents involves visual inspection. Consider the test positive if obvious bile or fecal matter is obtained. If there is blood in the fluid (a common finding), hold the intravenous bag against printed material. If the print cannot be read through the DPL fluid, the test is considered grossly positive. Diagnostic peritoneal lavage samples also can be sent for laboratory analysis. Send the fluid for the following tests:

- Hematocrit and red blood cell count
- White blood cell count
- Bile
- Amylase
- Culture and Gram stain

Any significant quantity of bacteria indicates intestinal perforation, bile is indicative of hepatic injury, and amylase is associated with pancreatic trauma. Red blood cell counts greater than 500 cells/mm^3 generally are considered significant, but the level at which surgery is indicated depends on institutional policy.

THE PREGNANT PATIENT WITH ABDOMINAL TRAUMA

Trauma in the pregnant patient is addressed specifically in Chapter 42. Nonetheless, a few considerations related to abdominal injury follow:

- Trauma in pregnancy is relatively unusual. However, blunt abdominal injury frequently produces placental abruption and may cause uterine rupture.
- Penetrating abdominal injuries produce highly variable degrees of damage to the uterus, placenta, and fetus.[3] For the mother, the pregnant uterus is protective; most women who sustain penetrating trauma to the gravid uterus will not have other intraabdominal injuries.
- Fetal survival is highly dependent on maternal survival. Therefore resuscitative efforts must always focus on the mother.
- After 20 weeks of gestation, the combined weight of the fetus, placenta, and amniotic fluid is sufficient to compress the abdominal vena cava and produce obstructive hypovolemia when the patient is supine. Whenever possible, elevate the woman's right hip, tilt the backboard to the left, or manually displace the uterus to promote venous return to the right heart.
- Remember to shield the uterus with a lead apron as much as possible during radiologic procedures. However, never defer necessary studies for fear of fetal irradiation.

References

1. Emergency Nurses Association: Abdominal trauma. In *Trauma nursing core course,* ed 5, Des Plaines, Ill, 2000, The Association.

2. Smith JK Kenny PJ: Imaging of renal trauma, *Radiol Clin North Am* 41(5):1019–1035, 2003.
3. Marx JA et al: Abdominal trauma. In Marx JA, Hockberger R, Walls R, editors: *Rosen's emergency medicine: concepts and clinical practice*, ed 5, St Louis, 2002, Mosby.
4. Hahn DD, Offerman SR Holmes JF: Clinical importance of intraperitoneal fluids in patients with blunt intra-abdominal injury, *Am J Emerg Med* 20(7):595–600, 2002.
5. Asensio JA et al: Abdominal vascular injuries: injuries to the aorta, *Surg Clin North Am* 81(6): 1395–1416, 2001.
6. EAST Practice Management Guidelines Workgroup: *Practice guidelines for the evaluation of blunt abdominal trauma,* 2001, Eastern Association for the Surgery of Trauma.
7. Orlinsky M et al: Current controversies in shock and resuscitation, *Surg Clin North Am* 81(6): 1217–1262, 2001.
8. Hsieh C et al: Diagnosis and management of bladder injury by trauma surgeons, *Am J Surg* 184(2):143–147, 2002.
9. Demetriades D et al: Pelvic fractures: epidemiology and predictors of associated abdominal injuries and outcomes, *J Am Coll Surg* 195(1):1–10, 2002.
10. American College of Surgeons Committee on Trauma: Abdominal trauma. In *Advanced trauma life support course for doctors: manual,* ed 6, Chicago, 1997, The College.
11. Jehle DV, Stiller G, Wagner D: Sensitivity in detecting free intraperitoneal fluid with pelvic views of the FAST exam, *Am J Emerg Med* 21(6):476–478, 2003.
12. EAST Practice Management Guidelines Workgroup: Practice management guidelines for the non-operative management of blunt injury to the liver and spleen, 2003, Eastern Association for the Surgery of Trauma.
13. Lynn-McHale DJ, Carlson KK: Performing percutaneous peritoneal lavage. In American Association of Critical Care Nurses: *AACN procedure manual for critical care,* ed 4, Philadelphia, 2001, WB Saunders.

39

Musculoskeletal Emergencies

Chris M. Gisness, RN, MSN, FNP, CEN

Musculoskeletal injuries are the chief complaint of a large portion of emergency department patients. These injuries are seldom life threatening, but can potentially result in significant long-term disability, loss of income, disfigurement, and pain. The general goal of care is to restore and preserve function. Musculoskeletal complaints can be associated with fractures, sprains, ligamentous tears, tendon lacerations, and joint dislocations. In any orthopedic injury or complaint, neurologic and vascular status must be evaluated carefully.[1]

COMPONENTS OF THE MUSCULOSKELETAL SYSTEM

Bones

The human skeleton is composed of approximately 206 bones (the actual number varies) that form the framework of the body. The bones function to support and protect vital organs; they provide leverage and a means of movement. Bone contains its own blood and nerve supply and is usually capable of healing itself.[1] The two basic types of bone are (1) cancellous (spongy) bone, which is found in the skull, vertebrae, pelvis, and long-bone ends; and (2) cortical (dense) bone, which is found in the long bones.

Ligaments

Ligaments are fibrous connective tissues that connect bone to bone. They provide joint stabilization and facilitate movement.

Tendons

Tendons are fibrous connective tissues that join muscle to bone, permitting flexion and extension of muscle groups.

690

Cartilage

Cartilage is dense connective tissue found in the nasal septum, external ear, larynx, trachea, and bronchi and between the vertebrae, between the ribs, and on the articulating surfaces of bones. Cartilage has no vascular supply.

Joints

A joint is the site where two bones connect to provide mobility or stability. Some joints (e.g., in the cranium) do not move. Other joints flex, extend, rotate, abduct, or adduct. A moving joint consists of articulating bone surfaces (covered with cartilage), a two-layered bursal sac (containing synovial membranes to provide lubrication), and a capsule that thickens and becomes a ligament. Muscles overlying joints attach the bone surfaces one to another and provide movement.

GENERAL GUIDELINES FOR EMERGENCY MANAGEMENT

Because of the disfiguring and sometimes gruesome nature of orthopedic trauma, the tendency is to evaluate the specific injury and not the patient as a whole. Nevertheless, as is true for all emergency care, initial management of individuals with musculoskeletal complaints begins with an assessment of airway, breathing, and circulatory status. Unless otherwise indicated, the following general patient management guidelines should be applied to all persons with an acute musculoskeletal complaint[2]:

- Perform a primary assessment (airway, breathing, circulation, disability) and initiate appropriate interventions. (See Chapter 34.)
- Evaluate the neurovascular status of each injured extremity.
- Secure any impaled objects.
- Remove rings, other jewelry, and tight clothing (e.g., boots) from injured extremities.
- Immobilize extremities beyond the joints above and below the site of injury.
- Reevaluate neurovascular status after repositioning or immobilization.
- Cover open wounds with a sterile dressing.
- Apply ice packs to areas of swelling.
- Avoid putting any cleaning solutions (e.g., hexachlorophene, hydrogen peroxide, isopropyl alcohol, or povidone-iodine) directly in a wound. (See Chapter 12.)
- Elevate injured extremities.
- Obtain radiographs as indicated.
- Assess the patient's tetanus immunization status and vaccinate as needed.
- Manage pain.
- Hold all oral food, fluids, and medications if emergency surgery is probable.
- Repeat radiographs after any manipulation.
- Obtain orthopedic surgical consultation.

Neurovascular Assessment

Any patient who has extremity trauma is at risk for potential neurovascular injuries and tissue ischemia. Use the five *P*'s to evaluate limb circulation, sensation, and motor function:

Pain: A description of the pain is helpful. Is the pain diffuse or tender at a specific point ("point tenderness")? Ischemic pain usually is described as burning or throbbing. Did the pain occur immediately upon injury or develop later? What are the precipitating and relieving factors? Have the patient rate the pain on a scale of 0 to 10 so that changes can be tracked. (See Chapter 14.)

Pallor: What is the color of the injured extremity? Is there mottling? Check capillary refill and skin temperature.

Pulses: How strong are proximal and distal pulses? How do these pulses compare with those on the unaffected side?

Paresthesia: Does the patient have two-point discrimination in the toes or fingers of the affected extremity? The unaffected extremity? Is there tingling, numbness, burning, or another abnormal sensation?

Paralysis: What is the general mobility of the limb? Was there loss of movement after the initial injury? Does the patient have extremity weakness?

Inspection

Inspect the injured area for the following:
- Color
- Disrupted skin integrity
- Extremity position
- Edema, swelling, or ecchymosis
- Range of motion
- Symmetry, alignment, deformity

Palpation

Palpate the injury to identify the following:
- Skin temperature
- Pain, point tenderness
- Bony crepitus, joint instability
- Peripheral nerve function: Sensory and motor

Age-Related Characteristics

Pediatrics

Musculoskeletal injuries in children frequently are related to recreational activities. The incidence of orthopedic trauma increases as the child's environment expands to encompass bicycles, skateboards, trampolines, and motorized vehicles. Specific physiologic phenomena pertinent to pediatric injuries include the following:
- The epiphyseal growth plate does not close until after adolescence. Growth plate injuries may arrest healing and bone formation.
- The child's incomplete calcification renders bones more pliable than those of adults. This results in greenstick fractures that do not extend through the cortex.
- Fractures, lacerations, abrasions, or other trauma not consistent with the reported mechanism of injury should be evaluated for the possibility of child maltreatment.
- In children with joint effusion and no fracture, repeat an examination in 7 to 10 days if symptoms are still present.
- The majority of dislocations are associated with fractures, not ligamentous laxity.

Geriatrics

Falls are the most frequent mechanism of musculoskeletal trauma in the elderly. The incidence of fractures, especially of the hip and wrist, increases with age. Consider also the possibility of elder abuse. Risk factors for orthopedic and soft tissue injury in the elderly include the following:

- Chronic diseases such as diabetes
- History of extensive smoking or steroid use
- Gait and balance disturbances
- Osteoporosis
- Muscle mass loss because of atrophy
- Arthritis (limits mobility and joint flexibility)
- Subcutaneous tissue loss (less protection for underlying structures)
- Decreased bone density
- Reduced skin elasticity
- Increased healing time
- Poor nutritional status

Splinting of Orthopedic Injuries

Splinting is done to decrease pain, limit further bone and soft tissue injury, and minimize damage to nerves, arteries, and veins. Always immobilize extremities by splinting beyond the joints above and below the site of injury. For patient teaching regarding splints, see Patient Education and Discharge Instructions at the end of this chapter.[3]

A variety of splint materials is available, from commercial products to household items, but splints can be divided into four basic types:

- *Soft splints:* Nonrigid, such as a pillow
- *Hard splints:* A firm, rigid surface such as a board
- *Air splints:* Inflatable splints, which provide rigidity without being hard
- *Traction splints:* Splints that support fractures, decrease angulation, and provide traction

General Splinting Principles

Follow these general splinting principles:

- First, assess neurovascular status to determine a baseline for future comparisons.
- Remove all jewelry and (preferably) clothing from the injured area.
- Assemble equipment and padding before moving the injured part.
- Solicit adequate personnel to assist with splint application.
- Immobilize the joints proximal and distal to the injury.
- Correct severe angulation only if it is impossible to apply a splint in the current position or if neurovascular compromise is present. Otherwise, splint them as they lie.
- Ensure that splints are well padded.
- Secure the injured part to the splint. Do not impair circulation by securing too tightly.
- Reassess neurovascular status after splinting or moving the injured site.
- Avoid snug splints or casts when the risk of compartment syndrome is high.
- Careful consideration is required before splinting or casting infected wounds.

SOFT TISSUE INJURIES

See Chapter 12.

JOINT AND MUSCLE INJURIES

Strains

Strains are caused by muscle stretching or tearing. First-degree strains usually result when a muscle is stretched with excessive force. The cause of second-degree strain is similar but involves disruption of a greater amount of muscle tissue. In third-degree strain, complete disruption of the muscle fibers and possible rupture of the overlying fascia occurs. Commonly strained muscle groups are the gastrocnemius, biceps, hamstrings, and quadriceps.

Signs and symptoms

First-Degree Strains

- Local pain aggravated by movement
- Point tenderness
- Spasm
- Ecchymosis

Second-Degree Strains

- Same as those for first-degree strain but usually more severe

Third-Degree Strains

- Point tenderness, severe pain
- Swelling
- Discoloration, hematoma formation
- Snapping noise at the time of injury
- Loss of muscle function at the time of injury

Therapeutic Interventions

First- and Second-Degree Strains

- See General Guidelines for Emergency Management.
- Apply a compression bandage (e.g., Ace wrap)
- Elevate for 48 hours.
- Apply cold packs for 48 hours; heat after 72 hours.
- Immobilize the injured muscle as needed.
- Avoid active or passive stretching.
- Begin light weight bearing when pain is resolved.

Third-Degree Strains

- See General Guidelines for Emergency Management.
- Splint the affected part.
- Elevate for 48 hours.
- Apply cold packs for 48 hours.
- Do not permit weight bearing.
- Refer patient to an orthopedic surgeon for evaluation.

Sprains

Sprains can occur in any movable joint and are among the most common complaints treated in emergency departments. Sprains result from the stretching or tearing of the supporting ligaments of a joint. Sprains are rare in children whose epiphyseal plates are still open. Ankle sprains generally are caused by inversion stress.

Categories

Sprains are categorized as follows:

First-degree: Disruption of a few ligament fibers; no joint instability; minimal swelling and discoloration

Second-degree: Partial ligamentous tear; intact joint; increased swelling and ecchymosis

Third-degree: Complete ligamentous disruption; joint unstable when stressed; significant swelling and ecchymosis

Signs and symptoms

First-Degree Sprains

- Slight pain, swelling
- Patient may not complain of pain for up to 24 hours after injury.

Second-Degree Sprains

- Point tenderness, local pain
- Swelling, discoloration
- Short-term disability

Third-Degree Sprains

- Pain (may be painless with complete rupture)
- Point tenderness
- Diffuse swelling
- Discoloration
- Joint instability
- An egg-shaped swelling develops within 2 hours of injury.

Therapeutic interventions

- See General Guidelines for Emergency Management.
- Provide posterior splint, air splint, or gel splint.
- Use crutches as needed.
- Refer patient to an orthopedic surgeon for evaluation.[4]
- Range of motion should be reassessed every 2 to 3 weeks until healing is complete.

PERIPHERAL NERVE INJURIES

Peripheral nerve injuries can be produced by trauma (mechanical, chemical, or thermal), toxins, malignancy, metabolic disorders, or collagen diseases. In the setting of acute trauma, peripheral nerve injuries usually are associated with lacerations, fractures, dislocations, or penetrating wounds. Emergency department diagnosis of peripheral nerve injury is based on clinical evaluation. Diagnostic tests such as electromyography, nerve conduction studies, and electrical stimulation are of little or no value for urgent evaluation. Repair of peripheral nerves requires expert surgical intervention and should not be undertaken in an emergency department. Table 39-1 lists major peripheral nerves, common associated injuries, and clinical assessment techniques.

Table 39-1   Modes for Assessing Common Peripheral Nerve Injuries

Nerve	Frequently Associated Injuries	Assessment Technique*
Radial	Fractures of the humerus, especially the middle and distal thirds	Inability to extend the thumb in a "hitchhiker's sign"
Ulnar	Fractures of the medial humeral epicondyle	Loss of pain perception in the tip of the little finger
Median	Elbow dislocation; wrist or forearm injury	Loss of pain perception in the index finger
Peroneal	Tibia or fibula fracture; dislocation of the knee	Inability to extend the great toe or foot; also may be associated with sciatic nerve injury
Sciatic and tibial	Occurs infrequently with fractures; associated with dislocation of the knee	Loss of pain perception in the sole of the foot

*Tests may be invalid if extension tendons are severed or severe muscle damage is present. Sensation testing is subjective and can be inaccurate.

Table 39-2   Types of Fractures

Type	Etiology
Transverse	Angulation force or direct trauma
Oblique	Twisting force
Spiral	Twisting force with a firmly planted foot
Comminuted	Severe direct trauma, such as crush injuries and high-velocity bullets; more than two bone fragments are present
Impacted	Severe trauma causing fracture ends to jam together
Compressed	Severe force to the top of the head or from an acceleration/deceleration injury
Greenstick	Compression force; usually occurs in children under 10 years of age
Avulsion	A muscle mass contracts forcefully, causing a bone fragment to tear off at the muscle insertion site; ligaments also can tear fragments from bone
Depressed	Blunt trauma to a flat bone; usually involves extensive soft tissue damage

See Figure 39-1 for illustrations.

FRACTURES

Several types of fractures occur (Table 39-2; Figure 39-1). These can be divided into two general categories:

1. *Closed (simple):* The bone is broken but the skin is intact.
2. *Open (compound):* The bone is broken and the skin is disrupted by the following:
   • A bone that has punctured through from the inside
   • An object that has penetrated from the outside at or near the fracture site

SPECIFIC UPPER EXTREMITY INJURIES

Clavicular Fractures

Clavicular fractures are the most common childhood fractures; 80% occur in the middle one third of the clavicle (Figure 39-2). (See Chapter 37.)

Mechanism of injury

• Fall on an extended arm or shoulder
• Direct blow to the lateral shoulder

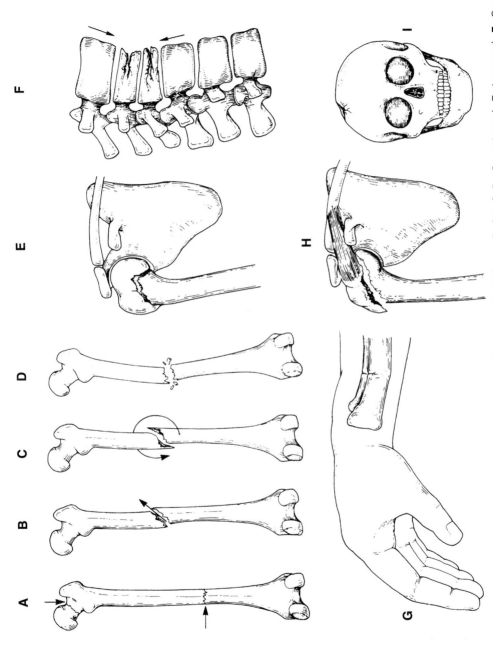

Figure 39-1. Types of fracture: transverse through depressed. **A,** Transverse. **B,** Oblique. **C,** Spiral. **D,** Comminuted. **E,** Impacted. **F,** Compressed. **G,** Greenstick. **H,** Avulsion. **I,** Depressed. See Table 39-2 for descriptions.

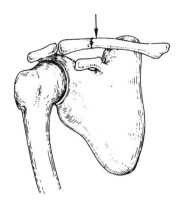

Figure 39-2. Clavicular fracture.

Signs and symptoms

- Pain in the clavicular area, point tenderness
- Swelling, deformity, bony crepitus
- Patient refuses to raise the affected arm

Therapeutic interventions

- See General Guidelines for Emergency Management.
- Immobilize shoulder.
- Use a figure-of-eight splint (controversial)

Complications

- Brachial plexus injury
- Subclavian vascular injury
- Ligamentous damage
- Malunion

Special note

When splinting, pad the axilla well to avoid damage to the brachial plexus and artery.

Shoulder and Proximal Humeral Injuries

Fractures to the proximal humerus include all injuries involving the humeral head and neck. Shoulder fractures occur more commonly in the elderly because of bone decalcification and weakened musculature. More than 80% of proximal humeral fractures are nondisplaced (Figure 39-3).

Mechanism of injury

- Fall on an outstretched arm
- Direct trauma to the shoulder from a blunt instrument or fall

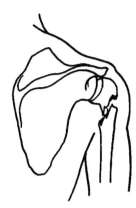

Figure 39-3. Displaced fracture of the proximal humerus.

Signs and symptoms

- Pain in the shoulder area
- Point tenderness
- Inability to move the affected arm
- Posterior rotation
- Adduction of the humerus
- Abduction of the humerus (this finding is associated with a higher incidence of neurovascular compromise)
- Gross swelling and discoloration that may extend to the chest wall

Therapeutic interventions

- See General Guidelines for Emergency Management.
- Immobilize the arm in a sling and swath.
- Surgery may be required for impacted, comminuted, or displaced fractures, especially of the humeral neck.

Complications

- Laceration of the axillary artery
- Brachial plexus injury
- Avascular necrosis of the humeral head
- Frozen shoulder syndrome
- Nonunion

Scapular Fractures

Scapular fractures are a relatively uncommon injury. A great deal of force is necessary to break a scapula. Because of the force required, look for associated injuries such as rib fractures, pulmonary contusions, and neurovascular compromise (Figure 39-4).

Mechanism of injury

- Direct trauma, blunt or penetrating

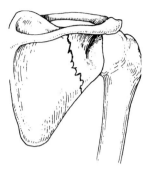

Figure 39-4. Scapular fracture.

Signs and symptoms

- Pain on shoulder movement
- Point tenderness
- Swelling, ecchymosis
- The arm usually is held in adduction, with resistance to abduction.
- Palpable bony displacement

Therapeutic interventions

- See General Guidelines for Emergency Management.
- Immobilize the arm in a sling and swath.
- Pad the axilla well to avoid damage to the brachial plexus and artery.

Complications

- Underlying injury to the ribs
- Pneumothorax, hemothorax
- Compression fractures of the spine

Upper Arm Fractures (Humeral Shaft)

Suspect abuse when humeral shaft (diaphyseal) fractures are found in the very young or very old. Because of its proximity to the shaft, the radial nerve is susceptible to injury when the humerus fractures. Assess for neurovascular impairment of the median, ulnar, and radial nerves (Figure 39-5).

Mechanism of injury

- Fall on the arm or a direct blow
- Twisting or throwing of the arm

Signs and symptoms

- Pain, point tenderness
- Swelling, bruising

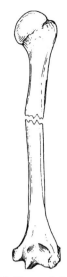

Figure 39-5. Humeral shaft fracture.

- Inability or hesitance to move the arm
- Severe deformity or angulation
- Bony crepitus

Therapeutic interventions

- See General Guidelines for Emergency Management.
- Immobilize the arm in a sling and swath.
- Prepare for surgical intervention for the following:
  - Shaft fractures with vascular compromise
  - Spiral fractures of the distal third of the humerus with radial nerve palsy
  - Fractures extending into the elbow

Complications

Stretching or laceration of the radial nerve can cause neuropraxia (failure of nerve conduction in the absence of structural changes).

Elbow Fractures (Supracondylar, Epicondylar, and Intercondylar)

Mechanism of injury

- Fall on an extended arm (Figure 39-6)
- Fall on a flexed elbow

Signs and symptoms

- Severe pain, point tenderness
- Rapid swelling

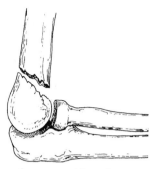

Figure 39-6. Elbow fracture.

- Shortening of the arm, deformity
- Delayed capillary refill

Therapeutic interventions

- See General Guidelines for Emergency Management.
- Splint the arm in the presenting position, "as it lies."
- If neurovascular compromise is noted, try flexing the arm.
- Refer patient to an orthopedic surgeon for evaluation.
- Admit patient for observation of neurovascular status.
- Perform an arteriogram if vascular compromise is noted.

Complications

- Brachial artery laceration
- Nerve damage (median, radial)
- Volkmann's ischemic contracture

Forearm Fractures (Radius or Ulna)

Although isolated radial fractures are not unusual, it is more common for injuries severe enough to fracture the radius to fracture the ulna as well (Figure 39-7). Monteggia's fracture is a break at the junction of the proximal and middle thirds of the ulna. This fracture is associated with anterior dislocation of the radial head. Because of its proximity to the radial nerve, assess neurovascular function carefully.

Mechanism of injury

- Fall on an extended arm
- Direct blow ("nightstick fractures")
- Forced pronation of the forearm

Signs and symptoms

- Pain, point tenderness
- Swelling
- Deformity, angulation, shortening

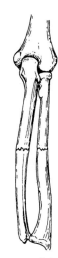

Figure 39-7. Fracture of the radius and ulna.

Therapeutic interventions

- See General Guidelines for Emergency Management.
- Assist with closed reduction.
- Assist with casting.
- Refer patient to an orthopedic surgeon for evaluation.
- Prepare for possible open reduction and internal fixation.

Complications

- Paralysis of the radial nerve
- Malunion
- Volkmann's ischemic contracture

Special note

A fracture of the ulnar can be a defensive wound inflicted by a blunt object, hence the name "nightstick" fracture. Examine the patient for concomitant injuries.

Wrist Fractures (Distal Radius, Distal Ulna, and Carpal Bone)

The bones of the wrist are frequently fractured. These injuries are particularly common in unsteady, osteoporotic, elderly patients who fall. Always examine the opposite extremity; bilateral wrist fractures are not unusual.[5]

Mechanism of injury

- Dorsiflexion, generally following a fall on an extended arm and open hand

Signs and symptoms

- Pain
- "Snuff box" tenderness if the navicular bone (scaphoid) is fractured (Figure 39-8)

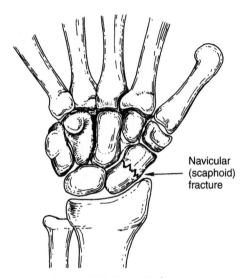

Figure 39-8. Navicular fracture.

- Swelling
- Deformity (may be severe with a Colles' fracture)
- Limited range of motion
- Numbness, weakness

Therapeutic interventions

- See General Guidelines for Emergency Management.
- Prepare for closed reduction of displaced fractures.
- Place a rigid splint or a thumb spica cast.
- Refer patient to an orthopedic surgeon for evaluation.

Complication

- Rare aseptic necrosis

Special notes

- Navicular (scaphoid) bone fractures may not be radiographically apparent for 4 to 6 weeks.[6] Patients who have pain in the "anatomical snuff box" following trauma should be splinted and referred to an orthopedic surgeon for evaluation and repeat radiographs in 2 weeks.
- A combined fracture of the distal radius and ulna is known as a Colles' fracture, or "silver fork" deformity. This type of fracture usually occurs in the distal one third of the ulna. Investigate the mechanism of injury. The patient (particularly younger patients) may have fallen from a height. Check for associated lumbodorsal compression fractures and calcaneal (heel) fractures.

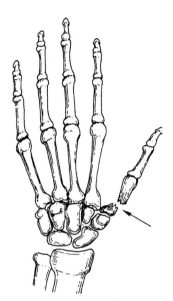

Figure 39-9. Finger fracture.

Hand and Finger Fractures (Carpals, Metacarpals, and Phalanges)

Distal phalanx fractures are the most frequent hand fractures (Figure 39-9). Because no other body part plays a greater role in the activities of daily life, hand injuries should be evaluated promptly. Nondisplaced or impacted fractures are often not apparent on initial radiographs; lucency at the fracture site will be visible within 10 to 14 days.[6] When caring for individuals with hand injuries, consider the patient's hand dominance, occupation, and other factors that may influence recovery.[7]

Mechanism of injury

- Forceful hyperextension
- Direct trauma
- Crush injury

Signs and symptoms

- Pain
- Severe swelling
- Deformity
- Inability to use the hand
- Open fractures (common)

Therapeutic interventions

- See General Guidelines for Emergency Management.
- Prepare for closed reduction of displaced fractures.

- Apply finger traction.
- Splint distal phalanges with a padded aluminum guard.
- "Buddy tape" an injured digit to the adjacent finger.
- Antibiotics are indicated for open fractures.
- Internal fixation rarely is required.

Complications

- Malunion
- Osteomyelitis
- Subungual hematoma

Special note

A fractured fourth and/or fifth metacarpal head routinely is referred to as a "boxer's" fracture. These fractures commonly are caused by punching an object. If the punch was to a human mouth, any open wounds should be considered a human bite; this makes an otherwise minor injury an open, contaminated fracture.

High-Pressure Injection Injuries

See Chapter 12.

Subungual Hematoma

See Chapter 12.

Pelvic Fractures

Pelvic fractures can be classified as stable or unstable. Stable pelvic fractures do not transect the pelvic ring and are not associated with significant hemorrhage. Unstable pelvic fractures result when the posterior elements or the integrity of the ring are disrupted (Figure 39-10). These fractures may be open or closed, and this is a potentially life-threatening injury. Pelvic fracture mortality is 6% to 19%.[4]

Most pelvic fractures are associated with a significant mechanism of injury, and 65% of patients also will have trauma to other body areas. The pelvic region is highly vascular and can accommodate large quantities of blood. Because hemorrhage is the leading cause of early death from pelvic fractures, aggressive resuscitation and management of patients with this major trauma is crucial.[8] See Chapters 22 and 34.

Mechanism of injury

- Motor vehicle collision
- Fall from a height
- Crush injury
- Direct trauma

Signs and symptoms

- Tenderness when the pubis or iliac wings are compressed
- Paraspinous muscle spasm

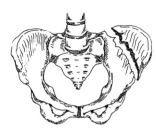

Stable fracture not
involving the ring

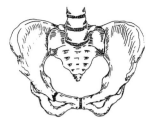

Stable fracture; minimal
displaced fracture of the ring

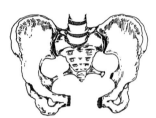

Rotationally unstable,
vertically stable "open
book" fracture

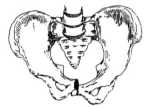

Rotationally unstable,
vertically stable lateral
compression (ipsilateral)

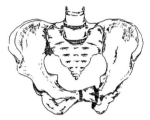

Rotationally unstable,
vertically stable lateral
compression (contralateral
bucket handle)

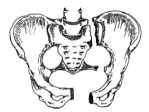

Rotationally and vertically
unstable bilaterally

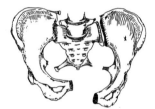

Rotationally and vertically
unstable associated with
acetabular fracture (not shown)

Figure 39-10. Various pelvic fractures. From Kozin S, Berlet A: Pelvis and acetabulum. In *Handbook of common orthopaedic fracture*, ed 2, Chester, Pa, 1992, Medical Surveillance.

- Sacroiliac joint tenderness
- Paresis or hemiparesis
- Pelvic ecchymosis
- Hematuria
- Groin pain
- Inability to bear weight
- Inability to void
- Blood at the urethral meatus
- Perineal hematomas
- Prostate displacement, loss of sphincter tone

Therapeutic interventions

Open or Unstable Pelvic Fractures

- See General Guidelines for Emergency Management.
- Provide aggressive resuscitation: Oxygen, crystalloids, blood (massive transfusion may be required).[8]
- Immobilize the spine and legs (long board). Flexing the knees may decrease pain.
- Perform frequent (every 5 minutes) vital sign assessment.
- Consult an orthopedic surgeon for evaluation.
- Provide pelvic stabilization, which decreases fracture mobility, limits pelvic ring expansion, and reduces hemorrhage:
  - Pneumatic antishock garment (Inflate the abdominal section.)
  - Pelvic binder: Commercial device or a tightly tied sheet
  - External fixation
  - Internal fixation
- Prepare for pelvic computed tomography scan.[9]
- Prepare for angiography with possible embolization.[10]
- Prepare for peritoneal lavage, abdominal computed tomography scan, or possible laparotomy (to explore intraabdominal injuries). (See Chapter 38.)
- Administer antibiotics.

Stable Pelvic Fractures

- See General Guidelines for Emergency Management.
- Treat patient symptomatically.
- Encourage bed rest for 2 to 3 weeks.
- Apply a pelvic belt, strap, or traction.
- Provide crutches or walker.
- Administer laxatives.

Complications

- Hemorrhage, shock, death
- Bladder, genital, or lumbosacral trauma
- Ruptured internal organs; gastrointestinal tract injury
- Pulmonary or fat emboli
- Chronic pain
- Compartment syndrome
- Osteomyelitis

Hip Fractures (Acetabulum, Greater Trochanter, and Femoral Head)

Mechanism of injury

- Frequently seen in pedestrian trauma (Figure 39-11)
- Direct blow or fall (common in the elderly; osteoporosis is a major risk factor)
- Axial transmission of force from the knees (knee-to-dashboard injuries)

Signs and symptoms

- Pain in the hip or groin area
- Severe pain with movement

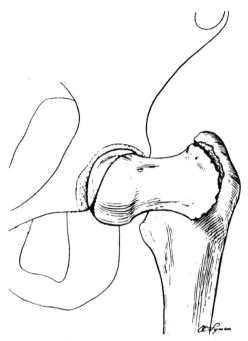

Figure 39-11. Hip fracture.

- Inability to bear weight
- External rotation of the affected hip and leg
- Shortening of the affected limb (minimal)
- If injury is extracapsular and associated with a trochanteric fracture, then look for the following:
  - Pain in the lateral hip
  - Increased shortening
  - Greater external rotation

Therapeutic interventions

Interventions depend largely on the mechanism of injury. Is this a pedestrian hit by a speeding motor vehicle? (Manage as a major trauma patient.) Or is this an elderly, osteoporotic individual with a ground-level fall? (Manage symptomatically.)

Consider the following interventions for hip fractures:
- See General Guidelines for Emergency Management.
- Immobilize in a position of comfort. Backboards and other splinting materials will require padding, especially for elderly patients.
- Apply traction.
- Consult an orthopedic surgeon for evaluation.
- Prepare for surgical intervention.

Complications

- Avascular necrosis of the femoral head
- Phlebitis of the femoral vein

- Osteoarthritis
- Sciatic nerve injury
- Fat emboli syndrome
- Hypovolemic shock

Femoral Shaft Fractures

Femoral shaft fractures occur between the subtrochanteric and supracondylar regions of the femur (Figure 39-12). Fractures may be open or closed. Look for associated injuries, especially of the knee, hip, pelvis, and lower leg. The thigh can accommodate large volumes of blood; assess for hemorrhagic shock. In the young child, consider the possibility of maltreatment. Seventy percent of femoral fractures in children younger than 3 years are the result of nonaccidental trauma.[4]

Mechanism of injury

- Indirect force transmitted upward through a flexed knee
- Direct trauma
- Motor vehicle and automobile-pedestrian trauma
- Gunshot wounds
- Falls

Signs and symptoms

- Angulation, deformity
- Limb shortening
- Severe muscle spasm

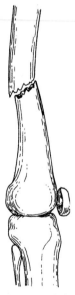

Figure 39-12. Femoral shaft fracture.

- Bony crepitus
- Severe pain
- Swelling of the thigh
- Hematoma formation in the thigh
- Inability to bear weight on the affected leg

Therapeutic interventions

- See General Guidelines for Emergency Management.
- Provide aggressive resuscitation: Oxygen, crystalloids, blood (massive transfusion may be required).
- Perform frequent (every 5 minutes) vital sign assessment.
- Immobilize thigh with a traction splint, (e.g., Sager, Fernotrac, or Hare).
- Refer patient to an orthopedic surgeon for evaluation.
- Prepare for open reduction with internal fixation.

Complications

- Hemorrhage (Average blood loss is 1000 mL.)
- Severe muscle damage
- Knee trauma (often overlooked at the time of injury)

Knee Sprains and Strains

Mechanism of injury

Knee injuries are caused by extreme rotation, hyperextension, or hyperflexion.

Common types

- Medial meniscus injury: Rotational trauma
- Collateral ligament injury: Medial injuries result from valgus stress; lateral ones from varus stress.
- Anterior and posterior cruciate ligament injury: Hyperextension trauma

Signs and symptoms

- Swelling, effusion, ecchymosis
- Pain, tenderness
- Joint instability

Therapeutic interventions

- See General Guidelines for Emergency Management.
- Apply a compression bandage (e.g., Ace wrap).
- Apply a knee immobilizer.
- Provide crutches.
- Ensure no weight bearing.
- Refer patient to an orthopedic surgeon for evaluation.

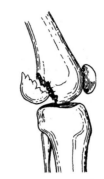

Figure 39-13. Knee fracture.

Knee Fractures (Supracondylar or Intraarticular Femur Fracture or Tibial Fracture)

Mechanism of injury

- High-velocity vehicular trauma (Figure 39-13)
- Pedestrian trauma: "Bumper" or "fender" fractures
- Fall from a height onto a flexed knee
- Hyperabduction

Signs and symptoms

- Bony crepitus
- Tense swelling in the popliteal area
- Hemarthrosis, swelling around the joint
- Knee pain, tenderness
- Inability to bend or straighten the knee

Therapeutic interventions

- See General Guidelines for Emergency Management.
- Apply a non–weight-bearing cast.
- Refer patient to an orthopedic surgeon for evaluation.
- Prepare for open reduction and internal fixation.
- Apply traction.
- Provide crutches.

Complications

- Popliteal nerve or artery injury
- Fat emboli
- Rotational deformities
- Traumatic arthritis

Patellar Fractures

Mechanism of injury

- Usually caused by direct trauma (dashboard impact or a fall; Figure 39-14)
- Indirect trauma following quadriceps muscle pull or contraction

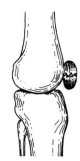

Figure 39-14. Patellar fracture.

Signs and symptoms

- Knee pain
- Open fracture (common)
- Hemarthrosis
- Inability to extend the knee actively

Therapeutic interventions

- See General Guidelines for Emergency Management.
- Injury may require surgery for quadriceps repair.
- Antibiotics are indicated for open fractures.
- Inpatient admission is required.

Complications

- Avascular necrosis

Tibia-Fibula Fractures

The tibia is the most frequently fractured long bone and the most common open fracture. The lateral tibial plateau has the highest incidence of fractures. Examine the lateral condyle for associated knee injuries, especially in older individuals. The fibula frequently is broken in association with the tibia; isolated fibular shaft fractures are uncommon. The fibula is a non–weight-bearing bone, but the distal portion is essential for ankle stability (Figure 39-15).

Mechanism of injury

- Rotational or twisting forces
- Direct trauma
- Fall with compression forces
- Fall with the foot fixed in place (e.g., ski injury)

Signs and symptoms

- Pain, point tenderness
- Swelling

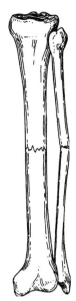

Figure 39-15. Tibia-fibula fracture.

- Deformity
- Bony crepitus

Therapeutic interventions

- See General Guidelines for Emergency Management.
- Check for any puncture that may have been caused by the tibial bone (open fracture).
- Perform wound debridement and irrigation.
- Assist with casting.
- Provide crutches.
- Open reduction and internal fixation is indicated for displaced or complicated fractures.

Complications

- Compartment syndrome: Usually occurs within 24 to 48 hours of injury
- Infection
- Osteomyelitis
- Nonunion

Special note

Tibial plateau fractures generally require individuals to be non–weight bearing for 6 months.

Ankle Fractures

The ankle bears more weight than any other joint in the body, and it is the joint most commonly injured (Figure 39-16). The majority of ankle injuries occur with the foot planted or fixed on the ground. The extent of injury varies greatly depending on the position of the foot

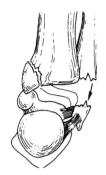

Figure 39-16. Ankle fracture.

Box **39-1**   Ottawa Ankle Rules

An ankle series is required only for patients with pain in the malleolar zone
AND
Bone tenderness at the posterior edge or tip of either the lateral or medial malleolus
OR
A total inability to bear weight immediately after the injury and for four steps in the emergency
  department.
A foot x-ray series is required only if the patient has some pain in the midfoot
AND
Bone tenderness at the base of the fifth metatarsal
OR
Navicular bone tenderness
OR
An inability to bear weight immediately and in the emergency department.
These criteria exclude patients who are pregnant, who are less than 18 years old, and whose injuries occurred
  10 days or more prior.

From Stiell IG et al: Implementation of the Ottawa Ankle Rules, *JAMA* 271(11):827–32, 1994.

(fixed, supinated, pronated, or inverted) and the direction of force applied (eversion, inversion, or rotation). The Ottawa Ankle Rules (Box 39-1) are evidence-based guidelines used to predict malleolar and foot fractures. They have been shown to be nearly 100% sensitive. Nonetheless, specificity is low; 77% of patients who meet the Ottawa criteria have no fracture.[9]

Mechanism of injury

- Direct trauma
- Indirect trauma
- Torsion, inversion, or eversion

Signs and symptoms

- Patients may report a popping sound at the time of injury (torn ligaments).
- Ecchymosis
- Bony crepitus
- Pain upon ambulation or altered gait
- Inability to bear weight if the injury is unstable

Therapeutic interventions

- See General Guidelines for Emergency Management.
- Assist with closed reduction.
- Apply a posterior splint.
- Prepare for possible open reduction and internal fixation.
- Assist with casting.
- Provide crutches.

Complications

- Nonunion (primarily following closed reduction)
- Infection
- Posttraumatic arthritis
- Sudeck's atrophy: A form of sympathetic dystrophy characterized by rapidly developing osteoporosis, burning pain, and trophic changes in the foot

Achilles Tendon Rupture

Mechanism of injury

This injury most commonly occurs during stop-and-start sports (e.g., tennis, racquetball, and basketball) when the patient steps abruptly on the forefoot, with the knee forced into extension. Diagnosis is based on clinical findings.

Signs and symptoms

- Deformity along the Achilles tendon (a palpable deficit)
- Complete tears that cause a severe, sharp pain in the lower calf (a sensation of being "kicked in the back of the leg")
- Inability to walk

Therapeutic interventions

- See General Guidelines for Emergency Management.
- Apply a compression dressing (e.g., Ace wrap).
- Refer patient to an orthopedic surgeon for evaluation.
- Prepare for possible walking cast application.
- Prepare for possible surgical repair.
- Provide crutches.
- Splint the foot in plantar flexion.

Foot Fractures (Metatarsals)

The foot contains 28 bones and 57 articulating surfaces. Because foot injuries often are associated with ankle trauma, the foot and ankle should always be assessed together (Figure 39-17). Certain systemic disorders, such as diabetes and peripheral vascular disease, may influence the severity of foot injuries and the extent of treatment.

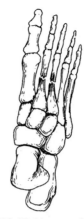

Figure 39-17. Metatarsal fracture.

Mechanism of injury

- Similar to ankle injury mechanisms
- Athletic injuries
- Direct trauma

Signs and symptoms

- Deep pain, point tenderness
- Ecchymosis, swelling
- Subungual hematoma
- Hesitance to bear weight
- Deformity

Therapeutic interventions

- See General Guidelines for Emergency Management.
- Bulky dressing
- Orthopedic shoe
- Posterior splint
- Cane or crutches
- Early weight bearing in most cases

Complications

- Avascular necrosis
- Malunion
- Gait abnormalities

Heel Fractures (Calcaneus)

Twenty-five percent of all calcaneal fractures are associated with other injuries to the lower extremity; 10% are bilateral (Figure 39-18). Look for concomitant leg, lumbar, or lower thoracic fractures in patients with heel trauma.

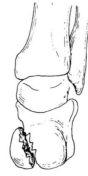

Figure 39-18. Calcaneal fracture.

Mechanism of injury

- Fall from a height

Signs and symptoms

- Pain increases with hyperflexion
- Point tenderness and pain in the hindfoot
- Soft tissue ecchymosis
- Superficial skin blistering
- Deformity

Therapeutic interventions

- Pay special attention to the mechanism of injury and look for associated trauma.
- See General Guidelines for Emergency Management.
- Apply a bulky compressive dressing.
- Ensure non–weight bearing or partial weight bearing.
- Provide crutches.
- Heels are not routinely casted for 2 days to 2 weeks following injury.
- Closed reduction is indicated for displaced fractures.

Complications

- Chronic pain
- Nerve entrapment

Toe Fractures (Phalanges)

Mechanism of injury

- Direct trauma such as kicking or toe stubbing (Figure 39-19)
- Crush injuries
- Athletic injuries

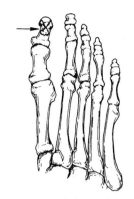

Figure 39-19. Phalangeal fracture.

Signs and symptoms

- Subungual hematoma
- Deformity
- Pain
- Discoloration

Therapeutic interventions

- See General Guidelines for Emergency Management.
- Apply a compression dressing.
- "Buddy tape" the injured digit to the toe next to it.
- Provide orthopedic shoe.
- Suggest cane use as needed.

DISLOCATIONS AND SUBLUXATIONS

Dislocations and subluxations result when a joint exceeds its range of motion. The difference between the two injuries is one of degree. A dislocation (or separation) is a complete joint disruption in which the articular surfaces are no longer in contact. Subluxations are less severe disruptions; some contact between articular surfaces remains. These injuries can damage adjacent vessels and nerves. Therefore dislocations should be reduced as soon as possible. Severe muscle spasm around the joint is common, and intravenously administered muscle relaxants (benzodiazepines) often are needed for successful reduction. Table 39-3 summarizes dislocation and subluxation injuries.

Signs and Symptoms

Signs and symptoms of dislocations and subluxations are as follows:
- Severe pain
- Deformity at the joint
- Inability to move the joint

Table 39-3   **Common Dislocations**

Body Area	Typical Mechanism of Injury	Clinical Findings	Treatment
Shoulder	Anterior fall on an outstretched arm or a direct blow to the shoulder	Arm abducted, cannot bring the elbow down to the chest or touch the hand of the affected side to the opposite ear	Splint in a position of comfort; reduce as soon as possible.
Posterior	Rare; strong blow to the front of the shoulder; violent convulsions or seizures	Arm held at the side, unable to externally rotate the arm	Same as for shoulder
Elbow Radius and ulna	Fall on an outstretched hand with the elbow in extension	Arm shortened pain with motion; rapid swelling; nerve injury may occur	Same as for shoulder Surgical repair is required if the dislocation is associated with fracture of the radial head or olecranon.
Radial head (children)	Sudden longitudinal pull, jerk, or lift on a child's wrist or hand ("nursemaid's elbow")	Pain; patient refuses to use the arm; limited supination; can flex and extend at the elbow; may have no deformity	Reduce; place in a sling; advise parents that this may recur until the age of 5 years.
Hip (usually posterior)	Blow to the knee while the hip is flexed and adducted (sitting with crossed knees); common in front seat passengers in a motor vehicle collision	Hip flexed, adducted, internally rotated, and shortened; may have an associated fracture of the femur; sciatic nerve injury (this nerve lies posterior to the femoral head)	Splint in a position of comfort; reduce as soon as possible.
Patella	1. Spontaneous	The knee is flexed; the patella can be palpated lateral to the femoral condyle	Reduce dislocation (may occur spontaneously) or immobilize with a cast or splint.
	2. Associated with other trauma	Excessive swelling, tenderness, and a palpable soft tissue defect	Surgical repair of soft tissue injury or fractures is required.
Knee (rare)	Severe direct blow to the upper leg or forced hyperextension of the knee	Ligamentous instability; inability to straighten the leg; peroneal nerve and popliteal artery injury are common; assess distal neurovascular function	Immediate neurovascular assessment is necessary; reduce dislocation.
Ankle	The ankle is a complex joint, with multiple ligaments providing stability; dislocation usually is associated with other injuries such as fractures and soft tissue trauma	Swelling, tenderness; loss of alignment and function	Splint ankle; ankle dislocation usually requires open reduction because the joint is complex and must be realigned accurately.

From Kozin S, Berlet A: Pelvis and acetabulum. In *Handbook of common orthopaedic fractures*, ed 2, Chester, Pa, 1992, Medical Surveillance.

- Swelling
- Point tenderness

Therapeutic Interventions for Dislocations

Therapeutic interventions for dislocations include the following:
- See General Guidelines for Emergency Management.
- Carefully assess neurovascular status distal to the dislocation.
- Evaluate for concurrent fractures.
- Administer analgesic and muscle relaxant medications.
- Consult an orthopedic surgeon for evaluation.
- Reduce the dislocation/subluxation.
- Reevaluate neurovascular status following relocation.
- Obtain postreduction radiographs to verify relocation.

SPECIFIC DISLOCATIONS AND SUBLUXATIONS

This section discusses dislocations of the acromioclavicular joint, shoulder, elbow, wrist, hand or finger, hip, knee, patella, ankle, and foot.

Acromioclavicular Separation

Mechanism of injury

Acromioclavicular separation (Figure 39-20) is a common athletic injury produced by a fall or a direct blow to the point of the shoulder. The injury is common in cyclists.

Signs and symptoms

- Great pain in the joint area
- Inability to raise the arm or bring it across the chest
- Deformity
- Point tenderness or general area tenderness
- Swelling, hematoma formation

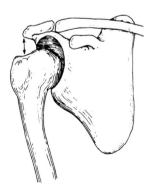

Figure 39-20. Acromioclavicular separation.

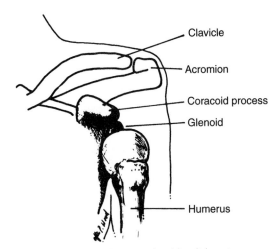

Figure 39-21. Anterior shoulder dislocation.

Therapeutic interventions

- See Therapeutic Interventions for Dislocations.
- Immobilize joint using a sling.

Shoulder Dislocation

More than half of all shoulder dislocations involve the glenohumeral joint, and 95% of dislocations are anterior (Figure 39-21).

Mechanism of injury

- *Anterior dislocation:* Usually an athletic injury resulting from a fall on an extended arm, which is abducted and externally rotated, forcing the head of the humerus anterior to the shoulder joint. In many individuals, this is a recurrent injury.
- *Posterior dislocation:* A rare dislocation sometimes seen in tonic-clonic seizure patients when an extended arm has been forcefully abducted and internally rotated.

Signs and symptoms

- Severe pain in the shoulder area
- Visible deformity (difficult to see in posterior dislocations)
- Palpable head of the humerus
- Inability to move the arm or touch the ear on the opposite side
- The arm is held in slight abduction and external rotation.

Therapeutic interventions

- See Therapeutic Interventions for Dislocations.
- Support arm in the position in which it was found or in the position of greatest comfort.
- Immobilize the arm in a sling and swath.

Complications

- Soft tissue damage
- Axillary nerve damage
- Rarely, axillary artery and brachial plexus damage

Elbow Dislocation

Mechanism of injury

- Fall on an extended arm (Figure 39-22)
- Young children: A sudden longitudinal pull on the arm with the forearm pronated (radial head subluxation or "nursemaid's elbow")[4]

Signs and symptoms

- Pain
- Swelling
- Deformity or lateral displacement
- Elbow that feels "locked"
- Severe pain produced by movement

Therapeutic interventions

- See Therapeutic Interventions for Dislocations.
- Immobilize the arm in a sling and swath.
- Provide prompt reduction when neurovascular compromise is present.
- Prepare for possible surgical repair.

Complications

The median nerve and brachial artery are at risk for compromise.

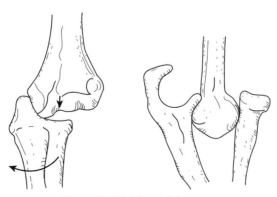

Figure 39-22. Elbow dislocation.

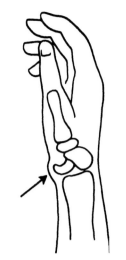

Figure 39-23. Wrist dislocation.

Wrist Dislocation

Mechanism of injury

- Fall on an outstretched hand (Figure 39-23)

Signs and symptoms

- Pain, point tenderness
- Swelling, deformity

Therapeutic interventions

- See Therapeutic Interventions for Dislocations.
- Splint the wrist.
- Immobilize the arm in a sling and swath in 90-degree flexion.

Complications

- Median nerve damage (an inability to pinch and loss of sensation in the index and middle fingers)[1]

Hand or Finger Dislocation

Mechanism of injury

- Fall on an outstretched hand or finger (Figure 39-24)
- Direct blow or a jamming force to the fingertip

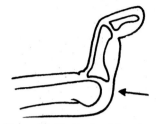

Figure 39-24. Finger dislocation.

Signs and symptoms

- Pain
- Inability to move the joint
- Swelling, deformity[7]

Therapeutic interventions

See Therapeutic Interventions for Dislocations.

Hip Dislocation

Mechanism of injury

- Usually associated with major trauma (e.g., frontal motor vehicle collision with the leg extended on the brake pedal or the knee hits the dashboard; Figure 39-25)
- Falls

Signs and symptoms

- Pain in the hip area
- Pain in the knee
- Pain that may radiate to the groin
- Hip that is flexed, adducted, and internally rotated (posterior dislocation)
- Hip that is slightly flexed, abducted, and externally rotated (anterior dislocation; this is a rare injury)
- Feeling that joint is "locked"
- Inability to move the leg

Therapeutic interventions

- See Therapeutic Interventions for Dislocations.
- Prepare for emergent reduction.

Complications

- Sciatic nerve damage
- Femoral artery and nerve damage
- Necrosis of femoral head, which can occur if the hip is not relocated within 24 hours

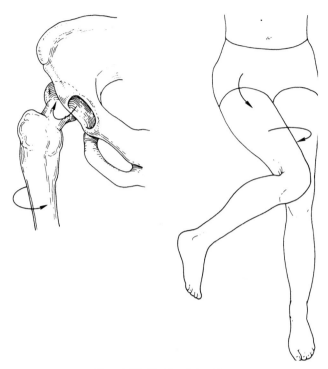

Figure 39-25. Hip dislocation.

Knee Dislocation

Knee dislocation is a true orthopedic emergency. Urgent reduction is needed to ensure limb salvage (Figure 39-26).

Mechanism of injury

- Major trauma
- High-speed motor vehicle collision
- Sports activities

Signs and symptoms

- Severe pain
- Gross swelling, deformity
- Inability to move the joint

Therapeutic interventions

- See Therapeutic Interventions for Dislocations.
- Splint knee in the position of comfort.
- Refer patient to an orthopedic surgeon for evaluation.
- Prepare for immediate reduction (within 6 hours) to avoid neurovascular damage.
- Inpatient admission is required.

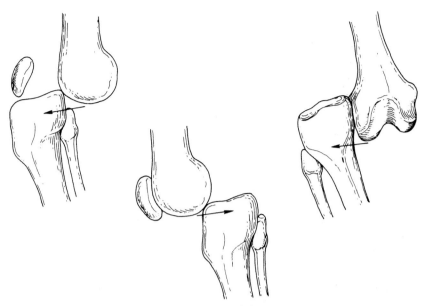

Figure 39-26. Knee dislocation.

Complications

- Peroneal nerve damage
- Posterior tibial nerve damage
- Popliteal artery damage

Patellar Dislocation

Mechanism of injury

- Spontaneous (patients often have a history of previous patellar dislocations; Figure 39-27)
- Direct trauma
- Rotation on a planted foot

Signs and symptoms

- Pain
- The knee is in a flexed position.
- Loss of function
- Tenderness, swelling

Therapeutic interventions

- See Therapeutic Interventions for Dislocations.
- Reduction may occur spontaneously.
- Apply splint, or cast, or some type of knee immobilizer that will keep the knee in full extension. Provide crutches for ambulation. Patient must wear splint or cast for 3 to 4 weeks.

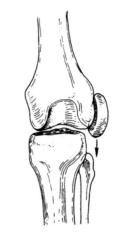

Figure 39-27. Patellar dislocation.

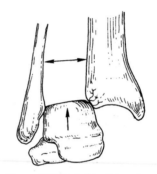

Figure 39-28. Ankle dislocation.

Complications

- Bleeding into the knee joint (hemarthrosis)

Ankle Dislocation

Mechanism of injury

- Usually associated with a fracture (Figure 39-28)
- Often a pedal injury in drivers involved in a motor vehicle collision

Signs and symptoms

- Pain
- Swelling, deformity
- Inability to move the joint

Therapeutic interventions

- See Therapeutic Interventions for Dislocations.
- Splint ankle in a position of comfort.
- Prepare for possible surgical reduction.
- Apply splint or cast and provide crutches.

Complication

- Neurovascular compromise

Foot Dislocation

Mechanism of injury

- A rare injury, generally resulting from an automobile or motorcycle crash
- Usually associated with an open wound

Signs and symptoms

- Pain, tenderness
- Swelling, deformity
- Inability to use the foot

Therapeutic interventions

- See Therapeutic Interventions for Dislocations.
- Apply sterile dressing to the open wound.
- Prepare for possible surgical reduction.
- Apply splint or cast and and provide crutches.

Complication

- Neurovascular compromise

REPETITIVE MOTION DISORDERS

Tendinitis

Tendinitis is a painful inflammation of the tendinous insertions into the bone. Tendinitis frequently occurs in the shoulder (rotator cuff tendinitis), elbow (lateral epicondylitis), wrist (de Quervain's tenosynovitis), knee, and heel (Achilles tendinitis).

Mechanism of injury

- Excessive continued stress
- Sudden hyperextension
- Idiopathic
- Acute or chronic inflammation

Signs and symptoms

- Aching pain that increases with motion
- Swelling
- Point tenderness with palpation

Therapeutic interventions

- Avoid activities that cause pain.
- Immobilize and elevate the affected area.
- Apply ice acutely; heat may be beneficial in the chronic phase.
- Apply a compression dressing (e.g., Ace wrap).
- Administer nonsteroidal antiinflammatory drugs.
- Radiographs may show calcification.
- Anesthetic and corticosteroid infiltrations may be necessary for chronic pain (but are never used in Achilles tendinitis).

Complications

- Synovitis
- Muscle tears
- Arthritis
- Nerve entrapment

Bursitis

Bursitis is an inflammation of the bursa, the fluid-filled sac that covers the prominences between bones, muscles, and tendons. Bursitis usually involves the elbow, shoulder, knee, heel, or hip.

Mechanism of injury

- Trauma (a direct blow or a chronic injury)
- Infection
- Chronic occupational stress
- Repetitive athletic stress
- Degenerative changes

Signs and symptoms

- Gradual onset of symptoms
- Red and warm skin over the affected area
- Aching pain that increases with motion
- Gross swelling in acute trauma
- Pain that radiates
- Joint crepitus

Therapeutic interventions

- Pad and immobilize the affected area.
- Apply ice to acute traumatic injuries.

- Apply local heat in cases in which pain is chronic.
- Administer steroid injections.
- Prepare for bursal injection or incision if infection is present.
- Prepare for aspiration of bursal fluid if infection is suspected; send for Gram stain and culture.

Complications

- Synovitis
- Muscle tears
- Arthritis
- Nerve entrapment

Nerve Entrapment Syndrome

Carpal tunnel syndrome is the most common nerve entrapment syndrome. It involves compression of the median nerve. Diagnosis is based on clinical findings.

Mechanism of injury

- Overuse of an extremity
- Repetitive use of the extremity
- Occupational or athletic stresses

Signs and symptoms

- Pain along the nerve pathway
- Pain that may radiate to the shoulder
- Paresthesia, numbness
- Limited range of motion
- Atrophy of surrounding muscles, extremity weakness
- Positive Phalen's test (Flex the wrist for 1 minute. The test is positive if flexion causes paresthesia in the nerve's distribution.)
- Positive Tinel's sign (Percussion of the median nerve causes pain and paresthesia in the nerve's distribution.)

Therapeutic interventions

- Avoid aggravating activities.
- Splint the wrists in a neutral or slightly extended position.
- Administer nonsteroidal antiinflammatory drugs.
- Administer local steroid injections.
- Electrodiagnostic studies may be performed.
- Prepare for surgical relief of nerve entrapment.

Complications

- Synovitis
- Muscle tears
- Arthritis
- Nerve entrapment

TRAUMATIC AMPUTATIONS

Cause

Traumatic amputations are often industrial injuries incurred by persons who work with machines such as farmers, industrial laborers, and mechanics. However, a substantial number of traumatic amputations are caused by automobile and motorcycle collisions. Amputations often occur along with multiple other injuries that must be addressed and may take precedence. (See Chapter 34.) Life-saving procedures are always the priority, but emergency personnel also must take steps to enhance the viability of the severed part.

Care of the Stump

Care of the stump may include the following:
- See General Guidelines for Emergency Management.
- Control bleeding by direct pressure, elevation, or a slightly inflated blood pressure cuff.
- Do *not* use clamps or tourniquets (unless bleeding cannot be controlled by any other means).
- Remove gross debris; do *not* scrub or put any cleaning solutions in the wound.
- Apply a splint.
- Obtain radiographs of the stump and the severed part.
- Administer antibiotics.
- Prepare the patient for surgery for stump debridement, repair of vascular damage, and possible replantation (also called reimplantation) of the severed part.

Management of the Severed Part

Management of the severed part consists of the following procedures:
1. Attempt to locate the severed part. Do not delay transport of the patient while attempting to locate the severed part.
2. Using sterile gloves, remove any gross foreign matter.
3. Wrap the part in sterile gauze (digits, ears); use a towel or clean sheet for limbs.
4. Rinse the part with saline or moisten the wrapping with a sterile isotonic solution (normal saline or lactated Ringer's solution). Do *not* use water or cleaning agents and do *not* soak or saturate the amputated part.
5. Place the part in a suitably sized plastic bag or container and seal it shut.
6. Place the sealed bag or container inside another container filled with an ice and water mix or refrigerate it (4° C). *Never* place the part directly on ice, in a freezer, or in ice water.
7. Label the bag with the patient's name, the date, and the time.
8. Transport severed parts with the patient, if possible.[4]

Survival Time

Never make a judgment as to the viability of a severed part; this is the surgeon's decision. Appropriate preservation of an amputated part greatly influences its survival time. A well-preserved part, without a large amount of muscle tissue (which necroses quickly), can be replanted up to 24 hours after amputation. However, nonpreserved parts still may be viable for up to 6 hours. Replantation tends to be more successful in children than in adults.

COMPLICATIONS OF ORTHOPEDIC INJURIES

Fat Embolism Syndrome

Fat embolism syndrome is a potentially life-threatening complication of long bone trauma, blunt trauma, and intramedullary manipulation. This syndrome manifests anywhere from 4 hours to several days after injury or orthopedic surgery. Fat globules, released from bone marrow, can embolize and occlude blood vessels in the brain, kidneys, lungs, and other tissues.

Signs and symptoms

General

- Elevated temperature
- Tachycardia
- Restlessness

Pulmonary

- Chest pain
- Dyspnea, cough
- Petechiae over the anterior chest and neck
- Crackles, pulmonary edema

Cerebral

- Decreased level of consciousness
- Hemiparesis
- Quadriplegia (tetraplegia)

Therapeutic interventions

- Aggressive oxygenation and ventilatory support
- Monitoring of arterial blood gases
- Immobilization of the injured part to reduce further marrow release
- Controversial therapies include the following:
  - Steroids

Osteomyelitis

Osteomyelitis is an infection of the bone, most commonly a result of direct contamination from open fractures, penetrating wounds, or surgical procedures. The longer the surgical procedure, the greater the risk of osteomyelitis. Organisms also can be spread hematogenously to the bone. It takes 10 to 14 days from the time of infection exposure before radiographs will demonstrate visible changes. The most common causative organism in osteomyelitis is *Staphylococcus aureus*.

Signs and symptoms

- Fever
- Pain and tenderness over the infected area
- Edema, erythema

- Exudate drainage
- Elevated sedimentation rate (late finding) and white blood cell count

Therapeutic interventions

- Immobilize the extremity.
- Culture any drainage.
- Initiate intravenous antibiotic administration.
- Bone scan may be performed.
- Prepare for surgical incision and drainage.
- Prepare for debridement.

Complications

- Septic arthritis
- Growth disturbances (in children)
- Chronic osteomyelitis
- Pathologic fractures

Compartment Syndrome

Compartment syndrome develops when the pressure in a muscle compartment exceeds the intraarterial hydrostatic pressure, causing collapse of capillaries and venules, which leads to ischemia and tissue necrosis. The exact pressure at which this develops is unclear, but intracompartmental pressures greater than 30 mm Hg generally are considered greatly elevated. A grace period of about 6 hours exists before irreversible soft tissue damage occurs. It is important to suspect compartment syndrome early. The first clue, in the alert patient, is pain out of proportion to the injury, unrelieved by standard interventions. Various techniques are available for measuring compartment pressure. The Stryker intracompartmental pressure monitoring system, a handheld device, is the most widely used. A mercury manometer or an arterial/venous pressure monitoring system and transducer also can be used. Box 39-2 summarizes compartment pressure measurement with a mercury manometer.[10]

Mechanism of injury

External

- Prolonged or inappropriate application of a pneumatic antishock garment, casts, splints, or tight dressings
- Skeletal traction
- Lying on a limb for prolonged periods

Internal

- Crush injury
- Burns, frostbite
- Envenomation
- Fractures, contusions
- Excessive muscle use during exercise or tonic-clonic seizures
- Bleeding into a muscle
- Extravasation of fluids into a fascial compartment

Box **39-2** Measuring Compartmental Pressure

Equipment

2 18-gauge needles
2 Sets of extension tubing
1 Three-way stopcock
1 Vial of bacteriostatic normal saline
1 20-mL syringe
1 Mercury manometer

Procedure

1. Prepare the patient for a sterile procedure.
2. Insert an 18-gauge needle to the side port of the three-way stopcock.
3. Connect the 18-gauge needle to the distal end of the first extension tubing set.
4. Aspirate 15 mL of air into the 20-mL syringe and attach the syringe to the middle stopcock port.
5. Insert an 18-gauge needle in the normal saline vial and inject 2 mL of air into the vial. Aspirate normal saline until the extension tubing is half filled (must be able to visualize the saline meniscus).
6. Connect the second extension tubing set to the third stopcock port.
7. Connect the tubing to the mercury manometer.
8. Insert the needle into the fascial compartment and turn the stopcock so that all ports are open.
9. Gently depress the syringe plunger while watching the fluid meniscus and manometer.
10. Document the pressure at which the meniscus falls.
11. Repeat the procedure to verify results.

Modified from Frankel NR, Villarin LA: Compartment syndrome. In Roberts JR, Hedges JR, editors: *Clinical procedures in emergency medicine,* ed 4, Philadelphia, 2004, Saunders.

Signs and symptoms

- The most reliable symptom is pain with passive movement or stretching (e.g., toe dorsiflexion).
- Pain upon palpation of the compartment
- Delayed capillary refill
- Decreased distal sensation, paresthesias, "burning"
- Decreased function, weakness
- Pallor, although pinkness may persist in the extremity tips despite proximal muscle ischemia
- Pulse presence or absence does not reliably identify tissue necrosis.
- Myoglobinuria (late sign)
- Renal failure (very late sign)
- Compartment pressures greater than 30 mm Hg, or only 30 mm Hg less than the diastolic pressure

Therapeutic interventions

- Remove all constrictive dressing, casts, and splints.
- Do not elevate the affected extremity; place it in a neutral position.
- Do not apply ice.
- Emergent fasciotomy and surgical débridement are required.

Volkmann's Ischemic Contracture

Though usually associated with supracondylar fractures, Volkmann's ischemic contracture can occur with fractures of the forearm, wrist, tibia, and femur. The cause and pathophysiology of this condition are similar to that of compartment syndrome. In addition, an ischemic fibrosis develops, causing contracture of the extremity. If left untreated, Volkmann's contracture produces permanent nerve damage, pain, and deformity and even may require extremity amputation.

Signs and symptoms

- Pain characterized as deep and poorly localized
- Pain aggravated by stretching
- Sensory loss distal (and sometimes proximal) to the injury
- Distal pulse is rarely obliterated.
- Wrist drop or foot drop
- Contractures can form within 12 hours of symptom onset.

Therapeutic interventions

- Do *not* elevate the extremity; maintain it in a neutral position.
- Do *not* apply cold.
- Immediate decompressive fasciotomy.

PATIENT EDUCATION AND DISCHARGE INSTRUCTIONS

Aftercare Instructions for Patients With Splints or Casts

Provide the following aftercare instructions to patients with splints or casts:
- Return to the emergency department, the orthopedic clinic, or your private physician in 24 hours for follow-up care.
- Keep the cast or splint dry.
- Elevate the injured limb above heart level for the first 24 hours.
- Do not place sharp objects (e.g., coat hangers or knitting needles) inside the cast.
- If the skin under a cast itches, blow cool air (from a fan or hair dryer) down the cast or try scratching the opposite extremity.
- Wiggle the digits at least once each hour.
- Seek urgent medical care for the following:
  - Digits that are cold or hot
  - Digits that are blue or mottled
  - Numbness, tingling, or decreased digital sensation
  - Foreign objects in the cast
  - Cast that becomes too tight
  - Foul odor coming from the cast[3]

Crutch and Cane Fitting

Fit crutches with the patient wearing a shoe on the unaffected side, preferably a low-heeled, rubber-soled, tied shoe. Canes are used on the side contralateral to the injury to minimize hip strain. Unlike a cane, crutches reduce weight-bearing stress on the upper extremities while augmenting balance and stability. Crutches offer more support than do canes but less support than a walker.

Axillary crutches

- Adjust crutch length as follows:
  - The arm pieces are 2 inches below the axilla (no weight on the axilla)
  - The crutch is at a 25-degree angle when the tips are 6 to 8 inches to side and in front of the foot
- Adjust crutch hand pieces so that the elbow has a 30-degree angle of flexion.

Lofstrand (forearm) crutches

- Adjust crutch length so that the crutch is at a 25-degree angle when the tips are 6 inches to the side and in front of the foot.
- Adjust crutch hand pieces so that the elbow has a 30-degree angle of flexion.

Gait training

- Assist the patient to stand and balance.
- Have the patient position the crutch tips 4 inches to the side and 4 inches in front of the foot.
- All weight should be carried on the hands by straightening the elbows. Instruct the patient *not* to place any weight on the axillas, even while resting.
- In the emergency department, a three-point gait is usually taught. This gait is used when little or no weight bearing is desired.
- Be sure to include instructions for stair climbing, sitting, and standing.

INJURY PREVENTION STRATEGIES

Emergency nurses are in a position to be at the forefront of the injury prevention movement. Nurses have countless ways to become involved in hospital, community, and legislative initiatives designed to reduce death and disability related to musculoskeletal trauma. The following are just a few prevention strategies that can decrease the number of orthopedic injuries significantly:

- Encourage parental supervision of infants and young children.
- Promote motor vehicle restraint and child passenger safety laws.
- Encourage firearm injury prevention education.
- Support helmet laws (motorcycle, bicycle, skiing)
- Encourage enforcement of existing alcohol and drug laws.
- Take an hourly break from repetitive activities to avoid strain.
- Support traffic safety enforcement.
- Do not wear loose clothing or jewelry around machinery.
- Support playground redesign.
- Encourage the use of wrist guards, kneepads, and helmets in sporting activities such as skating, skiing, and bicycling.
- Maintain Occupational Safety and Health Administration and workplace safety standards.
- Support lawn mower and snow blower redesign.

References

1. Emergency Nurses Association: Musculoskeletal trauma. In *Trauma nursing core course manual,* ed 5, Des Plaines, Ill, 2000, The Association.

2. Sponseller P, et al, editors: *The 5-minute orthopaedic consult,* Philadelphia, 2001, Lippincott Williams & Wilkins.

3. Davis D: Splinting. In Rosen P et al, editors: *Atlas of emergency procedures,* St Louis, 2001, Mosby.

4. Schaider J et al, editors: *Rosen and Barkin's 5-minute emergency medicine consult,* ed 2, Philadelphia, 2003, Lippincott Williams & Wilkins.

5. Hills S, Wasserman E: Wrist injuries: emergency imaging and management, *Emerg Med Pract* 11(3): 1-24, 2001.

6. Rogers LF: *Radiology of skeletal trauma,* ed 3, New York, 2002, Churchill Livingston.

7. Lang J, Counselman F: Common orthopaedic hand and wrist injuries, *Emerg Med* pp 20-35, 2003.

8. Wolfson AB et al, editors: Pelvic fractures. In *Harwood-Nuss' clinical practice of emergency medicine,* ed 4, Philadelphia, 2005, Lippincott Williams & Wilkins.

9. Wasserman E, Hill S: Ankle injuries in the emergency department: how to provide rapid and cost-effective assessment and treatment, *Emerg Med Pract* 5(4):1-28, 2002.

10. Frankel NR, Villarin LA: Compartment syndrome. In Roberts JR, Hedges JR, editors: *Clinical procedures in emergency medicine,* ed 4, Philadelphia, 2004, Saunders.

40

Facial, Ocular, ENT, and Dental Trauma

Anne Marie E. Lewis, RN, BSN, BA, MA, CEN

Because of the vital structures involved, patients with facial trauma are at risk for severe morbidity and mortality from airway obstruction, respiratory distress, and hemorrhage. Emergent assessment and intervention are required to identify and manage potentially life-threatening injuries to the face and the adjacent cervical spine and brain.

Blunt, penetrating, blast, burn, and crush mechanisms can produce trauma, but the most common cause of severe facial injuries in the United States today is the motor vehicle accident. In a collision the face readily strikes the dash, steering wheel, windshield, hood, or even the pavement (Figure 40-1). Fortunately, the use of airbags has reduced significantly the incidence of serious facial trauma in minor crashes. Fewer maxillofacial injuries occur with airbag deployment than with no restraint system or with seat belt use alone.[1,2]

Other common mechanisms of facial trauma include falls, athletic injuries, or physical assaults. Interpersonal and intimate partner violence accounts for many injuries to the face. Because of the right-handedness of most attackers, assaults to the face occur more frequently on the left side.[3] Victims of intimate partner violence are often reticent to report assault for fear of reprisal from the abuser. Consider the possibility of intimate partner violence whenever facial trauma patients recount an improbable history of injury (e.g., "I walked into a door").

ASSESSMENT

Begin assessment of facial trauma patients with the basics: airway (with cervical spine stabilization), breathing, circulation, and disability (Table 40-1). After identifying and managing life-threatening conditions, complete a focused assessment of the patient's injuries, and then initiate treatment. Box 40-1 summarizes general treatment recommendations for all patients with facial trauma.

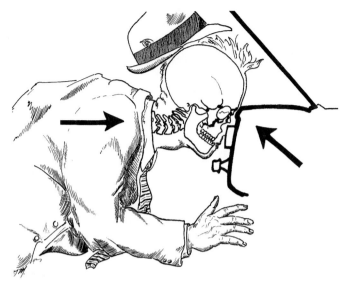

Figure 40-1. Common mechanism of facial injury in motor vehicle collisions. (From Schultz RC: *Facial injuries,* ed 2, St. Louis, 1997, Mosby.)

Table **40-1**   **Primary Assessment of the Patient With Facial Trauma**

Category	Assessment/Intervention
Airway and cervical spine	Ensure the airway is patent. Avoid tilting the head; assume concurrent cervical spine injury until proved otherwise. Use a jaw-thrust or chin-lift maneuver to open the airway.
	Noisy breathing indicates partial airway obstruction. The tongue, broken teeth, dentures, other foreign material, emesis, blood, avulsed tissue, edema, or a mandibular fracture can cause airway obstruction.
	Suction the airway to remove blood, vomit, and other debris. Consider invasive airway management, such as tracheal intubation or cricothyrotomy, if the airway cannot be opened and secured with basic maneuvers. See Chapter 19.
	Immobilize the cervical spine while opening and clearing the airway. Check the neck for a laryngeal fracture.
Breathing	Evaluate rate and quality of breathing, chest rise and fall, skin color, use of accessory muscles, and other indicators of respiratory effectiveness.
	Administer supplemental oxygen. Ventilate with a bag-valve-mask device as necessary.
Circulation	Control obvious bleeding with direct pressure and elevation (if possible). Initiate intravenous access. Give a bolus of isotonic crystalloids if bleeding is severe or signs of hypovolemia are present.
Level of consciousness	Evaluate the patient's level of consciousness and pupillary response.

Box **40-1** **General Care of the Facial Trauma Patient**

Elevate the head of the bed at least 30 degrees to reduce facial swelling and enhance airway clearance. If the spine has not yet been cleared, tilt the stretcher into a reverse Trendelenburg position (head up, feet down.
Keep suction equipment readily available.
Do *not* insert airways, suction catheters, gastric tubes, tracheal tubes, intranasal balloons, or packing into the nose of a patient with potential nasal or basilar skull fractures.
Apply cold packs to areas of swelling but do not chill the patient.
Consider prophylactic antibiotic administration.
Evaluate tetanus immunization status and immunize as indicated.
Provide emotional support and explain all procedures and instructions.

Focused Assessment

Eyes

Check each eye individually. Note any loss of vision. Evaluate eye movement in all visual fields, looking for restricted gaze or diplopia (double vision). Assess for subconjunctival hemorrhage, blood in the anterior chamber (hyphema), or globe penetration.

Dental malocclusion

Assess the patient's bite. Ask the patient to bite down on the back molars. Do the teeth fit together the same way they did before the injury?

Point tenderness

Assess for specific points of palpable tenderness.

Asymmetry

Evaluate for areas of facial asymmetry. Perform a side-to-side comparison of the eyebrows, infraorbital rims, zygomatic arches, anterior sinus walls, jaw angles, and lower mandibular borders.

Cerebrospinal fluid leak

Check for a cerebrospinal fluid (CSF) leak indicated by drainage from the nose (rhinorrhea) or ears (otorrhea), or a salty taste in the mouth.

Body piercing

Jewelry on the face, mouth, tongue, and ears may be caught or pulled during a motor vehicle collision, assault, or recreational activity. This can tear surrounding structures. Facial hardware also can impale patients in the ear, tongue, pallet, head, or face.[4] For specific information related to complications of piercing and facial jewelry removal, see Table 33-3 and Figure 33-8 in Chapter 33.

FACIAL SOFT TISSUE TRAUMA

Facial lacerations present as torn, ragged wounds. Animal and human bites exhibit characteristic teeth or bite marks, whereas blunt or crushing trauma produces irregular lacerations. Sharp objects such as glass, metal, and knives create incisions. Avulsions involve the tearing away of skin, with or without its underlying structures. Facial wounds can bleed profusely and may cause severe disfigurement. Evaluate for concomitant injuries to bones and nerves, particularly the superficial facial nerve.

Therapeutic Interventions

Therapeutic interventions for facial soft tissue trauma include the following:
- Elevate the head of the bed at least 30 degrees to reduce facial swelling and enhance airway clearance.
- Exert direct pressure on wounds that are actively bleeding.
- Place cold packs on areas of swelling.
- Apply a topical anesthetic to wounds or assist with local or regional parenteral anesthesia.
- Use copious amounts of normal saline to irrigate all bites, grossly contaminated injuries, and wounds more than 8 hours old.
- Assist with wound cleaning, debridement, and foreign body removal.
- Apply a sterile dressing.
- Close wounds by applying adhesive strips; assist with application of wound glue or suture placement (scalp wounds can be stapled).

Age/Developmental Considerations

Procedural sedation may be necessary for pediatric wound repair.

Patient Education and Discharge Instructions

Instruct the patient to do the following:
- Cleanse the wound 1 to 2 times per day with soapy water to avoid infection. Apply a topical ointment and cover the wound as directed.
- To prevent hyperpigmentation, avoid exposing recent wounds to sunlight for 2 to 12 months.[5]
- Have staples and sutures removed in 5 to 7 days.

Instruct patients with wounds closed with wound glue as follows:
- Do not scrub the wound site.
- Do not apply antibiotic to the wound site.
- Monitor the site for signs of infection.
- In 7 to 14 days, most of the adhesive will come off on its own. The remainder may be removed with soap and water.

Special Notes

Consider the following for facial soft tissue trauma:
- Plastic surgery consultation is appropriate for extensive trauma, special types of injuries, or when the patient or family requests it.
- When the lip is lacerated, the vermilion border must be reapproximated carefully.
- Trauma to the eyelid also may involve the eye or the nasolacrimal duct. Treat eye injuries before lid injuries. Ophthalmologic consultation may be indicated.
- Eyebrows should be approximated carefully and *never* shaved.

Facial Abrasions and Contusions

See Chapter 12 for a detailed description of wound types.

Therapeutic interventions

- Anesthetize large abraded areas with a topical anesthetic.
- Cleanse the wound with normal saline. Carefully remove foreign bodies to avoid permanent tattooing.
- Assist with debridement of devitalized or grossly contaminated tissue.
- Dress the wound with a topical antibiotic ointment and sterile gauze if indicated. Stretchy mesh dressings can be used to hold gauze in place without taping the face or hair.
- Consider oral antibiotics for severely contaminated wounds and wounds greater than 24 hours old.
- Apply a cold pack and elastic bandage to contusions (e.g., a forehead "goose egg") as needed.

Patient education and discharge instructions

- Cleanse the abrasion 1 to 2 times per day to remove old antibiotic ointment.
- Reapply new ointment and cover the wound as directed. (Many facial wounds are left open to air.)
- Seek medical care for signs of infection: redness, swelling, drainage, or a foul odor.
- Intermittently apply a cold pack to contusions for the first 48 hours. Place a thin towel between the cold pack and the skin.

FACIAL FRACTURES

When evaluating a patient for facial fractures, assess for concomitant injuries to the airway, eyes, and brain. Treatment of facial fractures commonly is delayed to address more serious injuries and allow facial edema to subside. Computed tomography (CT) scans have largely replaced plain radiographs of the face for diagnosis and evaluation of fractures.[6]

Nasal Fractures

Nasal fractures generally result from blunt nasal trauma. Be sure to identify and treat septal hematomas. Unexcised hematomas of the nasal septum can become infected and necrotic and will result in permanent deformity.

Signs and symptoms

- Nasal deformity
- Nasal and periorbital edema and ecchymosis; swelling may be extensive
- Bony crepitus
- Point tenderness
- Internal and external nasal bleeding
- Subconjunctival hemorrhage
- Flattening, twisting, or broadening of the nose
- CSF drainage if the fracture extends through the ethmoid bones

Diagnostic aids

- CT scan or nasal bone radiographs (Waters' view) if deformity is present

Therapeutic interventions

- Apply a cold pack.
- Control external bleeding with direct pressure; control internal bleeding by compressing the nares.
- Assist with anesthetic administration.
- Splint the nose, as indicated.
- Consider oral antibiotic, decongestant, and analgesic administration.
- Closed or open reduction may be necessary if the fracture is displaced, but surgery usually is performed after swelling has abated.

Patient education and discharge instructions

- Keep the splint in place for 1 week (simple fractures).
- Manage epistaxis as directed (see Chapter 33 for epistaxis interventions).
- Follow up with an ear, nose, and throat (ENT)/otolaryngology specialist in 5 to 7 days.

Zygomatic Fractures

The zygomatic bone may be fractured along the infraorbital rim, at the zygomatic suture line, or on the arch itself (Figure 40-2). A trimalar fracture refers to breaks in the zygoma in three specific points. These injuries are caused by blunt force to the front or side of the face. Fractures of the zygoma frequently are associated with orbital fractures and may involve trauma to the eye.

Signs and symptoms

- Use the TIDES mnemonic as a guide to assessment:
  - *T*rismus (if there is impingement on the coronoid process of the mandible)
  - *I*nfraorbital hyperesthesia

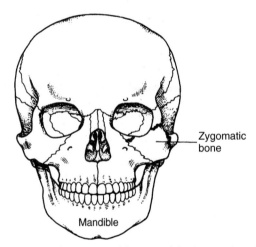

Figure 40-2. A, Depressed fracture of the zygomatic arch.

- *D*iplopia with impaired upward gaze
- *E*pistaxis of the naris on the affected side
- *S*ymmetry, absence of (may be obscured by edema)
- Possible CSF rhinorrhea
- Periorbital and facial edema and ecchymosis
- Subconjunctival hemorrhage
- Palpable step defect and point tenderness
- Facial flattening
- Anesthesia of the cheek, upper lip, side of the nose, teeth, and gums

Diagnostic aids

- Radiographs (submental vertex, Waters', and Caldwell's views)
- Facial CT scan

Therapeutic interventions

- See Box 40-1.
- Apply a cold pack to the affected cheek.
- Obtain ophthalmologic consultation as needed.
- Open reduction and internal fixation may be necessary if a cosmetic or functional deformity exists.

Orbital Rim Trauma

Orbital rim trauma typically follows blunt force to the face. Drivers and front seat passengers in frontal impact motor vehicle collisions routinely are injured by the steering wheel or windshield. The incidence of these injuries drops dramatically with airbag deployment.[7]

Fractures of the medial wall or floor of the orbit can occur as a result of blow-out injuries. When a portion of the orbit breaks and extrudes *into* the orbital space, it is known as a blow-in fracture. Intracranial trauma and CSF leaks are associated with orbital roof fractures. Assess all patients with orbital rim trauma for concomitant injury to the brain, globe, and cranial nerves III, IV, and VI.

Orbital Blow-out Fractures

A fracture of the very thin orbital floor (i.e., the roof of the maxillary sinus) results when a blunt object larger than the opening of the orbit strikes the eye and forces the globe inward (Figure 40-3). The most common mechanisms of orbital blow-out fractures include motor vehicle collisions, physical assaults (fist to the eye), and sports-related injuries (e.g., softball to the eye).[8] The incidence of serious ocular trauma is higher with blow-out fractures than with other types of orbital rim trauma.[9]

Signs and symptoms

- Impaired upward gaze (following entrapment of the inferior rectus muscle)
- Diplopia (usually on upward gaze)
- Enophthalmos (sunken eyeball)
- Infraorbital paresthesia
- Periorbital edema and ecchymosis
- Subconjunctival hemorrhage

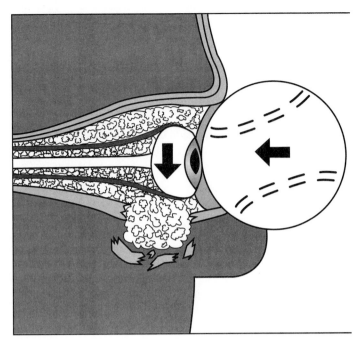

Figure 40-3. Mechanism of a blow-out fracture caused by the impact of a ball. The periorbital fat is forced through the floor of the orbit.

Diagnostic aids

- Mechanism of injury suggestive of a blow-out fracture
- Clinical assessment, including examination of visual acuity and ocular movement
- Plain radiographs (Waters' view)
- Facial CT scan

Therapeutic interventions

- Apply a cold pack to the affected eye.
- Obtain ophthalmologic consultation.
- Open reduction and internal fixation may be necessary if a cosmetic or functional deformity exists.

Patient education and discharge instructions

- Limit activity for 3 to 6 weeks to prevent reinjury.
- Avoid blowing the nose for 4 to 6 weeks to inhibit orbital emphysema formation.
- Wear protective eyewear for contact sports.
- Follow up with an ophthalmologist.

Maxillary (Midface) Fractures

In 1901, French pathologist René Le Fort observed that blunt trauma produced three specific facial bone fracture patterns. These injuries have been categorized as Le Fort I (horizontal), Le Fort II (pyramidal), and Le Fort III (craniofacial dysjunction) (Figure 40-4). Damage may

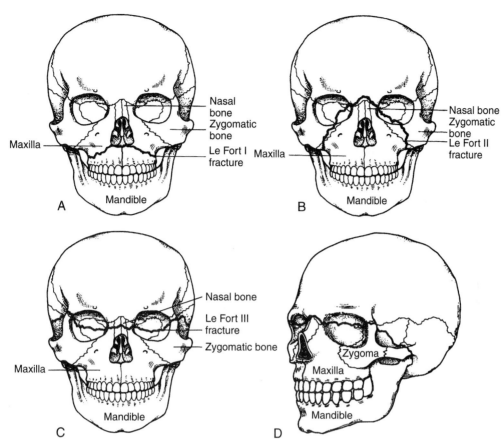

Figure 40-4. A, Le Fort I; **B,** Le Fort II; **C,** Le Fort III fractures; and **D,** Le Fort III, lateral view. (From March K: Head and neck trauma. In Cohen SS, editor: *Trauma nursing secrets,* Philadelphia, 2003, Hanley & Belfus.)

be unilateral or bilateral with varying levels of Le Fort fractures on either side of the face. Table 40-2 lists assessment findings associated with each level of injury.

Diagnostic aids

- Mechanism of injury suggestive of major facial trauma
- Clinical examination
- Facial CT scan
- Head CT scan for patients with a decreased level of consciousness
- Facial radiographs with lateral, Waters', and Caldwell's views (if CT is not available)
- A chest radiograph to rule out tooth aspiration, if any teeth are unaccounted for

Therapeutic interventions

- See Box 40-1.
- Maintain a patent airway. Suction secretions as needed. Consider oral tracheal intubation for Le Fort II and III fractures. Assist with cricothyrotomy when oral intubation is not possible.

Table 40-2　Assessment Findings for Le Fort Fractures

Fracture	Description	Assessment Findings
Le Fort I	A horizontal fracture through the maxilla that separates the entire upper jaw from the rest of the face	Malocclusion of the teeth A movable maxilla (hard palate) (The upper teeth move when pulled.) Epistaxis Facial edema and ecchymosis An elongated midface
Le Fort II	A pyramidal fracture that starts at the nasal bone and extends down through the zygomaticomaxillary suture	Nose and dental arch move together when manipulated. Epistaxis Periorbital and facial edema, ecchymosis Subconjunctival hemorrhage Infraorbital paresthesia Malocclusion of the teeth Cerebrospinal fluid rhinorrhea
Le Fort III	A major fracture that starts at the nasal bridge and extends through the orbits, separating the facial bones from the skull; may involve the maxilla, zygoma, mandible, nasal bones, ethmoids, and orbits	Massive bleeding Loss of consciousness is routine Cerebrospinal fluid rhinorrhea Epistaxis Periorbital and facial edema, ecchymosis Subconjunctival hemorrhage Infraorbital paresthesia Malocclusion of the teeth; anterior open bite Mobility of all facial bones (separated from the skull) "Dish face" deformity; an elongated and flattened facial appearance

- Administer analgesics as needed.
- Apply cold packs to the face but avoid hypothermia.
- Administer antibiotics intravenously for open fractures.
- Obtain ophthalmologic consultation for Le Fort II and III fractures.
- Neurosurgical consultation is indicated if a CSF leak is present.
- Urgent or delayed (possibly for several days) surgery is required for reduction and internal fixation.

Mandibular Fractures

Mandibular fractures are among the most common facial fractures. Because of its arch shape, the mandible often breaks in two places on the same or opposite side (Figure 40-5). Open fractures are associated with obvious intraoral bony fragments or bleeding around the teeth.

Signs and symptoms

- Malocclusion of the teeth
- Trismus (tonic contraction of the jaw muscles)
- Edema, ecchymosis
- Possible lacerations in the mouth
- Sublingual hematoma
- Point tenderness, especially with palpation
- Intraoral bleeding may or may not be present.

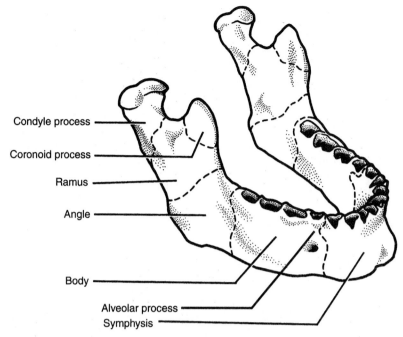

Condyle process

Coronoid process

Ramus

Angle

Body

Alveolar process

Symphysis

Figure 40-5. Fracture sites of the mandible (Modified from Rosen P et al: *Emergency medicine,* ed 3, St Louis, 1992, Mosby.)

Diagnostic aids

- Clinical examination
- Facial CT scan
- Panoramic topography radiographs
- Plain radiographs: mandibular series with a reverse Towne's view

Therapeutic interventions

- See Box 40-1.
- Maintain a patent airway.
- Apply a cold pack to the jaw.
- Give analgesics as needed.
- Administer antibiotics intravenously for open fractures.
- Assist with closed reduction. Treatment should occur as soon as possible to minimize the risk of infection. Patients who are mentally impaired, alcoholics, and persons with psychiatric or seizure disorders may require open reduction.

Patient education and discharge instructions

- Take antibiotics and analgesics as directed.
- If reduction was not required or if fixation was accomplished with a surgical plate, maintain the patient on a soft diet during healing.
- Leave intermaxillary fixation wires or rubber bands in place for 3 to 6 weeks. During this time, maintain appropriate oral intake. Consume high-calorie, high-protein liquids

through a straw. Brush the teeth and wires and rinse out the mouth several times per day. Carry wire cutters at all times to open the jaws in case of an airway emergency.
- Avoid strenuous exertion because this makes it more difficult to breathe and places strain on the wires or bands.
- Follow up with a maxillofacial surgeon.

OCULAR TRAUMA

In developed nations, trauma is the second leading cause of blindness.[10] Always consider the possibility of ocular trauma in any patient who has an injury to the eyelid, orbit, or surrounding structures. In unconscious individuals, check for and remove contact lenses to prevent corneal ulcerations. (Refer to Chapter 33, Figure 33-3, for information on hard and soft contact lens removal.)

Wearing standard eyeglasses does not influence the incidence of injury.[11] However, patients who wear protective eyewear are less likely to sustain serious ocular trauma. For example, paint balls can cause severe eye injuries and permanent vision loss if the eyes are unshielded.[12] Encourage patients to use protective eyewear when engaged in contact sports, work, or other hobbies in which the eye may be damaged.

Despite the sometimes dramatic nature of eye injuries, treatment of life-threatening injuries must always take priority over management of ocular trauma. See Box 33-1 and Table 33-1 in Chapter 33.

Subconjunctival Hemorrhage

A subconjunctival hemorrhage is a collection of blood under the conjunctiva. These injuries appear as a red blotch and may involve only a portion of the sclera or the entire white of the eye. Subconjunctival hemorrhage is common after ocular trauma. This disorder rarely requires treatment and generally resolves in about 2 weeks. Although usually benign, significant subconjunctival hemorrhage can be a sign of a globe rupture.[13]

Other causes of subconjunctival hemorrhage include forceful coughing, sneezing, or straining, high blood pressure, and bleeding disorders. Subconjunctival hemorrhages frequently occur in patients with bulimia who vomit repeatedly.

Patient education and discharge instructions
- Treat the underlying cause as indicated.
- Avoid aspirin or nonsteroidal antiinflammatory drugs unless approved by a physician.
- Follow up with a primary care provider if the condition recurs or does not resolve in 2 weeks or if there are indications of a serious underlying disorder.

Eyelid Laceration

Early repair of lid lacerations has been shown to decrease the incidence of infection. Nonetheless, repair sometimes is delayed for a variety of reasons.

Therapeutic interventions
- Save any avulsed eyelid pieces.
- Apply a cold pack to the lid.

- Assist with wound irrigation but remember that extensive irrigation can increase lid edema.
- Suturing may require an ophthalmologic surgeon, especially if the lacrimal duct is involved.
- If a section of tissue is missing, consult a plastic surgeon for reconstruction. Repair is required to protect the cornea.

Patient education and discharge instructions

- Keep the head elevated.
- Apply antibiotic ophthalmic ointment as directed.
- Follow up with an ophthalmologist.

Hyphema

Bleeding in the anterior chamber of the eye (hyphema) occurs in association with blunt or penetrating trauma. All or part of the chamber may be filled with blood. In patients with a partial hyphema, head elevation encourages blood to pool in the lower part of the iris. This makes the hyphema easier to visualize. Rebleeding can cause corneal staining, secondary glaucoma, and visual loss. Most uncomplicated hyphemas resolve within 5 to 6 days. An "8-ball hemorrhage" is a condition in which old, clotted blood fills the anterior chamber.

Signs and symptoms

- Visible blood in the anterior chamber
- Blurred vision
- Pain
- Photophobia
- Possible intraocular pressure elevation

Therapeutic interventions

- Raise the head of the bed 30 to 45 degrees (once the spine has been cleared).
- Maintain bed rest.
- Administer antiemetics and analgesics as needed.
- Patch the affected eye with a rigid eye shield.
- Avoid aspirin and nonsteroidal antiinflammatory drugs to minimize the risk of rebleeding.
- Consider administering cycloplegics and corticosteroids.
- Hospitalize patients in whom intraocular pressure is elevated and those with a hyphema involving more than one third of the anterior chamber.
- Surgery is required to remove the clot of an 8-ball hemorrhage.

Patient education and discharge instructions

- Restrict activity.
- Wear a shield over the affected eye.
- Apply ophthalmic medications as ordered.
- Seek medical care for any change in visual disturbances.
- Follow up with an ophthalmologist.

Extraocular Foreign Bodies

Common foreign bodies on the surface of the eye include eyelashes, dirt, sand, environmental debris, metal, glass, and wood.

Signs and symptoms

- Reddened conjunctiva
- Tearing
- Photophobia
- Pain
- Foreign body sensation

Diagnostic aids

- Perform a clinical examination; foreign body or a rust ring may be visible.
- Perform and document a visual acuity examination.

Therapeutic interventions

- Administer a topical anesthetic agent.
- For nonembedded foreign bodies, irrigate the eye with normal saline or lactated Ringer's solution. If flushing does not remove the object, assist with gentle extrication using a sterile foreign body removal device or needle. Rust rings can be eliminated with a rust ring spud.
- Administer topical antibiotics.

Patient education and discharge instructions

- Apply antibiotics as directed.
- Follow up with an ophthalmologist.
- Do not rub the eyes when the hands are contaminated with dirt, metal, and debris.
- Wear protective eyewear when engaged in high-risk activities.

Intraocular Foreign Bodies

Intraocular foreign bodies usually are caused by a small object (often metallic) that penetrates the eyeball at high speed and comes to rest somewhere within the posterior chamber. Pain may be minimal, and the entrance wound can be small and difficult to locate. Finding these wounds requires careful assessment and a high index of suspicion. This condition is a vision-threatening emergency.

Diagnostic aids

- Radiographs of the eye
- Slit lamp examination
- β-Scan ultrasound (ultrasound biomicroscopy)
- CT scan

Therapeutic interventions

- Consider antibiotic administration.
- Surgical intervention is required.

Eye Impalement Injuries/Ruptured Globe

Severe penetrating injuries to the eye occur most often with motor vehicle collisions (in which the occupant was unrestrained) or with gunshot wounds.[14] A ruptured globe is an ophthalmologic emergency that can cause permanent loss of vision or even loss of the eye.

Signs and symptoms

- Significant decrease in vision (or complete visual loss) in the affected eye
- Pain
- Vitreous humor leakage from the eye
- Diplopia and enophthalmos
- Obvious impaled object (if present)

Diagnostic aids

- CT scan
- Radiographs of eye if CT scanning is unavailable. Include Waters' and Caldwell's views to rule out associated orbital fracture(s).
- Obtain a magnetic resonance imaging examination. (Contraindicated if metallic foreign bodies are present.)

Therapeutic interventions

- Provide analgesia and sedation.
- Minimize manipulation of the eye (even for evaluation or medications).
- Secure the impaled object, if present.
- Apply a rigid shield *without* an underlying patch; do not put pressure on the ruptured globe.
- Give antiemetics as needed.
- Administer antibiotics parenterally.
- Obtain emergent ophthalmologic consultation. Surgical intervention will be necessary.

Conjunctival and Corneal Lacerations

Suturing may be required for corneal lacerations. Conjunctival lacerations generally heal well and require supportive care only.

Signs and symptoms

- Photophobia
- Tearing
- Pain
- Impaired vision

Diagnostic aids

- Perform visual acuity testing.
- Prepare for a slit lamp eye examination.
- Stain the eye with fluorescein dye and then evaluate the cornea with a cobalt light.
- Assess for foreign bodies in the wound.

Therapeutic interventions

- For patients with corneal lacerations, place a rigid shield over the eye; avoid pressure on the globe.
- Administer antibiotics parenterally.
- Give analgesics.
- Obtain ophthalmologic consultation.
- Assist with corneal laceration suturing as needed.

Patient education and discharge instructions

- Take antibiotics and analgesics as directed.
- Follow up with an ophthalmologist.

Corneal Abrasions

A corneal abrasion occurs when a foreign object, such as contact lens or fingernail, scrapes the epithelium of the eye. The cornea also can be damaged or disrupted by corneal disease. Uncomplicated abrasions generally heal quickly.

Signs and symptoms

- Tearing
- Pain on the surface of the eye (a foreign body sensation)
- Photophobia
- Reddened eye

Diagnostic aids

- Perform visual acuity testing.
- Stain the eye with fluorescein dye and then assess the cornea with a cobalt light.

Therapeutic interventions

- Administer topical and/or oral analgesics.
- Instill a topical antibiotic.

Patient education and discharge instructions

- Apply topical antibiotics as directed.
- Follow up with an ophthalmologist as needed.

Ocular Burns

Burns to the eye are caused by chemicals (acids and alkalis) and by radiant energy (thermal, ultraviolet, or infrared). Regardless of the cause, the patient experiences severe pain.

Chemical burns

Immediate irrigation takes precedence over assessment in the patient with a chemical eye injury; never delay irrigation to identify the chemical or perform a detailed assessment.

Once irrigation with normal saline or lactated Ringer's solution has been initiated, specific information about the involved substance can be obtained. Follow irrigation with careful eye examination.

Alkali burns

Ocular burns caused by alkaline agents are a true emergency. Alkalis cause extensive tissue destruction through a process of liquefaction necrosis. These chemicals can burn into the anterior chamber in as little as 5 to 15 minutes, causing internal damage to the eye. Burning continues until the chemical is removed.

Acid burns

Acid burns coagulate tissues and tend to be self-limiting. Damage generally is restricted to the superficial structures of the eye. The exception is hydrofluoric acid, which can cause a severe, penetrating burn. Car batteries contain sulfuric acid and are a common source of acid eye injuries.

General signs and symptoms

- Pain
- Photophobia
- Tearing
- Reduced vision
- Reddened eye (the eye may appear white and cloudy in severe burns)
- Foreign body sensation
- Possible eyelid edema
- Possible burns around the eye(s)

Therapeutic interventions

- Perform a visual acuity examination *after* irrigation so that vision-saving treatments are not delayed.
- Apply a topical anesthetic agent.
- Irrigate the eye with 1 to 2 L of normal saline or lactated Ringer's solution. See Chapter 33, Box 33-2.
- After initial irrigation, check the pH of the conjunctival sac.
- Continue irrigation until the pH is consistently 7.
- Fluorescein staining may be performed following irrigation to evaluate the extent of injury.
- Attempt to determine chemical type, amount, concentration, degree of penetration, duration of exposure, time since exposure, and any first aid the patient received. A material safety data sheet or your regional poison control center can help identify the properties of industrial chemicals.
- Administer topical antibiotics and cycloplegics.
- Give systemic analgesics as needed.
- Vaccinate for tetanus as indicated.
- Obtain an ophthalmologic consultation for patients with significant corneal damage.

Complications of acid and alkali burns

- Permanent visual impairment
- Adhesion of the globe to the eyelid
- Corneal ulceration
- Entropion (eyelashes that turn in toward the eyeball)
- Glaucoma

Patient education and discharge instructions
- Continue topical medications as directed.
- Follow up with an ophthalmologist.
- Wear protective eyewear when working with chemicals.
- Keep hazardous materials out of the reach of children.

Thermal burns

Thermal burns to the eye typically result from cigarettes, steam, hot liquids, fire, curling irons, and molten metal. Victims trapped in burning buildings sustain thermal ocular injuries by keeping their eyes open while trying to escape.

Therapeutic interventions
- Apply a topical anesthetic.
- Remove debris if present.
- Give systemically effective analgesics as needed.
- Administer antibiotics and cycloplegics.
- If the lid is burned, lubricate the eye and apply a cool, sterile saline compress.
- Consider eye patch(es).
- Obtain an ophthalmologic consultation.
- Vaccinate for tetanus as indicated.

Patient education and discharge instructions
- Apply antibiotics as directed.
- Follow up with an ophthalmologist.

Radiation burns

Two common types of radiation burns are ultraviolet and infrared.

Ultraviolet burns

Ultraviolet burns are seen in welders, snow skiers, ice climbers, persons who read on the beach, and persons whose eyes are unprotected under sunlamps. Symptoms develop 6 to 10 hours after exposure.

Infrared burns

Typically more severe than ultraviolet burns, infrared burns can damage the cornea, lens, and even the retina. Common causes are sun viewing (e.g., during a solar eclipse) arc welding, glassblowing, and exposure to certain lasers. The incidence of infrared burns decreases substantially with the use of protective eyewear. Repeated injury may cause cataracts.

Signs and symptoms
- Severe pain; foreign body sensation
- Reddened eye
- Blurred vision
- Photophobia
- Tearing

Diagnostic aids
- Stain the eyes with fluorescein and assess the corneas using a cobalt light.
- Perform a slit lamp examination.

Therapeutic interventions

- Administer topical antibiotics, analgesics, and cycloplegics.
- Give systemic analgesics as needed.
- Consider eye patches.
- Vaccinate for tetanus as indicated.
- Symptoms should improve with 1 to 2 days of therapy.

Patient education and discharge instructions

- Continue medications, as directed.
- Follow up with an ophthalmologist.
- Wear eye protection such as sunglasses, ski goggles, and welder's masks to protect the eyes.
- Avoid looking directly into laser lights, the sun, tanning lamps, and other sources of ultraviolet and infrared light.

Optic Nerve Trauma

The incidence of optic nerve damage in patients with a closed head injury approaches 5%.[15] Early administration of high doses of methylprednisolone may resolve optic nerve edema and improve vision, but this treatment is controversial.[16] Full or partial avulsion of the optic nerve or its blood supply usually results from severe trauma to the orbit and causes sudden and severe vision loss.

EAR, NOSE, AND THROAT TRAUMA

Auricular Lacerations

Therapeutic interventions

- Cleanse the wound.
- Assist with careful debridement and approximation of the wound edges (to avoid deformity). The skin must be pulled over any exposed cartilage. To avoid further cartilage damage, sutures should extend only through the skin and perichondrium.

Ear Amputations

Therapeutic interventions

- Remove dirt and debris.
- Administer antibiotics intravenously.
- Prepare the patient for surgical intervention.
- Postoperatively, leeches may be used to relieve vascular congestion and maintain blood vessel patency at the surgical site.

Hematomas of the Pinna

Undrained hematomas of the pinna can cause a permanent deformity known as cauliflower ear.

Therapeutic interventions

- Assist with anesthesia to the area.
- Assist with hematoma aspiration using a large-bore needle or a small stab incision. Drain placement may be necessary.

- Apply a pressure dressing to control bleeding and prevent blood reaccumulation. Vaseline gauze packed on both sides of the pinna can be used.

Ruptured Tympanic Membrane

A ruptured tympanic membrane (eardrum) can result from blunt, penetrating, or blast trauma. This condition is associated with loud noise or a slap over the ear (pressure from the outside), diving injuries (vacuum from the inside), aircraft travel or other rapid altitude changes (expanding air inside), skull fractures (direct tears), ear infections (internal fluid accumulation), or self-instrumentation (puncture).

Signs and symptoms

- Sharp ear pain, usually sudden in onset
- Blood or other fluid drainage from the ear
- Hearing impairment is proportional to the size of the perforation.
- Possible tinnitus and vertigo

Diagnostic aid

- Otoscopic examination

Therapeutic interventions

- Give analgesics.
- Administer antibiotics if there is a history of ear contamination.
- Consult an otolaryngologist. Most small perforations heal spontaneously within a few weeks. Large perforations may require surgical repair.

Patient education and discharge instructions

- Avoid water in the ear and any additional trauma during the healing process.
- Take acetaminophen or ibuprofen for pain.
- In the future, wear ear protection as needed.
- Do not put any instruments in the ear.

TRAUMA TO THE NECK

The neck contains a variety of vital structures vulnerable to injury (Table 40-3). Gunshots and stabbings, hanging and strangulation, motor vehicle collisions, assaults, and sports-related trauma can cause neck injury, vascular damage, and potential airway compromise.

Signs and Symptoms of Great Vessel Injury

Great vessel injury may be evident by the following:
- Hemorrhage: External or occult
- Cervical or supraclavicular hematoma formation
- Weak or absent pulses in the neck
- Hemothorax

Table 40-3   Structures That May Be Involved in Injuries to the Neck

Zone of Injury	Structures at Risk
Zone I (base of the neck)	Great vessels (subclavian vessels, brachiocephalic veins, common carotid arteries, and jugular veins), aortic arch, trachea, esophagus, lung apices, cervical spine, spinal cord, cervical nerve roots
Zone II (midportion of the neck)	Carotid and vertebral arteries, jugular veins, pharynx, larynx, trachea, esophagus, cervical spine, spinal cord
Zone III (superior aspect of the neck)	Salivary and parotid glands, esophagus, trachea, cervical spine, carotid arteries, jugular veins, major nerves (including cranial nerves IX-XII)

Modified from Levy D, Buckman R: *Neck trauma.* http://www.emedicine.com/emerg/topic331.htm. Accessed July 24, 2003.

- Pulsus paradoxus (systolic blood pressure decreases with inspiration)
- Upper extremity ischemia
- Hemiparesis
- Decreased level of consciousness
- Respiratory distress caused by tracheal compression

Signs and Symptoms of Cranial Nerve Injury

Cranial nerve injury may be evident by the following:
- Cranial nerve IX (glossopharyngeal nerve): Dysphagia
- Cranial nerve X (vagus nerve): Dysphagia, vocal changes
- Cranial nerve XI (spinal accessory nerve): Inability to shrug the shoulders or turn the head against resistance
- Cranial nerve XII (hypoglossal nerve): Tongue deviation

Signs and Symptoms of Esophageal or Pharyngeal Injury

Esophageal or pharyngeal injury may be evident by the following:
- Dysphagia
- Bloody saliva
- Pain
- Subcutaneous emphysema

Fractured Larynx

Direct blows to the neck or a strangulation event are the usual causes of fractured larynx. Because patients often have multiple trauma, these injuries are easy to overlook. A fracture of the larynx produces edema that can obstruct the upper airway.

Signs and symptoms

- History of neck trauma
- Throat pain
- Shortness of breath
- Respiratory stridor
- Vocal changes; hoarseness
- Subcutaneous air in the neck tissues

Diagnostic aids

- Clinical examination
- Direct, fiberoptic laryngoscopy
- Neck CT scan (Emergent treatment should not be delayed for imaging.)

Therapeutic interventions

- If the patient's airway is compromised, assist with emergent cricothyrotomy or tracheostomy.
- Administer analgesics as needed.
- Elevate the head of the bed 30 to 45 degrees (once the spine is cleared).

DENTAL TRAUMA

Following major trauma, check all patients for false teeth, partial plates, and bridges. Remove these items to avoid potential airway obstruction.

Chipped (Broken) Teeth

The six center, upper teeth are the dental structures most frequently injured. Assess the patient for associated maxillary or mandibular fractures. Inspect the mouth and pharynx for tooth fragments and debris that could obstruct the airway. Also check for pieces of teeth impaled in the gums. Cracks through the teeth that extend beyond the enamel can be stabilized with a calcium hydroxide paste. Bleeding from the tooth pulp requires emergency dental consultation.

Avulsed Teeth

An avulsed tooth is one that has been dislodged completely from the socket. Teeth that are reimplanted within 30 minutes have the best chance of survival (Box 40-2). Primary teeth are not reimplanted. A partially avulsed tooth should be repositioned and then stabilized. Administer antibiotics and vaccinate for tetanus as needed.

Box **40-2**　**Caring for an Avulsed Tooth**

Hold the avulsed tooth by the crown, not by the root.
Rinse the tooth with an isotonic solution; do not scrub.
The tooth may be reinserted in the socket or held between the cheek and the gum of a conscious, cooperative patient.
If the patient is unconscious or uncooperative, place the tooth in saline solution, milk, or Hank's solution to prevent further tooth damage (preferably in a suspension device such as a Save-A-Tooth kit).
Water is hypotonic and does not serve as a good tooth storage medium.
Consult a dentist or oral surgeon.

References

1. Major MS, MacGregor A, Bumpous JM: Patterns of maxillofacial injuries as a function of automobile restraint use, *Laryngoscope* 110(4):608-611, 2000.
2. Mouzakes J et al: The impact of airbags and seat belts on the incidence and severity of maxillofacial injuries in automobile accidents in New York State, *Arch Otolaryngol Head Neck Surg* 127(10): 1189-1193, 2001.
3. Le BT et al: Maxillofacial injuries associated with domestic violence, *J Oral Maxillofac Surg* 59(11): 1277-1283, 2001.
4. Meyer D: Body piercing: old traditions creating new challenges, *J Emerg Nurs* 26(6):612-614, 2000.
5. Leach J: Proper handling of soft tissue in the acute phase, *Facial Plast Surg* 17(4):227-238, 2001.
6. Holland AJ et al: Facial fractures in children, *Pediatr Emerg Care* 17(3):157-160, 2001.
7. Duma SM, Jernigan MV: The effects of airbags on orbital fracture patterns in frontal automobile crashes, *Ophthal Plast Reconstr Surg* 19(2):107-111, 2003.
8. Tong L, Bauer RJ, Buchman SR: A current 10-year retrospective survey of 199 surgically treated orbital floor fractures in a nonurban tertiary care center, *Plast Reconstr Surg* 108(3):612-621, 2001.
9. Brown MS, Ky W, Lisman RD: Concomitant ocular injuries with orbital fractures, *J Craniomaxillofac Trauma* 5(3):41-46, 1999.
10. Larian B et al: Facial trauma and ocular/orbital injury, *J Craniomaxillofac Trauma* 5(4):15-24, 1999.
11. Lehto KS, Sulander PO, Tervo TM: Do motor vehicle airbags increase risk of ocular injuries in adults? *Ophthalmology* 110(6):1082-1088, 2003.
12. Hargrave S, Weakley D, Wilson C: Complications of ocular paintball injuries in children, *J Pediatr Ophthalmol Strabismus* 37(6):338-343, 2000.
13. Rodriguez JO, Lavina AM, Agarwal A: Prevention and treatment of common eye injuries in sports, *Am Fam Physician* 67(7):1481-1488, 2003.
14. Smith D, Wrenn K, Stack LB: The epidemiology and diagnosis of penetrating eye injuries, *Acad Emerg Med* 9(3):209-213, 2002.
15. Spoor TC: Traumatic optic neuropathies. In Yanoff M, Duker JS, editors: *Ophthalmology,* Philadelphia, 1999, Mosby.
16. Steinsapir KD: Traumatic optic neuropathy, *Curr Opin Ophthalmol* 10(5):340-342, 1999.

41

Burns

Janice R. Sisco, RN, BSN

In the United States, about 2 million persons a year suffer burns significant enough to seek medical care. The majority of these injuries are relatively minor and can be treated in clinics and emergency departments (EDs). Nonetheless, about 70,000 burn victims per annum require hospitalization, and 6000 eventually die.[1,2] Although thermal injuries are by far the most common, there are a number of other burn causes. Table 41-1 lists types of burns and their energy sources.[2]

The severity of a burn is determined by the following:
- *Extent:* The amount of body surface area involved
- *Depth:* The depth (or "degree") of tissue destruction

Table **41-1** **Causes of Burns**

Type of Burn	Energy Source
Thermal	Flame
	Contact
	Steam
	Scald
	Flash
Chemical	Acids
	Alkalis
	Other chemicals (e.g., petroleum products)
Electrical	AC current
	DC current (including lightning)
Radiation	Infrared
	Ultraviolet
	Ionizing
Friction	Friction

Data from Jacobs B, Hoyt K, editors: *Trauma nursing core course provider manual,* ed 5, Des Plaines, Ill, 2000, Emergency Nurses Association.

- *Type:* Such as thermal, chemical, electrical
- *Location:* Special burn sites are at higher risk.
- *Patient factors:* Age, current medical status, associated trauma
- *Complications:* Such as inhalation injury, infection, compartment syndrome

BURN CLASSIFICATION

Depth

Signs and symptoms

First-Degree Burns (Superficial Partial Thickness) (Figure 41-1, A)
- Only the epidermis is involved.
- Local redness and pain occur.
- Minimal or no edema and no blistering occur.
- Skin blanches with pressure and refills when pressure is removed.
- Wound heals within 7 days.

Second-Degree Burns (Deep Partial Thickness) (Figure 41-1, B)
- The epidermis and some portion of the dermis are involved.
- Sweat glands, hair follicles, capillaries, and nerves remain.
- Burn appears mottled with pink, red, white, and tan areas.
- The wound is moist and may form large, wet blisters.
- Pain is intense.
- Skin blanches with pressure and refills when pressure is removed.
- Healing time is 5 to 35 days.
- Wound can convert to a full-thickness injury if undertreated or infected.

Third-Degree Burns (Full Thickness) (Figure 41-1, C)
- Burn involves the epidermis, the dermis, and the subcutaneous tissues.
- Burn can extend to muscles, tendons, ligaments, cartilage, vessels, nerves, and bone.
- Charred vessels may be visible under the eschar.
- Burn appearance depends on the cause; it can be white, brown, charred, or leathery.
- Wound is dry; no blister formation occurs.
- No blanching occurs with pressure.
- Full-thickness burns usually are surrounded by painful partial-thickness burns.
- Wound requires excision and grafting.

Extent

Rule of nines

The extent of a burn is calculated as a percentage of the total body surface area (BSA). A simple but imprecise system of determining burn extent in emergency situations is the rule of nines. Figure 41-2 shows adult and pediatric versions of this commonly used method. The Lund and Browder chart (Figure 41-3) provides a more accurate estimate of burn extent. However, this formula is complicated and rarely is used outside of burn centers.[3] Neither the rule of nines nor the Lund and Browder chart can estimate the extent of electrical burns accurately.

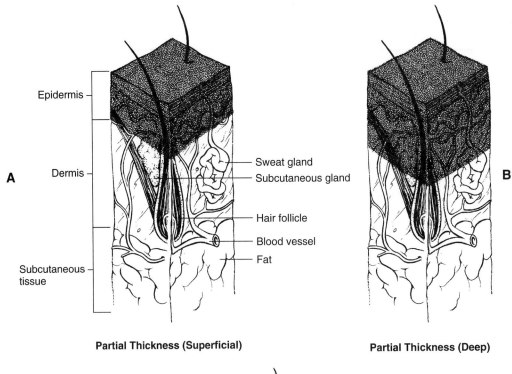

Epidermis

Dermis

Subcutaneous tissue

Sweat gland
Subcutaneous gland

Hair follicle

Blood vessel
Fat

A

B

Partial Thickness (Superficial)   **Partial Thickness (Deep)**

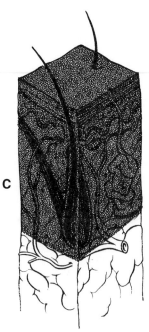

C

Full Thickness

Figure 41-1. First-, second-, and third-degree burns. Stippled areas indicate depth of burn injury. **A,** Superficial partial-thickness burn. **B,** Deep partial-thickness burn. **C,** Full-thickness burn injury. (From Edlich R, Bailey T, Bill T: Thermal burns. In Marx J, Hockenberger R, Walls R, editors: *Rosen's emergency medicine: concepts and clinical practice,* ed 5, St Louis, 2002, Mosby.)

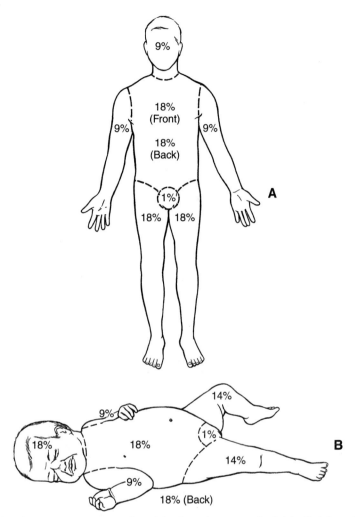

Figure 41-2. Rule of nines: percentages of total body surface area. **A,** Adult. **B,** Infant. (From Edlich R, Bailey T, Bill T: Thermal burns. In Marx J, Hockenberger R, Walls R, editors: *Rosen's emergency medicine: concepts and clinical practice*, ed 5, St Louis, 2002, Mosby.)

Severity

The American Burn Association has established a burn classification system that categorizes all burns as major, moderate, or minor.[2]

Major burns

Adults

- Second-degree burns 25% BSA or greater
- Third-degree burns 10% BSA or greater

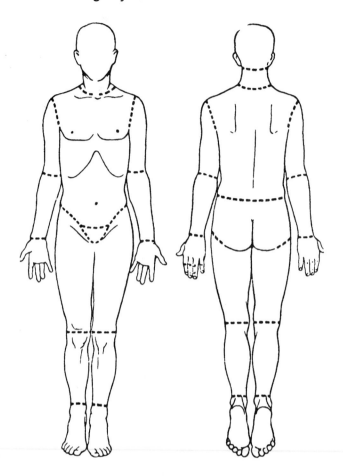

Percent Surface Area Burned

Area	1 Year	1-4 Years	5-9 Years	10-14 Years	>15 Years	Adult	2"	3"
Head	19	17	13	11	9	7		
Neck	2	2	2	2	2	2		
Ant. Trunk	13	13	13	13	13	13		
Post. Trunk	13	13	13	13	13	13		
R. Buttock	$2\frac{1}{2}$	$2\frac{1}{2}$	$2\frac{1}{2}$	$2\frac{1}{2}$	$2\frac{1}{2}$	$2\frac{1}{2}$		
L. Buttock	$2\frac{1}{2}$	$2\frac{1}{2}$	$2\frac{1}{2}$	$2\frac{1}{2}$	$2\frac{1}{2}$	$2\frac{1}{2}$		
Genitalia	1	1	1	1	1	1		
R. U. Arm	4	4	4	4	4	4		
L. U. Arm	4	4	4	4	4	4		
R. L. Arm	3	3	3	3	3	3		
L. L. Arm	3	3	3	3	3	3		
R. Hand	$2\frac{1}{2}$	$2\frac{1}{2}$	$2\frac{1}{2}$	$2\frac{1}{2}$	$2\frac{1}{2}$	$2\frac{1}{2}$		
L. Hand	$2\frac{1}{2}$	$2\frac{1}{2}$	$2\frac{1}{2}$	$2\frac{1}{2}$	$2\frac{1}{2}$	$2\frac{1}{2}$		
R. Thigh	$5\frac{1}{2}$	$6\frac{1}{2}$	8	$8\frac{1}{2}$	9	$9\frac{1}{2}$		
L. Thigh	$5\frac{1}{2}$	$6\frac{1}{2}$	8	$8\frac{1}{2}$	9	$9\frac{1}{2}$		
R. Leg	5	5	$5\frac{1}{2}$	6	$6\frac{1}{2}$	7		
L. Leg	5	5	$5\frac{1}{2}$	6	$6\frac{1}{2}$	7		
R. Foot	$3\frac{1}{2}$	$3\frac{1}{2}$	$3\frac{1}{2}$	$3\frac{1}{2}$	$3\frac{1}{2}$	$3\frac{1}{2}$		
L. Foot	$3\frac{1}{2}$	$3\frac{1}{2}$	$3\frac{1}{2}$	$3\frac{1}{2}$	$3\frac{1}{2}$	$3\frac{1}{2}$		
TOTAL								

Figure 41-3. Lund and Browder formula. (From Artz CP, Moncrief JA: *The treatment of burns*, ed 2, Philadelphia, 1969, Saunders.)

Children

- Second-degree burns 20% BSA or greater
- Any third-degree burn

All Patients

- Burns involving the hands, face, eyes, ears, feet, or perineum
- Inhalation burns
- Electrical burns
- Deep, circumferential burns
- Caustic chemical burns
- Burns with associated major trauma
- Burns in patients older than 55 years of age
- Patients with significant underlying medical problems (e.g., diabetes, heart diseases, renal failure, and neuromuscular disorders)

Moderate burns

Adults

- Second-degree burns 15% to 25% BSA

Children

- Second-degree burns 10% to 20% BSA

Minor burns

Adults

- Second-degree burns 15% BSA or less
- Third-degree burns 2% BSA or less

Children

- Second-degree burns 10% BSA or less
- Third-degree burns 2% BSA or less

Burn center admission is recommended for the following:
- Second- or third-degree burns to 10% BSA or greater
- Burns of special areas (Box 41-1)

Box **41-1**   **Special Burn Areas**

Ears
Eyes
Face
Feet
Fingers
Hands
Perineum
Burns to certain complex and functionally important body areas require special handing if optimal results are to be achieved. Refer these patients to a burn specialist.

- Circumferential burns
- Electrical or chemical burns
- Burns associated with multiple or significant trauma
- Burns associated with suspected child maltreatment

BURN CARE

Assessment

Signs and symptoms

- Obvious burns to the skin and (possibly) deeper structures
- Signs of inhalation injury, which include the following:
  - Singed eyelashes, brows, nasal hair, and other facial hair
  - Soot in or around the lips, mouth, or nostrils
  - Vocal changes, hoarseness
  - Drooling, stridor, cough
  - Progressive swelling and airway obstruction

Diagnostic aids

- Look for clinical signs of respiratory distress.
- Bronchoscopy may be performed to diagnose inhalation injury.
- Use the rule of nines to estimate burn extent quickly.
- Visually inspect wounds to calculate burn depth.

Therapeutic interventions

Immediate therapy

- Stop the burning process by cooling the area with liberal amounts of water or isotonic saline.
- Remove any smoldering material.

Airway/breathing

- Establish airway control if facial or inhalation injuries are present. Promptly intubate any patient with early signs of respiratory embarrassment.
- Postburn edema of the face and airways can develop rapidly. Many severely burned patients are awake on arrival to the ED yet require aggressive airway management.
- Assist with cricothyrotomy if a surgical airway is necessary (rarely indicated).
- Administer 100% oxygen, preferably humidified.
- Consider drawing samples for arterial blood gases and a carboxyhemoglobin level. (See Chapter 28 for information on carbon monoxide poisoning.)

Circulation

- Establish intravenous access with two (or more) large-bore (14- to 16-gauge) catheters.
- Fluid resuscitation should be based on the following guidelines[4]:
  - Calculate fluid requirements (Box 41-2).
  - Infuse half of the total amount in the first 8 hours *from the time of the burn.*
  - Divide the remaining amount over the next 16 hours.
  - Use the formulas as a rough estimate of fluid requirements. Always tailor volume replacement to individual patient needs based on urine output, laboratory values, and hemodynamic response.

Box **41**-2 Calculation of Fluids

Adults: Lactated Ringer's solution 2 to 4 mL × kg body weight × percent burn
Children: Lactated Ringer's solution 3 to 4 mL × kg body weight × percent burn
Infants and Young Children: Infants and young children should receive fluid with 5% dextrose at a maintenance rate *in addition to the resuscitation fluid noted above for children.*

- Aggressive fluid resuscitation is indicated for patients with greater than 20% body surface area burns. However, avoid overhydration.
- Frequently reassess the distal circulatory status in burned extremities. This may require a Doppler ultrasound to detect pulsations.[1]
- Place an indwelling urinary catheter in patients with the following:
  - Burns greater than 20% BSA
  - Perineal burns

Additional interventions

- Remove restrictive clothing and jewelry.
- Do not apply ice to burns.
- Do not put wet dressings on burns greater than 10% BSA.
- Maintain normothermia; burn patients chill easily.[3]
- Place a gastric tube, and attach it to suction:
  - In patients with burns greater than 20% BSA[1]
  - In intubated patients
  - If nausea or vomiting are present
- Provide generous doses of analgesics.
  - Use intravenous narcotics.
  - Because of poor perfusion, do not give analgesics intramuscularly.
  - Morphine sulfate is the drug of choice for pain control.
- Determine tetanus immunization status; administer as necessary.
- It is important to monitor glucose levels in children because they are more prone to hypoglycemia because of their limited glycogen stores.
- Do not administer antibiotics prophylactically.
- Arrange for admission to a burn center if the patient meets the criteria listed previously.

Burn Wound Care

When possible, elevate burned areas above the patient's heart to minimize edema formation.[1] Care of a burn wound consists of the following:
- Cover minor burns with dressings dampened with sterile normal saline.
- Cover burns greater than 10% BSA with a *dry* towel or sheet (does not have to be sterile).
- Once a minor burn has been evaluated, a variety of ointments can be applied such as bacitracin, silver sulfadiazine (Silvadene), or mafenide acetate (Sulfamylon). Cover the site with a dry, sterile dressing. Alternatively, apply a transparent dressing, hydrocolloid dressing, or Xeroform to keep the wound clean and moist.
- If a patient is being transferred to a burn center, always consult the center's specialist before debriding wounds or applying topical agents. Most burn centers prefer to receive patients without debridement or ointments.

Emergency Wound Procedures

Escharotomy

An escharotomy is performed when full-thickness, circumferential burns constrict underlying structures, impairing circulation or causing respiratory compromise. Common escharotomy sites are the arms, chest, fingers, hand, legs, and toes. This procedure may be performed in the ED by simply slicing through dead eschar with a scalpel. Pain and bleeding are minimal. This allows the underlying tissue to swell, reestablishing circulation or facilitating chest wall expansion. Incisions are made along the "seam lines" of the body (Figure 41-4).

Fasciotomy

A fasciotomy may be necessary if the burns are deep and substantial swelling is present in any fascial compartments. This is particularly common in patients with electrical burns.

Long-Term Wound Coverings

A variety of temporary and permanent grafts are available for wound closure, including allografts, homografts, xenografts, and heterografts. None of these are appropriate for ED use.

MANAGEMENT OF NONTHERMAL BURNS

Chemical Burns

Wear personal protective equipment during the decontamination procedure. (See Chapter 13 for information on decontamination following chemical exposure.)

Therapeutic interventions

- Remove the patient's contaminated clothing.
- Brush any powdered chemicals off the skin and hair.
- Immediately irrigate chemical burns with copious amounts of water.
- Hydrofluoric acid burns require complex management. Contact your regional poison control center for assistance.
- For chemical burns to the eye, see Chapter 40.

Tar Burns

Tar burns commonly occur in roofers and road construction workers. These burns usually involve the face, head, neck, hands, or arms.

Therapeutic interventions

- Initiate measures to cool the tar immediately.
- Do not attempt to peel off the tar; this removes skin as well.
- Soften and loosen tar with mineral oil, Vaseline, mayonnaise, or a tar solvent.
- Treat the resultant burns as thermal burns.

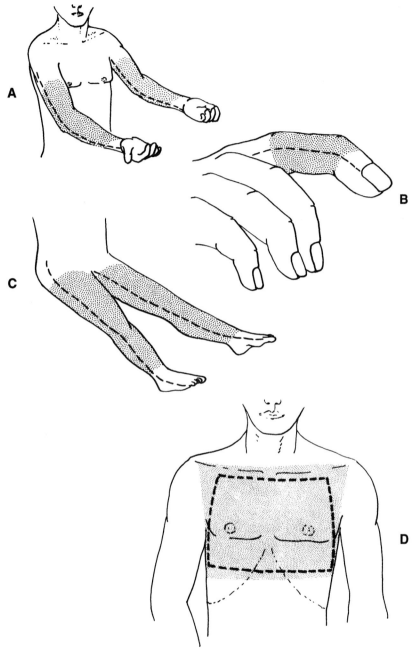

Figure 41-4. Escharotomy sites. **A,** Arms. **B,** Fingers. **C,** Legs. **D,** Anterior thorax.

Friction Burns

Friction burns are also known as "brush burns," "floor burns," and "road burns." This type of wound is the result of abrasion and the heat produced by friction. Friction burns frequently are seen in athletes who fall on gymnasium floors, tennis courts, artificial-turf fields, or running tracks. Motorcycle riders who fail to wear protective clothing are also subject to friction injuries with road contact. These wounds are rarely full thickness and are treated like partial-thickness burns or abrasions.

Electrical Burns

Evaluation of the extent of an electrical burn is difficult because the majority of the damage is internal. Entrance and exit sites are often small, but destruction of underlying tissue can be extensive. This destruction is the result of intense heat generated by the passage of electric current through the tissues. The full extent of an electrical burn may not be evident for 7 to 10 days following injury. Common complications of electrical burns include rhabdomyolysis, ventricular fibrillation, seizures, and compartment syndrome. Watch for the development of dark urine, dysrhythmias, and compartment tenseness. (See Chapter 39 for compartment syndrome information.)

References

1. Edlich R, Bailey T, Bill T: Thermal burns. In Marx J, Hockenberger R, Walls R, editors: *Rosen's emergency medicine: concepts and clinical practice,* ed 5, St Louis, 2002, Mosby.
2. Emergency Nurses Association: Burn Trauma. In Jacobs B et al, editors: *Trauma Nursing Core course provider manual,* ed 5, Des Plaines, Ill, 2000, The Association.
3. Wraa C: Burns. In Newberry L, editor: *Sheehy's emergency nursing principles and practice,* ed 5, St Louis, 2003, Mosby.
4. American Burn Association: *Advanced burn life,* Chicago, Ill, 2005, The Association.

42

Obstetric Trauma

Mara S. Kerr, RNC, MS

Trauma is the primary cause of morbidity and mortality among females in their childbearing years. Approximately 1 in 12 women will be treated for trauma during pregnancy. Motor vehicle collisions, falls, and intimate partner violence are the leading mechanisms of injury to childbearing women.[1]

Care of the pregnant trauma patient is complicated by the normal physiologic changes of pregnancy and the presence of a second patient, the fetus (Table 42-1). Stabilization of the mother is always the first priority; achieving a stable maternal condition provides the fetus with the best possible chance of survival. All interventions to resuscitate the fetus are directed at the mother.[2]

The emergency nurse must understand that pregnancy should never interfere with the rapid identification or management of injuries based on a perceived risk to the fetus.[1] Any test or procedure that routinely would be used for trauma care can be used in the management of the pregnant patient, with the addition of a few modifications and simple safety measures. This includes imaging studies (plain films, computed tomography, magnetic resonance imaging, angiography, intravenous pyelography) and invasive procedures (e.g., diagnostic peritoneal lavage, emergent thoracotomy, needle decompression, and exploratory laparotomy). Even pneumatic antishock garments can be applied for stabilization of lower extremity fractures as long as the abdominal compartment is not inflated.

ASSESSMENT OF THE OBSTETRIC TRAUMA PATIENT

Primary

The primary survey of the pregnant trauma patient is performed in the same manner as that of any other patient. (See Chapter 34.) Airway, breathing, and circulatory evaluation should

Table 42-1 Maternal Cardiovascular and Respiratory Changes During Pregnancy

Cardiovascular		Respiratory	
• Cardiac output	↑ 30%	• Tidal volume	↑ 40%
• Heart rate	↑ by 15 to 20 beats/min	• Vital capacity	↑ by 100 to 200 mL
• Blood pressure	↓ by 15 to 15 mm Hg	• Respiratory rate	↑ Slightly
• Venous pressure	CVP varies	• $PaCo_2$	↓ to 30 mm Hg (4.0 KPa)
	Increased in lower extremities	• Pao_2	↑ to 101 to 104 mm Hg (13.5-13.9 KPa)
• Hematocrit	↓ to 31 to 34%	• Arterial pH	↑ Slightly
• White blood count	Increased to 15,000/mm³	• Serum HCO_3	↓
	Normal differential		
• Electrocardiogram	Flattened of inverted T waves in III, AVF, AVL		
• Fibrinogen and clotting factors VII, VIII, IX	Increased		

From Emergency Nurses Association: *Trauma nursing care course*, ed 5, Des Plaines, Ill, 2000, The Association.

Table **42-2**   **Impact of Physiologic Changes of Pregnancy on the Trauma Patient**

Airway	Risk of aspiration caused by cardiac sphincter laxity, stomach compression, and gastric hypomotility is increased.
	Intubation is difficult because of increased upper airway vascularity.
Breathing	The pregnant patient's normal state of compensated metabolic alkalosis masks the signs of metabolic acidosis (shock) until the condition is advanced.
	Reduced oxygen reserves (because of diaphragm elevation) and high metabolic demands predispose the patient to hypoxia.
Circulation	Because of a 40% increase in circulating volume, signs of shock may not be evident until the patient has lost 1500 mL of blood.
	The pregnant patient (normally hot and flushed) may never develop the cool, clammy skin typical of shock.
	The physiologic anemia of pregnancy makes interpreting hemoglobin/hematocrit results difficult.
	The normal hypotension and tachycardia of pregnancy make interpreting vital signs difficult.
	After 20 weeks' gestation, the combined weight of the fetus, uterus, placenta, and amniotic fluid will compress the vena cava and decrease blood pressure when the patient is supine.
	In the presence of hypovolemia the body considers the uterus a nonvital organ and the fetus is hypoperfused very early.
	As a result of the increase in circulating volume, the pregnant patient may appear to be in congestive heart failure.
	Most clotting factor levels are elevated in pregnancy, making patients prone to clots and bleeding disorders.
	Because of a large circulating volume and hormonal changes, the pregnant patient does not concentrate urine efficiently and will continue to have a high output with dilute urine in the face of hypovolemia.
	Massive uterine blood flow predisposes pregnant patients to major hemorrhage if the uterus or its vessels are damaged.

occur simultaneously with interventions when any potentially life-threatening condition is identified.

Importantly, the changes of pregnancy can mask normal physiologic responses to trauma, and these changes must be considered carefully when caring for a gravid patient. Table 42-2 summarizes the effects of these changes on the trauma patient.

Secondary

Secondary assessment of the pregnant trauma patient includes the usual head-to-toe examination and a detailed evaluation of the abdomen and pelvis. Assess for uterine activity by palpating the uterus and noting fundal height and resting tone, as well as contraction frequency, intensity, and duration. The contraction pattern may indicate several conditions that will affect fetal outcome adversely if interventions are not provided quickly.

Fetal Assessment and Management

Gestational age and fetal injuries can be identified by ultrasound. The ultrasound examination also can be used to determine whether cardiac activity is present or absent. For ongoing assessment of the fetal response to interventions, use Doppler ultrasound to auscultate the fetal heart rate intermittently (<20 weeks' gestation) or initiate continuous electronic fetal monitoring (>20 weeks' gestation). Any patient with a viable pregnancy should be monitored for at least 4 hours after injury. To detect late onset complications, continue monitoring for up to 48 hours if the woman is symptomatic. Collaboration with the obstetric nursing staff is imperative. Interpretation of electronic fetal monitor tracings requires extensive training and practice to identify fetal distress and provide appropriate interventions.[3] Emergency nurses rarely have the requisite skill level and should not be expected to perform this task.

Signs and symptoms of fetal stress/distress

- Fetal heart rate is greater than 160 or less than 110 beats/min.
- No fetal heart rate accelerations are present.
- Periodic fetal heart rate decelerations occur.
- No beat-to-beat variability is present.
- Decreased fetal movement is noted by the mother.

Therapeutic interventions for fetal distress

- Administer oxygen by tight-fitting face mask at 10 to 15 L/min.
- Position the patient on her left side or displace the uterus to the left with a wedge under the right hip. Even patients on a backboard can be tilted readily.
- Infuse a bolus of lactated Ringer's solution or normal saline solution.
- Consider emergent cesarean delivery of a potentially viable fetus.

SPECIFIC OBSTETRIC EMERGENCIES

Abruptio Placentae

Abruptio placentae (also called placental abruption) can occur when the mother experiences a sudden, rapid deceleration or blunt abdominal impact. This trauma completely or partially detaches the placenta from the uterine wall, disrupting the maternal-fetal circulation. Fetal effects depend on the amount of functional placenta remaining. Placental bleeding is associated with the development of disseminated intravascular coagulation, making early identification of this condition important. Abruptio placentae is the most common cause of fetal demise following trauma.[2]

Signs and symptoms

- Abdomen is tender.
- Uterine rigidity is felt on palpation.
- Fetal heart rate may indicate distress or may be absent.
- Mother has a backache.
- Vaginal bleeding may or may not be present.
- A clot is visible behind the placenta on ultrasound.
- The amniotic fluid is port wine colored.
- Maternal shock develops.

Therapeutic interventions

- Administer oxygen by tight-fitting face mask at 10 to 15 L/min.
- Infuse a bolus of lactated Ringer's solution or normal saline solution.
- Obtain obstetric consultation to evaluate for possible emergent cesarean delivery.

- Draw and send laboratory studies including a complete blood count, Kleihauer-Betke test, type and crossmatch, and coagulation studies (prothrombin time [international normalized ration], activated partial thromboplastin time, fibrinogen, andD-dimer).

Preterm Labor

Regular contractions occurring before 37 completed weeks of gestation put the fetus at risk for preterm birth. Preterm labor is the most common obstetric complication following trauma.

Signs and symptoms

- Uterine contractions that occur every 10 minutes or less
- Abdominal cramping
- Backache
- Pelvic pressure
- An increase or change in vaginal discharge or onset of vaginal bleeding

Therapeutic interventions

- Assist with a pelvic examination (sterile speculum) to assess for ruptured membranes and evaluate the cervix.
- Initiate tocolytic therapy (drugs that stop contractions) for patients with a live fetus between 20 and 35 weeks of gestation.
- Admit the patient to an obstetric unit for continuous electronic fetal monitoring and ongoing assessment of uterine activity

Uterine Rupture

Uterine rupture is a rare injury that occurs in less than 1% of pregnant patients with major trauma. The uterus is a strong, flexible muscle that requires a great deal of force to rupture. This condition is seen in cases of sudden deceleration or severe abdominal compression (e.g., run over by a vehicle). Rupture is more likely in women with prior uterine scarring. The fetus is almost invariably dead.

Signs and symptoms

- Sudden onset of severe abdominal pain
- Vaginal bleeding (may be minimal or concealed)
- Fetal parts that can be palpated outside of the uterus
- Fetal bradycardia or asystole
- Maternal hypovolemic shock

Therapeutic interventions

- Volume replacement: Crystalloids and blood
- Emergent cesarean delivery; hysterectomy may be required

Perimortem Cesarean Delivery

A perimortem cesarean delivery should be considered when a mother has suffered cardiac arrest or is deteriorating rapidly and death appears imminent. The fetus must be alive and at least 26 weeks of gestation. Cesarean section performed within 5 minutes of the mother's death offers the greatest chance of delivering a neurologically intact infant. In rare instances, maternal resuscitation efforts are enhanced by fetal removal.[4] Perimortem delivery can occur in the emergency department. However, a team capable of resuscitating and stabilizing the neonate must be present with the appropriate equipment and supplies. In most cases, a large abdominal (classical) incision is performed so that the fetus can be accessed quickly. Continue maternal cardiopulmonary resuscitation until the fetus is delivered.

References

1. American Academy of Pediatrics, American College of Obstetricians and Gynecologists: Obstetric and medical complications. In Gilstrap L, Oh W, editors: *Guidelines for perinatal care,* ed 5 Washington, DC, 2002, The College.
2. Weiss HB, Songer TJ, Fabio A: Fetal deaths related to maternal injury, *JAMA* 286(15):1863-1868, 2001.
3. Mandeville LK, Troiano NH: *High-risk and critical care intrapartum nursing,* ed 2, Philadelphia, 1999, Lippincott.
4. Cunningham FG et al: Medical and surgical complications in pregnancy. In Cunningham FG et al, editors: *William's obstetrics,* ed 21, New York, 2001, McGraw-Hill.

43

Pediatric Trauma

Jeff Solheim, RN, CEN

In developed countries, traumatic injuries kill more children than all other diseases combined, accounting for more than 50% of total pediatric deaths. For every child that dies, four survive but are permanently disabled. Sadly, nearly all morbidity and mortality from pediatric trauma is preventable. The most common mechanisms of death in this population are motor vehicle collisions (33%), homicides (12.8%), suicides (9.6%), drownings (9.2%), pedestrian injuries (8%), and burns (7.2%).[1] The vast majority of children sustain blunt trauma (about 80%) as opposed to penetrating wounds (about 20%). Emergency nurses must always be alert to the possibility that pediatric trauma may be related to child maltreatment. Clinicians should be aware of patterns of injury suggestive of abuse. (See Chapter 47.)

The principles of trauma assessment and management are the same for children and adults (see Chapter 34). However, health care providers need to be familiar with a number of issues unique to children (e.g., differences in airway and breathing) (Tables 43-1, 43-2, and 43-3). The injured child is best cared for in an emergency department prepared with the appropriate personnel and supplies to meet their special needs. A quick reference method for identifying the right-sized equipment can save precious minutes. Length-based resuscitation guides (e.g., Broselow tape) and color-coded supply boxes, packs, or carts are the most frequently used systems (Figure 43-1).[3]

PRIMARY SURVEY

As with adults, the primary survey is used simultaneously to identify and immediately treat life-threatening injuries.[4]

Table **43-1** **Pediatric Airway Considerations**

Developmental and Anatomic Considerations	Clinical Significance
Children's tongues are large compared with the size of their oral cavities.	The tongue easily obstructs the airway. Proper head positioning is crucial; use a jaw-thrust maneuver to establish and maintain an open airway.
Children have smaller upper and lower airways; the infant's tracheal diameter approximates the diameter of the little finger.	Even small amounts of mucus, edema, or blood can cause airway obstruction.
Infants under 3 months of age are obligate nasal breathers.	Trauma to the nose that results in bleeding or secretions can lead to respiratory distress. Frequent nasal suctioning or tracheal intubation may be required in these cases.
The narrowest portion of a child's airway is the cricoid cartilage.	Children under 8 years of age should be intubated with an uncuffed tracheal tube. The narrow cricoid cartilage will provide an adequate seal. Cuff inflation can produce tracheal tissue ischemia.
The small child's larynx is higher and more anterior; the trachea is shorter	Tracheal intubation is more difficult, and right main stem bronchus intubation is common. Careful and ongoing assessment of tube placement is vital.

Table **43-2** **Pediatric Breathing Considerations**

Developmental and Anatomic Considerations	Clinical Significance
Infants breathe predominantly by using their abdominal muscles.	Abdominal distention or restriction can contribute to respiratory distress. Inserting a gastric tube to decompress the stomach may improve respiratory function and reduce the risk of aspiration.
Children's chest walls are thinner, softer, and more compliant.[2]	Children are more prone to visceral injuries. Lack of rib fractures does not rule out underlying organ damage, and the presence of rib fractures strongly suggests intrathoracic or abdominal injury.
The child's intercostal muscles are poorly developed. Children have less respiratory reserve than do adults.	Children are at increased risk for respiratory fatigue and compromise, leading to respiratory distress.
The infant's metabolic rate is about 2 times that of the adult.	Every attempt should be made to minimize metabolic stressors: treat pain, reduce fever, provide comfort measures, maintain normothermia and involve the family.

Airway (With Full Spinal Stabilization)

Assessment

- Ensure airway patency.
- Look for oral fluids and foreign bodies.
- Maintain full spinal stabilization.

Therapeutic interventions

- Use the jaw-thrust maneuver to open the airway of an unconscious child.
- Suction any blood, emesis, or secretions from the airway.

Table **43-3**   **Pediatric Circulation Considerations**

Developmental and Anatomic Considerations	Clinical Significance
The child's circulating blood volume is proportionally greater than that of the adult (Infants: 90 mL/kg; children: 80 mL/kg; adults: 70 mL/kg).[3]	Volume losses can produce hypovolemia more quickly than in adults.
Neonates have an incompletely developed sympathetic nervous system and are sensitive to parasympathetic stimulation. (e.g., suctioning and rectal stimulation)	Avoid procedures that stimulate the parasympathetic system. Monitor and manage bradycardia as needed.
Because the pediatric myocardium is incompletely developed, the small child's heart is unable to increase contractility significantly. In the event of hypovolemia, heart rate—rather than stroke volume—must rise to maintain cardiac output.[3]	Elevated heart rates are an early indicator of circulatory failure in the pediatric patient.
Because of excellent sympathetic compensatory responses, hypotension is a late sign of shock in children, usually occurring only after a circulating blood loss of at least 25%.	To provide adequate assessment and intervention, personnel caring for the pediatric patient must be aware of normal vital sign parameters for various age-groups. (See Table 7-5.)

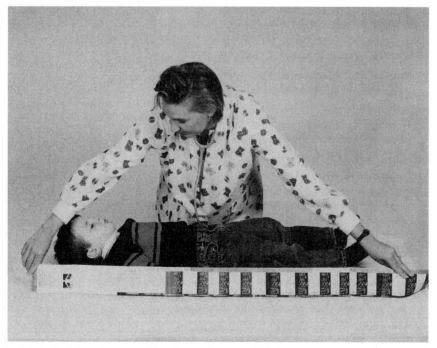

Figure 43-1. The Broselow tape system is one way to organize pediatric resuscitation equipment. The child's length is measured against the tape. This leads the team to a color-coded pack or code cart drawer containing equipment sized appropriately for the child. (Courtesy Armstrong Medical Industries, Lincolnshire, Ill.)

- If the child is unable to maintain a patent airway, place a nasopharyngeal airway (in the conscious patient) or an oropharyngeal airway (in unconscious patients and those with possible basilar skull fractures).
  - Select the appropriate sized oropharyngeal airway by measuring from the corner of the mouth to the angle of the jaw.[3]
  - Using a tongue blade to depress and displace the tongue forward, gently insert the oral airway.
  - Do not invert the oropharyngeal airway and then rotate it 180 degrees as is commonly done in adults. This practice can traumatize the child's oral soft tissues.
- Tracheal intubation is recommended for any child with respiratory distress, poor ventilation, or a Glasgow Coma Scale score of 8 or less.
- In children younger than 8 years old, use an uncuffed tube to avoid cord trauma, subglottic edema, and pressure necrosis.
- Choose an appropriately sized tube using one of the following methods:
  - Measure the patient with a length-based resuscitation guide (e.g., Broselow tape).
  - Select a tube that is approximately the diameter of the child's fifth finger.
  - Calculate tube size using the following formula:

$$\text{Tube size (mm)} = \frac{\text{Age in years} + 16}{4}$$

- Carefully assess for proper tube placement immediately after intubation by the following means:
  - Auscultate over the epigastrium and then over both lung fields. Epigastric gurgling indicates esophageal intubation. Breath sounds should be noted equally on both sides of the chest.
  - Inspect the chest for symmetrical rise and fall with assisted ventilation.
  - Confirm tracheal placement with a carbon dioxide detection device.
- Maintain cervical spine precautions using size-appropriate equipment and collars. Because the occiput of the infant and toddler is large and protruding, place a small towel roll under the shoulders to lift them to the level of the external auditory meatus. This simple practice aligns the spine and assists with airway maintenance[4] (Figure 43-2).

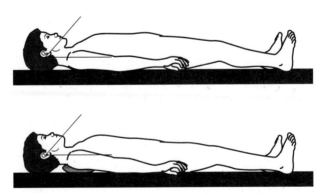

Figure 43-2. The head of a child is large in proportion to the rest of the body, resulting in forward flexion of the head when in the supine position. A small towel roll placed under the shoulders of the child on a backboard will bring the shoulders in line with the external auditory meatus and assist with airway maintenance. (From Emergency Nurses Association: *Trauma nursing core course provider manual*, Des Plaines, Ill, 2000, The Association.)

Breathing

Assessment

- Observe respiratory rate, depth, symmetry, and quality.
- Watch for signs of increasing respiratory effort or distress ("air hunger") such as grunting, nasal flaring, chest wall retractions, head bobbing, or shoulder lifting.
- Check the integrity of the chest wall, looking for open wounds and bony injuries.
- Auscultate breath sounds for equality and the presence of adventitious sounds. Because the child's chest wall is smaller and thinner, breath sounds can be transmitted easily from one location to another (e.g., sounds may be heard over an area of pneumothorax).
- Gently palpate the position of the trachea; note the presence of subcutaneous air and any deviation from midline.

Therapeutic interventions

- During the initial phase of care, administer 100% oxygen to all children.[2]
- Using a pulse oximeter, monitor oxygen saturation.
  - Digital readings are difficult to obtain in children with poor peripheral perfusion; try a nasal bridge or ear lobe probe.
- Provide positive-pressure ventilation with a bag-mask device or a mechanical ventilator.
- Assist with decompression of a suspected tension pneumothorax with a needle thoracostomy and then prepare for immediate chest tube insertion.
- Assist with tracheal intubation for ongoing control of airway, ventilation, and oxygenation.

Circulation

Assessment

- Evaluate the patient's level of consciousness.
- Check capillary refill time. Less than 2 seconds is considered normal; immediate refill is ideal.
- Observe for obvious external hemorrhage.
- Palpate the quality and effectiveness of central and peripheral pulses.
- Observe skin color and feel for temperature.

Therapeutic Interventions

- If the child's heart rate is less then 60 beats/min and perfusion is ineffective, initiate cardiopulmonary resuscitation (CPR) following the American Heart Association's Pediatric Advanced Life Support (PALs) guidelines.[2]
- Apply direct pressure to areas of uncontrolled external hemorrhage.
- If a pulse is present but circulation is inadequate, do the following:
  - Obtain vascular access by inserting two large-bore intravenous catheters or intraosseous needles.
  - Administer a 20 mL/kg bolus of warmed lactated Ringer's solution or normal saline.
  - If circulation remains inadequate, repeat the bolus.
  - After two boluses, consider switching to type-specific or O-negative packed red blood cells (10 mL/kg) for further fluid resuscitation.[2]

Disability (Neurologic Evaluation)

Developmental and Anatomic Considerations

- The relatively large head and lax neck muscles of pediatric patients make them more susceptible to head injuries.
- Intracranial trauma is the leading cause of death and disability in children.
- Because the anterior fontanelle does not close until 12 to 18 months of age, it can be used as an assessment tool. A bulging fontanelle may indicate increased intracranial pressure; a depressed fontanelle suggests dehydration.

Assessment

- Assess pupillary size, shape, and response to light.
- Determine the patient's level of consciousness using the pediatric Glasgow Coma Scale (see Chapter 7, Table 7-8) or the AVPU scale:
  A: alert
  V: responds to verbal stimuli
  P: responds to painful stimuli
  U: unresponsive

Therapeutic interventions

- Keep the head in neutral alignment (nose and navel in line).[5]
- Assist with tracheal intubation of any patient with a Glasgow Coma Scale less than or equal to 8.
- Consider pharmacologic intervention to improve mental status using naloxone (Narcan), dextrose, or mannitol as indicated.[2]

SECONDARY SURVEY

After completing the primary survey (with concomitant resuscitation), conduct a secondary examination to identify any other injuries. Reassess the child's respiratory, circulatory, and neurologic status frequently, and intervene as appropriate. Because injuries identified on the secondary survey are not immediately life threatening, finish the entire examination and then prioritize and perform interventions.[2,4]

The secondary survey consists of the following:
- Completely undress and expose the patient.
- Warm the child. An immature thermoregulatory system makes pediatric patients more susceptible than adults to hypothermia.[6] Establish and maintain normothermia with the use of blankets, radiant heaters, convective air warmers (e.g., Bair Hugger), and warmed intravenous fluids.
- Get a full set of vital signs, including blood pressure, oxygen saturation, and a rectal temperature.
- Obtain a history from the caregiver, witnesses, or emergency medical services personnel. The history should include mechanism of injury, treatments before arrival, medical history, allergies, current medications, tetanus immunization status, and the time of last oral intake.
- Perform a detailed head-to-toe assessment, inspecting and palpating the anterior and posterior body surfaces.
- Identify and prioritize all injuries.

Interventions after the secondary survey may include the following:

- Send blood and urine specimens for laboratory testing.
- Prepare the patient for imaging studies (e.g., plain radiographs, computed tomography, ultrasound, and angiography).
- Clean, debride, and dress wounds. Assist with repair as indicated.
- Splint, elevate, and place ice on suspected sprain or fracture sites.
- Insert an indwelling urinary catheter (Foley) and maintain output between 1 and 2 mL/kg per hour.
- Place a nasogastric or orogastric tube and attach it to suction to decompress the stomach.
- Provide analgesics and other comfort measures.
- Consider the unique psychosocial needs of the pediatric population and encourage caregiver involvement, when possible and appropriate.

SELECTED PEDIATRIC INJURIES

Head Trauma

Head injuries are common in children primarily because of their proportionally large head size and weak skull bones.[3] Head injuries are present in nearly 80% of all significant pediatric trauma cases, and most are blunt injuries. (See Chapter 35.) When caring for these patients, always consider the potential for child maltreatment.

Care considerations

- The injured brain is profoundly sensitive to hypoxia and hypotension. Ensure that the child is well oxygenated and volume resuscitated.[2,5]
- A great deal of blood can be lost via a scalp laceration. Control bleeding with direct pressure. Transfuse blood products as indicated.
- Unlike adults and older children, the infant's skull can accommodate a blood volume sufficient to cause hypotension and shock. Observe the infant for bulging anterior fontanelles (up to age 12 to 18 months).[3]
- Herniation is less common in small children than in the older child.
- Palpate the skull for depressed fractures and other injuries. A boggy, crepitant swelling— associated with subgaleal hematoma—often can be felt over linear skull fractures.
- Seizures following head injuries are common. Children with significant intracranial bleeds or diffuse cerebral edema may be given anticonvulsant medications prophylactically.[6]
- Administer benzodiazepines to control active seizures.
- Facilitate computed tomography scans of the head.
- Children often suffer cerebral hyperemia following significant head injuries. The precise cause of this increased cerebral blood flow is unknown.
- Hyperventilation is no longer considered an appropriate, routine practice when caring for the brain-injured patient.
- Facilitate pediatric neurosurgical consultation and admission to a specialty care facility.
- Once the child has been volume resuscitated and is hemodynamically stable, restrict intravenous fluids to two thirds of the usual maintenance rate.

Blunt Abdominal Trauma

Because of an immature cartilaginous rib cage and weak abdominal musculature, a child's intraabdominal organs are less protected than those of the adult.[6] (See Chapter 38.)

Care considerations

- The most commonly injured intraabdominal organs are the liver, spleen, and intestines.
- Blunt abdominal trauma in children is difficult to assess clinically; use computed tomography scans and ultrasound.
- Swallowing air while crying distends the child's stomach. Early placement of a gastric tube will decompress the stomach, reduce pressure on the diaphragm, and improve respiratory status.
- In the absence of blood at the urinary meatus, insert an indwelling catheter to monitor hourly urine output closely.
- Serial measurement of abdominal girth, at the level of the umbilicus, helps detect subtle abdominal distention.

Extremity Trauma

Sprains, strains, and limb fractures are among the most frequent childhood injuries. See Chapter 39 for further information.

Care considerations

- Extremity assessment is facilitated by comparison with the uninjured extremity. When performing radiographic studies, views of the injured and uninjured sides can be helpful.
- Fractures occurring near the epiphyseal (growth) plates require specialized attention.
- Because young children are not able to pinpoint pain and to communicate well, obtain radiographs of the joint above and below a suspected fracture site to assess the extent of injury.
- Perform and document a peripheral neurovascular assessment before and after any manipulation or splinting of an injured extremity.

COMMON DIAGNOSTIC TESTS IN INJURED CHILDREN

Laboratory Tests

Most modern laboratories can run all of the listed tests using a total of only 7 to 10 mL of blood:

- Type and crossmatch (this is the single most important laboratory study in the care of the major trauma patient)
- Complete blood count, with or without a differential
- Coagulation studies (e.g., prothrombin time [International Normalized Ratio], activated partial thromboplastin time, fibrinogen, platelets, and D-dimer)
- Serum electrolytes
- Renal function: Blood urea nitrogen and creatinine
- Glucose
- Amylase
- Arterial, venous, or capillary blood gases

Imaging Studies

Not all patients need all radiographic studies, but one should assume automatically that major trauma patients will receive cervical spine, chest, and pelvis radiographs unless a good argument can be made for omitting any of these films.

- Always obtain an image of injured extremities.
- Obtain thoracic and lumbar spine films when indicated.
- Plain radiographs of the skull and face, once a common practice, now have largely been replaced by computed tomography.
- Consider computed tomography scans of the neck, thorax, abdomen, and pelvis.
- Children are prone to spinal cord injuries without radiographic abnormalities.[3] Magnetic resonance imaging may be necessary to detect this type of trauma.

References

1. Chameides L, Hazinski M, editors: *Pediatric advanced life support course student manual,* Dallas, 2002, American Heart Association.
2. Rupp L, Day M: Children are different: differences and the impact on trauma. In Maloney-Harmon P, Czerwinski S, editors: *Nursing care of the pediatric trauma patient,* St Louis, 2003, Saunders.
3. Liebman M: Initial resuscitation of the pediatric trauma victim. In Maloney-Harmon, Czerwinski S, editors: *Nursing care of the pediatric trauma patient,* St Louis, 2003, Saunders.
4. Emergency Nurses Association: *Emergency nursing pediatric course provider manual,* ed 3, Des Plaines, Ill, 2004, The Association.
5. Vernon-Levett P: Traumatic brain injury in children. In Maloney-Harmon P, Czerwinski S, editors: *Nursing care of the pediatric trauma patient,* St Louis, 2003, Saunders.
6. Moore E, Mattox K, Feliciano D, editors: *Trauma manual,* ed 4, New York, 2003, McGraw-Hill.

44

Geriatric Trauma

Andrea Novak, MS, RN, CEN

THE GERIATRIC PATIENT

Elderly persons represent the fastest growing portion of the population in the United States today. Different definitions of *geriatric* have been proposed, but for the purposes of this chapter, individuals over the age of 65 years will be considered elderly. Currently, the elderly compose 13% of the population (25.5 million persons), a number that is expected to reach 20% (78 million) by the year 2030. These statistics are significant for emergency nurses because in the next few years, it is predicted that one out of every four patients seen will be aged 65 years or over. Caring for the elderly requires not only knowledge of the ABCs of emergency care (airway, breathing, circulation) but also an understanding of the normal physiologic changes associated with aging. Today, geriatric patients account for only 15% of emergency department (ED) visits but constitute 48% of all hospital admissions and 46% of admissions to critical care units. Alarmingly, these numbers have increased by 5% just since this text was last published. The average length of stay in the ED for an elderly patient is nearly 20% longer than that of other adults. Older persons also consume more health care resources than do their younger counterparts.[1]

Elderly individuals exist in a tenuous state of homeostasis. They are prone to infections, are likely to have atypical myocardial infarctions, and have abdominal pain that is difficult to assess. More diagnostic tests are necessary in this population because of the increased likelihood of problems and the importance of accurate diagnosis. The special challenges associated with caring for a geriatric trauma patient are related to the general effects of the aging process on the body, comorbidities, polypharmacy, and atypical presentations that frequently complicate diagnosis.

THE ELDERLY TRAUMA PATIENT

Trauma is the number four cause of mortality in persons older than 55 years and the seventh leading cause of death for those over the age of 75 years.[2] Geriatric trauma patients have a substantially higher mortality rate than younger patients with comparable injuries.[3] Even minor trauma may result in a substantial loss of pretrauma function for elderly persons. In addition, geriatric patients may not exhibit the same signs, symptoms, or level of pain found in their younger counterparts. In this population, pain intensity is an unreliable indicator of injury severity, and it is not uncommon for pain to be referred to another site.[4]

An aggressive approach to resuscitation is recommended because shock represents the primary cause of death in the injured elderly.[5] The physiologic changes of aging and concomitant medication use can limit the geriatric patient's ability to compensate, making it difficult to interpret vital signs. For example, the healthy young patient in shock will exhibit tachycardia; the elderly patient, with compromised cardiac function and daily beta-blocker or calcium channel blocker use, may be unable to mount a tachycardic response. The same is true for blood pressure and body temperature. A 1990 study by Scalea et al[5] found that, when hemodynamic derangements were aggressively monitored and treated, trauma mortality in high-risk geriatric patients fell from 85% to 47%.

ASSESSMENT

Medical History

When one is caring for an elderly individual, a thorough history and physical assessment are crucial. Special attention should be paid to the patient's medical and surgical history, preexisting conditions, and current medications. The list of each may be extensive. A spouse, family member, friend, or caretaker can assist with obtaining this information if the patient is not a reliable historian. Obtain old medical records if they are available.

Physical Assessment

The elderly patient seen in the ED for a traumatic condition challenges the nurse's ability to assess, treat, and evaluate care accurately. Normal aging, chronic health conditions, and medication use can affect treatment strategies by exacerbating or negating typical clinical findings. A head-to-toe assessment is performed on all trauma patients, but it is particularly important in the geriatric trauma population. Inspection, auscultation, and palpation are sometimes the only ways to identify an abnormality.

The hallmarks of aging are (1) a general decline in the functional reserve capacity of major organs and systems and (2) a limited range of adaptability.[1]

Primary survey

Begin with a standard primary survey. Assess the patient's ABC, and perform a brief neurologic examination, evaluating pupil size and reaction to light. Use the AVPU mnemonic to determine level of consciousness quickly[2]:

A: Alert
V: Responds to verbal stimuli
P: Responds to painful stimuli
U: Unresponsive

Table **44-1** **Structural and Functional Changes as a Result of Aging**

Body System	Alteration
Tissues	Decreased number of active cells
	Reduced tissue elasticity
Cardiovascular	Decreased distensibility of blood vessels
	Increased systolic blood pressure
	Increased systemic vascular resistance
	Decreased cardiac output
	Slow response to stress
Pulmonary	Decreased respiratory muscle strength
	Limited chest expansion
	Decreased number of functioning alveoli
	Decreased elastic recoil, small airway collapse
	Decreased resting oxygen tension
	Diminished protective mechanisms (cough)
Neurologic	Decreased number of functional neurons
	Decreased nerve conduction velocity
	Short-term memory loss
	Reduced cerebral blood flow
	Decreased visual acuity and darkness adaptation
	Decreased pupillary response and accommodation
	Increased auditory tone threshold
	Diminished sensation and touch sensitivity
Gastrointestinal/genitourinary	Decreased peristalsis
	Diminished acid secretion
	Decreased total nephron count
	Decreased glomerular filtration rate
	Diminished urine concentrating ability
Musculoskeletal/integumentary	Narrowing of the intervertebral disks
	Bone loss, increased risk for fracture
	Increased wear on joints
	Decreased number of muscle cells
	Loss of muscle strength
	Loss of skin thickness

From McQuillan K et al, editors: *Trauma nursing from resuscitation* through rehabilitation, ed 3, Philadelphia 2002, Saunders; and Greenhalgh DG: *Preexisting facts that affect care.* In Carrougher GH, editor: *Burn care and therapy,* St Louis, 1998, Mosby.

Gather information regarding the following:
- Mechanism of injury
- Events surrounding the injury (such as light-headedness, confusion, and palpitations)
- Medical history
- History of previous trauma
- Current medical conditions
- Current medication use
- Treatment at the scene
- Level of pain

Secondary survey

On completion of the primary survey, conduct a secondary assessment. This is a quick but thorough head-to-toe examination performed to identify all injuries.[2] (See Chapter 34 for details.)

Head

- Inspect the scalp and face.
- Palpate for pain, bleeding, hematomas, or bony deformities.
- Inquire about recent falls, changes in mental status, neurologic deficits, or a history of loss of consciousness.
- Prepare the head-injured patient for computed tomography, surgery, or intensive care unit admission.

Special Note

- As a result of the anatomic changes associated with aging, subdural hematomas are common in the elderly. These may be acute, subacute, or chronic.

Spinal cord and spinal column

- Assess motor and sensory status by checking for movement, motor strength, numbness, and tingling in the extremities. Compare sides.
- Palpate the entire spine for any deformities, step-off defects, pain, or swelling.
- Maintain spinal immobilization until injury is ruled out.

Special Note

- The elderly are prone to intravertebral disk and ligamentous injuries that are not readily apparent on routine radiographs.[5]
- The elderly are more prone to central cord syndorme.

Chest

- Inspect the thorax for symmetry, respiratory excursion, defects, and abnormalities.
- Auscultate the chest for diminished, absent, or adventitious breath sounds. Assess heart tones.
- Palpate the chest wall for areas of pain, fractures, bony crepitus, or subcutaneous emphysema.
- Monitor oxygen saturation; levels in the low 90s may be normal.
- Observe for accessory muscle use.
- Assess respiratory rate, depth, and effort; hypoventilation may be the patient's norm.
- Check for the presence of gag and cough reflexes.
- Evaluate the patient's ability to clear secretions effectively.
- Inspect the neck for jugular venous distention.

Special Note

- Injury resulting in the fracture of two or more ribs is an indication for hospitalization in the elderly.[5]

Abdomen/genitourinary

- Abdominal pain in geriatric patients is often vague but may reflect a serious pathologic condition.
- Observe for surgical scars and abdominal distention.
- Auscultate bowel sounds; slowed peristalsis is associated with aging, predisposing the elderly to constipation.
- Obtain a urine specimen for urinalysis; note the amount, color, specific gravity, and any unusual odors. Send for cultures as indicated.
- Assess for pain, guarding, or tenderness with abdominal palpation.
- Check the skin around the perineum for evidence of excoriation or breakdown.

- Perform rectal and prostate examinations. Test stool for occult blood (Hemoccult).
- Prepare the patient for abdominal imaging studies (ultrasound, plain radiographs, computed tomography, intravenous pyelogram, angiography).

Extremities

- Inspect all extremities for deformities, bruising, and normal and abnormal coloring.
- Assess limbs for pain, tenderness, and guarding.
- Look for leg shortening and external rotation of the foot when a hip fracture is suspected.
- Evaluate capillary refill, skin temperature, and skin condition; palpate distal pulses.
- Assess range of motion.
- Monitor vital signs frequently; fractures cause bleeding that can progress to shock in the elderly.

Special Notes

- Age-related changes in bone structure often make nondisplaced fractures difficult to diagnose on routine radiographic studies.[5]
- Consider the possibility of elder abuse if a patient has a fracture inconsistent with the history offered.

Skin

- Assess for skin turgor, temperature, and color. Identify areas of skin tears, bruising (old and new), burns (old or recent), rashes, and breakdown.
- Pad bony areas to protect the skin. Remove splints, backboards, and collars as soon as injuries are ruled out to minimize skin breakdown and discomfort.
- Gently clean areas of nonintact skin; apply protective ointments and dressings.
- Use paper tape and nonstick dressings on patients prone to skin tears.

Special Note

- If bruising and tears appear suspicious, ask who cares for the patient. Adopt a nonjudgmental approach and contact social services if elder abuse is suspected.

General Observations and Pertinent Questions

In addition to the usual care, when evaluating the geriatric trauma patient, assess for the following:

- Speech or hearing impairments; sensory deficits
- Mood disturbances or difficulty with thought processes
- Differences between the patient's and the family's interpretation of the chief complaint
- Living arrangements, activities of daily living, socioeconomic circumstances, and the physical layout of the home
- Fall history; use of assistive devices such as a walker or cane
- Dietary history: Smell or taste impairments, problems with chewing or swallowing, and the presence or absence of dentures
- Urinary or fecal incontinence
- Alcohol use
- Depression or anxiety: Poor appetite, changes in sleep patterns, and constipation are common findings in the elderly but also may be symptoms of depression. Inquire about suicidal thoughts and crying spells.
- Over-the-counter medications and alcohol intake: Alcohol and over-the-counter drugs can interact (together and with prescribed medications) to cause physiologic and psychological problems.

- Medication review: Once the patient is stabilized, perform a thorough review of all current medications. Look for possible adverse reactions, drug interactions, and toxic or subtherapeutic levels. Many elderly patients are taking numerous medications, and polypharmacy may be the underlying cause of their traumatic event. Medication dosing, interactions, and scheduling should be discussed with the patient or the patient's care provider.

Diagnostic Studies

Diagnostic procedures for evaluation of the elderly trauma patient include all standard laboratory tests (complete blood count, electrolytes, glucose, blood urea nitrogen, creatinine) but also may include magnesium and calcium levels, arterial blood gases, and troponin I. Consider coagulation studies, especially if the patient takes an anticoagulant medication such as aspirin or warfarin (Coumadin). Check the serum level of any medication that might be considered a contributing cause or precipitating factor (such as digoxin toxicity). Perform drug and alcohol screens as indicated. Elderly patients should have a 12-lead electrocardiogram. Obtain computed tomography scans, ultrasound, and other diagnostic studies as warranted.

General Nursing Interventions

In addition to the foregoing interventions, the emergency nurse should consider the following:
- Because the elderly may be less able to hear high-pitched sounds, health care workers should lower the pitch of their voices and speak clearly.
- Determine whether the patient has completed an advance directive.
- Administer intravenous fluids cautiously to prevent volume overload.
- Measure the patient's temperature; decreased amounts of body fat and muscle make the elderly prone to hypothermia.
- Keep the patient warm; infuse warmed intravenous fluids and apply warm blankets to the patient.
- Monitor vital signs, ABCs, level of consciousness, and urine output frequently.
- Check for hypoglycemia in patient; with altered level of consciousness or history of diabetes.
- Administer pain medications and other drugs as prescribed.
- Give a diphtheria/tetanus immunization, if needed.
- Perform meticulous wound care.
- Provide psychosocial support; minimize distracting stimuli, and frequently reorient confused patients.
- Encourage family members to be with the patient (as appropriate).
- Prepare the patient for discharge, admission, or transfer.[2]

SPECIFIC INJURIES IN THE GERIATRIC PATIENT

Falls

Falls are the leading cause of death in elderly trauma victims; more than half involve persons aged 75 years or older. Of all fall-related deaths in the United States, 70% occur among the elderly, and one out of seven falls results in a fracture. Fifty percent of patients over age 75 years will die within 1 year of breaking a hip.[1] Predisposing factors are poor vision and hearing, gait disturbances, diminished muscle strength, osteoporotic bones, altered balance, and associated fragility. Many medical conditions contribute to the incidence of falls, including cardiac dysrhythmias, dizziness, seizure disorders, alcoholism, and arthritis. Environmental

Box **44-1**　**Injury Prevention Activities for the Elderly**

Remove or tack down all scatter rugs.
Check staircases for stability; install handrails whenever possible.
Apply nonslip strips to stairways.
Carpet areas that are prone to spills or slipperiness.
Reduce clutter and open clear pathways through all rooms.
Pad wooden or metal furniture edges.
Install bright lights in hallways and entrances.
Place nonslip mats in the bathtub and shower.
Install grab bars near all bathrooms.
Install smoke detectors, and check them at regular intervals.
Obtain assistance with cooking, as needed. Extra care is required when using gas stoves.
Use assistive cooking devices, such as burner shields, long-handled utensils, and protective hand gear.
Do not wear loose-fitting garments while cooking.
Use rear stove burners rather than front ones, and avoid storing goods you may need over the stove.
Check central furnaces and space heaters frequently to ensure proper functioning.
Reduce thermostat settings on water heaters and clearly label all hot water faucets.
Annually review the directions for operating major appliances.
Wear short sleeved, nonsynthetic shirts and pajamas.
Do not smoke, especially while resting.
Keep easy-to-operate fire extinguishers readily accessible.
Use hot water bottles and heating pads only at low temperatures.
Know how to access 9-1-1.
Eliminate night driving if patient is affected by night blindness.
Wear seat belts.
Drive only in familiar locations, avoiding highly congested areas and roadways under construction.
Contact your state vehicle licensing agency to inquire about an "Over 75 Refresher Course."

Modified from Andrews JF: Trauma in the elderly. In *Forum Medicum, Postgraduate Studies in Trauma Nursing,* 1990; and McQuillan K et al, editors: *Trauma nursing: from resuscitation* through rehabilitation, ed 3, Philadelphia, 2002, Saunders.

factors—loose carpets, improper footwear, inappropriate furniture, awkward stairways, poor lighting, and unfamiliar surroundings—also promote falling.[6] Falls are the proximate cause of fractures, head trauma, and internal organ damage such as splenic rupture. These injuries can seriously compromise previously healthy and not-so-healthy individuals.

Burns

Diminished neurologic sensation, impaired vision and hearing, and psychomotor delays may leave the elderly unable to escape the hazards of heat and flames. Resuscitation and treatment of the elderly burn victim is the same as for younger patients. (See Chapter 41 for further information.) Nonetheless, this population deserves careful consideration because the physiologic changes of aging significantly compromise recovery time. Additionally, burns may be more severe than they initially appear because of thin, aging skin; diminished blood flow; and poor healing abilities. Following a burn, geriatric patients have a substantially higher mortality rate than do other patient populations.[2]

Motor Vehicle Collisions

Motor vehicle crashes account for 21.5% of injuries in the elderly population.[3] Limited vision, decreased hearing, slowed reaction time, and high traffic volumes affect the incidence of collisions involving elderly drivers.

Patient assessment and care priorities remain essentially the same as for younger individuals. However, the structural and functional changes associated with aging affect patient management strategies and recovery. In contrast to younger drivers, the older driver crashes more often at intersections, in good weather, during daylight hours, with another vehicle, and close to home. The incidence of automobile vs. pedestrian collisions peaks in the 65-plus age-group.[5]

Elder Abuse

Elder abuse can entail physical, emotional, verbal, financial, and sexual components. The possibility of abuse, maltreatment, or neglect must always be considered when treating older patients.[7] Although assessment of elder abuse may be difficult and time consuming, its importance cannot be overstressed. As the first person an elderly patient generally encounters in the ED, the emergency nurse plays a significant role in abuse screening. A sympathetic, nonjudgmental approach will go a long way toward eliciting this information. Patients may be hesitant to speak about maltreatment because they rely on the abuser for care and shelter. Frustration, economic difficulties, lifestyle changes, and an inability to care for the elderly patient are a few of the reasons elder abuse exists. If maltreatment is suspected, the social services division of the hospital should be notified for follow-up care or referral.

Clues

- Unexplained fractures, bruising, burns, or internal injuries
- "Noncompliance" with medications or treatment plans
- History of being "accident prone," or multiple ED visits
- Apparent fear of the patient's caregiver
- Malnutrition, dehydration, inadequate hygiene, and poor skin care
- Signs of confinement or restraint
- Unexplained delays in seeking treatment and differing accounts of what happened
- Unusual injury locations
- Distinct pattern injuries
- Unusual patient-family interactions
- Lack of caregiver interest
- Evidence of overmedication
- Alcohol or drug abuse in the client or caregiver

Elder Abandonment

Elder abandonment is an alarming and growing phenomenon in EDs. When caregivers find it frustrating and difficult to meet the needs of a chronically ill or disabled family member, they find ways to "dump" the patient. Because of 24-hour-a-day, 7-day-a-week access, EDs are a logical site for abandonment. Overwhelmed caregivers come to the ED for support, compassion, and a break from their caregiving responsibilities.

With the advent of diagnosis-related groupings from Medicare, hospitals are not predisposed to admit the elderly for "social reasons." Yet when patients are abandoned on the premises, hospitals have little choice. Facilitate early involvement of social services staff members to intervene with caregivers and discuss other options for services, respite care, or long-term placement.

References

1. The John A Hartford Foundation Institute for Geriatric Nursing, Geriatric Seminar, 2002.

2. Emergency Nurses Association: Geriatric trauma. In *Trauma nurse core course provider manual,* Des Plaines, Ill, 2000, The Association.
3. DeKeyser F, Carolan D, Trask A: Suburban geriatric trauma: the experiences of a level I trauma center, *Am J Crit Care* 4(5):379-382, 1995.
4. Eliopoulos C: *Gerontological nursing,* ed 3, Philadelphia, 1993, Lippincott.
5. Scalea TM et al: Geriatric blunt trauma: improved survival with early invasive monitoring, *J Trauma* 30:129, 1990.
6. Loftis P, Glover T: *Decision making in gerontologic nursing,* St Louis, 1993, Mosby.
7. Emergency Nurses Association: *Care of older adults in the emergency setting,* Des Plaines, Ill, 2003, The Association.

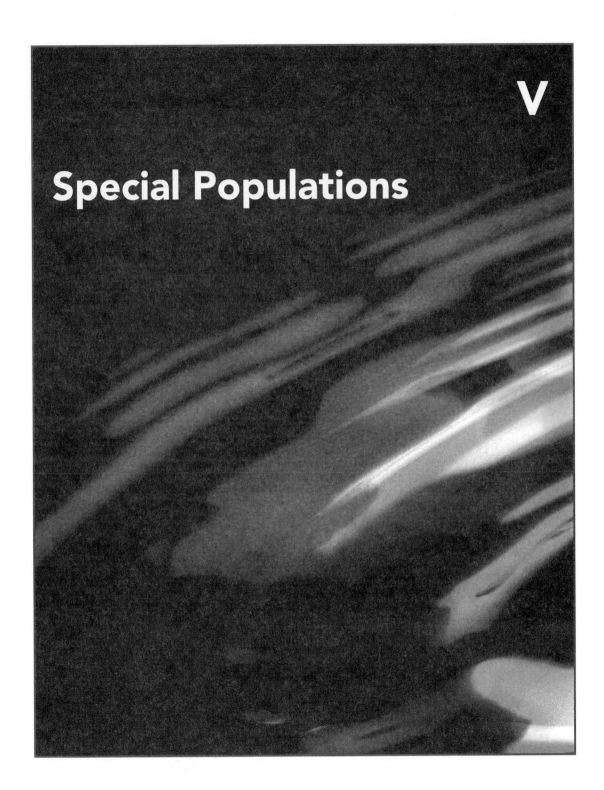

V

Special Populations

45

Obstetric and Gynecologic Emergencies

M. Lynn Herman, RN, MSN

Patients with obstetric and gynecologic problems are routine visitors to emergency departments (EDs). Several of the most prevalent obstetric and gynecologic disorders are presented in this section. For additional information, refer to one of the many references listed at the end of the chapter.

Nurses and patients frequently are confused by some of the terminology used to describe obstetric and gynecologic conditions. Box 45-1 provides key definitions.

COMPLICATIONS OF PREGNANCY

Ectopic Pregnancy

Two percent of all pregnancies in the United States are ectopic. An ectopic pregnancy occurs when a fertilized egg implants outside the endometrial cavity, usually in a fallopian tube (95% of the time). Cervical, abdominal, and ovarian implantation account for the remaining 5%. If the fetus continues to grow, the fallopian tube inevitably will rupture.[1] Symptoms commonly present around the sixth week of gestation.

Signs and symptoms

- Late or irregular period
- Abnormal vaginal bleeding
- Severe sudden onset of unilateral pelvic pain
- Abdominal tenderness and guarding
- Palpable pelvic mass
- Positive pregnancy test
- Sensation that a bowel movement would help relieve discomfort

Box **45-1**   **Obstetric and Gynecologic Definitions**

> *Labor:* The process by which the fetus, placenta, and membranes are expelled from the uterus. This usually occurs 40 weeks after conception.
>
> *Spontaneous abortion:* The natural termination of pregnancy before viability (less than 20 weeks gestation). The term *miscarriage* commonly is preferred by laypersons who use *abortion* to denote induced pregnancy loss.
>
> *Gravida:* The total number of pregnancies, including a current pregnancy.
>
> *Para:* The number of pregnancies that have gone to at least 20 weeks of gestation, regardless of whether the infant was dead or alive at birth.
>
> *Primigravida:* Pregnant for the first time.
>
> *Nullipara:* A woman who has not carried a pregnancy to viability.
>
> *Primipara:* A woman who has carried one pregnancy to viability.
>
> *Multipara:* A woman who has carried more than one pregnancy to viability.
>
> **Examples**
>
> *Gravida 3, Para 1:* A woman who has been pregnant 3 times and delivered one viable child.
>
> *Gravida 4, Para 0:* A woman who has been pregnant 4 times but has carried none of them to viability.
>
> *Gravida 2, Para 2:* A woman who has been pregnant 2 times and has delivered two viable children.
>
> *Gravida 1, Para 2:* A woman who has been pregnant 1 time but has delivered two viable children (twins).

If a rupture has occurred, additional signs and symptoms are as follows:
- Shoulder pain (Kehr's sign; see Chapter 38)
- Signs of hemorrhagic shock
  - Tachycardia
  - Cold, clammy skin
  - Hypotension, delayed capillary refill, narrowed pulse pressure
  - Decreasing level of consciousness

Diagnostic aids

- Human chorionic gonadotropin (hCG) level (pregnancy test)
- Complete blood count (CBC) and type and crossmatch with Rh
- Pelvic ultrasound
- Culdocentesis rarely done

Therapeutic interventions

- Provide high-flow oxygen.
- Initiate intravenous (IV) therapy with lactated Ringer's solution or normal saline.
- Administer antibiotics.
- Give Rh$_o$ (D) immune globulin (human RhoGAM) if the mother is Rh negative.
- Prepare the patient for surgery if rupture is suspected.
- Consider intramuscular injection of methotrexate for unruptured ectopic pregnancies.
- Refer the patient for follow-up care with a gynecologist.

Abortion

The term *abortion* is defined as the death or expulsion of the fetus (or products of conception) before the age of viability. About 10% to 15% of all known pregnancies end in spontaneous abortion. The major complications are hemorrhage and infection. Pregnancy loss in the first trimester is largely the result of embryonic chromosomal defects. Later loss more frequently is associated with infections, maternal endocrine disorders, or anatomic abnormalities of the mother's reproductive tract. Spontaneous abortions are classified as threatened, inevitable, incomplete, complete, missed, and septic.

Threatened abortion

A threatened abortion is possible in cases in which early symptoms of abortion—such as episodic, painless uterine bleeding, and mild cramping—are present. The cervical os is closed and the uterus is enlarged and soft. A quantitative β-HCG (serum) test provides a better indicator of fetal development than a qualitative β-HCG (urine) test.

Therapeutic interventions
- Bed rest
- Pelvic rest
- Mild sedatives
- Ultrasound confirmation of pregnancy

Inevitable abortion

A threatened abortion may progress to inevitable abortion. Findings include increased pain, cramping, and bleeding. The cervical os is dilated 3 cm or more.

Therapeutic interventions
- Bed rest
- Analgesics
- Uterine evacuation (dilation and curettage or dilation and evacuation) may be performed at the provider's and patient's discretion.
- Administration of Rh$_o$ (D) immune globulin if indicated

Incomplete abortion

In an incomplete abortion, bleeding is heavy, cramping is severe, and the cervical os is open. The patient has a positive pregnancy test and an enlarged uterus. Tissue has been passed, but some products of conception are retained.

Therapeutic interventions
- Obtain IV access and infuse Ringer's lactate.
- Infuse oxytocin (Pitocin, Syntocinon) 20 units per 1000 mL of lactated Ringer's solution to induce uterine contractions.
- Facilitate surgery for uterine evacuation (dilation and curettage or dilation and evacuation).
- Administer Rh$_o$ (D) immune globulin as needed.

Complete abortion

In a complete abortion a small amount of bleeding occurs, cramping is mild, all tissue has been passed (often in an intact amniotic sac), and the cervical os is closed.

Therapeutic intervention
- Observation
- Ultrasound as indicated

Missed abortion

A missed abortion is a pregnancy loss in which the products of conception remain in the uterus for an extended period after fetal demise. The characteristic symptoms of bleeding and cramping are absent.

Therapeutic interventions
- Uterine evacuation may be performed.
- Some providers will send the patient home for expectant management or scheduled evacuation.

Septic abortion

Infection after abortion occasionally occurs in patients who have had a complete abortion without surgical uterine evacuation. More frequently, infection is seen in patients who delay treatment of an incomplete abortion or become infected as a result of an elective abortion. Bacteria commonly responsible are alpha- and beta-hemolytic streptococci, gram-negative aerobes such as *Escherichia coli,* and occasionally *Clostridium perfringens,* all of which are considered normal vaginal flora.

Patients with *Clostridium* infection are of particular concern. This anaerobic organism is capable of producing gas gangrene, tissue necrosis, and uterine tissue sloughing. To avoid significant morbidity and mortality, treatment of septic abortion must be immediate and aggressive. If improvement does not occur after dilation and curettage, hysterectomy is indicated.

Signs and symptoms
- Foul vaginal discharge
- Constant pelvic pain
- Uterine tenderness
- Fever, chills

Therapeutic interventions
- Initiate an oxytocin infusion to expel uterine contents.
- Administer appropriate antibiotics.
- Prepare the patient for dilation and curettage.
- Observe for signs of toxic shock: Hypotension, renal failure, and tachycardia. See Toxic Shock Syndrome.

General postabortion care

Education
- Many women (and men) find the loss of their child devastating, even when it occurs early in pregnancy.
- Comfort the patient as appropriate. (See Chapter 15.)
- Determine what information is needed regarding the cause of abortion. Refer the patient to experts (e.g., obstetrician or geneticist) for evaluation, as indicated.
- If procedural sedation was administered for uterine evacuation, ensure that the patient is fully recovered before discharge. Explain potential medication effects.
- Provide the names of local support groups such as Compassionate Friends or SHARE. The hospital obstetric unit may have a list of resources.

- Refer patients for psychological counseling as needed, especially if the patient who has a history of depression or significant concurrent stressors.

Discharge instructions

- Vaginal bleeding may last 1 to 2 weeks. The bleeding should get progressively lighter until it subsides.
- Slight cramping for several days is normal.
- Avoid douching, tampons, or intercourse for at least 2 weeks (or until after a follow-up visit with the gynecologist).
- Rest for 2 to 3 days.
- Monitor body temperature in the morning and evening for 5 days.
- Seek medical care for the following:
  - Temperature above 37.7° C (100° F)
  - Chills
  - Severe nausea and vomiting
  - Severe cramps
  - Excessive bleeding

Pregnancy-Induced Hypertension

Preeclampsia

Pregnancy-induced hypertension (PIH) is the second leading cause of maternal mortality. The mildest form of PIH is preeclampsia. This condition is far more than just chronically elevated blood pressure. Preeclampsia is a multisystem disorder associated with hypertension, protein-uria, edema, and central nervous system irritability. At times, coagulopathies and liver function abnormalities are present as well.

Signs and symptoms

- Elevated blood pressure
  - Systolic blood pressure greater than 140 mm Hg *or*
  - Diastolic blood pressure greater than 90 mm Hg *or*
  - An increase in systolic blood pressure greater than 30 mm Hg, with a diastolic blood pressure increase 15 mm Hg above the first trimester baseline
- Albuminuria (2+ on a dipstick; catheter or clean catch specimen)
- Oliguria
- Edema of the face, hands, and sacrum
- Weight gain of 2 lb or more per week
- HELLP syndrome (defined in the following section)
- Visual changes
- Headaches
- Nausea
- Epigastric or right upper quadrant pain
- Increased deep tendon reflexes with clonus

Therapeutic interventions

- Provide supportive care.
- Obtain urgent obstetric consultation.
- Give hydralazine (Apresoline) or labetalol (Normodyne, Trandate) IV for hypertension.
- Infuse magnesium sulfate IV to prevent seizures.
- Arrange for admission to an obstetric care unit.

Eclampsia

In the continuum of PIH disorders, eclampsia simply represents preeclampsia that has progressed to the convulsive phase. HELLP syndrome is a variant of severe preeclampsia characterized by hemolysis (H), elevated liver enzymes (EL), and a low platelet (LP) count. A diagnosis of HELLP syndrome is made from laboratory studies.[2] Ultimately, delivery is the only cure for eclampsia. Nonetheless, patients are at risk for this disorder for up to 3 weeks postpartum; those with late presentation eclampsia often have atypical presentations.[3]

Signs and symptoms

- Symptoms of preeclampsia (see the foregoing)
- Generalized seizures with an associated postictal period that may last as long as 15 to 20 minutes
- Significantly elevated blood pressure (systolic blood pressure 140 to 200 mm Hg, diastolic blood pressure greater than 90 mm Hg)
- Decreased fetal heart rate, particularly during seizures

Therapeutic interventions

- Maintain a patent airway.
- Provide high-flow oxygen.
- Place the patient in a left lateral position.
- Administer a 4- to 6-g IV bolus of magnesium sulfate over 15 minutes, then begin a maintenance drip at 1 to 3 g/hr.
- Give hydralazine (Apresoline) or labetalol (Normodyne, Trandate) IV for hypertension.
- Monitor blood pressure, respiratory rate, and deep tendon reflexes every hour or as indicated.
- Arrange for admission to a high-risk obstetric care unit.
- Anticipate cesarean section (depending on gestational age).

Bleeding in Pregnancy

Placenta previa

Placenta previa is defined as implantation of the placenta in the lower uterine segment, over the internal os. The incidence of placenta previa is about 1 in every 200 births.[4] Placenta previa is categorized based on the extent of internal cervical os involvement; the os can be totally, partially, or only marginally covered (Figure 45-1). As the fetus grows, the area thins and bleeds (usually in the third trimester). Placenta previa is associated with potentially life-threatening hemorrhage and fetal loss.

Signs and symptoms

- Sudden *painless* bleeding (usually after 7 months of gestation)
- Bright red (vs. dark) blood from the vagina
- Maternal hemorrhagic shock (hypotension, tachycardia, poor capillary refill)

Therapeutic interventions

- Insert one or more large-bore IV catheters and give the patient a bolus of lactated Ringer's solution or normal saline solution.
- Send blood for the following: CBC and type and crossmatch with Rh.
- Keep the patient in a left lateral recumbent position to increase blood return to the heart.

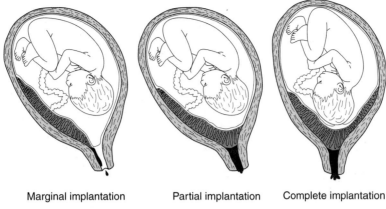

Marginal implantation   Partial implantation   Complete implantation

Figure 45-1. Placenta previa.

- Defer a vaginal examination until an ultrasound has indicated the placental location. (Manual examination can disrupt the placenta further.)
- Anticipate cesarean section, depending on the gestational age, extent of bleeding, and maternal condition.

Placental abruption

Placental abruption (abruptio placentae) is a major cause of obstetric hemorrhage and hypovolemic shock. Placental abruption is the most common cause of fetal demise following maternal trauma. The rupture of small arterial vessels causes separation of the placenta from the uterine wall. This ultimately inhibits the supply of oxygen and nutrients to the fetus. The area of separation can be small or large. If separation occurs at the placental margin, vaginal bleeding will be present. However, areas of separation toward the placental center are concealed and do not cause obvious blood loss. Maternal and fetal death can occur as a result of this condition.

Signs and symptoms
- Backache
- Painful uterine contractions
- Uterine rigidity
- Sudden, colicky abdominal pain
- Frank, dark red vaginal bleeding *or* bleeding concealed behind a partially separated placenta
- Maternal hemorrhagic shock (hypotension, tachycardia, poor capillary refill)
- If a large portion of the placenta has separated, fetal heart tones will be absent.
- Patients with small, concealed bleeds may be asymptomatic.

Therapeutic interventions
- Administer high-flow oxygen.
- Insert one or more large-bore IV catheters and give the patient a bolus of Ringer's lactate or normal saline solution.

- Consider transfusion with crossmatched or O-negative packed red blood cells.
- Draw a mark on the abdomen at the level of the uterine fundus; reassess fundal height frequently.
- Send blood for CBC and type and crossmatch with Rh.
- Rapidly transport the patient to an operating room or obstetric unit (depending on fetal viability and the degree of maternal shock).
- Unless the patient is delivered emergently, continuous electronic fetal monitoring is required. This procedure must be performed by skilled obstetric nurses.

Trauma in Pregnancy

See Chapter 42 for information on trauma in the pregnant patient.

EMERGENT DELIVERY

Although one of the most natural processes on earth, childbirth is by definition an emergent condition. Add any complications and the process can jeopardize two (or more) lives. This chapter provides a concise, step-by-step approach to caring for the delivering mother and her baby. Table 45-1 outlines the stages of labor; Box 45-2 lists information to elicit from the laboring mother or a family member.

If the following signs and symptoms are present, prepare for immediate delivery. Birth in a sterile environment is desirable. However, if delivery is imminent, do not risk endangering the mother and infant while attempting to create a sterile situation.

Table **45-1**   **Stages of Labor**

		Average Duration	
		---	---
Stage	*Description*	*Primipara*	*Multipara*
Stage 1: Dilation	From the onset of regular uterine contractions to complete cervical dilation.	12½ hours	7 hours
Stage 2: Expulsion	From the time of complete dilation until the baby is delivered.	80 minutes	30 minutes
Stage 3: Placental	From the time immediately following delivery of the baby until expulsion of the placenta.	5-30 minutes	5-30 minutes

Box **45-2**   **Questions to Ask the Laboring Patient**

How many weeks along are you? What is your due date?
When did your labor (pain) start?
How close together are your contractions?
Has your water broken?
Are you bleeding now?
Have you had any complications with this pregnancy?
How many babies have you delivered before?
Is there more than one baby?
Do you feel the need to push or move your bowels?
Have you taken any medications?

Signs and Symptoms of Impending Delivery

The following are indications of impending delivery:
- Findings that can occur days or minutes before delivery:
  - Bloody show: A mucous discharge that is tinged pink or brown with blood
  - Ruptured amniotic membranes ("my water broke"): A trickle or gush of amniotic fluid
  - Frequent contractions
- A desire by the mother to bear down
- The mother states that she is going to defecate or that "the baby is coming."
- Bulging membranes are visible at the vulva
- Crowning of the fetal head (Figure 45-2)

Equipment

Except for the isolette, the following equipment can be stored together easily in an emergent delivery kit for ready access. Consider having a kit in the triage area and in the ED treatment rooms:
- Basin or plastic bag
- Scissors or a scalpel (sterile)
- 2 cord clamps or 2 Kelly clamps (sterile)
- 1 bulb syringe
- Fluid-absorbent pads (large)
- Sterile gloves
- Clean baby blankets
- Sanitary pad or towel
- 1 infant hat (stockinette material can be used to make a hat)
- Identification bands for the mother and infant
- Heated isolette (if possible) or warm blankets
- Copy of the Apgar score can be helpful.

Procedure

1. Place the mother supine, with the knees bent up, or in a side-lying position (Figure 45-3). Delivery of the anterior shoulder is often easier if the mother is side-lying. However, this position requires someone to support the mother's upper leg.
2. Check vital signs (including fetal heart tones) if time permits.
3. Offer ongoing verbal support and explanations.
4. Place a fluid-absorbent pad under the mother.

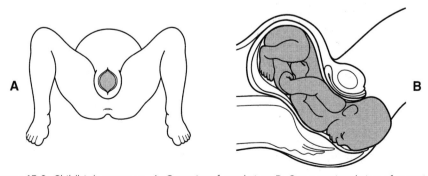

Figure 45-2. Childbirth sequence. **A,** Crowning, frontal view. **B,** Cross-sectional view of crowning.

5. Put on sterile gloves.
6. Have the mother pant with each contraction or lightly push.
7. When the head appears, place gentle pressure on the crown to prevent rapid fetal expulsion. Support the perineum to reduce tearing (Figure 45-4).
8. Hold the infant's head with both hands, and allow it to rotate naturally (Figures 45-5 and 45-6).

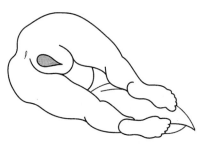

Figure 45-3. Side-lying position.

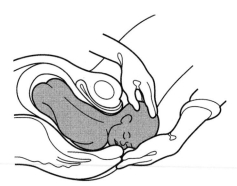

Figure 45-4. Perineal support

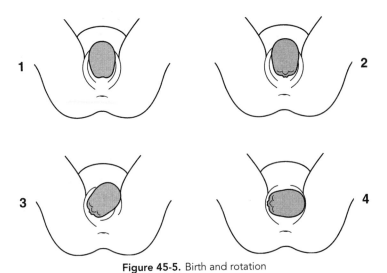

Figure 45-5. Birth and rotation

9. Feel for the cord around the infant's neck. If the baby is entangled, do the following:
   - Attempt to slip the cord over the infant's head.
   - If the cord is wound too tightly, immediately clamp the cord in two places and cut between the clamps.
10. If the amniotic sac is still intact, make a quick snip at the baby's nape, and peel the membranes away from the face.
11. Suction the fluids from infant with a bulb syringe (or wall suction on a low setting). Clear the mouth and oropharynx first and *then* suction the nares. Remember, newborns are obligate nose breathers. Nasal suctioning often stimulates gasping and the mouth needs to be cleared before this happens.
12. Deliver the shoulders by guiding the head downward (to deliver the anterior shoulder) and then upward (to free the posterior shoulder).
13. Once the head and shoulders are free, the remaining parts will deliver quickly. You may need to apply gentle traction (Figure 45-7).
14. Note the time of birth.
15. After delivery, the infant should be held at the level of the uterus and the oropharynx should be suctioned again to prevent aspiration.[5]

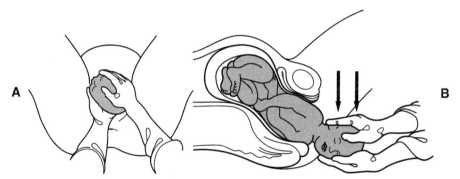

Figure 45-6. A, Delivery of the head. **B,** Cross-sectional view of delivery of the head.

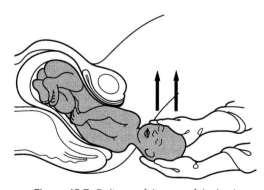

Figure 45-7. Delivery of the rest of the body.

Table 45-2   Apgar Score Chart

	0	1	2
Appearance (color)	Blue, pale	Pink body, blue extremities	Pink
Pulse (heart rate)	Absent	<100 beats/min	>100 beats/min
Grimace (muscle tone)	Limp	Some flexion	Good flexion
Activity (reflex irritability)	Absent	Some motion	Good motion
Respiratory effort	Absent	Weak cry	Strong cry

From Rita S, Reed B: Obstetric emergencies. In Newberry L, editor: *Sheehy's emergency nursing: principles and practice*, ed 5, St Louis, 2003, Mosby.

16. Clamp the cord at two sites 4 to 5 cm from the baby. Be sure the clamps are closed firmly. Using sterile scissors, cut between the clamps.[6]
17. Dry the neonate immediately and thoroughly. While drying the baby, assess for evidence of respiratory effort. Discard wet blankets or towels.
18. The infant should make an effort to breathe by crying spontaneously. If spontaneous breathing does not occur following gentle stimulation (back rub, foot tapping), initiate positive-pressure ventilation with 100% oxygen.
19. Check the neonate's heart rate after 30 seconds of positive-pressure ventilation. If the rate is less than 80 beats/min and not rising, initiate chest compressions and continue ventilations.
20. Determine Apgar score at 1 minute and again at 5 minutes (Table 45-2).
21. Keep the infant warm by placing the neonate in a heated isolette. If a prewarmed isolette is not readily available, the mother can hold the infant on her chest/abdomen to provide skin-to-skin body heat. Wrap the mother and baby well. If available, place a hat on the child.

Delivery of the Placenta

Placental separation generally occurs within minutes of birth but can be delayed as long as 30 minutes. There is no reason to hurry this process. Allow the placenta to expel naturally. Never tug on an umbilical cord to speed expulsion because it may cause uterine inversion. Gentle fundal massage can aid placental separation from the uterine wall.[5]

Signs and symptoms of impending placental delivery

- The umbilical cord will advance 2 to 3 inches further out of the vagina
- The fundus rises upward in the abdomen
- The uterus becomes firm and globular
- A large gush of blood comes from the vagina (this bleeding is normal)

Procedure

1. Instruct the mother to bear down.
2. Do *not* exert traction on the umbilical cord. Allow the placenta to deliver spontaneously.
3. Massage the fundus immediately after placental delivery.
4. After the placenta is expelled, inspect it for missing sections.
5. Save the placenta in a basin or plastic bag and send it with the mother to the obstetric unit.
6. Closely observe the mother for signs of hemorrhage. Once the placenta has delivered, bleeding should slow significantly.

Box **45-3** Normal Newborn Vital Sign Range

Pulse: 100-160 beats/min
Respirations: 40-60 breaths per minute
Temperature: >36.5° C

Care of the Mother

Perform the following care for the mother:
- To involute the uterus and expel clots, massage the fundus while applying moderate suprapubic pressure.
- Gently wipe the perineal area with a clean towel.
- Remove the soiled fluid-absorbent pad and any soiled linen from underneath the mother.
- Place a sanitary pad or towel over the perineum.
- Infuse IV fluids (usually lactated Ringer's solution or lactated Ringer's solution with 5% dextrose) at approximately 150 mL/hr (faster if bleeding is excessive).
- Administer oxytocic agents as indicated. Oxytocin (Pitocin, Syntocinon) 20 units per 1000 mL of lactated Ringer's solution (250 to 500 mL/hr) can reduce bleeding effectively.[5]
- Keep the mother warm.
- Observe the mother closely; monitor vital signs frequently (every 15 minutes) until they are stable.
- Put an infant identification band on the mother's wrist.

Care of the Infant

Perform the following care for the newborn:
- Dry the infant.
- Keep the infant warm. If a preheated isolette is not available, place the infant directly on the mother's skin. If this is impractical (e.g., resuscitation is in progress), a large chemical warming pad works well. However, *never* place a neonate directly on a warming pad. Always put several layers of blanket between the chemical pack and the baby. Check the temperature of the pad frequently to avoid burns.
- Once the baby is pink and breathing well, maintain the airway by placing the infant on its side.
- Observe the cord stump for bleeding. Ensure that the clamp is closed tightly.
- Put an identification band on the baby's wrist or ankle (or both).
- Observe the infant closely and monitor vital signs (Box 45-3).
- Prepare to transfer the mother and baby to an obstetric/neonatal unit.

COMPLICATIONS OF DELIVERY

Meconium-Stained Fluid

The goal of intervention for the infant with meconium-stained amniotic fluid is to prevent aspiration of the fluid into the lungs. All efforts are directed at clearing the airway before the baby takes a first breath. This procedure requires a rapid sequence of events best performed by those with experience. Unless delivery is imminent, transfer the mother to an obstetric unit or page obstetric staff members to the ED.

Signs and symptoms

- Meconium-stained amniotic fluid (Fluid will be green or dark yellow. It may be "pea soup" thick.)
- Possible signs of fetal distress (bradycardia, decreased movement)

Therapeutic interventions

- Apply oxygen to the mother.
- If possible, have a neonatal nurse, respiratory therapist, and physician present.
- Prepare the equipment:
  - Use 3.5- or 4-mm tracheal tubes for term infants. Select an appropriately sized tube for preterm neonates.
  - Use 10 French or larger suction catheters attached to wall suction (not to exceed 100 mm Hg).
  - Use a meconium aspirator (designed to attach to the tracheal tube). Tracheal tube/aspirator combinations are commercially available.
  - Attach a bag-valve-mask device (or anesthesia bag) to 100% oxygen.
- When the equipment and personnel are ready, encourage the mother to push with each contraction, but only until the head is delivered.
- When the baby's face is visible, use a 10-French or larger suction catheter to clean out the mouth, pharynx, and nose thoroughly.
- As soon as the infant has been delivered, before drying or stimulation, suction any residual meconium from the hypopharynx.
- If the infant's heart or respiratory rate is depressed or the meconium is thick and particulate, assist with immediate tracheal intubation. If meconium is visible below the cords, a tracheal tube (with a meconium aspirator attached) is inserted under direct visualization. Suction is applied as the tube is removed. This process essentially uses the tracheal tube as a large suction catheter.
- Repeat this procedure as needed before encouraging the baby to breathe (no longer than 20 to 30 seconds).
- After this process, many infants will do well on their own; others require intubation and mechanical ventilation and, possibly, resuscitation.

Fetal Bradycardia

Fetal distress is best monitored and managed in an obstetric unit or operating room. Unless delivery is imminent, immediately transfer the mother to an appropriate site with experienced personnel and electronic fetal monitoring capabilities.

Signs and symptoms

- Decreased fetal heart rate (less than 100 beats/min)

Therapeutic interventions

- Administer high-flow oxygen.
- Place the mother in a side-lying position.
- Check for a prolapsed cord.
- Notify obstetric/neonatal specialists.
- Insert an IV catheter and infuse lactated Ringer's solution.

- Encourage the mother to push if she feels the urge.
- Follow the steps for normal vaginal delivery or transport the mother for rapid cesarean section.
- Be prepared to resuscitate the neonate.

Breech Position of the Fetus

Three percent of all fetuses present in the breech position. This can be the buttocks first (frank or full breech) or foot first (footling breech) (Figure 45-8). These positions are dangerous for the fetus because of the increased likelihood of a difficult delivery and cord prolapse. Optimally, breech fetuses will be delivered by cesarean section. Nevertheless, a woman may have an obvious breech delivery in progress.

Therapeutic interventions

- Notify obstetric/neonatal specialists.
- Support the baby's legs and buttocks. Do not allow them to hang freely.
- Do *not* pull on the baby. This may cause the cervix to clamp tighter around the baby's head. Work with the mother's contractions.
- When the mother has a contraction, place gentle traction on the fetus. Wrapping a towel around the baby makes the infant easier to grasp.
- Insert a gloved finger into the vagina to help deliver first one shoulder and then the other (Figure 45-9).

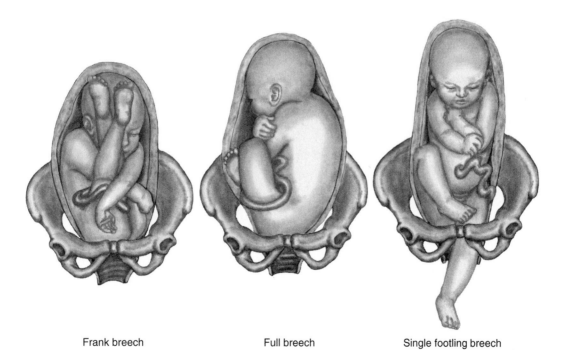

Frank breech   Full breech   Single footling breech

Figure 45-8. Three variations of breech presentation. Frank breech is most common. Footling breeches may be double or single. (From Gorrie TM, McKinney ES, Murray SS: *Foundations of maternal-newborn nursing*, Phildelphia, 1998, WB Saunders.)

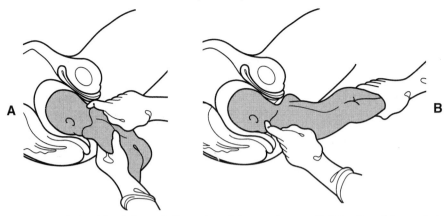

Figure 45-9. Breech-shoulder delivery. **A,** Extraction of the anterior arm. **B,** Extraction of the posterior arm.

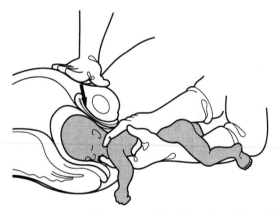

Figure 45-10. Delivery of the arms and shoulders. Breech-head delivery.

- To deliver the head, do the following:
  - Support the fetus's chest with your arm and hands.
  - Place a finger into the posterior vagina and find the infant's mouth.
  - As the mother pushes with contractions, reach into baby's mouth, grasp the chin and apply gentle upward pressure to head and shoulders (Figure 45-10).
  - Have an assistant apply pressure to the suprapubic area to aid head expulsion.

Prolapsed Cord

A prolapsed cord is a state in which the umbilical cord precedes the infant out the vagina. This is an acute emergency because the cord will be compressed between the fetus's and mother's bodies, reducing or eliminating blood flow (Figure 45-11).

A   B   C

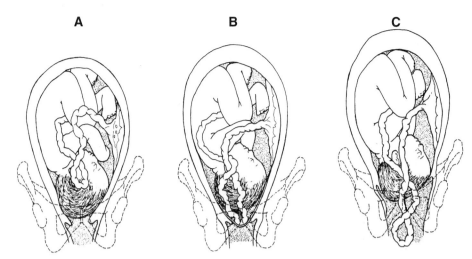

Figure 45-11. Prolapse of the umbilical cord. Note pressure of presenting part on umbilical cord, which endangers fetal circulation. **A,** Occult (hidden) prolapse of cord. **B,** Complete prolapse of cord. Note membranes are intact. **C,** Cord presenting in front of fetal head may be seen in vagina. (Modified from Lowdermilk DL, Perry SE, Bobak IM: *Maternity and women's health care,* ed 7, St Louis, 2000, Mosby.)

Signs and symptoms

- Visible cord protruding from the vagina
- Fetal heart rate frequently less than 100 beats/min (palpate the cord to check for pulsations)

Therapeutic interventions

- Notify obstetric/pediatric specialists.
- Place the mother in a knee-chest position (face and knees on the stretcher, buttocks in the air).
- Administer high-flow oxygen.
- Keep the mother warm.
- Put a gloved hand into the vagina and elevate the fetus's head (or other body part) to relieve pressure on the cord; *once this has been accomplished, leave the hand in place.*
- Do not attempt to return the cord to the vagina.
- Feel for cord pulsations, but handle it as little as possible to prevent spasm of the cord vessels.
- Transport the patient for immediate cesarean section. If transport time is prolonged, keep the cord moist.

Postpartum Hemorrhage

Postpartum hemorrhage is defined as excessive vaginal bleeding any time after delivery (or abortion), for up to 6 weeks. Blood loss with delivery is normal and the mother has an excess blood supply available. However, losses in excess of 500 mL are considered postpartum hemorrhage. Hemorrhage that occurs within 24 hours is called primary postpartum hemorrhage.

Signs and symptoms

- Steady flow of bright red blood
- Nausea
- Pale, clammy skin
- Signs of hypovolemia and hemorrhagic shock (See Chapter 22.)

Therapeutic interventions

- Massage the uterus while applying suprapubic pressure to promote involution and expel clots.
- Apply manual pressure to perineal tears, if present.
- Provide appropriate interventions care for hemorrhagic shock.
  - Administer high-flow oxygen.
  - Insert two large-bore IV catheters and give the patient a bolus of Ringer's lactate or normal saline.
  - Draw blood for type and crossmatch. Transfuse blood products as indicated.
- Give oxytocic agents. Oxytocin (Pitocin, Syntocinon) 20 units per 1000 mL of Ringer's lactate (250 to 500 mL/hr) can reduce bleeding effectively.[5]

GYNECOLOGIC EMERGENCIES

Vaginal Bleeding

Abnormal uterine bleeding is one of the most common gynecologic complaints. Blood loss ranges from acute, life-threatening hemorrhage to occasional spotting. Causes of uterine bleeding are many and varied, often involving abnormalities of the patient's hormonal patterns. A thorough patient history will help identify the cause. For information on bleeding during pregnancy (abortion, abruption, placenta previa), see the previous discussion. Patients also may experience bleeding caused by cancer, trauma, lesions, polyps, fibroids, or infections. Emergency treatment focuses on identifying issues that present an immediate threat to the patient's well-being. Dysfunctional uterine bleeding and other non–life-threatening causes generally are best addressed with follow-up gynecologic consultation.

Consider the following interventions:

- Is the patient hemodynamically stable? If not, intervene immediately.
  - Obtain a CBC and type and crossmatch.
  - Transfuse lactated Ringer's solution or normal saline as indicated.
  - Consider the need for surgical intervention.
- What is the color and volume of the blood (bright red, dark)?
- When was the last menstrual period?
- Has the patient delivered or had an abortion recently?
- Does the patient have a clotting disorder or take anticoagulant medications?
- Does the patient have an intrauterine device in place?
- Is the patient currently pregnant?
- If the patient is not pregnant or is under 20 weeks' gestation, perform a vaginal examination.
- Before performing a vaginal examination on a bleeding pregnant patient (>20 weeks), rule out placenta previa with an ultrasound.
- Is the cervical os open or closed?
- If no emergency exists, recommend follow-up gynecologic consultation.

Ruptured Ovarian Cyst

Ovarian cysts may be asymptomatic until hemorrhage, rupture, or torsion occurs. A ruptured ovarian cyst can be confused with an ectopic pregnancy because signs and symptoms are similar. Appendicitis, diverticulitis, ovarian torsion, and pelvic inflammatory disease also must be considered. Cysts occur at anytime in life but are most common during the child-bearing years. A ruptured cyst may leak serous fluid or can be hemorrhagic. Symptoms range from mild abdominal pain to hypovolemic shock.

Signs and symptoms

- Lower abdominal pain: sudden, sharp, unilateral
- Nausea, vomiting
- Peritoneal irritation
- Irregular menstrual cycle
- Palpable adnexal mass
- Low-grade fever
- Hemoperitoneum
- Signs of hemorrhagic shock

Therapeutic interventions

- Provide high-flow oxygen.
- Initiate IV therapy with lactated Ringer's solution.
- Administer analgesics.
- Give antibiotics.
- Prepare the patient for surgical intervention if the patient is hemodynamically unstable.

Gestational Trophoblastic Disease

Two kinds of gestational trophoblastic tumors are hydatidiform moles and choriocarcinoma. These are rare forms of cancer found only in women of childbearing age. A hydatidiform mole (molar pregnancy) occurs when conception takes place. However, instead of a baby, a cystic tumor is formed, which resembles a bunch of grapes. Hydatidiform moles do not metastasize. More than 80% of hydatidiform moles are benign.

Choriocarcinomas may originate from a hydatidiform mole or from tissue that remains in the uterus following abortion or normal delivery. These tumors can spread from the uterus to other parts of the body. Fortunately, choriocarcinoma is among the most sensitive cancers to chemotherapy, and even with metastasis the cure rate is 90% to 95%.

In the early stages the clinical manifestations of these diseases cannot be distinguished from those of normal pregnancy. Later, vaginal bleeding occurs in most cases.

Signs and symptoms

- Bright red or brownish bleeding that is intermittent or continuous
- Enlarged uterus (often greater than appropriate for gestational age)
- High β-HCG levels
- Absent fetal heart tones
- "Snowstorm" pattern on ultrasound; no evidence of a fetus
- Signs of preeclampsia that may appear at an early gestational age
- Hyperemesis gravidarum

Therapeutic interventions

- If bleeding is heavy, monitor vital signs and give a fluid bolus.
- Draw blood for CBC, type and crossmatch, and β-HCG.
- Prepare for uterine evacuation (dilation and curettage or dilation and evacuation) if bleeding is heavy.
- Observe for signs and symptoms of preeclampsia.

GYNECOLOGIC INFECTIONS

Pelvic Inflammatory Disease

Pelvic inflammatory disease is a term commonly used to describe infections of the uterus, fallopian tubes, ovaries, pelvic peritoneum, or some combination of these sites. The three clinically identifiable subgroups of pelvic inflammatory disease are endometritis-salpingitis, pelvic peritonitis, and tuboovarian abscess.

Pelvic inflammatory disease occurs as a result of upward migration of bacteria from the vagina. Pelvic inflammatory disease can be caused by sexually transmitted organisms or by flora indigenous to the lower genital tract. The bacteria most often isolated are gonococci (25% to 80% of cases), *Chlamydia*, streptococci, *E. coli, Proteus, Klebsiella/Enterobacter,* and clostridia. Predisposing factors include trauma, multiple sexual partners, recent abortion, and use of an intrauterine device. Pelvic inflammatory disease can lead to chronic abdominal pain, ectopic pregnancy, or infertility. Table 45-3 outlines the presenting symptoms and treatment options.

Toxic Shock Syndrome

Toxic shock syndrome is a gynecologic form of staphylococcal sepsis characterized by high fever (>38.8° C, 102° F), headache, sore throat, and myalgias. In addition to these finding, a diffuse rash with edema and blanching erythema develops. Less frequent symptoms include

Table 45-3   Diagnosis and Management of Symptomatic Pelvic Inflammatory Disease

History and Pelvic Examination	Laboratory Tests	Treatment
Pain and tenderness	Gram stain and cultures Complete blood count Possible culdocentesis or laparoscopy	Pelvic examination Pain medications Oral antibiotics
Pain, tenderness, and temperature <39° C (102.5° F)	As above	As above; also may need hospitalization and intravenously administered antibiotics
Pain, tenderness, and temperature >39° C (102.5° F) Possible nausea and vomiting	As above, plus blood cultures	Hospitalization and intravenously administered antibiotics
All the above plus pelvic mass	As above, plus culdocentesis if the cul-de-sac is bulging	Surgery if the mass does not resolve with antibiotics
Septic shock in addition to any of the above findings	As above	As above, plus critical care for management of septic shock (See Chapter 22.)

vomiting, diarrhea, and hypotension. The causative organism is usually *Staphylococcus aureus*, which can be isolated from local sites of skin disruption.

Historically, toxic shock syndrome most often was preceded by the use of hyperabsorbent tampons or contraceptive sponges. When these products were removed from the market, the incidence of toxic shock syndrome dropped dramatically. Contraceptive sponges are once again available in the United States. Toxic shock syndrome also has been associated with tubal ligation, hysterectomy, and carbon dioxide laser vaporization of genital condyloma. Treatment is like for any other cause of septic shock. For more information, see Chapter 22.

Therapeutic interventions

- Initiate contact isolation.
- Support the patient's airway, breathing, and circulation.
- Provide supplemental oxygen to maintain a Pao$_2$ greater than 60 mm Hg; intubate as necessary.
- Restore intravascular volume with IV crystalloids.
- Identify and remove potential sources of infection.
- Begin timely antibiotic administration. Antibiotics may exacerbate symptoms initially as dying bacteria release even more endotoxins.
- Closely monitor the patient's hemodynamic status.
- Facilitate admission or transfer to a critical care unit.
- Anticipate insertion of an arterial line to track blood pressure changes. (See Chapter 11.)
- Consider administration of drotrecogin alpha (Xigris), a new agent for the treatment of sepsis.
- Give antipyretic agents to patients with a body temperature above 38° C (101° F).
- Positive inotropic medications (e.g., dobutamine) may be needed to increase cardiac contractility and output.
- After volume replacement, consider vasopressor use to constrict dilated blood vessels.

Infections of the External Genitalia

Diagnosis of external genitalia infections is made through visual inspection. Table 45-4 lists some of the more common infections. See Chapter 30, Table 30-2, for more specific information on several of these infestations and infections. Figure 45-12 is a Word catheter, which is inserted for treatment of a Bartholin cyst.

Vulvovaginitis

When the ecology of the vagina is disturbed (such as by antibiotic use or diabetes), vaginal infection can occur. Some sexually transmitted diseases cause vulvovaginitis, as do various chemicals found in bubble baths, soaps, and perfumes. Factors such as poor hygiene and allergens contribute to the proliferation of organisms that thrive in warm, damp, dark environments. Sexual abuse should be considered in children with unusual infections and recurrent episodes of unexplained vulvovaginitis.

Vulvovaginitis is not an emergency. Nonetheless, because the condition is annoying, patients with such infections frequently come to the ED. These individuals are more appropriately treated in gynecologic offices and clinics where they can receive follow-up care. Several causes of vulvovaginitis are described next.

Table **45-4**   Infections of the External Genitalia

Infection	Therapeutic Interventions
Scabies	Lindane (Kwell) lotion or shampoo
Vulvar abscess	Incision and drainage
	Antibiotics
	Sitz baths
Simple cyst	Sitz baths
Bartholin cyst (infected)	Antibiotics
	Sitz baths
	Later, incision and drainage
	Word catheter placement
	Indwelling urinary catheter (Foley) placement
	Culture for gonorrhea
Condyloma (genital warts)	Local application of podophyllin
	Local application of trichloroacetic acid
	Large lesions may be surgically removed or treated with laser
Herpes simplex	Acyclovir
	Analgesics

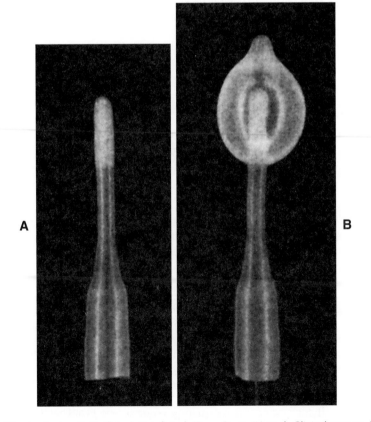

Figure 45-12. Word catheter. **A,** Uniflated. **B,** Inflated. (From Davis JH et al: *Clinical surgery*, St Louis, 1987, Mosby.)

Candida albicans

Candida albicans, a yeast, is one of the most common pathogenic organisms to produce this condition in women of all ages. Antibiotic use can lead to yeast infections by killing the normal antifungal bacteria that live in the vagina. Yeast infections typically cause genital itching and a thick, white vaginal discharge.

Bacterial vaginosis

Another source of vulvovaginitis is bacterial vaginosis, an overgrowth of certain types of bacteria in the vagina. Bacterial vaginosis may cause a thin, grey, vaginal discharge and a fishy odor.

Trichomonas vaginalis

Trichomonas vaginalis, a sexually transmitted infection, is another common precipitant of vulvovaginitis. This infection is associated with genital itching, vaginal odor, and a heavy discharge that may be yellow-grey or green.

Nonspecific vulvovaginitis

Nonspecific vulvovaginitis (where no causative agent can be identified) is seen in all age-groups, but its frequency is greatest in prepubertal girls. Following menarche, the vagina becomes more acidic, which tends to help prevent infections. Nonspecific vulvovaginitis can blossom in anyone with poor genital hygiene and is characterized by a foul smelling, brownish-green discharge and irritation of the labia and introitus. This condition often is associated with an overgrowth of *E. coli.*

Signs and symptoms
- Irritation and/or itching of the genital area
- Inflammation of the labia majora, labia minora, or perineal area
- Possible lesions
- Vaginal discharge
- Foul vaginal odor
- Dysuria

Diagnostic aids
- Assist with a pelvic examination.
- Microscopic evaluation of the vaginal discharge is performed to identify offending organisms.
- Cultures of the discharge may be indicated.

Therapeutic interventions
- For infections, antimicrobial therapy is prescribed.
- In patients with noninfectious vulvovaginitis, treatment is symptomatic.

ABDOMINAL/PELVIC PAIN

Endometriosis

Endometriosis occurs when endometrial tissue cells migrate and grow outside the uterus. This tissue reacts to hormonal changes in the same manner that uterine endometrial tissue does. When menstruation occurs, the tissue sloughs, causing pelvic pain. Symptomatology is highly dependent on the extent of the disease.

Table **45-5**   **Contraceptive Emergencies**

Type	Problem	Therapeutic Intervention
Unprotected sex or contraceptive failure	Potential pregnancy	Emergency contraception with levonorgestrel (Plan B, Preven), a "morning after pill," is effective for up to 72 hours after unprotected intercourse. This oral agent prevents ovulation, disrupts fertilization, and inhibits implantation.
Diaphragm	Unable to remove	Remove with ring forceps
Intrauterine device (IUD)	Unable to remove	Remove with ring forceps
	Lost string	Use abdominal radiographs or ultrasound to determine IUD position; may be removed with an IUD hook.
	Partial expulsion	Remove; advise an alternate form of contraception.
	Abdominal cavity migration	Use abdominal radiographs or ultrasound to determine IUD position; may require exploratory laparotomy.
Oral contraceptives	Thrombophlebitis	Encourage bed rest and local heat application; administer anticoagulant therapy.
	Pulmonary embolus	ABCs, administer oxygen, intravenous fluids, analgesia, bronchodilators, and heparin; provide reassurance.
	Stroke	ABCs, provide oxygen, intravenous fluids, and stroke care.

Signs and symptoms

- Dysmenorrhea
- Episodic pelvic pain
- Dysuria, hematuria
- Dyspareunia (painful intercourse)
- Infertility

Diagnostic aids

- Laparoscopic visualization (by a gynecologist)
- Biopsy (by a gynecologist)

Therapeutic interventions

- Analgesia
- Gynecologic referral for the following:
  - Hormonal therapy
  - Danazol (Danocrine)
  - Oral contraceptive agents
  - Surgery

SEXUAL ASSAULT

Sexual assault is described in Chapter 51.

CONTRACEPTIVE EMERGENCIES

Occasionally, a patient with a contraceptive emergency will present to the ED. Table 45-5 lists some of the more common contraceptive emergencies.

References

1. Fylstra D: Tubal pregnancy: a review of current diagnosis and treatment, *Obstet Gynecol Surv* 53(5): 320-328, 1998.
2. Kidner MC, Flanders-Stepans MB: A model for the HELLP syndrome: the maternal experience, *J Obstet Gynecol Neonatal Nurs* 33(1):44-53, 2004.
3. Martin J, Sidman R: Late postpartum eclampsia: a common presentation of an uncommon diagnosis, *J Emerg Med* 25(4):387-390, 2003.
4. Clark S: Placenta previa and abruptio placenta. In Creasy R, Resnik R, editors: *Maternal-fetal medicine,* ed 4, Philadelphia, 1999, WB Sanders.
5. Schaider J et al: *Rosen and Barkin's 5-minute emergency medicine consult,* ed 2, Philadelphia, 2003, Lippincott Williams & Wilkins.
6. Doan-Wiggins L: Emergency childbirth. In Roberts J, Hedges J, editors: *Clinical procedures in emergency medicine,* ed 4, Philadelphia, 2004, Saunders.
7. Rita S, Reed B: Obstetric emergencies. In Newberry L, editor: *Sheehy's emergency nursing: principles and practice,* ed 5, St Louis, 2003, Mosby.

46

Pediatric Emergencies

Colleen Andreoni, APRN, BC, NP, CCNS, CEN

This chapter covers a broad range of pediatric problems commonly seen in emergency departments (EDs). Children present a unique challenge to the emergency nurse because assessment must include their growth and developmental level and their physical symptoms. Table 46-1 provides information about physical and psychosocial characteristics of the growing child along with guidelines for nursing assessment.[1]

PEDIATRIC TRIAGE

Consider the child's developmental level when performing a triage assessment and allow the parent to remain with the patient, as appropriate. The pediatric assessment triangle is a simple technique for performing a rapid, visual, across-the-room assessment of children presenting to the ED.[2] The pediatric assessment triangle consists of the following three components:
- *Appearance:* Muscle tone, consolability, spontaneous movements, speech/cry, distress level
- *Breathing:* Respiratory distress, abnormal airway sounds
- *Circulation:* Skin color, such as pale, mottled, cyanotic, or flushed

Primary Assessment

Following the quick visual "once over," the next step in the initial assessment is the primary survey, which includes the following:

Airway

- Patency

Breathing

- Rate: fast, slow, normal
- Quality: Effective, ineffective
- Breath sounds: Wheezing, stridor, diminished, absent
- Mechanics: Retractions, grunting, nasal flaring

Circulation

- Skin color: Mottled, ashen, cyanotic, dusky, flushed
- Capillary refill time: Delayed more than 2 seconds
- Skin temperature: Hot, warm, cool, cold
- Central nervous system perfusion: Response to parents, threatening stimuli (nurse), pain

Vital Signs

Once the primary assessment has identified the presence or absence of immediate life-threatening conditions, obtain a baseline set of vital signs, as well as a weight in kilograms, looking for any deviations from normal. Table 46-2 is a chart of age-appropriate vital signs.[3] "Red flag" findings include the following:

Temperature

- Fever associated with abnormal activity, respiratory patterns, or dermal warning signs
- Any temperature greater than 40.5° C (105° F)
- Hypothermia
  - Infant: Less than 35.5° C (96° F)
  - Toddler or child: Less than 35° C (95° F)

Heart Rate

- Infant: Greater than 200 beats/min
- Toddler: Greater than 180 beats/min
- Child: Greater than 160 beats/min
- Significant bradycardia in any age-group

Respiratory Rate

- Infant: Greater than 60 breaths/min
- Toddler: Greater than 40 breaths/min
- Child: Greater than 30 breaths/min

Blood Pressure

- Any blood pressure value in the presence of poor capillary refill
- Systolic blood pressure
  - Infant: Less than 50 mm Hg
  - Toddler: Less than 60 mm Hg
  - Child: Less than 70 mm Hg

Weight

- Less than the 5th percentile for age

Table 46-1   **Pediatric Growth and Development**

	Physical	*Motor Skills*	*Psychosocial*
Infant (Birth-1 yr)	Period of the most rapid growth Weight doubles by 6 mo; triples by 12 mo Head circumference is 1-2 cm larger than the chest The posterior fontanelle closes by 2-3 mo Can distinguish odors, including mother's scent Visual acuity is 20/400 at birth but nears adult acuity levels by 8 mo The neonatal bladder capacity is ≤15 mL	3 mo—lifts head while prone 5 mo—turns from abdomen to back 7 mo—turns from back to abdomen; transfers objects from one hand to the other 9 mo—sits unsupported 12 mo—walks with one hand; crawls quickly; sits from a standing position; uses pincer grasp; eats with fingers	Trust vs. mistrust 6 mo—fears separation and strangers Coping skills: sucking, crying, cooing, babbling, thrashing
Toddler (1-3 yr)	Growth slows Average weight gain is ≤5 lb/yr Brain is 90% of adult size by age 2 yr The anterior fontanelle closes by 18-24 mo	12 mo—learning to walk 15 mo—able to walk alone, begins climbing Has a wide-based gait 24 mo—can dress self with simple clothing Can kick a ball without losing balance 2½ yr—can build a tower of six blocks; draws stick figures	Autonomy vs. shame and doubt Expresses independence as "no!" Possessive of toys and parents Temper tantrums are common Transitional objects may help decrease separation anxiety Spends most of the time playing Focuses on potty training Very curious Fears: separation, loss of control, pain, altered rituals
Preschool (3-5 yr)	Gains <5 lb/yr Limbs grow more than the trunk	Dresses and undresses self Coordination and muscle strength increase rapidly Jumps rope, skips, plays catch Learns to ride a bike Uses scissors, prints name, can tie shoes	Initiative vs. guilt Greater independence Imitates parents and other adults Age of discovery Trial and error leads to learning Magical thinking May see injury or illness as a punishment Fears: mutilation, loss of control, death, dark, ghosts Coping skills: denial, somatization, regression, displacement, projection, fantasy

Communication	Pain and Reflexes	Assessment Guidelines

Cries in response to needs
Is most interactive during the quiet-alert stage
12 mo—uses a three-word vocabulary, one-word sentences
Touch is important
Responds to rocking, holding, patting
	Experiences pain
	Withdraws from pain
	Reflexes present at birth:
	Babinski's reflex
	  Fans toes up and outward (disappears at 9 mo)
	Moro (startle)
	  Sudden extension of the arms with return to midline when startled (disappears at 4 mo)
	Rooting reflex
	  Turns head toward the stimulated side when the face is stroked
		Allow a parent to hold the child or maintain eye contact (when possible)
		Allow the infant to keep a security object
		Approach gently and quietly
		Use distraction techniques
		Obtain a rectal temperature at the end of the examination

2 yr—can almost communicate verbally Attention span is ~2 min at 2 yr Literally believes what is heard Uses short, concrete terms when describing or explaining	No formal concept of pain, may react as intensely to painless procedures as to painful ones Reacts with resistance, aggression, and regression Is rarely able to fake pain Gives unreliable answers when questioned about pain	Approach gradually; establish a relationship Allow the toddler to remain with the parent as much as possible Allow the child to handle equipment before use Use play to interact with the child Keep skin exposures minimal Praise the child for cooperating and when the assessment is finished
Beginning to understand cause and effect >2100 word vocabulary Uses five-word complete sentences Counts to 10; knows the days of the week, name, and address May benefit if given the chance to ask questions Attention span: ~10 min at 3 yr ~30 min at 5 yr	May think pain is a punishment Does not understand that painful procedures are necessary to get better All pain is perceived as "bad pain" Reacts to pain with aggression and often, "I hate you"	Allow the child to be close to caregivers Allow the child to handle equipment before use Allow the child to undress self; respect the child's modesty Expose skin only as necessary for assessment Use play and games to elicit cooperation

Continued

Table 46-1   **Pediatric Growth and Development—cont'd**

	Physical	*Motor Skills*	*Psychosocial*
School-age (6-12 yr)	Gains ~5$\frac{1}{2}$ lb/yr Lymph tissue grows until age 9 Frontal sinuses develop at age 7 Puberty may begin in late school age Increased myelinization improves fine motor skills	Musculoskeletal growth allows greater coordination and strength Involved in active play, sports, and games Performs activities requiring balance and strength Beginning team sports Improved eye-hand coordination Learning new skills	Industry vs. inferiority Takes pride in accomplishments Interacts best with same sex, same age friends Becoming competitive in games Remains dependent on parents for love and security Beginning to take responsibility Fears: separation from friends, loss of control, physical disability
Adolescent (12-21 yr)	Final growth spurt Experiences puberty Sweat gland function increases; acne is common Increased muscle mass Weight problems and eating disorders often develop at this age	Greater coordination of gross and fine motor skills	Identity vs. role confusion Transition from child to adult Peers are important and provide a sense of belonging Moody Developing own values Very private Seeks independence Family dissent is common Involved in risk-taking behaviors Developing sexual orientation Thinking of vocational goals, college Fears: changes in physical appearance or functioning, dependency, loss of control

Modified from Andreoni C, Klinkhammer B: *Quick reference for pediatric emergency nursing*, Philadelphia, 2000, Saunders.

Table 46-2   **Pediatric Vital Signs**

Age	Heart Rate (beats/min)	Systolic Blood Pressure (mm Hg)	Respiratory Rate (breaths/min)	Mass (kg)
Preterm	120-180	40-60	55-65	2
Newborn	90-170	52-92	40-60	3
1 month	110-180	60-104	30-50	4
6 months	110-180	65-125	25-35	7
1 year	80-160	70-118	20-30	10
2 years	80-130	73-117	20-30	12
4 years	80-120	65-117	20-30	16
6 years	75-115	76-116	18-24	20
8 years	70-110	79-119	18-22	25
10 years	70-110	82-122	16-20	30
12 years	60-110	84-128	16-20	40
14 years	60-105	84-136	16-20	50

Modified from Barkin R et al: *Pediatric emergency medicine: concepts and clinical practice*, ed 2, St Louis, 1997, Mosby.

Communication	Pain and Reflexes	Assessment Guidelines
Attention span >30 min Learns to write in cursive Begins to think logically Understands past, present, and future Growing vocabulary allows description of feelings and thoughts May be unable to verbalize the need for parental support	Reactions to pain are often guided by past experiences Able to talk about pain in simple, descriptive terms May exaggerate pain because of fears of more pain or death	Help foster self-esteem by frequent and sincere praise Opinions of health care are often guided by past experiences Allow privacy and time to compose oneself Explain the purpose of the assessment, relating it to the child's illness or injury Diagrams and teaching aids are helpful Give the older school-age child the choice of having parents remain during the assessment
Memory fully developed Able to project to the future Can see the consequences of actions Uses language to convey ideas, beliefs, values Language includes slang	Accurately locates and describes pain May be hyperresponsive to pain Associates pain with possible changes in appearance or function Usually has good self-control during painful procedures	Give the child the choice of having parents remain during assessment Explain the purpose of the examination and all equipment Allow the child to undress in private Provide feedback, especially normals, during the assessment

Secondary Assessment

The purpose of the secondary survey is to develop a complete picture of the child's problem. This allows the clinician to examine the entire patient and focus on specific complaints.[2]

The secondary assessment consists of the following:

- While maintaining privacy, undress the child as much as the triage area will allow.
- Assess for rashes, surface trauma, bruising, unusual marks, deformities, and signs of previous medical care (surgical scars, shunts, baldness, vascular access devices, feeding tubes).
- Evaluate the child's pain (if present) by using a scale appropriate to the patient's developmental level. Provide comfort measures as indicated. (See Chapter 14.)
- Systematically obtain a history that includes the following:
  - Presenting complaint
  - Immunizations
  - Allergies
  - Current medications
  - Medical history (include birth history for infants and young children)

MEDICATION ADMINISTRATION AND INTRAVENOUS THERAPY

Because virtually all pediatric medications are dosed according to a child's weight, an accurate measurement should be obtained as part of the initial assessment. If this is not possible, use a length-based resuscitation tape to calculate estimated body mass.

Oral Medications

Children who cannot, or will not, swallow pills present a nursing challenge. Tips for successful oral medication administration include the following:
- Mix or dilute medications in a minimal amount of fluid, applesauce, or chocolate syrup to encourage the child to ingest the entire dose.
- Demonstrate to parents how to use a syringe to administer medications in the young child's buccal cavity.

Intramuscular Medications

Table 46-3 provides information regarding intramuscular injections in children.

Intravenous Therapy

Establishing and maintaining vascular access in the young patient is one of the most difficult and stressful emergency nursing tasks. Tips for successful intravenous (IV) therapy include the following:
- Provide emotional support to patients and their caregivers; this procedure is anxiety-provoking for both.
- Young children tend to have deep veins that are well covered with subcutaneous tissue. In these patients, scalp veins are an excellent alternative to extremity sites.
- In the presence of volume depletion, small children may have no visible peripheral veins, even after a tourniquet has been applied.
- Scalp veins and the veins on the dorsum of the hand or foot are the preferred sites for over-the-needle IV catheter insertion (24 gauge or larger).
- Quickly consider an intraosseous site if the child is critically ill or injured and requires emergent vascular access. Intraosseous lines offer many benefits and few drawbacks. Refer to Chapter 8 for more information.
- When selecting a site, try to avoid the antecubital fossa, veins over joints, or the dominant hand.

Table 46-3   Intramuscular Medications in Children

Site	Considerations	Volume
Vastus lateralis	The preferred site for children <3 years old.	Can accommodate volumes of 0.5-2 mL.
Ventrogluteal	Consider this site for children >3 years old.	Can tolerate large injection volumes.
Dorsogluteal	Contraindicated in children who have not been walking for at least 1 year.	Can tolerate large injection volumes. Risk of injury to the sciatic nerve exists.
Deltoid	Consider this site for all ages, infant through adult .	Give only small injection volumes (0.5-1 mL). Risk of radial nerve injury exists in young children.

- Once access is obtained, be sure to secure the device well.
- Always use an infusion pump to control the volume of fluid delivered.
- Volume loss is treated by administering isotonic crystallized fluid boluses (lactated Ringer's solution or normal saline). The amount of the bolus is usually calculated at a rate of 20 mL/kg and may be repeated based on the patient's response.
- After any volume losses have been replaced, run the child's IV at maintenance rate. This rate is calculated based on the patient's age and weight. Table 46-4 provides pediatric maintenance formulas.

PEDIATRIC CARDIOPULMONARY ARREST

The child in respiratory failure or shock is at high risk for further decompensation and subsequent cardiopulmonary arrest. Advanced life support interventions must be implemented emergently. Begin with basic life support maneuvers by immediately opening the airway, assisting ventilations, and initiating cardiac compressions as needed. Table 46-5 summarizes the ABCs (airway, breathing, and circulation) of pediatric resuscitation.[4]

Table 46-4   Maintenance Intravenous Fluid Rates in Children

Weight	Amount/Hour (mL)
1-10 kg	100 mL/kg/24 hr
10-20 kg	1000 mL *plus* 50 mL/kg for each additional kilogram over 10 (up to 20 kg), given over 24 hr
≥21 kg	1500 mL *plus* 20 mL/ kg for each additional kilogram over 21, given over 24 hr

Table 46-5   Summary of ABC Maneuvers

Maneuver	Child (1-8 Years Old)	Infant (<1 Year Old)
Airway	Head tilt-chin lift (If trauma is present, use jaw thrust.)	Head tilt-chin lift (difficult to perform in younger patients because of large occiput). To maintain airway, place padding under child's shoulders. (If trauma is present, use jaw thrust.)
Breathing		
Initial	2 breaths at 1-1$\frac{1}{2}$ sec/breath	2 breaths at 1-1$\frac{1}{2}$ sec/breath
Subsequent	~20 breaths/min	~20 breaths/min
FBAO	Heimlich maneuver	Back blows and chest thrusts
Circulation		
Pulse check	Carotid	Brachial or femoral
Compression landmarks	Lower half of sternum	1 finger width below the intermammary line
Compression method	Heel of 1 hand	2 thumbs-encircled hands (for 2 providers) or 2 or 3 fingers
Compression depth	Approximately one third to one half depth of chest	Approximately one third to one half depth of chest
Compression rate	100/min	≥100/min
Compressions/ventilation ratio	5:1 (Pause for ventilation until the trachea is intubated.)	5:1 (Pause for ventilation until the trachea is intubated.)

Data from American Heart Assocation *PALS pocket reference card*, 2003, The Association.

Pediatric Advanced Life Support Measures

Advanced life support measures for children include the following:
- Early recognition of the child in distress is essential for the best outcome.
- Administer 100% oxygen via a non-rebreather mask or bag-valve-ventilation.
- Attach the patient to a monitor/defibrillator and analyze the cardiac rhythm.
- Refer to the appropriate algorithm for pediatric bradycardia (Figure 46-1), pediatric tachycardia with poor perfusion (Figure 46-2), or pediatric pulseless arrest (Figure 46-3).
- Postresuscitation care involves ongoing stabilization based on the patient's status:
  - Persistent hypotension (decompensated): Consider additional fluid boluses and epinephrine (0.1 to 1 mcg/kg/min), dopamine (up to 20 mcg/kg/min), or norepinephrine (0.1 to 2 mcg/kg/min) infusions.
  - Normotensive (compensated): Consider additional fluid boluses and dobutamine (2 to 20 mcg/kg/min), dopamine (2 to 20 mcg/kg/min), epinephrine (0.05 to 0.3 mcg/kg/min), amrinone, or milrinone infusions.
- Facilitate family presence at the bedside.
- Arrange for admission to a pediatric intensive care unit (ICU). Start this process early.

Sudden Infant Death Syndrome

Sudden infant death syndrome (SIDS) is the sudden death of a child (generally less than 12 months old) that remains unexplained after postmortem examination, investigation of the death scene, and review of the patient's case history. The peak SIDS incidence is between 2 and 4 months of age.

Causes

- Many theories have been posited, but no consensus exists.
- There is general agreement that more than one causative factor contributes to the sudden death of infants.
- Theories include the following:
  - Brainstem abnormalities
  - Prone sleeping position (affects oropharyngeal patency)
  - Small airway occlusion
  - Cardiovascular abnormalities
  - Metabolic defects
  - Infections
  - Abnormal sleep and arousal states

Therapeutic interventions

- Implement basic life support and pediatric advanced life support resuscitation guidelines.
- Because of the poor prognosis, prehospital protocols may allow the pronouncement of death at the scene, without initiation of futile resuscitation efforts.
- Most therapeutic interventions are directed at the grieving family.
- Permit the family to say goodbye before discontinuing resuscitation.
- Allow family member to hold the deceased infant; do not rush them.
- Provide mementos such as a lock of hair, footprints, or handprints (these also can be obtained from the funeral home).
- Explain to the family that it is unlikely they did anything to cause the infant's death and that there was nothing they could have done to prevent it.
- Describe what will happen next: Autopsy, release to the funeral home.

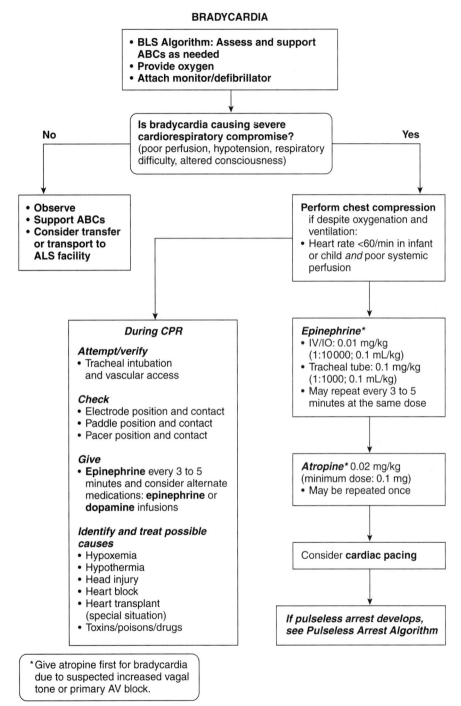

BRADYCARDIA

- **BLS Algorithm: Assess and support ABCs as needed**
- **Provide oxygen**
- **Attach monitor/defibrillator**

Is bradycardia causing severe cardiorespiratory compromise? (poor perfusion, hypotension, respiratory difficulty, altered consciousness)

No / Yes

- **Observe**
- **Support ABCs**
- **Consider transfer or transport to ALS facility**

Perform chest compression if despite oxygenation and ventilation:
- Heart rate <60/min in infant or child *and* poor systemic perfusion

During CPR

Attempt/verify
- Tracheal intubation and vascular access

Check
- Electrode position and contact
- Paddle position and contact
- Pacer position and contact

Give
- **Epinephrine** every 3 to 5 minutes and consider alternate medications: **epinephrine** or **dopamine** infusions

Identify and treat possible causes
- Hypoxemia
- Hypothermia
- Head injury
- Heart block
- Heart transplant (special situation)
- Toxins/poisons/drugs

Epinephrine*
- IV/IO: 0.01 mg/kg (1:10000; 0.1 mL/kg)
- Tracheal tube: 0.1 mg/kg (1:1000; 0.1 mL/kg)
- May repeat every 3 to 5 minutes at the same dose

Atropine* 0.02 mg/kg (minimum dose: 0.1 mg)
- May be repeated once

Consider **cardiac pacing**

If pulseless arrest develops, see Pulseless Arrest Algorithm

*Give atropine first for bradycardia due to suspected increased vagal tone or primary AV block.

Figure 46-1. Pediatric bradycardia algorithm. *ABCs*, Airway, breathing, circulation; *ALS*, advanced life support; *BLS*, basic life support; *CPR*, cardiopulmonary resuscitation; *IO*, intraosseous; *IV*, intravenous. (From American Heart Association: *PALS pocket reference card*, Dallas, 2003, The Association.)

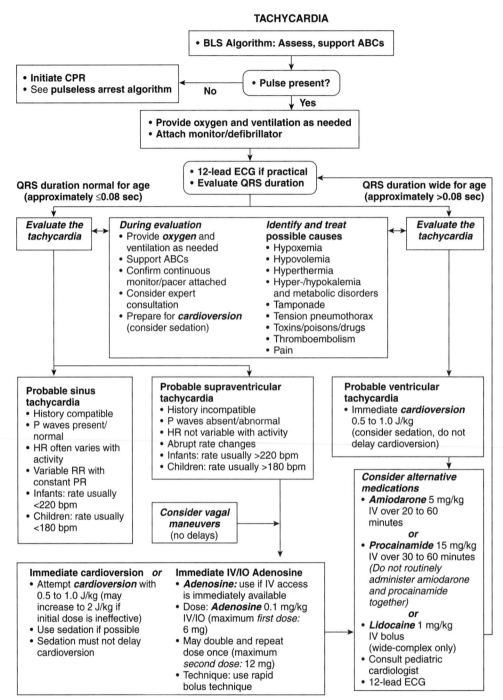

Figure 46-2. Algorithm for pediatric tachycardia with poor perfusion. *ABCs,* Airway, breathing, circulation; *BLS,* basic life support; *CPR,* cardiopulmonary resuscitation; *ECG,* electrocardiogram; *HR,* heart rate; *IO,* intraosseous; *IV,* intravenous. (From American Heart Association: *PALS pocket reference card,* Dallas, 2001, The Association.)

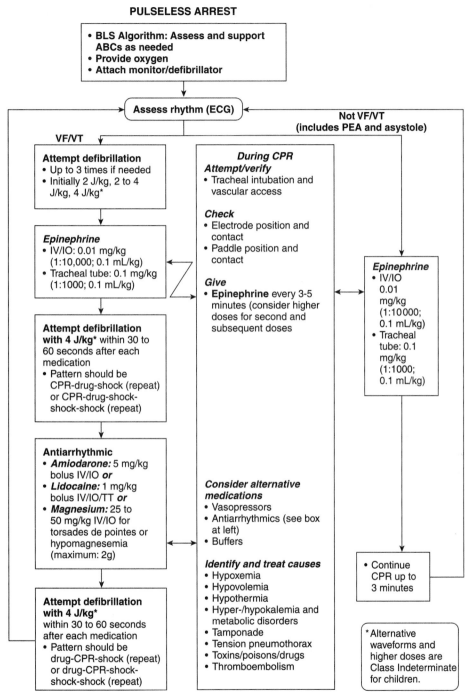

PULSELESS ARREST

- **BLS Algorithm: Assess and support ABCs as needed**
- **Provide oxygen**
- **Attach monitor/defibrillator**

Assess rhythm (ECG)

VF/VT

Not VF/VT (includes PEA and asystole)

Attempt defibrillation
- Up to 3 times if needed
- Initially 2 J/kg, 2 to 4 J/kg, 4 J/kg*

Epinephrine
- IV/IO: 0.01 mg/kg (1:10,000; 0.1 mL/kg)
- Tracheal tube: 0.1 mg/kg (1:1000; 0.1 mL/kg)

Attempt defibrillation with 4 J/kg* within 30 to 60 seconds after each medication
- Pattern should be CPR-drug-shock (repeat) or CPR-drug-shock-shock-shock (repeat)

Antiarrhythmic
- *Amiodarone:* 5 mg/kg bolus IV/IO *or*
- *Lidocaine:* 1 mg/kg bolus IV/IO/TT *or*
- *Magnesium:* 25 to 50 mg/kg IV/IO for torsades de pointes or hypomagnesemia (maximum: 2g)

Attempt defibrillation with 4 J/kg*
within 30 to 60 seconds after each medication
- Pattern should be drug-CPR-shock (repeat) or drug-CPR-shock-shock-shock (repeat)

During CPR
Attempt/verify
- Tracheal intubation and vascular access

Check
- Electrode position and contact
- Paddle position and contact

Give
- **Epinephrine** every 3-5 minutes (consider higher doses for second and subsequent doses

Consider alternative medications
- Vasopressors
- Antiarrhythmics (see box at left)
- Buffers

Identify and treat causes
- Hypoxemia
- Hypovolemia
- Hypothermia
- Hyper-/hypokalemia and metabolic disorders
- Tamponade
- Tension pneumothorax
- Toxins/poisons/drugs
- Thromboembolism

Epinephrine
- IV/IO 0.01 mg/kg (1:10000; 0.1 mL/kg)
- Tracheal tube: 0.1 mg/kg (1:1000; 0.1 mL/kg)

- Continue CPR up to 3 minutes

*Alternative waveforms and higher doses are Class Indeterminate for children.

Figure 46-3. Pediatric pulseless arrest algorithm. *ABCs,* Airway, breathing, circulation; *BLS,* basic life support; *CPR,* cardiopulmonary resuscitation; *IO,* intraosseous; *IV,* intravenous; *PEA,* pulseless electrical activity; *TT,* tracheal tube; *VF,* ventricular fibrillation; *VT,* ventricular tachycardia. (From American Heart Association: *PALS pocket reference card,* Dallas, 2003, The Association.)

- Encourage follow-up grief counseling.
- Many SIDS websites are available as resources for distraught families and staff members.

GENERAL PEDIATRIC EMERGENCIES

Pediatric Fever

An elevated temperature is probably the single most common complaint for which caregivers bring a child to the ED. Hyperthermia has a variety of causes, most commonly infection (fever), but it also can result from poisoning, dehydration, heat exposure, metabolic disorders, or collagen-vascular diseases.

Signs and symptoms

- Rapid pulse
- Flushed skin
- Tachypnea
- Agitation
- Diaphoresis

Therapeutic interventions

- Encourage oral intake (clear liquids) in the conscious child.
- Dress the child in a minimal amount of lightweight clothing.
- Administer antipyretic medications:
  - Acetaminophen 15 mg/kg initially *and/or*
  - Ibuprofen 10 mg/kg (avoid ibuprofen in the newborn (<6 months) and the child who has been vomiting)
  - Do not administer aspirin to a child under 12 years of age.
- Give the child a tepid bath or shower. Do *not* give isopropanol (rubbing alcohol) sponge baths.
- Identify and treat the cause of the elevated temperature.
- A fever of unknown cause in an infant under 3 months of age requires a septic workup that includes lumbar puncture, blood cultures, and urine culture.

RESPIRATORY EMERGENCIES

Airway Obstruction

A common cause of respiratory distress in children is airway obstruction. If the child is in distress but still moving some air, attempt to identify the cause of the obstruction. Perform a rapid assessment, checking for the following:
- Level of consciousness: Alert, irritable, lethargic
- Skin signs: Color, temperature, moistness
- Signs of hypoxia: Circumoral or general cyanosis, rapid respiratory rate
- Upper airway obstruction: Stridor, object in the mouth, oropharyngeal edema
- Nasal plugging (infants)
- Use of accessory muscles of respiration: Retractions, abdominal muscle use, nasal flaring
- Unusual breath odors: Ketones, chemicals, ethanol
- Decreased air movement

- Abnormal lung sounds: Wheezes, stridor, crackles, absent
- Tracheal deviation
- Neck vein distention
- Vital signs (be sure to include temperature)
- Evidence of dehydration: Poor skin turgor, dry mucosa, lack of tears, sunken fontanel
- Signs of trauma: Chest, neck, face, head

Nasopharyngeal Obstruction

Signs and symptoms

- Young infants are obligate nose breathers, and obstruction can be life-threatening.
- Respiratory distress
- Cyanosis

Causes

- Obstruction may be caused by the following:
  - A foreign body: Beads, beans, food, small toy parts
  - Impacted nasal secretions (especially in young infants)
  - Edema: Trauma, infection, swollen adenoids

Therapeutic interventions

- Administer high-flow oxygen by any means the child will tolerate.
- Assist with foreign body removal or nasal suctioning.
- Use airway adjuncts as indicated, based on level of consciousness and level of distress (an oral airway or a tracheal tube).

Oropharyngeal Obstruction

Signs and symptoms

- Noisy breathing: Gargling, snoring, stridor
- No air movement
- Neck extended and chin extended
- Insistence on a sitting position
- Cyanosis
- Difficulty speaking, hoarseness
- Dysphagia, drooling

Causes

Obstruction may be caused by facial trauma, swelling of the tongue, infection, burns, anaphylaxis, or foreign body aspiration.

Therapeutic interventions

- Administer high-flow oxygen by any means the child will tolerate.
- Keep the patient and caregiver calm.

- If the child is moving air, encourage the patient to cough, but do not attempt to remove the foreign body and do not force the patient to change position.
- If there is no air movement in a patient with a known foreign body obstruction, perform the following maneuvers:
  - Infant: Hold the patient prone, with head lower than the trunk; administer five back blows, followed by up to five chest thrusts (stop if the object is dislodged).
  - Child: Administer a series of up to five subdiaphragmatic abdominal thrusts (Heimlich maneuver).
  - Attempt to ventilate the patient.
  - Repeat the foregoing steps until the foreign body is expelled, or prepare to assist with a more invasive method of removal (i.e., direct laryngoscopy) or cricothyrotomy.

Croup Syndromes

Croup syndromes are upper airway conditions associated with varying degrees of obstruction and are characterized by hoarseness and inspiratory stridor. The disorders involved include acute epiglottitis, acute laryngotracheobronchitis, acute spasmodic laryngitits, and acute tracheitis. Of these, epiglottitis is the most life-threatening, but acute laryngotracheobronchitis is the croup syndrome most commonly encountered in the ED.

Epiglottitis

Epiglottitis is a state in which the epiglottis is inflamed. This condition occasionally is seen in connection with upper airway burns but most frequently is the result of a rapidly progressive, potentially lethal bacterial infection of the epiglottis and surrounding structures. *Haemophilus influenzae* type B is the usual causative organism. The number of cases of epiglottitis has declined sharply since childhood Hib vaccination has become routine. In fact, the incidence of epiglottis is now greater among adults than children.

Signs and symptoms
- Typically seen in unimmunized 2- to 5-year-old children
- Abrupt onset of symptoms
- History of an upper respiratory tract infection
- Temperature higher than 39.5° C (103.1° F)
- Sore throat, muffled voice, drooling, dysphagia
- Inspiratory stridor, respiratory difficulty
- Neck extended and chin extended
- Anxious appearance, agitation
- Absent cough
- Pallor, tachycardia
- Insistence on a sitting position

Diagnostic aids
- Diagnosis generally is based on history and examination.
- Lateral soft tissue neck radiographs will demonstrate massive epiglottal swelling, giving "it a thumb" shape.

Therapeutic interventions
- Administer high-flow oxygen by any means the child will tolerate.
- Patients require emergent endotracheal intubation.
- Keep the child as calm as possible; crying stimulates laryngospasm and airway obstruction.

- Do not attempt to look in the child's mouth; doing so may aggravate spasm and lead to complete airway obstruction.
- Delay invasive diagnostic tests and procedures (e.g., IV access) until the airway is secure.
- Ensure that the equipment for emergent tracheal intubation and cricothyrotomy are available at the child's bedside.
- The preferred location for definitive airway management is an operating suite, with a highly experienced clinician to perform the intubation.
- Antibiotics are administered as soon as the airway is secured.
- Corticosteroids may reduce swelling in the first 24 hours.

Acute laryngotracheobronchitis

Acute laryngotracheobronchitis, commonly referred to as "croup," is the most frequent cause of upper airway obstruction in children. Acute laryngotracheobronchitis is a viral infection of the trachea and larynx (which may extend to the bronchi) that causes edema and inflammation of the laryngotracheal mucosa. Transmission is by direct contact with respiratory secretions. The incidence of infection is highest in the fall and winter months, and severity ranges from mild (stage I) to severe (stage IV).

Signs and symptoms
- Patient age usually 3 months to 8 years
- Signs of an upper respiratory tract infection
- Several day history of increasing nocturnal respiratory distress
- Overall appearance of being active and well
- Low-grade fever
- Loud "barking" cough
- Hoarse voice, inspiratory stridor
- Tachypnea, sternal retractions
- Tachycardia

Diagnostic aids
- Diagnosis is based on history and examination.
- Subglottic narrowing ("steeple sign") may be present on lateral neck radiographs.

Therapeutic interventions
- Institute continuous cardiac monitoring.
- Provide cool, humidified oxygen to maintain saturation above 95%.
- To reduce swelling, administer nebulized racemic epinephrine.
  - Effects are seen within 30 minutes and last 2 hours.
  - Symptoms can return when the medication wears off.
- Corticosteroids may reduce swelling in the first 24 hours.

Apnea

Apnea is defined as the absence of breathing for more than 20 seconds. This condition most commonly is encountered in the emergency care setting among infants who arrive following an apparent life-threatening event (ALTE). The child may appear entirely normal or may be in cardiac arrest. A long list of conditions have been associated with apneic events, but often no cause is identified.

Signs and symptoms

- A history of cessation of respirations, color change, decreased muscle tone, choking, or gagging

Causes

- Sepsis
- Seizures
- Upper airway abnormalities
- Gastroesophageal reflux disease
- Hypoglycemia
- Poisoning
- Metabolic disorders
- SIDS (<7% of children with SIDS have a history of an apparent life-threatening event)

Diagnostic aids

- Complete blood count (CBC) with differential
- Platelet count
- Arterial blood gases (ABGs)
- Serum chemistry panel
- Chest radiograph
- 12-lead electrocardiogram
- Toxicologic studies

Therapeutic interventions

- Begin continuous cardiorespiratory monitoring.
- Initiate basic and advanced life support measures as indicated.

Disposition

Infants with an apparent life-threatening event are admitted for observation and further evaluation.

Bronchiolitis

Bronchiolitis is a viral infection of the lower respiratory tract that is particularly prevalent in children under 2 years of age. This condition is most pervasive in the winter months and early spring. Infants at highest risk are those who were less than 34 weeks' gestational age at birth and those with compromised cardiac, pulmonary, or immune systems.

Signs and symptoms

- History of mild respiratory infection, rhinorrhea
- Respiratory difficulty: Prolonged expiratory phase, dyspnea
- Diminished breath sounds, wheezing
- Frequent coughing
- Intercostal and subcostal retractions, nasal flaring

- Poor feeding
- Apneic spells

Causes

- Respiratory syncytial viruses are the most common infective organisms.
- Other pathogens include adenoviruses, parainfluenza, rhinovirus, and influenza.

Diagnostic aids

- Chest radiographs show hyperinflation, interstitial infiltrates, or atelectasis
- CBC
- Nasal swab or nasal washing for respiratory syncytial virus antigens
- Rapid immunofluorescent antibody testing
- Enzyme-linked immunoabsorbent assay
- Viral cultures (may take several days to get results)

Therapeutic interventions

- Place the patient on contact isolation.
- Institute continuous cardiac, respiratory, and oxygen saturation monitoring.
- Give humidified oxygen to keep saturation greater than 95%.
- Administer aerosolized bronchodilator therapy (patient response to this intervention varies).
- Corticosteroid administration has *not* been proved beneficial.
- For patients with severe tachypnea, provide IV rehydration.
- Tracheal intubation and positive-pressure ventilation are required for patients in moderate to severe distress.

Pneumonia

Pneumonia is an inflammation of the lung parenchyma caused by a variety of infectious agents, including viruses, bacteria, and mycoplasma. Overcrowded conditions predispose children to pneumonia; those from homes with smokers have twice the risk. Table 46-6 gives characteristics of various pneumonia types.

Therapeutic interventions

- Perform serial respiratory assessments.
- Place the patient in a position of comfort.
- Hydrate as necessary with oral and/or IV fluids.
- Provide humidified oxygen to maintain saturation greater than 95%.
- Administer antibiotics.
- Give antipyretics as needed.
- Treat bronchospasm with bronchodilators.

Disposition

- Most children with pneumonia can be treated and released from the ED.
- Consider admission for patients who meet the following criteria:
  - Apneic, cyanotic, or greatly fatigued

Table 46-6   Types of Pneumonia With Characteristic Features

	Viral	Bacterial	Mycoplasmal
Causative agent	Respiratory syncytial virus, parainfluenza, influenza, adenovirus, rhinovirus	*Streptococcus pneumoniae, Staphylococcus aureus, Haemophilus influenzae*	*Mycoplasma pneumoniae*
Age	All ages, most common in children <5 yr	All ages	Most common in children >5 yr
Onset	Gradual	Rapid	Gradual
Fever	Moderate	High, often with chills	Low
Cough	Dry	Productive	Dry, hacking, especially at night
Breath sounds	Few crackles, few wheezes	Decreased, crackles, rhonchi	Fine crackles, rare wheezes
Other signs or symptoms	Severity varies; myalgias Chest x-ray film: diffuse or patchy infiltrates White blood cells normal	Pleuritic pain, anorexia Chest x-ray film: diffuse or patchy infiltrates White blood cells increased, often with increased bands	Headache, pharyngitis, malaise, anorexia Chest x-ray film: may show areas of consolidation White blood cells normal
Specific emergency department treatment	Supportive care Susceptible to a secondary infection	Supportive care Antibiotics	Supportive care Antibiotics

Data from Andreoni C, Klinkhammer B: *Quick reference for pediatric emergency nursing*, Philadelphia, 2000, Saunders.

- At high risk for complications
- Have a concomitant pleural effusion
- Require supplemental oxygen

Asthma

Asthma is a recurrent reactive airway disease associated with reversible obstruction. The airways of asthmatic patients are hyperresponsive to a variety of triggers that stimulate the release of inflammatory mediators. The three pathologic components of asthma are bronchospasm, mucous gland hypertrophy, and mucous plugging. Hypoxia and hypercarbia result from a mismatch between ventilation and perfusion produced by these conditions. Children at high risk for life-threatening exacerbations include those with a history of the following:
- Prior intubation or ICU admission for asthma
- Two or more asthma hospitalizations in the past year
- Three or more ED visits for asthma within the last 12 months
- An ED or inpatient admission for asthma within the past month
- Daily oral corticosteroid use

Signs and symptoms

The following signs and symptoms depend greatly on the severity of the exacerbation:
- Shortness of breath, cough, dyspnea, tachypnea
- Use of accessory muscles, retractions
- Nasal flaring, grunting
- Chest discomfort

- Breath sounds
  - Prolonged expiration
  - Expiratory wheezes (also may have inspiratory wheezing)
  - No expiratory sounds (silent chest) if air movement is minimal
- Tachycardia
- Exercise intolerance
- Hypocapnia initially; hypercapnia develops as the patient decompensates

Triggers

- Allergens
- Environmental irritants
- Cold air
- Respiratory infections
- Exercise

Diagnostic aids

- Oxygen saturation (pulse oximetry)
- Serial peak expiratory flow rate measurements (before and after each intervention)
- Routine chest radiographs are *not* indicated. Obtain films only for patients with the following:
  - The first episode of wheezing
  - Suspected pneumonia, pneumothorax, or other respiratory disorder
  - Unilateral wheezing (to rule out foreign body)
  - Severe exacerbations unresponsive to treatment
- Chest radiographs predictably demonstrate hyperinflation, increased bronchial markings, and possible atelectasis.
- ABGs (for severe exacerbations only)

Therapeutic interventions

- Institute continuous cardiac, respiratory, and oxygen saturation monitoring.
- Provide supplemental oxygen to maintain saturation above 95%.
- Administer an inhaled beta$_2$-agonist (albuterol or levalbuterol). These drugs relax smooth airway muscles and have a 5-minute onset of action. Inhaled beta$_2$-agonists can be given using the following:
  - A multidose inhaler with spacer. Observe for correct technique. Administer every 20 minutes as needed.
  - A nebulizer. Administer continuously or every 20 minutes as needed.
- Initiate antibiotic therapy if indicated, but most exacerbations are associated with viral, not bacterial, infections.
- Give corticosteroids to any patient with a moderate to severe exacerbation.
  - Bronchodilators only treat the bronchospastic component of asthma. Antiinflammatory agents address the inflammatory component and have been shown to reduce the rate of relapse.
  - Oral steroid preparations are just as effective as parenteral (IV or intramuscular) steroid administration. All routes have an onset of action of about 6 hours, so initiation of therapy should not be delayed.

- Administer anticholinergics (e.g., ipratropium bromide).
  - Anticholinergic drugs decrease vagal stimulation of the airways.
  - Ipratropium bromide can be administered by multidose inhaler with a spacer or by nebulizer. The drug may be mixed with albuterol.

Disposition

- Admit any child who remains symptomatic, hypoxic, or fatigued.
- Discharge those with improved peak expiratory flow rates and minimal symptoms.
- Encourage follow up with a primary care provider in 3 to 5 days.

Patient education and discharge instructions

- Observe, coach, and correct patients' peak expiratory flow rate and multidose inhaler techniques.
- Emphasize the importance of routine peak expiratory flow rate monitoring and having a customized action plan.
- Discuss the appropriate use of corticosteroids (oral and inhaled) and beta$_2$-agonists (long-acting and short-acting).
- Emphasize early signs of exacerbation.
- Teach trigger avoidance strategies.

Status Asthmaticus

Status asthmaticus is asthma that fails to respond to conventional therapy. This condition can progress to respiratory failure without timely intervention.

Therapeutic interventions

- Institute continuous cardiac, respiratory, and oxygen saturation monitoring.
- Provide humidified oxygen to maintain saturation above 95%.
- Continuously administer an inhaled beta$_2$-agonist.
- Obtain vascular access.
- Give systemically effective corticosteroids (IV, intramuscular, or oral) as soon as possible.
- Consider administration of epinephrine, terbutaline, magnesium sulfate, ketamine, or heliox (although the effectiveness of most of these agents is not well supported in the literature).
- Consider noninvasive positive-pressure ventilation (e.g., biphasic positive airway pressure) or tracheal intubation and mechanical ventilation.
- *Do not allow asthmatics to become hypoxic, hypercarbic, or acidotic. Once patients have reached this state, intubation is associated with a high incidence of mortality.*

Disposition

Admit patient to a pediatric ICU.

NEUROLOGIC EMERGENCIES

The Unconscious Child

Evaluation of the child with a severely altered level of consciousness must be rapid, systematic, and thorough. Determining the cause is crucial, but immediate priority is given to supporting airway, breathing, and circulation. Refer to Chapter 43 for the child with unconsciousness related to injury.

Signs and symptoms

- Poor muscle tone
- Decreased level of responsiveness
- Loss of bladder or bowel control (in a toilet-trained child)
- Lack of awareness of the surroundings; poor interaction
- Pallor, mottling, cyanosis
- Delayed capillary refill
- Tachypnea, apnea
- Bradycardia, tachycardia
- Hypothermia, hyperthermia
- History may include metabolic or cardiovascular disorders or exposure to toxins. (Refer to Chapter 28.)

Possible causes of unconsciousness

Central nervous system

- Trauma
- Infection
- Seizures

Cardiovascular

- Heart failure
- Congenital heart disease
- Infection

Respiratory

- Acute respiratory failure, obstruction, or hypoxia
- Trauma
- Allergy
- Infection

Shock

- Septic
- Hypovolemic
- Neurogenic
- Cardiogenic
- Anaphylactic

Gastrointestinal

- Vomiting and diarrhea
- Dehydration

Metabolic

- Ketoacidosis
- Hypoglycemia
- Toxic exposure
- Reye's syndrome
- Renal or hepatic failure

Endocrine

- Addisonian crisis
- Diabetes mellitus

Diagnostic aids

- CBC
- Chemistry panel
- Glucose
- Ammonia level
- Toxicology screen, ethanol level
- ABGs
- Lumbar puncture
- Computed tomography (CT) scan of the brain
- Chest radiograph

Therapeutic interventions

- Initiate cardiorespiratory monitoring.
- Monitor oxygen saturation, administer oxygen as necessary, and consider tracheal intubation.
- Determine serum glucose. Treat hypoglycemia with dextrose.
- Measure a rectal temperature.
- Perform neurologic assessments, including serial pediatric Glasgow Coma Scale scoring (see Table 7-9).
- Obtain a history and description of events from the family, caregivers, or prehospital personnel.
- Initiate vascular access.
- Insert a gastric tube and decompress the stomach.
- Place an indwelling urinary catheter (Foley).
- Maintain normothermia; warm or cool as needed.
- Definitive treatment depends on the cause of unconsciousness.

Febrile Seizures

The most common cause of seizures in children is fever. Febrile seizures usually occur between the ages of 5 months and 5 years. These convulsions are associated with a febrile illness, most often viral. This is not a seizure disorder; two thirds of children who experience a febrile seizure never have another. However, other seizure causes must be excluded before a definitive diagnosis is made. Seizure causes include hypoglycemia, hypoxia, central nervous system infections, toxins, epilepsy, metabolic disorders, developmental defects, and head trauma. In addition, seizures in the pediatric population are frequently idiopathic. Refer to Chapter 23 for further information on seizure disorders.

Signs and symptoms

- History of a preceding illness with a rapidly elevating fever
- Self-limited, generalized, tonic-clonic motor activity
- Duration less than 15 minutes, usually followed by a postictal period
- Normal level of consciousness that returns after the postictal period

Diagnostic aids

- Check the serum glucose level.
- Consider a chemistry panel, CBC with differential, and blood cultures.
- Lumbar puncture is indicated only if the seizure cause is unclear, the patient is highly symptomatic, or a central nervous system infection is suspected.
- Send cerebrospinal fluid (CSF) to laboratory for cell count, Gram stain, culture, protein, and glucose.

Therapeutic interventions

Generally, patients with a febrile seizure will recover by the time they arrive at the ED. The presence of continued seizures or a prolonged postictal period strongly suggests a nonfebrile cause. Treatment is largely symptomatic and is focused on airway, breathing, circulation, and seizure control.

Interventions include the following:

- Protect seizing or postictal patients from injury.
- When possible, place the child in a lateral decubitus position.
- Suction secretions as needed to maintain airway patency. A nasopharyngeal airway can be inserted even in patients with a clenched jaw.
- Provide 100% oxygen by mask or blow-by during the seizure and postictal period to maintain saturation.
- Assist ventilations as indicated.
- If the seizure is prolonged, initiate vascular access for anticonvulsant infusion. Consider an intraosseous site.
- Anticonvulsants can be administered by intramuscular and rectal routes, but absorption is slow and unreliable.
- Prepare for tracheal intubation if there is a delayed return of spontaneous respirations. Rapid sequence induction intubation is necessary if the patient is still seizing. (See Chapter 19.)
- Correct hypoglycemia.

Disposition

- Discharge stable, postfebrile seizure patients who do not have a serious infectious cause.
- Admit patients who remain symptomatic and those with a first-time seizure of questionable cause.

Patient education and discharge instructions

- Administer antipyretics and antibiotics as directed.
- Follow up with a physician in 3 to 5 days.
- Prepare to manage seizures at home.

Meningitis

Meningitis is an acute inflammation of the meninges from a viral or bacterial infection. Continued inflammation leads to increases in intracranial pressure. Infection can progress rapidly and may invade the ventricles. The clinical presentation of meningitis varies with the age of the child and the severity of the illness. Viral meningitis is generally much less severe than bacterial. The most common bacterial organisms are *H. influenzae, Streptococcus pneumoniae,* and *Neisseria meningitidis.* Box 46-1 highlights signs and symptoms of bacterial meningitis by age-group.[1]

Like epiglottitis, the declining incidence of viral meningitis has been attributed to the introduction of routine Hib vaccination. Symptoms tend to be similar to those of bacterial meningitis but are considerably milder. Common findings include fever, stiff neck, and headache. Symptom severity dictates the extent of diagnostic studies and therapeutic interventions.

Diagnostic aids

- CBC
- Chemistry panel
- Glucose
- Urinalysis and urine culture
- ABGs
- Coagulation profile

Box **46-1** Signs and Symptoms of Bacterial Meningitis

Neonate

Symptoms are often vague.
Altered level of consciousness
Apnea
Bulging or tense fontanelle
Fever or hypothermia
Irregular respiratory patterns
Irritability
Meningeal signs possibly absent
Opisthotonus (head, neck and spine are arched backward)
Petechia or purpura
Poor feeding
Poor muscle tone
Seizures
Vomiting, diarrhea
Weak cry
Weak suck

Infant-Toddler

Altered level of consciousness
Ataxia
Bulging fontanelle
Fever (may be absent in neonates)

High-pitched cry
Irritability
Lethargy
Meningeal signs may be absent in child less than 2 years
Petechia or purpura
Poor feeding
Vomiting

Preschooler-Adolescent

Altered level of consciousness
Anorexia
Confusion
Fever
Headache
Meningeal signs:
  Positive Brudzinski's sign (Flexion of head produces flexion of the hips and knees.)
  Positive Kernig's sign (pain with extension of the leg and knee)
Myalgias
Photophobia
Purpura
Seizures
Vomiting and diarrhea

From Andreoni C, Klinkhammer B: *Quick reference for pediatric emergency nursing,* Philadelphia, 2000, Saunders.

- Blood cultures
- Lumbar puncture: Send CSF for cultures, Gram stain, protein, glucose, and cell count.
- CT scan of the brain
- Chest radiograph

Therapeutic interventions

- Initiate respiratory isolation.
- Maintain airway, breathing, and circulation.
- Administer supplemental oxygen.
- Obtain vascular access, and administer the following:
  - Fluid boluses (20 mL/kg) for hypotension and poor perfusion
  - Antibiotics: Do *not* hold antibiotics if the lumbar puncture or blood cultures are delayed.
  - Antipyretics
  - Analgesics
  - Dexamethasone IV for suspected *H. influenzae* meningitis.
- Perform ongoing neurologic assessments and document Glasgow Coma Scale score.
- Consider placing a gastric tube and indwelling urinary catheter.
- Institute seizure precautions.
- Assist with lumbar puncture after CT scan.
  - Arrange the older child or young infant in a sitting or side-lying position. Place small children in a lateral decubitus position to provide maximal control.[3,5]
  - Be careful to avoid airway obstruction during the procedure; continuously monitor heart rate and oxygen saturation.
  - Number CSF specimens as they are drawn and send the tubes for testing in the following order:
    1. Culture and Gram stain
    2. Protein and glucose
    3. Cell count
    4. Miscellaneous tests as ordered

Disposition

- Facilitate pediatric ICU admission for the child with an abnormal cardiorespiratory or neurologic status.
- Stable children with viral meningitis may be discharged.
- Provide caretakers with information regarding the disease course, symptomatic treatments, and comfort measures.

Meningococcemia

Meningococcemia is a systemic bacterial infection caused by *N. meningitidis*. Sepsis occurs with or without concomitant meningitis. Meningococcemia is a rapidly progressive disease capable of producing death from shock and coagulopathies within hours of symptom onset.

Signs and symptoms

- Fever (or hypothermia in the neonate and young infant)
- Chills

- Rash: Petechia, purpura
- Headache, irritability, altered level of consciousness, coma
- Hypotension
- Diffuse bleeding

Diagnostic aids

- Lumbar puncture: Send CSF for cultures, Gram stain, protein, glucose, and cell count.
- CBC with differential
- Chemistry panel
- Glucose
- Erythrocyte sedimentation rate
- Urinalysis, urine culture
- Coagulation profile/disseminated intravascular coagulation screen

Therapeutic interventions

- Immediate recognition and intervention.
- Implement isolation precautions.
- Institute continuous cardiorespiratory monitoring.
- Provide supplemental high-flow oxygen.
- Obtain vascular access and give isotonic crystalloid boluses (20 mL/kg) for hypotension and poor perfusion.
- Rapidly initiate antibiotic administration.
- Facilitate pediatric ICU admission.
- Consider antibiotic prophylaxis for family, friends, and staff members with potential droplet exposure.

Ventriculoperitoneal Shunt Emergencies

Children with hydrocephalus often are brought to the ED with a problem related to their ventriculoperitoneal shunt. These catheters are placed surgically to redirect CSF from the ventricles to the peritoneal cavity in patients with inadequate ventricular drainage. The two most common problems are shunt malfunction and shunt infection. Malfunction involves catheter obstruction, disconnection, or distal tip migration. Patients with shunt malfunction frequently require ICU admission and surgical shunt revision. Children with shunt-related infections are treated aggressively with antibiotic therapy in a pediatric ICU.

Signs and symptoms

Ventriculoperitoneal Shunt Malfunction in Infants

- Increased head circumference, separation of the cranial sutures
- Bulging or tense fontanelles
- Irritability, lethargy
- Vomiting

Ventriculoperitoneal Shunt Malfunction in Older Children

- Altered level of consciousness
- Vomiting
- Headache

- Ataxia
- Seizures

Diagnostic aids

- Radiographic views of the lateral neck, chest, and abdomen (shunt series)
- CT scan of the head
- Other tests may be performed in patients with a possible coexisting infection.

Signs and symptoms of ventriculoperitoneal shunt infection

- Most commonly occurs 1 to 2 months after catheter insertion
- Nausea
- Headache
- Fever
- Malaise, altered level of consciousness
- Signs and symptoms consistent with meningitis

GASTROINTESTINAL EMERGENCIES

Vomiting and Diarrhea

Vomiting and diarrhea in children are caused by a variety of conditions, the most common of which is self-limiting viral gastroenteritis. Intractable vomiting occurs with increased intracranial pressure, Reye's syndrome, gastroesophageal reflux, pyloric stenosis, toxicities, or bowel obstruction.

Diarrhea is defined as three or more liquid stools in a day. Viruses, bacteria, parasites, toxins, gastrointestinal bleeding, medications, malabsorption syndromes, certain diets, and bowel disorders can produce diarrhea. Regardless of the cause, diarrhea generally stops within a week. Serious episodes are characterized by voluminous stools, bloody diarrhea, and coexisting vomiting. Decompensation can progress rapidly. Although most cases of vomiting and diarrhea are mild and self-limiting, gastroenteritis is nonetheless the leading cause of childhood mortality in developing nations.

Signs and symptoms

- Diarrhea
- Vomiting
- Abdominal pain
- Fever
- Dehydration (Table 46-7)
  - Dry mucous membranes
  - Limited tearing
  - Decreased urine output
  - Concave anterior fontanelle
  - Sunken-appearing eyeballs
  - Weight loss
  - Thirst
  - Poor skin turgor
  - Listlessness
  - Hypovolemic shock
  - Prolonged capillary refill

Table **46-7**   **Dehydration Severity**

Signs and Symptoms	Mild (<5% Loss)	Moderate (5%-10% Loss)	Severe (10%-15% Loss)
Mucous membranes	Somewhat dry	Dry	Very dry
Skin turgor	Normal	Poor	Very poor
Anterior fontanelle	Normal	Sunken	Sunken
Eye appearance	Normal	Sunken	Sunken
Heart rate	Normal	Increased moderately	Increased greatly
Respiratory rate	Normal	Increased	Increased
Blood pressure	Normal	Minimally decreased	Decreased
Skin	Pale, warm	Very pale to mottled, cool	Mottled to cyanotic, cool
Capillary refill	Normal	Minimally delayed	Delayed
Urine output	Normal	Decreased	Decreased to none
Mental status	Normal	Normal to lethargic	Lethargic to unresponsive

Causes

- Infectious causes are viral, bacterial, or parasitic.
  - Transmission is by the oral-fecal route or person to person.
  - The incidence of viral gastroenteritis in highest during the winter months.
  - Bacterial gastroenteritis is more common in the summer.
- Noninfectious causes are toxins, gastrointestinal bleeding, malabsorption syndromes, certain diets, bowel disorders, cathartic abuse, and medications (e.g., antibiotics).

Diagnostic aids

The scope and extent of diagnostic testing in the child with vomiting and diarrhea depends on the duration and severity of symptoms and their probable cause.

Testing includes the following:

- CBC with differential
- Chemistry panel
- Urinalysis
- Stool for culture, ova, and parasites

Therapeutic interventions

- Support airway, breathing, and circulation.
- Institute oral rehydration in patients capable of drinking.
  - Give $1/2$ cup of an oral rehydration solution (Pedialyte, Rehydralyte, Infalyte, Ricelyte) every hour or after each diarrheal stool. Give the total volume in small amounts (sips of 1 to 2 tsp) to facilitate absorption and discourage vomiting.
  - Avoid sugary drinks and salty soups.
  - Encourage continuation of breast-feeding.
- In the presence of moderate or severe dehydration (>10%), establish vascular access.
  - Administer an isotonic crystalloid fluid bolus (20 mL/kg); reassess and give another bolus as needed. Several boluses may be required.

- Following rehydration, reduce IV fluid administration to maintenance levels (see Table 46-4).
- Closely monitor intake and output.

Pyloric Stenosis

Infants with pyloric stenosis have a history of projectile vomiting after feeding. Congenital hypertrophy of the pyloric muscles leads to obstruction at the pyloric sphincter. This results in forceful vomiting in which gastric contents can be spewed a distance of up to 4 feet. The force of vomiting intensifies as the extent of obstruction increases. The cause of pyloric stenosis remains controversial.

Signs and symptoms

- Age of the infant is usually 2 to 5 weeks
- Projectile vomiting after feedings
- Continued hungry behavior
- No indications of pain
- Poor weight gain
- Few stools
- Visible peristaltic waves on the abdomen
- Palpable abdominal mass above the umbilicus, in the right upper quadrant (about the size of an olive)
- Signs of dehydration may be present.

Diagnostic aids

- Diagnosis usually is based on history and examination.
- Abdominal ultrasound
- Barium swallow (after surgical consultation)
- CBC
- Chemistry panel
- Urinalysis

Therapeutic interventions

- Initiate IV fluid replacement. Patients may require potassium replacement as well.
- Monitor intake and output.
- Insert a gastric tube to decompress the stomach.
- Prepare for admission and surgical repair.

Appendicitis

Appendicitis is the most common cause of abdominal pain and abdominal surgery in children. This disease is rare in patients less than 2 years old. Symptoms can be difficult to interpret, and diagnosis is complicated in the very young child.

Signs and symptoms

- Pain originates in the periumbilical area and then localizes in the right lower quadrant (McBurney's point).

- The child's preferred position is supine with the legs flexed.
- Positive iliopsoas (or psoas) test: The psoas test is said to be positive if, when lying on the left side, hyperextension of the right hip produces pain.
- Loss of appetite: If anorexia is *not* present, appendicitis is unlikely.
- Nausea and vomiting occur.
- Right lower quadrant guarding and pain with movement are present.
- Peritoneal signs will be present if the appendix has ruptured:
  - Rebound tenderness
  - Abdominal rigidity
- Fever and tachycardia are present.

Diagnostic aids

- CBC
- Chemistry panel
- Urinalysis
- Abdominal ultrasound
- Abdominal CT scan
- Chest radiograph (to rule out lower lobe pneumonia as the cause of abdominal pain)

Therapeutic interventions

- Maintain NPO status.
- Establish vascular access.
- Administer the following:
  - Analgesics
  - Antipyretics
  - Antibiotics

Disposition

Prepare the patient for surgery and admission.

Intussusception

Intussusception is the telescoping of one segment of the bowel into another. This disorder is most common in children between 3 months and 5 years of age. The typical location is the ileocecal valve. Intussusception may follow a viral infection, especially in younger children.

Signs and symptoms

- Sudden, acute, episodic abdominal pain occurs.
- The knees are flexed.
- The patient is pain-free between episodes.
- Vomiting occurs after the onset of pain.
- Patient passes "currant jelly" stool with bloody mucous.
- Abdominal distention is present.
- A sausage-shaped mass is palpable in the right upper quadrant.
- Early examination may appear normal.
- Later signs include fever, tachycardia, lethargy, and dehydration.

Diagnostic aids

- Abdominal radiographs
- CBC
- Chemistry panel
- Barium enema can both diagnose and reduce an intussusception.
- CT scan of the abdomen may be obtained.

Therapeutic interventions

- Maintain NPO status.
- Establish vascular access.

Disposition

Admit for surgery if the barium enema failed to reduce the intussusception or if it reoccurs.

Volvulus

Malrotation of the bowel is a congenital anomaly involving abnormal bowel rotation and mesenteric attachment. This twisting (volvulus) of the small intestine can result in strangulation of the superior mesenteric artery and bowel infarction. Volvulus most commonly occurs in the first month of life but can appear later in childhood.

Signs and symptoms

- Bilious vomiting
- Signs of abdominal pain
- Abdominal distention
- Bloody stools
- Hematemesis
- Visible peristaltic waves
- Peritoneal signs if the bowel is perforated

Diagnostic aids

- CBC
- Chemistry panel
- Urinalysis
- Upper gastrointestinal series if the patient is stable
- CT scan of the abdomen may be obtained.

Therapeutic interventions

- Establish vascular access.
- Give analgesics as needed.
- Administer IV antibiotics.
- Insert a gastric tube to decompress the stomach.

Disposition

Prepare the patient for surgery and admission.

References

1. Andreoni C, Klinkhammer B: *Quick reference for pediatric emergency nursing,* Philadelphia, 2000, Saunders.
2. Emergency Nurses Association: *Emergency nursing pediatric course provider manual,* ed 3, Des Plaines, Ill, 2004, The Association.
3. Barkin R et al: *Pediatric emergency medicine: concepts and clinical practice,* ed 2, St Louis, 1997, Mosby.
4. American Heart Association: *PALS pocket reference card,* Dallas, 2003, The Association.
5. Lang S: Procedures involving the neurologic system. In Bernardo LM, Bove M, editors: *Pediatric emergency nursing procedures,* Boston, 1993, Jones and Bartlett.

47

Abuse and Neglect

Patricia L. Clutter, RN, MEd, CEN

Although child maltreatment has always existed, Western culture has recognized it only as a problem since the 1962 landmark publication, "The Battered Child Syndrome."[1] The actual incidence of maltreatment is nearly impossible to establish. In 2002 the National Clearinghouse of Child Abuse and Neglect Information reported about 3 million referrals to child protective services agencies, representing 5 million children. Of these referrals, 32% were determined to be actual cases of abuse or neglect. Several factors contribute to variation in the number of reported cases, but over the past decade, maltreatment prevalence rates have been calculated between 11.8 and 15.3 per 1000. Children from birth to 3 years have the highest incidence of any age group.[2,3] In the United States a child is reported as abused or neglected every 38 seconds.[4] In the year 2000, 1200 American children were estimated to have died of maltreatment. The actual number of deaths may be significantly higher because of an underreporting rate of as much as 60%.[5] Despite considerable negative publicity, only 2.7% of fatalities took place in a foster care environment.[3,6]

Abuse of elderly and dependent adults is discussed together because the issues involved for each group are so similar. Adults who are elderly (age 60 and over) or otherwise dependent have a limited ability to report their maltreatment or have compelling reasons not to report it. In 1996, about 450,000 cases of elder abuse and neglect were documented. Ninety percent of perpetrators are family members; two thirds are the victim's adult child or spouse.[7]

Handicapped individuals, especially those with mental deficiencies, are at risk for a variety of abusive situations, including physical, sexual, financial, emotional, or verbal abuse and neglect.[8] The extent of the problem is likely to be seriously underdocumented. In 2003, investigative journalists at the *Washington Post* identified 47 suspicious deaths of handicapped individuals that had gone unreported. Of the 116 deaths during the study period, only 69 were officially ruled as maltreatment; 8 autopsies were completed, but there was no documentation of death investigation.[9] Frequently, even if the dependent individual can describe the situation and identify the perpetrator, there is no arrest, prosecution, or conviction because the disabled victim is unable to testify effectively on his or her own behalf.[10]

Women with disabilities often are devalued and have poor support systems. This places them at considerably higher risk for abuse than their counterparts without disabilities. These victims remain largely invisible, rarely connecting with services that understand their needs or have the ability to meet them.[11,12]

CHILD MALTREATMENT

Child maltreatment is defined as any harm that occurs to a child as a result of physical, emotional, or sexual abuse or neglect. Maltreatment can take many forms, and minors are regularly the victims of more than one type of abuse.

Maltreatment Categories

Neglect

Neglect involves failure (intentionally or unintentionally) to provide basic needs such as food, shelter, clothing, schooling, and medical care. Figure 47-1 depicts failure to thrive as a consequence of negligence. Neglect commonly is subcategorized as follows:

Medical: This type of neglect consists of failure to provide medical care, including immunizations, necessary surgical procedures, or emergency interventions. Cases of alleged medical neglect because of a family's philosophical or religious beliefs may require resolution in court.

Physical: This type of neglect exists when caregivers either fail to protect the child from harm or do not provide for basic needs.

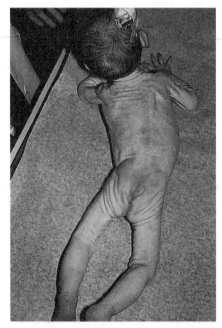

Figure 47-1. Psychological failure to thrive as a result of neglect. (From Newberry L: *Sheehy's emergency nursing: principles and practice*, ed 5, St. Louis, 2003, Mosby.)

Emotional: The caregiver fails to maintain a nurturing environment that will meet the emotional and developmental needs of the minor. This type of neglect is difficult to recognize and define.

Educational: Poor school attendance or failure to provide necessary specialized education constitutes educational neglect.

Mental health: Caregivers may fail to obtain necessary care for a child with emotional or behavioral problems.[5,13]

Physical abuse

Physical abuse, or nonaccidental trauma, is defined as injury intentionally inflicted on a child. This includes trauma that results from discipline, punishment, torture, maiming, or the use of unreasonable force.

Sexual abuse

Sexual abuse involves molestation or exploitation of a minor by an older child, adolescent, or adult. Abusive behaviors may be violent, coercive, or even nontouching (e.g., pornographic photography). (See Chapter 51.)

Emotional abuse

Unlike emotional neglect, in which the child's needs simply are not met, emotional abuse is deliberate. In reality, it may be difficult to draw a distinction between the two. Table 47-1 lists emotionally abusive strategies used by abusers and common responses to abuse. Box 47-1 describes factors that contribute to child maltreatment.

Duty to Report

The duty of health care providers to report actual or suspected child maltreatment exists in all 50 states. Local law enforcement or child welfare agencies must be notified of any suspicion of abuse or neglect. Persons who disclose suspected maltreatment in good faith are immune from prosecution. Be sure to document to whom this information was transmitted and the date and time the information was relayed. Importantly, the reporter is under no obligation to prove the allegation, only to describe it. Abuse laws vary from state to state; become familiar with regulations in your practice locale. Reporting procedures also vary by institution. Know how to access facility-specific protocols.

Table 47-1   Emotional Abuse

Abusive Action	*Children's Responses*
Verbal abuse	Withdrawal
Verbal threats	Eating disorders
Constant criticism	Head banging
Expectations that are outrageous	Rocking
Use of the child to manipulate other adults	Learning difficulties
Extreme behaviors (anger, passivity)	Enuresis
Lack of affection toward the child	Suicidal behavior
Use of the child as a bargaining tool between parents	Self-destructive or risk-taking behaviors

Box **47-1**	**Factors That Contribute to Child Maltreatment**

Sociological	Situational
Dangerous living environment	Alcohol or other drug abuse by the caretaker
Inadequate housing	Inadequate support systems
Poverty	Intimate partner abuse in the home
Social isolation	Many small children in the home
	Parental discord
Parent/Caretaker	
Unemployment	**Child**
A perception of the child as "different"	Child of a multiple birth
Attention-seeking behavior	Chronically ill
Belief in corporal punishment	Developmental delays
Female gender (62% of the time)[2]	Feeding difficulties
History of abuse as a child	Mental deficits
Inability to be nurturing	Physically disabled
Lack of self-control	Prenatal drug addiction
Low self-esteem	Preterm delivery
Physical or psychological illness	Psychosocial disabilities
Single parent	
Unmet emotional needs	
Unrealistic expectations of the child	

In general, the following information should be included in a maltreatment report:
- The child's name (and any other names the child may be using)
- The child's address and telephone number
- Where the child is living now (if this is different from the stated address)
- The child's birth date
- The name of the child's parents or other caretakers
- The reasons for your suspicions
- The alleged cause of injury or the nature of the neglect
- The circumstances surrounding the incident
- Where the alleged incident occurred
- A description of the child, including any injuries or other signs of maltreatment
- The extent of abuse or neglect
- The name or any description of the suspect(s)
- The suspect's address and telephone number
- Your name, work address, and work telephone number

Behavioral Signs of Child Maltreatment

Behavioral signs of child maltreatment include the following:
- The caregiver delays seeking treatment for illness or injury in the child.
- The caretaker is also a child.
- Evidence of caregiver ignorance or carelessness exists.
- Descriptions of events are confusing, conflicting, ever-changing, or improbable.
- The caregiver focuses on the child's behavior.
- The caregiver denies knowledge of how the injury occurred.
- A change in caregivers has occurred recently.

- The caregiver emphasizes unimportant details or minor problems not directly related to the present situation.
- The caregiver focuses on self-absorbed concerns rather than on the needs of the child.
- The caregiver bypassed a closer emergency department (ED) to seek treatment.
- Tension or outright hostility exists between caregivers.
- Caregivers exhibit tension, hostility, or aggressiveness toward ED staff members.
- The caregiver is uncooperative and demanding.
- The child has a history of multiple ED visits.
- Caregivers describe the child as clumsy or accident-prone.
- The child exhibits low self-esteem.
- The child displays attention-seeking behavior.
- The caregiver lacks any sense of guilt, remorse, or culpability for the incident ("If only I had …").
- The child appears fearful of adults or is unusually unafraid.
- The child is fearful of the caregiver.
- The caregiver displays anger toward the child regarding the injury or illness.
- Answers to questions are evasive.
- The caregiver refuses to leave a verbal child alone with health care providers.
- The child's age (chronological or developmental) does not correlate with the reported history of injury.

Physical Signs of Child Maltreatment

The list of physical manifestations suggestive of abuse or neglect is extensive. Table 47-2 describes many possible assessment findings. Figures 47-2 to 47-4 provide examples of retinal hemorrhage, cigarette burns, and pattern bruises related to abuse.

Munchausen Syndrome by Proxy

Munchausen syndrome by proxy is a psychiatric disorder occasionally seen in caregivers. This bizarre form of child abuse often is missed (or even unintentionally abetted) by health care providers. In Munchausen syndrome by proxy, an adult caregiver (almost always the mother) fabricates a child's illness or actually creates symptoms through a variety of mechanisms. Health care personnel too, particularly nurses, have been perpetrators of Munchausen syndrome by proxy. These individuals can operate in any setting in which the victim is vulnerable. After first causing or faking an illness, the clinician/perpetrator then can glory in the attention received from "saving" the child or the "kindness" bestowed on grieving parents.[15]

The traditional and most accepted explanation for Munchausen syndrome by proxy is the secondary gain (attention) received by the perpetrator. Attention is garnered from medical professionals, family members, and friends who laud the mother's care, devotion, and selflessness. Munchausen syndrome by proxy is a serious disorder than ends in the death of up to 10% of child victims. An additional 8% develop long-term medical problems.[16-18] Several rationales for Munchausen syndrome by proxy have been posited in the medical literature. The perpetrator may have the following characteristics:

- May believe that an ill child will bring about an improved relationship with her spouse (many of these children have distant, uninvolved fathers).
- May have had an emotionally deprived childhood and was physical abused herself.
- May injure her child to express anger and fear.
- May use the child's illness as a means of escaping the responsibilities and realities of life.
- May gain gratification and a sense of importance in the presence of medical professionals.[20]

Table 47-2   **Possible Manifestations of Physical Abuse and Neglect**

Area/Injury	Manifestations
Fractures	Ribs/scapulae/clavicular ends
	Fingers and femur in nonwalking children
	Fractures in various stages of healing
	Any fracture in a child less than 3 years of age
Head	Traumatic alopecia
	Uneven hair growth (various lengths in different spots)
	Subgaleal hematomas
	Head injuries
	Subdural hematomas
	Skull fractures
	Unexplained unconsciousness
	Unexplained cardiopulmonary arrest
Ear, eye, nose, throat	Displaced nasal cartilage
	Bleeding from the nasal septum
	Fractured mandible
	Lacerated frenulum
	Loose/missing teeth not appropriate for age
	Retinal hemorrhages
	Detached retina
	Hyphema
	Periorbital ecchymosis
	Ruptured tympanic membrane
	Postauricular hematoma (Battle sign)
	Petechiae around the head or neck (from choking)
Burns	Lips and tongue
	Rectum or perineum
	Cigarette burns
	Chemical burns
	Electrical burns
	Lines of demarcation, limited injury to protected areas, and uniform burn depth
	Burns in the shape of an object (e.g., iron, heating grate, and stove coils)
	Splash burns of nonuniform depth involving various body parts
Bruising, ecchymosis, lacerations	In various stages of healing
	In the shape of certain objects (e.g., handprint, extension cord, belt buckle)
	Human bite marks
Genitalia/perineal (See Chapter 51.)	Genital/perineal trauma
	Discharge: vaginal or rectal (may indicate sexually transmitted disease)
	Bleeding
	Pain
	Urinary tract infection symptoms
	Behavior associated with serious psychological or physical trauma
	Posttraumatic stress syndrome
	Attention deficit hyperactivity disorder
	Secondary enuresis or encopresis
	Nightmares
	Inappropriate sexual behavior
Poisoning	Ingestion of alcohol or other drugs
	"Morning-after" poisoning (ingestion of drinks left over from a party the night before)
	Intentional poisoning by a parent, caregiver, or other adult

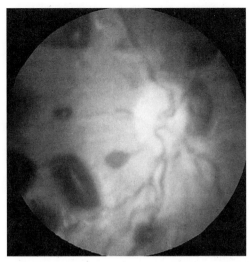

Figure 47-2. Retinal hemorrhages caused by shaken impact syndrome. (From Zitelli GJ, Davis HW: *Atlas of pediatric physical diagnosis,* ed 3, St Louis, 1997, Mosby. Courtesy Stephen Ludwig, Children's Hospital of Philadelphia.)

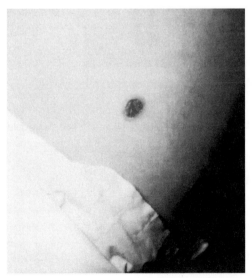

Figure 47-3. Cigarette burn. (From Zitelli GJ, Davis HW: *Atlas of pediatric physical diagnosis*, ed 3, St Louis, 1997, Mosby.)

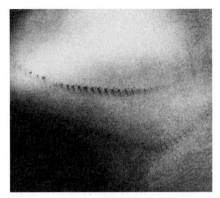

Figure 47-4. Child was struck with a chain, leaving a clear imprint of the links. (From Zitelli GJ, Davis HW: *Atlas of pediatric physical diagnosis,* ed 3, St Louis, 1997, Mosby.)

- May insist on being included in health care decision making, further reinforcing attention and support.[17]
- May develop a perverse relationship with clinicians that allows her to feel power over these important persons. The child's disease becomes a game in which the caregiver controls the script, provides clues, and manipulates health care professionals.[18]

Signs and symptoms

The caregiver may display any of the following signs and symptoms:
- Is extremely attentive and refuses to leave the child alone. She initially may appear to be the "perfect" mother.
- Demands an extensive workup and will not accept a minor diagnosis.
- Is unusually calm and is not as worried about the child as the staff is.
- Is knowledgeable about health care, uses medical terminology, and frequently has a health care background.
- Appears to enjoy the hospital environment, engaging in gossip with staff members and involving herself in the details of other patient's problems.
- Spends more time with the staff than with the child.
- Either highly supportive of medical personnel or is angry and devaluing, demanding more treatments and procedures.
- Is inordinately concerned about the personal and professional lives of staff members.
- Is emotionally distant from her spouse.
- May report a history of dramatic, negative events in her life.
- Brings the child to the ED frequently.
- Requires much adulation and may even seek public acknowledgment.
- Comes from a dysfunctional family setting.
- Works to form close relationships with staff and appears to have few other friends or support persons.
- May have a complex medical history.
- Is not concerned about subjecting the child to painful diagnostic tests or treatments.
- Is overly attached to the patient.
- Treats the child as if the child has a disability even when no true disability is present.

The child may have any of the following signs and symptoms:
- A medical course that is puzzling and unexplainable
- One or more medical problems unresponsive to therapy
- Seizures witnessed only by the caregiver and unresponsive to anticonvulsants
- Multiple "allergies"
- A general appearance that does not correspond with laboratory results
- Symptoms that manifest only in the presence of the caregiver
- A sibling with a similar illness or unexplained death
    Physical findings vary widely but tend to have the following characteristics:
- Unusual, bizarre
- Multisystem
- Prolonged
- Incongruent, inappropriate, and inconsistent with known pathophysiology
    Symptomatology associated with Munchausen syndrome by proxy involves many facets. The imagination of the perpetrator is the only limiting factor. Table 47-3 lists several common symptoms with possible causes.

Diagnostic aids

Making the diagnosis of Munchausen syndrome by proxy is always challenging. This disorder often is overlooked, but some argue that the label is applied too quickly whenever a caregiver is anxious, overly concerned, provides an inaccurate history, has unusual coping mechanisms, or knows more about a disease than the health care professionals.[19] Forensic Munchausen syndrome by proxy is a situation in which, as part of a divorce proceeding and custody battle, one parent falsely claims that the child has been sexually abused by the other. The child is forced to undergo physical examination and intensive interviewing as a result of these accusations.[20]

Approach to the Suspected Child Maltreatment Patient

The interview

In the patient with suspected maltreatment, the manner in which the initial ED interview is handled will set the tone for the rest of the evaluation process. The emergency nurse cannot possibly obtain the entire "story" in the triage area. Avoid excessive questioning at this time. Perpetrators who detect suspicion may flee with the child or become violent. Move suspected abuse patients into a treatment room as quickly as possible. The emergency nurse will find it much easier to calm and contain the victim and potential perpetrator in a patient room. Nonetheless, the triage nurse should document fully whatever the caregiver states to facilitate comparison of stories once a more thorough assessment and history have been obtained. The primary goals of therapeutic intervention in the ED are to identify and address the immediate needs of the child, prevent further harm, facilitate investigation of potential abuse, and assist the child and family to deal with the crisis.

    Methods of interviewing the child vary depending on the patient's developmental age. If possible, interview multiple caregivers separately and away from the child to check the consistency of the story.

    The following are tips for patient and family interviewing in a potential child maltreatment situation:
- Listen closely and watch interactions between the child and the caregiver.
- Evaluate the child's state of cleanliness, nutrition, and dress.

Table 47-3   Physical Findings in Patients With Munchausen Syndrome by Proxy

Symptoms	Possible Causes
Bleeding	Warfarin (Coumadin) poisoning
	Laxative abuse
	Bleeding exogenous to the child
	Use of colored substances
Poisoning	Phenothiazines
	Hydrocarbons
	Iron
	Salts
Central nervous system depression	Insulin
	Chloral hydrate
	Barbiturates
	Aspirin
	Diphenhydramine (Benadryl) or other antihistamines
	Tricyclic antidepressants
	Acetaminophen
	Hydrocarbons
	Diphenoxylate hydrochloride and atropine sulfate (Lomotil)
	Suffocation
Diarrhea/vomiting	Syrup of ipecac
	Laxatives
	Salt administration
	Lying (the symptom does not actually exist)
Rashes	Drug poisoning
	Scratching
	Caustics (e.g., oven cleaner)
	Skin painting
Seizures	Intoxication
	Suffocation
	Poisoning
	Carotid sinus pressure
	Lying (the symptom does not actually exist)
Infection	Needlesticks
	Intravenous line contamination
	Bladder catheterization
Apnea	Suffocation
	Poisoning
	Lying (the symptom does not actually exist)
Fever	Injection of contaminants into the blood (through an intravenous line)
	Falsifying temperatures on a chart

- Pay particular attention to patients with a history of multiple ED visits.
- Be nonjudgmental and nonaccusatory. Cooperation is more likely if discussions are held in a nonthreatening manner.
- Speak in easy-to-understand language.
- Be aware of cultural remedies and health care practices that can mimic abuse (e.g., cupping and coining; Box 47-2).
- Ask open-ended questions at first.
- Attempt to determine an event time line.

Box **47-2** Conditions That Mimic Child Maltreatment

Blood dyscrasias
Coagulation disorders
Coin rubbing
Complementary and alternative therapies that delay appropriate care or actually cause harm
Cultural/ethnic practices that produce physical marks
Cupping and moxibustion
Failure to thrive
Mongolian spots
Reye's syndrome
Scarring
Sudden infant death syndrome

- Establish whether similar situations have occurred in the past.
- Initially avoid questions that deal with the alleged assault.
- If possible, ask the child who the perpetrator is.
- If necessary, use role reversal to dialogue with the child.
- Inquire about other children within the family.
- Carefully document objective assessment findings and any statements made by the patient or caregivers.

The examination

Undressing the child completely for the examination is important in order to identify potential undisclosed injuries. Be sure to provide privacy and protect the child's modesty. Explain each part of the examination as you proceed. Physical assessment, diagnostic testing, and therapeutic interventions depend on the chief complaint, the child's general condition, and the type of abuse suspected. Consider each of the following components, as appropriate:

- Primary and secondary surveys
- Radiographic studies for patients with suspicious injuries (especially preverbal or nonverbal children)
- Laboratory studies: Complete blood count, glucose, serum chemistries, toxicologic screens, urinalysis, and pregnancy testing.
- Visual acuity testing, eye examination
- Neurologic examination
- Growth and developmental level (compare with normative charts)
- Inspection and palpation of the following:
  - Head
  - Chest
  - Abdomen
  - Pelvis (see Chapter 51)
  - Extremities
  - Back

Documentation

Documentation is an essential part of the medical-legal process in any case of suspected child maltreatment. Documentation by health care professionals is viewed as objective third-party evidence in legal proceedings. Unfortunately, these records are frequently incomplete, inaccurate, or illegibile.[21]

Tips for clinicians that will facilitate successful prosecution include the following:
- Write legibly.
- Place quotation marks around statements made by the victim or caregiver.
- Take and appropriately label instant camera photographs (date, time, child's name, medical record number, photographer's name). Obtain long-, medium-, and close-range shots, and place a color chart and ruler in the picture.
- Draw injuries on body maps to indicate their locations, size, and potential age.
- Put the words such as "patient states," "patient reports," "father states," "mother said" to identify who is being quoted.
- Use medical terms when charting. Avoid legal terms such as "alleged perpetrator" or "assailant."
- Objectively describe emotional and mental states, behaviors, and physical problems.
- Record dates and times accurately.
- Provide detailed descriptions of injuries.
- Document only facts.[27]

If any potential evidence is collected during the assessment process, strictly follow the institutional guidelines for evidence preservation and custody. Do not allow the chain of custody to be broken. (See Chapter 51.)

Prevention of Child Maltreatment

It is vital that health care professionals recognize and report instances of abuse and neglect to prevent future morbidity and mortality. Maltreatment that results in the death of a child is almost always preceded by prior instances of abuse. Early identification of at-risk children and appropriate referral is essential.[22] Many educational programs and informational materials are available that address parenting techniques, anger management, child abuse prevention, and intimate partner violence. Emergency departments can post information where it will be visible and make it and easily obtainable in waiting rooms and treatment areas.

ELDER/DEPENDENT ADULT ABUSE

Mistreatment Categories

In many ways, abuse of elders and dependent adults is similar to that of children. In addition to the types of maltreatment already listed, adults are subject to the following forms of abuse:
- Violation of personal rights
- Abandonment (for information on elder abandonment, see Chapter 44)
- Financial abuse

Financial abuse

Financial exploitation of an elder or dependent adult is difficult to determine. This practice can involve stealing money or other possessions. The older individual also may be coerced into signing a contract, changing a will, assigning durable power of attorney, and transferring assets to family members or caregivers. Financial abuse of elders is part of the marketing scheme of corporations that prey on those who simply do not understand things such as computer technology or complicated payment plans. Box 47-3 outlines risk factors for elder and dependent adult abuse.

Box **47-3**   **Risk Factors for Elder/Dependent Adult Abuse**

Exertion of power or control by a dominant spouse
Personal problems of the abuser or victim, such as alcoholism and drug abuse
Caregiver stress and burnout
Extensive care needs of persons with dementia, major physical deficits, or developmental limitations
Transmission of abuse from one generation to another
Caregiver inexperience
Financial distress
Caregiver mental illness
Lack of caregiver support systems
The sudden and unpredictable nature of the needs of elders/dependent individuals
Poor physical living conditions[5,23]

Signs and symptoms

Manifestations of elder and dependent adult abuse vary greatly and may include any of the following physical findings:
- Soft tissue trauma: bruises, welts, lacerations
- Sprains, dislocations, fractures
- Burns
- Untreated injuries and medical problems
- Sexually transmitted diseases, genital infections
- Vaginal or rectal bleeding
- Stained or bloody underwear
- Dehydration, malnutrition, decubitus ulcers
- Overdose, underdose
- Changes in mentation or personality
- Withdrawal, decreased communication
- Social isolation
- Lack of personal hygiene
- Signs of unsafe or unclean living conditions (e.g., lice, fleas, and soiled clothing)[5]

Reporting

Identifying and reporting abuse of elders and dependent adults is just as important as recognizing and intervening in cases of child abuse. Individuals who rely on others for their well-being deserve optimal care. Emergency nurses must be aware of state reporting laws and institutional policies and practices regarding elder and dependent adult abuse.

References

1. Kempe CH et al: The battered child syndrome, *JAMA* 181:17-24, 1962.
2. National Center for Victims of Crime: Statistics: child victimization. Retrieved August 27, 2003, from www.ncvc.org/STATS.
3. National Clearinghouse on Child Abuse and Neglect Information; Children's Bureau Administration on Children, Youth and Families: National Child Abuse and Neglect Data System (NCANDS) summary of findings from calendar year 2000. Retrieved August 27, 2003, from www.nlm.gov/medlineplus/childabuse.html.

4. National Center for Victims of Crime: 2001 crime clock. Retrieved August 27, 2003, from www.ncvc.org/vroom/crimeclock/.

5. Newberry L, editor: *Sheehy's emergency nursing: principles and practice,* ed 5, St Louis, 2003, Mosby.

6. US Department of Heatlh and Human Services, Administration for Children & Families, Children's Bureau: Child maltreatment 2000. Retrieved August 27, 2003, from www.acf.hhs.gov/programs/cb/publications/cm00/chapterone.htm.

7. The National Elder Abuse Incidence Study: Executive summary, October 31, 2002. Retrieved August 27, 2003, from www.aoa.gov/abuse/report/Cexecsum.htm.

8. Family violence and people with a mental handicap. Retrieved September 13, 2003, from www.phac-aspc.gc.ca/ncfv-cnivf/familyviolence/html/fvintecta.e.html.

9. Boo K: System loses lives and trust, *Washington Post* p A1, Dec 5, 1999. Retrieved September 13, 2003, from www.washingtonpost.com/wp-srv/local/invisible/deaths5.htm.

10. Mishra R: In attacks on disabled, few verdicts, *Boston Globe* June 10, 2001. Retrieved September 13, 2003, from www.boston.com/news/globe.

11. Feature issue on violence against women with developmental or other disabilities, *Impact* vol 13, No 3, Fall 2000, Institute on Community Integration and the Research and Training Center on Community Living, College of Education and Human Development, University of Minnesota. Retrieved September 13, 2003, from http://ici.umn.edu/products/impact/133/default.html.

12. Sobsey D: Faces of violence against women with developmental disabilities, *Impact* vol 13, No 3, Fall 2000, Institute on Community Integration and the Research and Training Center on Community Living, College of Education and Human Development, University of Minnesota. Retrieved September 13, 2003, from http://ici.umn.edu/products/impact/133/over2.html.

13. Stockman Reid K for Council for the Prevention of Child Abuse and Neglect: Child abuse and neglect, prevention strategies, and resources. Retrieved September 13, 2003, from www.capaa.wa.gov/childabuse.html.

14. Abuse, Health A to Z, Encyclopedia Index A. Retrieved September 13, 2003, from www.healthatoz.com/healthatoz/Atoz/ency/abuse.jsp.

15. Munchausen syndrome and Munchausen syndrome by proxy (MSBP). Retrieved May 16, 2002, from www.bullyonline.org/workbully/munchaus.htm.

16. University of Iowa Health Care, Physician Assistant Program: Munchausen's syndrome by proxy: prognosis and outcome. Retrieved May 16, 2002, from www.medicine.uiowa.edu/pa/sresrch/Huynh/Huynh.

17. Behrman R, Kleigman R, Jenson HB: *Nelson textbook of pediatrics,* ed 16, Philadelphia, 2000, WB Saunders.

18. Dowdell E, Foster K: Munchausen's syndrome by proxy: recognizing a form of child abuse, *Nursing Spectrum.* Retrieved May 16, 2002, from http://nsweb.nursingspectrum.com/ce/ce209.htm.

19. Mothers against Munchausen syndrome by proxy allegations. Retrieved May 16, 2002, from www.msbp.com.

20. Naegele T, Clark A: Forensic Munchausen syndrome by proxy: an emerging subspecies of child sexual abuse, *Forensic Examiner* pp 21-23, March/April 2001.

21. Isaac N, Pualani EV: Documenting domestic violence: how health care providers can help victims, Washington, DC, 2001, National Institute of Justice. Retrieved October 6, 2002, www.ncjrs.org/txt-files1/nij/188564.txt.

22. Emergency Nurses' Association: *Emergency nurse pediatric course provider manual,* ed 2, Des Plaines, Ill, 1998, The Association.

23. What are the major types of elder abuse? Retrieved October 6, 2002, www.elderabusecenter.org/basic/index.html.

48

Mental Health Emergencies

Jule Blakeley Monnens, RN, MSN

The emergency department (ED) is an important contact point for persons experiencing acute exacerbation of mental illness, problems of addiction, or other psychosocial crises. One in every five adults, or about 40 million Americans, experiences some type of mental disorder each year. Of these, 5% have serious illnesses such as schizophrenia, major depression, obsessive-compulsive disorder, or bipolar disease.[1,2] Emergency management of these individuals involves identifying the cause, intervening for acute distress, and referring the patient for ongoing therapy.

MENTAL HEALTH TRIAGE AND ASSESSMENT

The goal of mental health triage is to determine the severity of the presenting problem while protecting the patient, staff, and others. Mentally ill individuals commonly exhibit intense personal distress, suicidal ideation, and self-neglect that jeopardizes their health and safety. Those making threats or acting violently put others at risk as well.

Not all mental health emergencies result from psychotic conditions. Acute anxiety, panic attacks, severe depression, or substance abuse also can cause disordered or dangerous behavior. The Mini-Mental Status Examination is used to determine the patient's level of psychopathology. The Mini-Mental Status Examination is a brief, quantitative measure of cognitive status in adults (Box 48-1). The examination is used to screen for cognitive impairment, to estimate the severity of impairment, to follow the course of cognitive changes in an individual over time, and to document a patient's response to treatment.[3]

Evaluation of the patient with a mental health disturbance differs significantly from the typical triage history-taking process. Based on assessment of the following parameters, individuals are assigned a triage category (Table 48-1):

Box 48-1 Mini-Mental Status Examination Sample Questions

Orientation to time
"What is the date?"
Registration
"Listen carefully. I am going to say three words. You say them back after I stop.
Ready? Here they are ...
HOUSE (pause), CAR (pause), LAKE (pause). Now repeat those words back to me."
[Repeat up to 5 times, but score only the first trial.]
Naming
What is this?" [Point to a pencil or pen.]
Reading
"Please read this and do what it says." [Show examinee the words on the stimulus form.]
  CLOSE YOUR EYES

*Reproduced by special permission of the Publisher, Psychological Assessment Resources, Inc., 16204 North Florida
Avenue, Lutz, Florida 33549, from Mini-Mental State Examination, by Marshall Folstein and Susan Folstein,
Copyright 1975, 1998, 2001 by Mini Mental, LLC, Inc. Further reproduction is prohibited without permission
of PAR, Inc. The MMSE can be purchased from PAR, Inc., by calling (800) 331-8378 or (813) 968-3003.*

Table 48-1 Mental Health Triage Scale

Triage Code	Triage Category	Description	Typical Presentation
1	Emergent	Actively suicidal or homicidal Severe behavioral disturbance	Violent behavior Possession of a weapon Self-injurious behavior Extreme agitation Verbally aggressive Grave disability; greatly diminished self-care capacity Requires restraint Poor impulse control; fighting Drug/alcohol abuse with psychiatric symptoms
2	Urgent	Possible danger to self or others Moderate behavioral disturbance	Agitated; restless Intrusive behavior Confusion Withdrawn; uncommunicative Suicidal ideation without a plan Verbal or auditory hallucinations Delusions Paranoia Severe depression or anxiety Elevated or irritable mood
3	Semiurgent	Moderate distress	No agitation or restlessness Cooperative Gives a coherent history Suicidal ideation but is accompanied by a capable friend or family member No suicidal ideation Irritable without aggression
4	Nonurgent	No acute distress	Cooperative Communicative Compliant Known patient with chronic symptoms
5	Nonurgent	No distress	Medication request/refill

Modified from Broadbent M, Jarman H, Berk M: Improving compliance in mental health triage, *Accid Emerg Nurs* 10:
155-162, 2002.

Initial Assessment

The first step in assessment of patients with a mental health hold focuses on identifying those who require immediate care. Patients with any of these findings automatically are considered in need of emergent care:
- A prehospital mental health hold
- Suicidal ideation, suicidal gestures
- Homicidal ideation
- Grave disability or a greatly diminished self-care capacity
- Self-injurious or self-mutilating behaviors
- Poor impulse control or violence
- Bizarre and unexplained behavior
- Drug and alcohol use associated with psychiatric symptoms

Secondary Assessment

The second part of mental health triage consists of assessments for appearance and general body movements, ability to participate in an interview, speech, mood and affect, cognition and thought control, and insight and judgment.

Appearance and general body movements

Does the patient exhibit any of the following?
- Unkempt, unclean
- Slumped, tense, rigid
- Provocative, threatening
- Inappropriately dressed (e.g., shorts in the winter)

Ability to participate in an interview

Assess the patient for the following:
- Level of consciousness
- Orientation to person, place, and time
- Level of distraction
- Ability to cooperate vs. resistance
- Degree of guardedness or suspicion
- Level of agitation or hostility

Speech (rate, tone, fluency)

Is the patient's speech characterized by any of the following?
- Slurred, stammering
- Increased, loud
- Decreased, soft
- Pressured

Mood and affect

Is the patient's mood or affect characterized by any of the following?
- Depressed
- Euphoric
- Manic
- Labile

- Anxious
- Hostile

Cognition and thought control

Evaluate whether the patient has the following characteristics:
- Intellectual impairment
- Disorganized thinking
- Flight of ideas
- Loosening of associations
- Tangential thinking
- Thought blocking
- Delusions
- Disorientation
- Hallucinations

Insight and judgment

Does the patient have any of the following?
- An understanding of the problem and the need for help or treatment (insight)
- The ability to make sound decisions (judgment)

GENERAL MANAGEMENT TECHNIQUES

Quickly identify the general nature and severity of the presenting problem. Often the emergency nurse must rely on the patient's family or friends for this information. The emergency nurse should ask certain key questions, including the following:
- Why is this person coming for help *now?*
- Is the patient a danger to himself or herself or others?
- What were the events that led up to this condition?
- Was there some event or thing that triggered it?
- Who brought the patient in?
- What does the patient expect from this visit?
- What medications is the patient taking? Not taking?
  During the patient interview, do the following:
- Set firm limits, if necessary.
- Appear calm and nonjudgmental.
- Encourage the patient to remain as focused as possible.
- Be sure that help is nearby should the patient become physically dangerous.
- *Do not allow the patient to come between you and the door.*
- Try to decrease the patient's anxiety level.
- Do not argue with patients or try to talk them out of how they are feeling.
- Provide clear explanations to the patient.
- Be honest about the therapeutic plan.

General Approach to the Mentally Disturbed Patient

Individuals with psychiatric emergencies may lack self-control and be out of contact with reality. The primary concern of emergency care providers is not to specify a cause or label the presenting syndrome but rather to evaluate the degree of dysfunction and the extent of loss of contact with reality. Treatment involves immediate therapy to alleviate acute distress and help patients reestablish a sense of self-control. Once this is achieved, referral can be made for more extensive care.

When dealing with mentally ill patients, do the following:
- Attempt to establish good rapport.
- Use eye contact.
- Appear relaxed.
- Let the patient know that you care about the patient as a person.
- Listen well, but gently redirect the conversation when necessary to keep the interview focused.
- Establish the chief complaint.
  - What is the patient asking for?
  - Why is the patient asking for it at this time?
  - What precipitated this visit?
  - What has precipitated similar visits in the past?
  - What has helped in past episodes?
- Speak clearly and without using jargon.
- Recognize patient regression. Encourage independence and participation in decision making whenever possible.
- Be honest.
- Expect safe behavior and state this clearly.
- Anticipate the emotional component (such as anger, crying, or grief).
- Explain procedures to the patient.
- Take the patient seriously.
- Validate the individual's feelings.
- Do not hestitate to ask for help if you do not feel safe.
- Do not be afraid to admit to ignorance.
- Include the family or patient's significant others whenever possible.

NONPSYCHOTIC SITUATIONS

Anxiety

Anxiety is a diffuse response that alerts an individual to an impending threat, real or imagined. Fear, however, is a natural psychological and physiologic reaction to an actual threat. Fear is object-focused, whereas anxiety involves a faceless threat; no identifiable object can be isolated. About 19.1 million Americans (13.3% of the population) suffer from an anxiety disorder.[1] Panic disorder and obsessive-compulsive disorder fall into this category.

Panic disorder

Panic disorder affects 1% to 2% of the population; onset is usually before the age of 24. Women are twice as likely to be affected as men, and only 25% will seek any kind of psychiatric help.[5] Panic attack symptoms are so intensely physical that it simply does not occur to sufferers that the attack is the result of a neurochemical imbalance. Panic attacks begin without any warning, during activities that are routine and nonthreatening. Out of the blue a person will be seized by intense fear, palpitations, chest pain, shortness of breath, and dizziness. Individuals are overwhelmed by the certainty that they are going to die, go insane, or lose complete control. An attack typically peaks in less than 10 minutes and dissipates within half an hour.

Obsessive-compulsive disorder

Obsessive-compulsive disorder (OCD) is America's hidden mental health epidemic. One person in 40 will develop OCD in his or her lifetime, one third of these before age 15. More than

400,000 children have OCD. Morever, many patients with OCD have comorbidities: 66% suffer from major depression, and 26% experience anxiety attacks. Diagnostic criteria for OCD generally involve obsessions and compulsions. Obsessions are recurrent thoughts, images, and impulses that invade the mind, causing intolerable anxiety. These preoccupations make no sense, are repulsive, or revolve around themes of violence and harm.

Compulsions are devised to relieve the unbearable anxiety and doubt generated by an obsession. The patient will be driven to perform specific repetitive, ritualized behaviors calculated to reduce discomfort temporarily. These behaviors can take on a life of their own, literally imprisoning the individual in a pattern of peculiar activities. Common compulsions include hand washing, showering, or house cleaning; excessive ordering and arranging; incessant checking and rechecking; repetitive counting, touching, and activity rituals; excessive slowness in daily activities such as eating and tooth brushing; and constant demands for reassurance that the perceived threat has been removed. Persons with OCD are not delusional and are not having hallucinations, but they simply cannot control the compulsive responses to their anxiety.[5]

Acute Anxiety Attack

An acute anxiety attack typically lasts from a few minutes to several hours. The individual does not lose contact with reality, but judgment and insight are impaired. Patient management focuses on preventing future attacks by teaching self-management strategies.

Signs and symptoms

- Hyperactivity
- Dry mouth
- Fidgety movements of the hands, tremors
- Precordial discomfort (sense of pressure in the chest)
- Choking sensation
- Dysphagia (difficulty swallowing)
- Feelings of impending danger, dying, or going crazy
- Literal attempts to escape
- Hyperventilation: breathlessness, paresthesias, and acute restlessness
- Tachycardia, tachypnea
- Profuse sweating, sweaty palms
- Urinary frequency

Levels of anxiety

Mild: Mild anxiety is usually a productive state. Patients can benefit from information-sharing about the condition.

Moderate: Moderate anxiety may be productive but expends more energy than is necessary. Patients need a directive-supportive relationship.

Serious: Serious anxiety is usually nonproductive and even counterproductive; the caregiver must take control of the situation. Give direct commands in short, simple sentences, and focus on intellectual functioning.

Severe: Severe anxiety is crippling to witness and experience and rapidly becomes contagious. Isolate the individual from others (use physical restraints if needed). Do not leave the patient alone. Be supportive but firm.

Terror: Terror is a do-or-die situation; assume total responsibility for the patient.

Therapeutic interventions

The goal of emergency care for persons with acute anxiety is to promote an environment in which the individual can achieve an adequate degree of self-control.

To decrease feelings of anxiety, do the following:

- Provide general support.
- Identify and treat hyperventilation syndrome. Encourage slow, regular breathing.
- Keep calm and appear calm.
- Encourage the patient to talk.
- Direct the patient toward reality.
- Assist the patient with priority setting.
- Help the patient identify the anxiety source.
- Let the patient have some control over the situation.
- Avoid false or excessive reassurance; give supportive attention during the attack.
- Consider the use of antianxiety medications such as lorazepam (Ativan).
- After a thorough examination, if no physical cause is found, emphasize the importance of seeking mental health treatment on a nonemergency basis to work on the underlying source of anxiety.
- Use consultants and make referrals as necessary.

Acute Grief

Grief is the expected response to a significant loss, such as the loss of a loved one, one's health, a job, a way of life, or a major financial loss. Acute grief reactions are frequently seen in the ED following a patient's death. The grieving process is influenced by a one's cultural background, personality style, history of losses, and individual factors. Emergency nurses must anticipate psychological and physiologic grief reactions and be prepared to provide physical and emotional support to patients and family members.

Signs and symptoms

- Shock, disbelief, denial
- Emotional lability with overt tears, moaning, or wailing
- Diminished and slowed speech
- Inability to concentrate
- Anger, sadness, guilt
- Focus on the "lost object"
- Feelings of helplessness
- Anorexia or changes in appetite and weight
- Sleep disturbances

Therapeutic interventions

- Accept that the individual's response is normal and provide supportive dialogue.
- Encourage expression of feelings, especially sadness and loss.
- Provide privacy in a room with normal lighting but decreased environmental stimuli.
- Stress the importance of proper nutrition and fluid intake, even if the desire to eat is diminished.
- Encourage the individual to seek out a close friend, family member, or bereavement group to discuss feelings of grief.

Depression

Patients with depressive disorders are commonly encountered in emergency care settings. These conditions have a high prevalence in the general population and result in significant morbidity and mortality. About 18.8 million adults in the United States (9.5% of the population) suffer from clinical depression.[1] Normal sadness, grief, and emotional responses to life's difficulties must be distinguished from a depressive disorder. A sad or depressed mood is only one of the indicators of clinical depression.

Signs and symptoms

- Feelings of worthlessness, loneliness, helplessness, sadness
- Diminished interest in usual activities
- Guilt
- Physical fatigue, especially in the morning
- Psychomotor retardation or agitation
- Sleep disturbances
- Indecisiveness
- Weight change, loss of appetite
- Reduced facial animation
- Hand wringing
- Suicidal ideation
- Decreased libido
- Constipation
- Pacing, easy fatigability
- Psychotic symptoms (only in the most severe forms of depression)

Therapeutic interventions

- Do not isolate the patient.
- Provide safety and psychological security.
- Avoid excessive environmental stimuli or forced decision-making.
- Encourage the expression of feelings, especially underlying anger.
- Help the patient express grief over losses; point out that this is normal.
- Explore sources of emotional support.
- Involve family members and the patient's social network for continued support.
- Assess the risk for suicide.
- Refer the patient for psychiatric evaluation to include psychotherapy and medications, if indicated.

Suicide

Suicide took the lives of 29,350 Americans in 2000; an average of 1 person every 18 minutes. Overall, suicide is the eleventh leading cause of death in the United States and the third leading cause of death for those aged 15 to 24.[6]

Assessment of suicide potential

Gender

- Females attempt suicide 3 times more often than do males.
- Men are 4 times more successful at suicide than are women.

- Seventy-three percent of all suicide deaths involve white men.
- Females tend to prefer drug overdoses; males use firearms.

Age

- The potential for suicide increases with age, and the incidence is highest in white men over 65.
- Younger persons attempt suicide more often, but older individuals are more likely to be successful on their first attempt.

Race/Ethnic Groups/Minorities

- The suicide rate among foreign-born persons in the United States is greater than among natives.
- Homosexuals have a higher incidence of suicide than heterosexuals.
- Muslims have the lowest suicide rate of any major religious group in the United States. They are followed (in order) by Catholics, Jews, and Protestants.

Marital Status

- Persons who are married have the lowest suicide rate.
- Single persons kill themselves twice as often as do married persons.
- The suicide risk is high among widowed or divorced individuals.

Family History

- The risk of suicide is increased in persons with a family history of suicide attempts.
- The probability of success is high if the patient has a history of suicide attempts. Forty percent to 80% of those who die have made previous attempts.

Seasonal

- The incidence of suicide is highest in the spring and fall.
- More suicides occur on Wednesdays and Saturdays; the fewest on Sundays.

Other

- Substance abuse (alcohol, drugs) greatly increases suicide risk.
- The risk is more serious if the patient has a weapon or a well–thought out plan.
- Do *not* be afraid to ask directly if the patient is planning suicide.
- Mental illness increases the incidence of suicidal behavior.
- Debilitating physical illness increases suicide risk.
- History of serious emotional loss increases suicide risk, particularly on the anniversary of the loss.

Signs and symptoms

- Feelings of worthlessness, hopelessness, helplessness, confusion
- Restlessness, agitation, irritability
- Gastrointestinal complaints
- Indifference, fatigue, insomnia
- Decreased physical activity
- Actual suicide attempt that was unsuccessful

Approach to the suicidal patient

The goal of emergency care for suicidal patients is to provide a psychologically and physically protective environment and establish empathetic rapport. All patients presenting with suicidal ideation or a suicide attempt are considered to require emergent care and should be placed immediately in an examination room. Institute one-on-one observation, and document interventions using suicide precaution and intensive monitoring forms. Care of the patient who presents after overdose, wrist slashing, hanging, or other type of suicide attempt is focused initially on managing the immediate medical crisis. Once life-threatening issues have been addressed, direct care toward the mental health of the patient.

Problem solving

Suicidal thoughts are attempts by the patient to solve problems. Try to establish what it is the patient considers a problem. Problems commonly involve the following:

- Work
- Finances
- Family
- Interpersonal issues
- Illness (mental and physical)
- Substance abuse
- Unrelenting physical pain

Therapeutic interventions

- Chronic illness with little hope of improvement
- Evaluate the problem with the patient
- Help the patient look for alternatives.
- If the patient is unsure of possible alternatives or has no alternatives, hospitalization is mandatory.
- If there are alternatives, be specific about them.
- Try to involve family or friends in decision making and planning.
- When in doubt, obtain psychiatric consultation. If this is not possible, admit the patient to the hospital for observation.
- Sedation may be required.

Posttraumatic Stress Disorder

Posttraumatic stress disorder is a reaction to a witnessed or experienced catastrophic event, such as war, rape, or injury. Patients with posttraumatic stress disorder suffer from emotional, physical, behavioral, or psychological impairment.

Signs and symptoms

- Guilt, blame, self-punishment
- Flashbacks of the event
- Dissociation
- Depersonalization
- Psychogenic amnesia
- Psychogenic fugue (an altered state of consciousness in which the patient appears to perform acts in full awareness but upon recovery cannot recollect the deeds)
- Difficulty concentrating and problem solving
- Emotional lability
- Sleep disturbances
- Sexual dysfunction
- Suicidal ideations

- Substance abuse
- Impaired relationships (involving issues of mistrust, betrayal, or rejection)

Therapeutic interventions

- Remain calm and relaxed.
- Assess the risk for suicide.
- Evaluate the potential for violence.
- Identify the traumatic event.
- Help the patient identify and use a support system.
- Administer antidepressants and anxiolytics as indicated.
- Facilitate consultations and referral.

PSYCHOTIC SITUATIONS

Acute Psychotic Reactions

Acute psychosis is an emergency requiring rapid, accurate assessment and diagnosis. This condition must be differentiated quickly from psychosis resulting from organic causes such as dementia, delirium, brain tumor, or substance abuse. Individuals with medical reasons for their disorders are treated differently than the person suffering an acute schizophrenic episode. Psychosis is a bizarre state of profoundly altered thinking and behavior involving deterioration of thought processes, affective responses, and one's ability to maintain connection with reality. Deterioration continues to a point where the patient can no longer communicate with or relate to others.

Signs and symptoms

- Delusions
- Hallucinations
- Disorganized speech
- Grossly disorganized behavior

Therapeutic interventions

- Place the patient in a quiet, sparsely decorated room.
- Extremely violent (or potentially violent) patients require restraints or a locked room.
- Remove all of the patient's clothing. Check for concealed weapons.[7,8]
- Administer antipsychotics as indicated.

The Violent Patient

The acutely psychotic patient may present a hazard to self or others, especially when agitated. An immediate safety assessment must be conducted to determine whether this is an issue. *Threats of violence should always be taken seriously.* Box 48-2 lists patient factors that increase the risk for violent behavior.

Consider the following when evaluating a patient's safety risk:
- Is the patient directable?
- Is the patient agitated or irritable?
- Is the patient's posture threatening?

- Is the patient's behavior out of control?
- Is the patient verbally aggressive or abusive?

Patient factors that increase the risk for violent behavior are as follows:

Psychological

- Anxiety or fear for personal safety
- Feelings of being overwhelmed or unable to cope
- A history of physical or sexual abuse

Organic

- Alcohol or drug intoxication
- Medication side effects (sedation, akinesias (an inability to initiate movement), disequilibrium)
- Inadequate symptom control
- Delirium

Psychotic

- Delusional beliefs of persecution
- "Command" hallucinations to hurt others ("the voices in my head")
- Depression and acute suicidal intent

Therapeutic interventions

Threats of violence must be taken seriously. Care of the violent or potentially violent patient includes the following:

- Obtain unobstructed access to the patient. Clear away movable furniture and potential weapons. Ask bystanders to leave quietly.
- Do not hurry the patient. Most psychotic individuals can be "talked down" if given time. Engaging the patient in conversation and allowing verbalization of complaints may be all that is required.
- Speak calmly. Many psychotics are frightened of being out of control. Reassure patients you will help them regain self-control. Be clear, direct, nonthreatening and honest. Avoid confrontation.
- Stand sideways to the patient; this is less threatening and presents a smaller target. Keep your hands visible so that it is obvious you are not concealing a weapon.
- Do not try to cope with a violent patient alone. Obtain help as quickly as possible.

Schizophrenia

Schizophrenia is a devastating brain disease that always involves a psychotic episode in the acute stage. This common neurobiologic disorder affects 1 out of every 100 persons; onset is typically in the young adult years. The word *schizophrenia* means "to split the mind," a phrase that aptly describes the complete rupture between reality and psychotic though processes.[5]

Signs and symptoms

- Delusions
- Auditory hallucinations
- Difficulty making associations
- Disordered thoughts with a clear sensorium

- Combative or assaultive behavior
- Withdrawn or catatonic behavior
- Bizarre gesturing

Therapeutic interventions

Establish whether this is an initial event or a repeat episode. Has there been a history of psychiatric hospitalizations? Is the patient currently taking any antipsychotic medications? If medications were used in the past, was medication forcibly or voluntarily stopped or was the patient directed to stop?

- Use simple, concrete expressions and brief sentences.
- Avoid figures of speech that are subject to misinterpretation.
- Project a confident (but nonthreatening) manner to reassure the patient of your ability to control yourself and the environment.
- Listen as the patient talks of delusions to gain clues regarding thought distortions.
- If the patient is paranoid, avoid closed doors or blocked doorways; allow the patient to feel "uncornered."
- If antipsychotics are given, observe for postural hypotension and dystonic side effects.
- Consider hospital admission.

Paranoia

Paranoia is a symptom of schizophrenia and several other conditions. A paranoid person demonstrates loss of reality through a delusional thought system, generally involving persecution or excessive religious sentiments. Paranoid patients can be dangerous because of their belief that specific persons or unnamed forces are "out to get me."

Signs and symptoms

- Projective delusions
- Feelings of uniqueness going toward grandiosity
- Auditory hallucinations
- Difficulty with association
- Illogical thought processes
- Obsessive thinking
- Restlessness, agitation
- Combative or assaultive behavior

Therapeutic interventions

- Avoid psychological and physical threats or challenges.
- Establish limits.
- Use simple, concrete expressions.
- Remain calm and authoritative.
- Move slowly and quietly to avoid appearing intrusive.
- Sit or stand on the same level as the patient to avoid a "power" discrepancy.
- Allow the patient to be close to the slightly open door.
- Encourage patients to verbalize distorted or illogical thinking.
- Intended victims must be notified if the patient threatens violence or aggression against a particular person or group.
- Avoid trying to convince the patient that the delusions are erroneous, but do not validate false beliefs.

Hypomania/Manic Psychosis

Bipolar disorder occurs in 1.2% of the population, a rate slightly higher than that of schizophrenia. *Bipolar I* is characterized by at least one period of acute mania, usually accompanied by a minimum of one severe depressive event. Episodes follow a characteristic pattern for each person, and certain individuals tend more toward mania and others toward depression. Attacks of pure mania, distinct from depressive episodes, are much less common than the diagnosis of *Bipolar I, mixed.* In a mixed disorder, patients display symptoms of mania and depression simultaneously. Most exhibit a hyped-up depression, with feelings of sadness, irritability, agitation, and anxiety that may involve psychotic features and suicidal thinking. *Bipolar II* is characterized by recurrent severe depressive episodes that swing into hypomania.[5]

The prognosis in bipolar disease and depression is not good. For many, this is a lifelong chronic illness. More than half of all individuals with these disorders will have some functional disability that persists throughout their life. As a rule, the more episodes a person has, the more likely they are to experience future episodes. Patients with bipolar disorders have the highest completed suicide rates of any psychiatric diagnostic subgroup.

Ten percent to 25% of those with unipolar and bipolar depression become psychotic. This is the most serious form of depression, involving extreme suicidality and catatonia.[5]

Medication levels should be measured immediately in patients taking lithium, carbamazepine (Tegretol), or divalproex sodium (Depakote).

Signs and symptoms

- Elation or increased mental excitement that is unstable
- Irritability, irrational anger
- Pressured speech (it is difficult to interrupt the patient because speech is so rapid)
- Increased motor activity (restless, increased energy)
- Decreased need for sleep
- Demanding or euphoric manner
- Grandiose ideas
- Loud voice
- Sexual acting out or preoccupation with sex
- Bright-colored clothing, bright-colored (overdone) makeup

Therapeutic interventions

- Assume an authoritative, nonthreatening manner.
- Guard the patient, caregivers, and environment against physical harm.
- Decrease environmental stimulation.
- Provide an unencumbered, safe, and private room to allow pacing or ritualistic motor activity.
- Do *not* encourage the patient to talk; ask succinct questions.
- Respond in an unhurried, simple, speech pattern.
- Avoid mechanical restraints if possible.

HOMICIDAL AND ASSAULTIVE BEHAVIOR

Homicidal and assaultive behavior can be found in individuals who are acutely intoxicated, paranoid, manic, or sociopathic. Extreme caution must be used to protect oneself and others in the environment.

Therapeutic Interventions

- Approach the individual with an obvious show of force (a group of persons).
- Confiscate all real or potentially harmful objects.
- Apply physical restraints to establish psychological and physical control on behalf of the patient.
- Designate one person to act in a calm, authoritative, unhurried manner as the patient liaison.
- Speak in simple, direct sentences.
- Separate the individual from the family and any intended victims. If the target victim is not present, emergency personnel are responsible for ensuring that this person is warned of the patient's ideations.
- Observe for suicidal and homicidal attempts; suicide may follow a homicidal attempt because of impaired judgment.

MEDICAL OR NEUROLOGIC PSYCHIATRIC SYMPTOMS

When a patient comes an ED with what appears to be a psychiatric disorder, it is important to identify possible medical (organic) causes. Medical conditions capable of inducing psychosis include cerebral tumors, head injuries, epilepsy, migraine headaches, infections, endocrine and metabolic disorders, and hepatic or renal disease. A thorough medical and neurologic workup, including laboratory and radiographic studies, often is indicated. In addition, inclusion of the mini-mental status examination described previously is crucial (see Box 48-1). Unless the patient has a known history of psychiatric illness with psychosis, an organic cause should always be strongly considered. A key assessment finding in patients with organic disorders is the appearance of behavioral symptoms that are completely out of character or fluctuating. Dementia and delirium are two neurologic conditions frequently encountered in the ED that can mimic psychosis. These disorders may be seen separately or together.

Dementia

Behavioral and psychiatric disturbances are a common reason for the caregivers of patients with dementia to seek emergency treatment. Dementia involves a diffuse disruption and impairment of the functional capacity of the brain caused by a variety of pathologic conditions such as Alzheimer's disease, brain tumors, or vascular disorders. The deficits of dementia are generally chronic and irreversible. Neurologic consultation is necessary for patients with new or recent symptom onset.[9] Findings in the dementia patient include the gradual development of multiple cognitive deficits and at least one of the following symptoms:

- *Aphasia:* A defect or loss of the ability to speak or write; loss of the ability to understand spoken or written words
- *Apraxia:* An inability to execute a skilled or learned motor act (not related to paralysis or lack of comprehension) caused by a cortical lesion
- *Agnosia:* Loss of the ability to recognize objects, persons, sounds, shapes, or smells

Signs and symptoms

- Decreased orientation
- Decreased memory
- Decreased judgment

- Decreased ability to calculate, figure, plan, and organize
- Shallow affect

Acute Delirium

Unlike dementia, delirium is an acute, potentially reversible state of confusion with a rapid onset. Delirium is a frequent complication of acute medical conditions that often goes unrecognized and misdiagnosed, especially in older adults. Symptoms are generally worse at night, a state referred to as sundowning. Rapid diagnosis is critical because 15% to 30% of delirious individuals will die. Identification of the patient's baseline mental status is essential. Comprehensive physical and psychosocial assessments are also a requisite part of patient evaluation.[9]

Causes

- Biochemical disturbances: Electrolyte imbalance, hypoglycemia, uremia, porphyria, hepatitis
- Polypharmacy (more than three drugs) or recent changes in medication use
- Impaired nutritional status
- Bladder catheterization (associated with urosepsis)
- Systemic infection
- Cerebral hypoxia
- Drug withdrawal
- Hypothermia
- Head injury
- Metastatic neoplasms
- Heavy metal toxicity

Signs and symptoms

- Delusions, hallucinations, illusions
- Disorientation
- Frightening dreams
- The patient is highly distractible
- Fluctuating levels of consciousness (hyperactive and hypoactive states)
- Outbursts of rage, emotional lability
- Difficulty with retention and recall
- Hyperventilation, tachycardia
- Tremors, incoordination, restlessness
- Urinary incontinence

Therapeutic interventions

- Identify and treat any toxic exposures (see Chapter 28).
- Orient the patient to reality with simple, repetitive statements.
- Reduce environmental stimuli.
- Keep some light on at night and in windowless rooms.
- Ensure the patient's basic care needs are met.
- Ask a responsible person to stay with the patient.
- Avoid physical restraints, which only serve to increase confusion, disorientation, and general agitation.

Pediatric Psychiatric Emergencies

In the United States there are about 13.5 million children and adolescents (20% of all 9- to 17-year-olds) who have been diagnosed with mental illness; 5% are impaired to the extent that their ability to function socially, academically, or emotionally is severely disrupted. The prevalence of pediatric psychiatric problems is rising. Currently, four of the leading causes of disability for persons age 5 and older are mental disorders. The World Health Organization estimates that by 2020 neurobiologic diseases will be among the five most common causes of childhood morbidity.[1]

Suicidal ideation, feeling out of control, aggression, and drug-related antisocial behavior are the most common presenting problems for children with behavioral emergencies. The young psychiatric patient presents additional challenges for emergency nurses because of the following:

- The impulsiveness associated with the patient's age
- Involvement of other systems such as the family, school, courts, and social services
- A limited availability of inpatient care beds

The emergency nurse must identify who the child's legal guardian is before initiating treatment or determining disposition. Whether the child has been brought to the ED because of aggressive behavior or not, always ask about a history of violence. Inform the patient that aggressive behavior will not be tolerated; setting limits is essential. If the minor is unable to cooperate, use security personnel, a seclusion room, physical restraints, or sedation to protect the child and others. Provide support for the parents or caregivers who also may become extremely emotional.[10]

DRUG-RELATED PSYCHIATRIC EMERGENCIES

The function of emergency personnel in an acute, drug-induced crisis involves rapid intervention, critical observation, and supportive therapeutic communication. Clinical findings are as diverse as the substances to which a patient may be exposed.

Signs and Symptoms

Signs and symptoms of a drug-induced psychiatric crisis include the following:

- *Central nervous system:* Depression, tremors, confusion, decreased level of consciousness, agitation, seizures, coma
- *Respiratory:* Tachypnea, hyperpnea, hyperventilation, hypoventilation, apnea
- *Autonomic nervous system:* Increased or decrease temperature, pulse, and blood pressure
- *Pupil size:* increased or decreased
- *Behavioral/psychiatric:* Mood distortion, altered thought patterns, hallucinations, aggression
- *Gastrointestinal:* Anorexia, nausea, vomiting, diarrhea, bleeding, hepatic failure

Questions to Ask

The emergency nurse should ask the following questions of or about a patient experiencing a drug-induced psychiatric crisis:

- To what type of substance was the patient exposed?
- When? How much?
- What has happened (symptoms, interventions) since the drug was taken?

- Was there only one substance involved?
- Has the patient consumed alcohol?
- What is the patient's drug use history?
- Is this part of a chronic pattern of abuse or an isolated incident?
- How did the exposure occur (Orally or parenterally? By inhalation or absorption?)
- Where was the substance obtained (Over-the-counter? Prescription? Street drug?)

For information regarding specific drug and toxin-related emergencies, see Chapters 27, 28, and 49.

ADVERSE REACTIONS TO ANTIPSYCHOTIC DRUGS

Antipsychotic Dystonic Reactions

Occasionally, the drug of choice for treatment of a psychiatric condition produces more stress than relief for the patient. One such example is the severe extrapyramidal symptoms of some major tranquilizers (also referred to as EPS, dystonic, or phenothiazine reactions). Drugs that commonly produce these side effects include prochlorperazine (Compazine), trifluoperazine (Stelazine), chlorpromazine (Thorazine), fluphenazine (Prolixin), and most other common antipsychotic medications. Patients given haloperidol (Haldol) or droperidol (Inapsine) in the ED require careful monitoring for the development of extrapyramidal symptoms. Ziprasidone (Geodon), a relatively new neuroleptic agent, is associated with a much lower incidence of extrapyramidal symptoms.

Signs and symptoms

Physical examination findings may include any of the following:
- Dystonia (disordered tonicity of the muscles)
  - Oculogyric crisis (deviation of the eyes in all directions)
  - Blepharospasm (spasm of the eyelid muscles causing forced eyelid closure)
  - Buccolingual crisis (spasm of the face, jaw, and pharynx muscles producing trismus, tongue protrusion, grimacing, and difficulty speaking)
  - Opisthotonos (spasm of the paravertebral muscles forcing the trunk and neck into hyperextension)
  - Torticollis (spasm of the neck muscles with twisting of the neck to one side)
  - Tortipelvic crisis (forced spasm of the trunk and pelvic muscles causing bizarre body postures)
- Akathisia (an urge to move about constantly and an inability to sit still)
- Unaffected mental status
- Vital signs that are usually normal

When a patient arrives at the ED with any of these signs and symptoms, be sure to ask about a medication history. Extrapyramidal side effects commonly are mistaken for hypocalcemia, tetany, or seizures.[11] Akathisia often is misdiagnosed as psychotic agitation, and the patient is treated with a neuroleptic medication, which only worsens the condition.

Parkinsonism usually develops within 20 days of starting drug therapy. Symptoms include muscular rigidity, resting tremors, a masklike face, and drooling. Dystonic reactions are more likely to occur during the initial phase of psychotropic drug therapy (within 1 hour to 5 days). The appearance of extrapyramidal symptoms can be anxiety provoking and may be enough to convince patients to refuse all further prescribed medications. Emergency personnel can help these individuals understand that antipsychotic drug therapy requires patience and persistence to achieve a satisfactory response.

Therapeutic interventions

- Inform the patient that untoward symptoms are usually completely reversible, will rapidly disappear with proper medication, and generally resolve spontaneously even without treatment.
- In most instances, symptom reversal is achieved quickly by the administration of diphenhydramine (Benadryl) or an antiparkinsonian drug such as benztropine mesylate (Cogentin) or trihexyphenidyl (Artane).
- Propranolol (Inderal) is used to treat akathisias.
- Provide a quiet, darkened room where the patient can lie down until the antagonist drug takes effect.
- Have a nonthreatening person stay with the patient until the symptoms have subsided (generally within 1 hour of drug administration).

Neuroleptic Malignant Syndrome

Neuroleptic malignant syndrome is a life-threatening form of delirium and hyperthermia produced by the use of an antipsychotic agent. This condition requires immediate medical management. Neuroleptic malignant syndrome onset can occur within days or months of initiating neuroleptic therapy. The incidence is highest in the summer, and symptoms usually resolve in 1 to 2 weeks. Serotonin syndrome is another potentially fatal drug reaction that resembles neuroleptic malignant syndrome in presentation but does not involve a neuroleptic agent. Medication history is the most important factor in distinguishing between the two.[11,12]

Signs and symptoms

- Hallmark symptoms
  - Hyperthermia
  - Severe muscular rigidity
  - Autonomic instability (tachycardia, respiratory distress and hypoxia, labile or unstable blood pressure)
  - Changing level of consciousness
- Other symptoms, including the following:
  - Diaphoresis
  - Leukocytosis
  - Elevated creatine kinase levels (rhabdomyolysis)
  - Renal failure

Therapeutic interventions

- Initiate life support measures:
  - Stabilize blood pressure.
  - Normalize body temperature.
  - Correct hypoxia.
- Reduce muscular rigidity with bromocriptine (Parlodel) and dantrolene (Dantrium).
- Arrange for inpatient admission.

MENTAL HEALTH PATIENT DISPOSITION

The single most important question in the ED management of the psychiatric patient is, "Does the patient require hospitalization?" An important factor to consider is the presence or

absence of a solid support system. Does the patient have competent family members or friends willing to observe and supervise the individual? Patients who cannot be discharged safely must be placed on a psychiatric hold, usually by a psychiatrist. Mental health holds typically are limited to 72 hours in most states. Involuntary hold criteria differ from state to state, but most states require mandatory hospitalization if the patient meets the following criteria:
- A serious, imminent risk to health and safety exists because the patient is completely unable to provide self-care.
- The patient is a suicide risk.
- The patient is a physical threat to others.

References

1. US Department of Health and Human Services: *Mental health: a report of the surgeon general,* Rockville, Md, 1999, US Department of Health and Human Services, Substance Abuse and Mental Health Services Administration, Center for Mental Health Services, National Institutes of Health, National Institute of Mental Health.
2. US Department of Health and Human Services: *Healthy people 2010,* conference ed, Washington, DC, 2000, US Government Printing Office.
3. Huff SJ, Brady WJ: Confusion. In Marx J, Hockenberger R, Walls R, editors: *Rosen's emergency medicine: concepts and clinical practice,* ed 5, St Louis, 2002, Mosby.
4. Broadbent M, Jarman H, Berk M: Improving compliance in mental health triage, *Accid Emerg Nurs* 10:155-162, 2002.
5. Burland J: *Family to family teaching manual,* ed 2, rev, Arlington, Va, 2001, National Alliance for the Mentally Ill.
6. McIntosh J: USA suicide: 2000 official final data. Retrieved September 5, 2003, from www.suicidology.org/associations/1045/files/2000datapg.pdf.
7. Jensen L: Managing acute psychotic disorders in an emergency department, *Nurs Clin North Am* 38:45-54, 2003.
8. Green G: Guidelines for assessing and diagnosing acute psychosis: a primer, *J Am Psychiatr Nurs Assoc* 8:S31-S35, 2002.
9. Antai-Otong D: Managing geriatric psychiatric emergencies: delirium and dementia, *Nurs Clin North Am* 38:123-135, 2003.
10. Falsafi N: Pediatric psychiatric emergencies, *J Child Adolesc Psychiatr Nurs* 142:81-88, 2001.
11. Antai-Otong D: Adverse drug reactions associated with antipsychotic, antidepressants, and mood stabilizers, *Nurs Clin North Am* 38:161-176, 2003.
12. Weitzel C: Could you spot this psych emergency? *RN* 639:35-38, 2000.

49

Substance Abuse

Donna Mason, RN, MS, CEN

In 2002 the U.S. Department of Health and Human Services estimated that 19.5 million Americans—8.3% of the population aged 12 and older—were currently illicit drug users. Of these persons, about 166,000 abused heroin, 2 million consumed cocaine, and 567,000 smoked crack. The estimated number of users of hallucinogens was 1.2 million, a figure that includes 676,000 Ecstasy abusers. The percent of 12- to 17-year-olds who have ever smoked marijuana is believed to be nearly 21%. This amount more than doubles (53%) among persons 18 to 25 years old.[1]

Although young adults have the highest abuse rates (20.2%), the Department of Health and Human Services calculated that 11.6% of U.S. adolescents (12- to 17-year-olds) use some form of illegal substance.[2] Adults (aged 26 or older) have a 5.8% incidence of illicit drug use, and even 3.3% of pregnant women (ages 15 to 44) report substance abuse.

As staggering as these statistics are, the abuse of *legal* drugs is a considerably greater problem. An estimated 120 million Americans over the age of 12 report being current alcohol drinkers, and about 54 million have participated in binge drinking at least once in the past 30 days. Of this number, 15 million can be classified as heavy drinkers. In 2002, 30% of the U.S. population reported using a tobacco product within the past month. Roughly 61.1 million smoked cigarettes, 12.8 million smoked cigars, 7.8 million used smokeless tobacco, and 1.8 million smoked pipe tobacco.[3,4]

Currently popular drugs of abuse vary according to geography and can change frequently. Regional poison control centers are often the best source of information when a patient has an overdose of the latest "designer" drug. A respectful, nonjudgmental approach to the individual facilitates the process of substance identification and therapeutic intervention. Aggressive, unpredictable behavior is a common finding in those with acute drug and alcohol abuse or withdrawal. Ensuring a safe environment for the patient and the emergency department staff is a priority.

ALCOHOLS

Ethanol is the most popular drug of abuse because it is readily accessible and socially acceptable, and many persons do not view it as a drug. For information regarding the complications of ethanol abuse, see Chapter 27. The effects of toxic alcohols (methanol, isopropanol, and ethylene glycol) are discussed in Chapter 28.

COCAINE

Cocaine, a strong central nervous system stimulant, is a powerfully addictive drug. The National Institute on Drug Abuse reports that more than 30 million persons in the United States have tried cocaine; 5 million are regular users.[3] Cocaine frequently is cut with other substances (active and inert) to dilute it or increase its potency. Cocaine can be injected, ingested, smoked, inhaled (snorted), or rubbed on mucous membranes. Onset of action is dictated by the route of administration: the faster the absorption, the more intense the high. "Crack" is the street name for cocaine that has been converted to its free base form. When smoked, crack has an onset of action of mere seconds. Drug smugglers, or "body packers," transport the drug by swallowing large qualities of latex-wrapped cocaine. These balloons or condoms can rupture and leak, creating a medical emergency.[5]

Signs and Symptoms

Cocaine can affect virtually every organ or system in the body and is associated with a number of serious short- and long-term effects. Acute myocardial infarction has been reported up to 14 days after cocaine use in patients with and without preexisting cardiac disease, some as young as 19 years. In addition, cocaine readily crosses the placenta and is excreted in breast milk for up to 36 hours after use. Box 49-1 summarizes clinical manifestations of acute and chronic cocaine use.

Box **49-1**   **Clinical Manifestations of Cocaine Use**

Cardiovascular	Pneumomediastinum ("crack lung")
Contraction band necrosis	Pulmonary edema
Deep venous thrombosis	
Dysrhythmias	**Obstetric/Perinatal**
Hypertension	Abortion
Myocardial ischemia/infarction	Breast-feeding complications
	Neonatal cerebral infarction
Central Nervous System	Placental abruption
Agitation	
Cerebral infarction	**Other**
Headaches	Infectious diseases (tuberculosis, human immuno-
Seizures	deficiency virus, skin abscesses)
	Psychiatric: mania, aggression, paranoia, psychosis
Pulmonary	Renal failure
Cough	Rhabdomyolysis
Hemoptysis	

Therapeutic Interventions

Ingestion

- Abdominal radiographs may reveal latex packets in body packers.
- Ingestion of a single crack "rock" can be lethal to a small child. Aggressive management is required.
- Administer activated charcoal and a cathartic to treat ingestion.
- Use whole bowel irrigation to remove packets.
- Rarely, endoscopy or surgical removal of packets is required (when packets rupture and cause severe toxicity).

Inhalation

- Treatment is largely symptomatic.
- A chest radiograph may show pneumomediastinum from alveolar rupture (because of deep breath holding while inhaling cocaine). Significant amounts of mediastinal air require chest tube or mediastinal tube placement.
- Provide basic and advanced supportive care as indicated.
- Administer benzodiazepines for sedation and seizures.
- Treat hyperthermia with acetaminophen and external cooling.
- Obtain a 12-lead electrocardiogram, and initiate continuous cardiac monitoring.
- Draw a sample for a troponin I level in patients complaining of ischemic chest pain.
- Treat significant dysrhythmias. Lidocaine is *not* the first drug of choice because of its potential to increase the toxic effects of cocaine.[5]

HEROIN

Heroin is the most abused and the most rapid-acting of the opiates. Heroin is derived from morphine, a naturally occurring substance extracted from the seedpods of certain poppies. Heroin typically is processed into a white or brown powder for sale. Abuse of this agent continues to be a significant problem in the United States and throughout the world. Heroin can be injected, sniffed, snorted, ingested, or smoked. For a parenteral heroin abuser to inject up to 4 times in a day is not uncommon. Intravenous administration produces the most rapid onset of euphoria (7 to 8 seconds). Other routes of administration have a slower onset but longer duration of effect. Nearly all reported heroin-related fatalities involve parenteral use.

As with other illicit drugs, impurities and commixing with various substances may complicate a patient's presentation and clinical management. Individuals with significant heroin overdoses merit close observation and supportive care for 24 to 48 hours.

Signs and Symptoms of Chronic Abuse

Chronic abusers of heroin have the following signs and symptoms:
- Red or raw nostrils
- Scars or track marks on the arms or other locations
- Use or possession of syringes, bent spoons, bottle caps, eye droppers, and rubber tubing
- Infectious diseases such as human immunodeficiency virus infection (acquired immunodeficiency syndrome) and hepatitis B and C
- Collapsed veins
- Bacterial infections, skin abscesses

- Endocarditis
- Signs of withdrawal

Signs and Symptoms of Acute Narcosis

Signs and symptoms of acute narcosis include the following:
- Central nervous system depression
- Hypotension, bradycardia
- Miosis (pinpoint pupils)
- Nausea, vomiting
- Respiratory depression (the most critical problem)
- Slurred speech

Therapeutic Interventions

Therapeutic interventions for abusers of heroin include the following:
- Provide basic and advanced supportive care as indicated.
- Consider gastric lavage, activated charcoal, and cathartic administration for patients with recent oral ingestions. (See Chapter 28.)[6]
- Reverse the narcotic effects:
  - Naloxone (Narcan) is a rapid-acting narcotic antagonist that can be given intravenously, intraosseously, subcutaneously, intramuscularly, or sublingually. Titrate the dose to patient response. Give only enough to restore vital signs and gently rouse the patient. Up to 2 mg may be required. Naloxone has a short half-life; repeat as needed.
  - Nalmefene (Revex) is a newer narcotic antagonist with a considerably longer duration of effect than naloxone. Given intravenously in large doses (1.5 mg), nalmefene can block opioid activity for up to 8 hours. The usual starting dose is 0.5 mg; titrate to effect.[7]

INHALANTS

Inhalants are a common form of substance abuse, particularly among teenagers. Many routine household chemicals contain breathable vapors that have psychoactive effects. Although inhalant abuse is illegal, possession of these substances is not, making them an inexpensive and readily available high. The most commonly abused inhalants include glue, hair spray, deodorants, dry-cleaning fluids, gasoline, paint thinners, fabric protection sprays, air freshener, oven cleaners, nail polish remover, cooking sprays, aerosolized whipped cream, and felt-tipped pens.

Inhalants typically are classified into three categories: solvents such as paint thinner, paint removers, degreasers, gasoline, and glue; gases such as in butane lighters, propane tanks, whipping cream aerosols, refrigerator gasses, or spray paints; and nitrates (aliphatic nitrates), which are found in room deodorizers.

According to the American Association of Poison Control Centers, children as young as 4 years have been known to get high from sniffing, "bagging," "wanging," puffing, or "huffing" these products.[6] Huffing involves putting the substance in a bag or other closed container that can be held tightly to the face to maximize inhalation. Because inhalants are absorbed rapidly through the lungs, it takes only 10 to 15 seconds to achieve a high that can last for several minutes. Inhalation of these products causes dizziness, which can lead to syncope and, in some instances, sudden death. Inhalant-induced sudden death is unpredictable; this phenomenon can occur with the first use or any time thereafter. According to the American Academy of Pediatrics, sudden death is responsible for half of all reported inhalant-related mortality.

Each time toxins are inhaled, chemicals enter the lungs, pass from the bloodstream to the brain, and cause some degree of damage. Symptoms of chronic use include watery eyes, sores around the mouth, red or runny nose, loss of appetite, mood swings, headache, nausea, vomiting, impaired concentration, poor balance, slow or slurred speech, hearing loss, and hallucinations.[7]

Signs and Symptoms

Signs and symptoms of inhalant abuse include the following:
- Anxiety, irritability
- Behavioral changes
- Cardiotoxic and neurotoxic effects
- Nausea
- Red or runny nose and eyes
- Slurred speech, disorientation
- Unusual breath odor
- Ventricular fibrillation ("sudden sniffer's death")

Therapeutic Interventions

Therapeutic interventions for inhalant abuse include the following:
- Provide basic and advanced supportive care as indicated.
- Attempt to determine what substance(s) were inhaled.
- Provide symptomatic treatment.

NUTMEG

Nutmeg is a common household spice that has gained a reputation as a hallucinogen. Symptoms occur 3 to 8 hours after ingestion and can persist as long as 24 hours. Persons abusing nutmeg often experience flushing, an increased heart rate, and dry mouth. Treatment goals are (1) to keep the patient calm during hallucinations, (2) to maintain a normal blood pressure, and (3) to manage vomiting.[5]

Signs and Symptoms

Signs and symptoms of nutmeg abuse include the following:
- Anxiety
- Blurred vision
- Giddiness, euphoria
- Hallucinations, detachment from reality
- Headache
- Hypotension
- Nausea, vomiting
- Tingling

Therapeutic Interventions

Therapeutic interventions for nutmeg abuse include the following:
- Provide basic and advanced supportive care as indicated.
- Perform gastric lavage only for recent ingestions.
- Administer activated charcoal.
- Give antiemetics for nausea and vomiting.
- The sedatives most commonly used for management of severe agitation are diazepam (Valium) and chlorpromazine (Thorazine).

PHENCYCLIDINE (PCP)

Phencyclidine is a powerful sympathomimetic agent with dissociative anesthetic and hallucinogenic effects. Developed as an intravenous anesthetic, this drug was discontinued because of the negative side effects patients experienced while recovering. Phencyclidine is available as a white powder that is diluted readily in alcohol or water. Phencyclidine can be smoked, snorted, or ingested and is available in capsule, powder, or tablet form. Street names for this drug include angel dust, ozone, wack, rocket fuel, and killer joints (Box 49-2).

Frequently, a traumatic injury (not toxicity) ultimately brings the phencyclidine-using patient to the emergency department. Motor vehicle crashes, falls, and other injuries related to hallucinations are the primary cause of death from this drug. Many users experience violent and bizarre psychotic effects. The phencyclidine-intoxicated patient can be extraordinarily strong, has a sense of complete invulnerability, and easily can be a danger to self or others. Although extreme reactions are more common with repeated use, psychotic behavior has been reported after a single dose. Serum phencyclidine levels are not available or helpful.[5]

Signs and Symptoms

Signs and symptoms of phencyclidine abuse include the following:
- Agitation
- Amnesia to events
- Extreme image distortion

Box 49-2 Street Names for Various Illegal Substances

Phencyclidine (PCP)	M	Nitro
Angel dust	Roll	Soap
Crystal joint	X	Xyrem
Killer joint	XTC	
Ozone		Flunitrazepam (Rohypnol)
Rocket fuel	Ketamine	
Wack	K	Circles
	Special K	Mexican Valium
Ecstasy	Vitamin K	R2
		Roll
Adam	GHB	Roofies
Bean		Rope
Clarity	G	
Hug drug	Liquid ectasy	
Lover's speed	Liquid X	

- Hallucinations
- Hyperthermia
- Intense physical strength
- Loss of coordination
- Numbness, anesthesia to pain
- Nystagmus (horizontal, vertical, or rotary)
- Paranoia, self-destructive behavior
- Rhabdomyolysis
- Slurred or blocked speech
- Tachycardia, hypertension
- Violent behavior

Therapeutic Interventions

Therapeutic interventions for phencyclidine abuse include the following:
- Treatment is largely supportive and symptomatic.
- Provide basic and advanced supportive care as indicated.
- Physical restraint generally is required. Taking down the patient must be done with a large, coordinated group of skilled personnel to avoid injury to staff members or the patient.
- Place the patient in a low-stimulation environment.
- Try to calm and "talk down" the patient.
- Sedate the patient with a benzodiazepine (diazepam, lorazepam). Large amounts of these agents may be required to control agitation. Sedation prevents seizures as well.
- Control hypertension by treating agitation.
- Check the patient's temperature rectally. Cool hyperthermic patients aggressively.
- Fluid losses may be severe. Replace fluids with intravenously administered crystalloids. Keep urine output brisk.
- Observe for signs of rhabdomyolysis (dark urine, elevated creatine kinase level); treat as indicated.[5]

DATE RAPE OR CLUB DRUGS

Several substances fall into the "date rape" or "club drug" category. Agents in this broad grouping include Ecstasy, ketamine, GHB (gamma hydroxybutyrate), and flunitrazepam (Rohypnol).[8] The term *date rape drug* refers to central nervous system depressant substances that can be added easily to alcohol and ingested unknowingly. The resultant incapacitation leaves victims vulnerable to sexual assault. Other club drugs, such as ketamine and Ecstasy, are central nervous system stimulants and hallucinogenics.

Ecstasy (MDMA)

Ecstasy (3,4-methylenedioxymethamphetamine) is a relatively simple chemical that belongs to the amphetamine family. This drug, with stimulant and hallucinogenic properties, has become popularly associated with underground "rave" dance parties. Although Ecstasy does not cause true hallucinations, users commonly experience distorted time perception. Many researchers consider Ecstasy to be the fastest growing drug of abuse in the United States. According to the American Association of Poison Control Centers, in the year 2000 an estimated 1.3 million teenagers consumed this substance to produce feelings of intimacy, euphoria, and increased energy.[8] Ecstasy frequently is mixed with caffeine, dextromethorphan, ephedrine, or cocaine. Symptom onset typically begins 30 to 60 minutes after an oral dose and lasts anywhere from 8 to 12 hours. The powdered form of Ecstasy can be snorted for a more rapid onset of effects. Vick's inhaler or Vick's vapor rub are used to enhance effects when the drug is snorted.

Signs and symptoms

Most Common Symptoms on Emergency Department Arrival

- Agitation, anxiety, tachycardia, hypertension

Other Symptoms

- Atrioventricular blocks, dysrhythmias, asystole
- Confusion, delirium, paranoia, seizures, cerebral edema
- Headache
- Irritability, depression
- Muscle aches, muscle spasms, rigidity, teeth grinding (bruxism)
- Pulmonary edema

Therapeutic interventions

- Provide basic and advanced supportive care as indicated.
- Attempt to determine what substance(s) were used and when.
- Send a urine sample for qualitative drug testing. Ecstasy can be detected in the urine for 48 to 72 hours.
- Diagnosis is based on history and presenting symptoms.
- Administer activated charcoal for oral ingestions.
- Give benzodiazepines to control anxiety.
- No known antidote exists for Ecstacy.

Ketamine

Ketamine, chemically similar to phencyclidine, originally was developed as a veterinary anesthetic. Parenteral preparations of this agent routinely are used in many emergency departments for procedural sedation. Ketamine is available in parenteral, powdered, or tablet forms. Ketamine can be injected (intravenously or intramuscularly), ingested, smoked, or snorted. Powdered ketamine may be mixed and smoked with marijuana or tobacco. Effects last 30 to 60 minutes. Recreational abusers use ketamine to produce a dissociative sensation. Dreamlike states and hallucinations make ketamine popular in rave or club settings for recreational use and date rape.

Information regarding long-term effects are mainly anecdotal. Flashbacks and hallucinations have been reported. Some studies suggest that long-term ketamine use may be associated with visual damage and attentional disorders. Ketamine can cause a tremendous psychological dependence and may be physically addicting as well. Tolerance develops rapidly. Overdose may present as respiratory arrest.[8]

Signs and symptoms

- Confusion, aggression, delirium
- Hypertension
- Increased heart rate, palpitations

- Lack of coordination
- Respiratory depression, apnea

Therapeutic interventions

- Provide basic and advanced supportive care as indicated.
- No specific antidote is available for ketamine.
- Give midazolam (Versed) for agitation and combativeness.

Gamma Hydroxybutyrate (GHB)

The drug gamma hydroxybutyrate (also called gamma hydroxybutyric acid) more commonly is referred to simply as GHB. This drug was developed for the treatment of narcolepsy and alcohol or opiate withdrawal.[5] The combination of central nervous system depression, euphoria, and suppression of inhibitions makes GHB an excellent drug for sexual assault. Gamma hydroxybutyrate usually comes in a liquid form. Because of its salty taste, this drug often is hidden in fruity or sweet drinks to be given to the unknowing victim of robbery or rape.

Peak effects occur 30 minutes after ingestion and last 3 to 6 hours. The most distinctive and alarming feature of GHB overdose is its rapid time course. This drug can take effect in as little as 15 minutes, quickly causing respiratory depression and possible respiratory arrest.[8]

Signs and symptoms

- Bradycardia
- Dizziness, euphoria, drowsiness, decreased level of consciousness
- Drunken behavior without the odor of alcohol
- Hypotension
- Hypothermia
- Hypoventilation, respiratory distress, apnea
- In rare cases: Seizures, coma, and death
- Slurred speech, disorientation, impaired memory
- Vomiting

Therapeutic interventions

- Provide basic and advanced supportive care as indicated.
- A toxicologic test for GHB is not routinely available. However, in cases of suspected criminal activity (e.g., rape) samples should be collected for analysis at a specialized forensic laboratory.
- Consider gastric lavage if the patient arrives within 60 minutes of ingestion.
- Administer activated charcoal.
- No antidote exists for GHB.
- Give atropine for bradycardia.
- Treat seizures with a benzodiazepine such as diazepam (Valium).

Flunitrazepam (Rohypnol)

Flunitrazepam, more commonly known as Rohypnol, is a powerful benzodiazepine that is many times more potent than diazepam (Valium). This drug commonly comes in pill form. Sedation occurs within 30 to 60 minutes of ingestion, and effects peak in 2 to 3 hours. Rohypnol is illegal in the United States.

A well-publicized date rape drug, Rohypnol can be lethal when mixed with alcohol. Patients generally show signs of sedation, although Rohypnol has been known to produce excitability in certain individuals.[8]

Signs and symptoms

- Dizziness, confusion
- Hypotension
- Lack of muscle control
- Loss of consciousness
- Visual disturbances

Therapeutic interventions

- Provide basic and advanced supportive care as indicated, including supplemental oxygen and cardiac monitoring.
- Protect the airway with an oral, nasopharyngeal, or tracheal tube as needed.
- A toxicologic test for flunitrazepam is not routinely available. However, in cases of suspected criminal activity (e.g., rape) samples should be collected for analysis at a specialized forensic laboratory.
- Gastric lavage may be helpful if the patient arrives within 60 minutes of ingestion.
- Administer activated charcoal.
- Give the antidote flumazenil (Romazicon). The standard dose is 0.2 mg intravenously over 15 seconds. Repeat the dose every 1 minute as needed, up to a total of 2 mg.

PREVENTION STRATEGIES AND TREATMENT MODALITIES

As is true of so many conditions regularly treated in emergency departments, education and prevention are the ultimate solutions to the problem of substance abuse. Mental health and behavioral modification programs are available across the country to support abusers. Substance abuse prevention education, targeted at the elementary and middle school levels, can influence the incidence of future drug use.

References

1. US Department of Health and Human Services, Substance Abuse and Mental Health Services Administration: Retrieved March 27, 2003, from http://www.samhsa.gov.
2. National Institute on Drug Abuse: High school and youth trends. Retrieved March 27, 2003, from http://www.nida.nih.gov.
3. National Institute on Drug Abuse: Costs to society. Retrieved February 17, 2004, from http://www.drugabuse.gov.
4. Hanson G: Hearing before the Senate Caucus on International Narcotic Control: looking the other way—rave promoters and club drugs (Dec 4, 2001). Retrieved March 27, 2003, from http://www.drugabuse.gov.
5. Dart R et al, editors: *The 5 minute toxicology consult,* Philadelphia, 2000, Lippincott Williams & Wilkins.
6. Criddle L: Toxicologic emergencies. In Newberry L, editor: *Sheehy's emergency nursing: principles and practice,* ed 5, St Louis, 2003, Mosby.
7. Schaider J et al, editors: *Rosen and Barkin's 5-minute emergency medicine consult,* ed 2, Philadelphia, 2003, Lippincott Williams & Wilkins.
8. Smith KM, Larive LL, Romanelli F: Club drugs: methylenedioxymethamphetamine, flunitrazepam, ketamine hydrochloride, and gamma-hydroxybutyrate, *Am J Health Syst Pharm* 59(11):1067-1076, 2002.

50

Intimate Partner Violence

Susan Rolniak, RN, MSN, CRNP and Elizabeth Burke, BA

Intimate partner violence (IPV), also known as domestic violence, is defined as a pattern of assaultive and coercive behaviors by an individual against a current or former intimate partner. Intimate partners may be heterosexual or homosexual. Eighty five percent of the time, IPV involves a women being abused by a male partner.[1] However, violence against men by women and violence against a partner in a same-sex relationship also occur. Intimate partner violence is a global health problem. Worldwide, between one quarter and one half of all women have been abused physically by a current or former partner.[2] Numerous studies have reported that American women experience a similar incidence of physical or sexual abuse.[3] According to the National Violence Against Women Survey, 1 out of 4 U.S. women has been physically assaulted or raped by an intimate partner; 1 out of every 14 U.S. men has had a comparable experience.[4] Women are much more likely than men to be killed by an intimate partner. Intimate partner violence accounts for 33.5% of murders of women, but less than 4% of murders of men.[5] For many complex reasons, including embarrassment and fear, IPV is underreported. Underreporting is especially prevalent in same-sex relationships and among abused men.

The emergency nurse must understand that IPV can be found in all economic, racial, religious, educational, and age groups. Victims have no specific personality type, occupation, or sexual orientation profile. Factors that place women at increased risk for IPV include young age (16 to 25 years), low socioeconomic status, recent separation from a partner, young children (<12 years) in the home, and homelessness.[6] In the United States, blacks suffer domestic violence at rates higher than those of other racial groups.[7] Nearly one third of black American women experience IPV in their lifetimes compared with one quarter of white American females.[4] Most victims are not identified unless a health care provider directly and sensitively asks about the possibility of IPV.

TYPES OF INTIMATE PARTNER ABUSE

Intimate partner violence takes many forms, including physical, emotional, psychological, and sexual abuse and economic control. Although it is possible to experience only a single type of abuse, those in IPV situations commonly report multiple categories of abuse over time, particularly if the relationship remains unchanged.

IPV may manifest as follows:

Physical: Physical abuse is usually repetitive and increases in frequency and severity over time. Examples of physical abuse are pushing, shoving, slapping, kicking, choking, restraining, leaving the victim in a dangerous place, and refusing to help a sick or injured victim.

Emotional: Emotional abuse may occur before or along with physical violence.

Psychological: Psychological abusers control by means of fear or terror. Victims are made to feel guilty, responsible, alone, helpless, and powerless. Examples of psychological abuse include physical and social isolation from family and friends, threats of physical harm, extreme jealousy, economic deprivation, and acts of intimidation, humiliation, and degradation.

Sexual: Sexual abuse includes completed or attempted sexual acts against the victim's will and any form of nonconsensual physical contact.

Economic: Economic abuse involves excluding victims from access to family income, requiring victims to ask for money or an allowance, appropriating victims' assets, and preventing victims from getting or keeping a job.

IDENTIFYING INTIMATE PARTNER VIOLENCE

Victims of IPV present to emergency departments with a multitude of complaints ranging from major trauma to milder physical and mental health symptoms. Chronic medical and psychological conditions, minor and serious injuries, depression, suicidal behavior, sexually transmitted diseases, substance abuse, and even death are only a few of the health consequences of IPV. In addition to physical injuries, a number of stress-related conditions have been linked to IPV, such as chronic neck and back pain, recurrent headaches, chronic pelvic pain, indigestion, diarrhea, constipation, gastritis, and spastic colon.[3,8] Overall, victims of partner violence have more surgeries, medical visits, and hospitalizations than persons without a history of abuse.[3]

Signs and Symptoms Suggestive of Abuse

The following signs and symptoms suggest IPV:

- The patient describes the alleged "accident" in a hesitant, embarrassed, or evasive manner, or avoids eye contact.
- The extent or type of injury is inconsistent with the explanation offered by the patient.
- The victim has a history of traumatic injuries or frequent emergency department visits.
- The patient denies physical abuse but has unexplained bruises; areas of erythema or bruises in the shape of a hand or other object; lacerations, burns, scars, fractures, or multiple injuries in various stages of healing; mandibular fractures; or a perforated tympanic membrane.
- The patient expresses a fear of returning home or concern for the safety of her children.

- Injuries are in areas hidden by the clothing or hair (e.g., head, chest, breasts, abdomen, and genitals). Accidental trauma generally injures the extremities, whereas IPV often involves truncal and extremity injuries.
- The partner (or suspected abuser) accompanies the patient, insists on staying close to the victim, and tries to answer all questions directed at the patient.
- The patient admits to past or present physical or emotional abuse as a victim or as a child witness.
- The woman is pregnant. Homicide is the leading cause of death for pregnant women, and intimate partners are the most common perpetrators.[9,10]
- The victim shows evidence of sexual assault.
- The patient is the mother of an abused child.
- A substantial delay occurred between the time of injury and presentation for treatment. The patient may have been prevented from seeking medical attention sooner or had to wait for the batterer to leave.
- The patient has psychosomatic complaints such as panic attacks, anxiety, a choking sensation, or depression.
- A complaint of chronic pain (especially back or pelvic pain), with no substantiating physical evidence, often signifies fear of impending or actual physical abuse.

Assessment and Intervention

The Emergency Nurses Association recommends the development of routine protocols and procedures for the assessment and identification of IPV. Intervention goals for victims include the following:
- Treat presenting complaints or injuries.
- Offer emotional support.
- Help victims establish a safety plan and identify available options.
- Give victims information regarding legal protection, including assault documentation.
- Provide information about available support services and community resources.

Identification of IPV victims requires sensitivity, understanding, and a high index of suspicion. The psychological effects of battering are complex and can be difficult to understand. Victims are made to feel stupid and worthless. Abusers repeatedly tell their victims that no one cares and that, if the abuse is revealed, more violence will follow. For these reasons, it can be extremely difficult for victims to take the first step toward revealing abuse. However, breaking through the barrier of silence and denial will begin the process of physical and psychological healing. Many victims will acknowledge abuse openly if questioned in a nonjudgmental manner in a safe environment. When not asked directly, abused patients are generally hesitant to bring up the subject. Screening with explicit but nonthreatening questions increases disclosure rates (Box 50-1). Nonetheless, victims may require several visits and screenings before they can feel comfortable revealing abuse.

Therapeutic Interventions

Therapeutic interventions in cases of IPV include the following:
- Find a quiet, safe, private environment to assess the patient and screen for violence.
- Interview the patient privately, not in the presence of family members or other accompanying individuals.
- Universally screen all adult patients for IPV regardless of the presenting complaint.
- Have the patient undress completely so that any hidden injuries will be exposed.

Box **50-1** **Screening Questions for Adult Patients**

- Is anyone in your home being hurt, hit, threatened, frightened, or neglected?
- Do you feel safe in your current relationship?
- Do you ever feel afraid at home? Are you afraid for your children?
- Sometimes patients tell me that they have been hurt by someone close to them. Could this be happening to you?
- You seem frightened of your partner. Has he/she ever hurt you?
- Have there been times during your relationship when you have had physical fights?
- Do your verbal fights ever include physical contact?
- Have you been hit, punched, kicked, or otherwise hurt by someone within the past year? If so, by whom?
- You mentioned that your partner uses alcohol (drugs). How does he/she act when drinking (on drugs)?
- Does your partner consistently control your actions or put you down?
- Sometimes when others are overprotective and as jealous as you describe, they react strongly and use physical force. Is this happening in your situation?

- Take a careful history. Begin a domestic violence screen with a statement such as the following:

Domestic violence has come to be recognized as an important, often overlooked health issue in our society. So many persons are affected directly or indirectly. Sometimes they are even afraid to say anything. We care about our patients and want to help everyone in need. We screen every patient who comes to the emergency department for abuse because it is so common, so I would like to ask you a few questions. Does your current partner or a partner from a previous relationship make you feel unsafe now? Are you here today because of an illness or injury related to violence from a partner, or ex-partner? Has your partner ever controlled your actions? Threatened you? Hit, shoved, punched, kicked, or otherwise physically hurt you? Forced you to have unwanted sexual contact?

- Following these questions, ask patients if they want additional information on domestic violence or would like to discuss their situation with someone.[11]

Examples of other direct, nonthreatening questions are the following:
- You seem frightened of your partner. Has he/she ever hurt you?
- Sometimes patients tell me someone close to them has hurt them. Could this be happening to you?
- Your partner seems overly concerned and anxious. Is he/she responsible for your injuries?
- I noticed you have a number of bruises. Did someone hit you?

Assessment of the patient's safety is important in order to reduce the danger faced after discharge. Determine whether the patient has a safe place to go and the necessary resources (such as medications). Ask if the patient needs help locating a shelter. Offer to find a social worker or medical advocate to talk with the victim. Let patients know that IPV is against the law and that a police report can be made and a temporary restraining order can be obtained.

Explain to the patient the physical and emotional sequelae of chronic battering, for her and her children. Stress the importance of follow-up for medical, legal, and social support. Emphasize that the cycle of violence *can* be broken and that help is available.

ADVOCACY AND SUPPORT SERVICES

Intimate partner victim advocates have specialized training in abuse issues and are dedicated to providing victim assistance. Their role is to be available to help and support the patient whenever needed, from the initial emergency department visit through the critical days or months ahead.

The advocate offers a victim the opportunity to explore various available options, such as crisis intervention, a safe home network, and legal representation. Advocates work with the victim to support *her* choices, regardless of whether the advocate agrees with the decision. Many times a patient will choose to return to an unsafe and potentially violent environment. For a variety of complex reasons—low self-esteem, guilt, fear, loneliness, lack of support systems, insufficient funds—victims are frequently unprepared to separate from violent partners. The advocate's role is to provide *unconditional* support so that victims feel they are no longer alone.

With the patient's permission, notify a local advocacy service to initiate contact and support while the patient is still in the emergency department (if possible). Provide the patient with the telephone number of the abuse hotline in your area. Various social services can be contacted to help the patient identify programs and options available.

KNOW YOUR LEGAL OBLIGATIONS

The emergency nurse must be familiar with IPV reporting laws in the state or location in which the nurse is employed. Expectations vary between jurisdictions:
- Are you mandated to report nonfatal but life-threatening injuries (e.g., gunshot wounds or strangulation)?
- Is there an obligation to report non–life-threatening injuries?
- Does your facility have policies and procedures in place regarding IPV reporting?
  Every U.S. state has some form of legislation that offers protection to IPV victims. Be aware of state laws and services for abuse victims in your area.

DOCUMENTATION

Accurate and concise documentation of suspected IPV is essential from medical and legal perspectives. Your medical records can provide evidence of injury, escalating violence, or patterns of abuse. These records can be subpoenaed for subsequent criminal hearings.

The patient's injuries should be documented clearly in the medical record by licensed health care professionals. Record the size, pattern, estimated age, description, and location of all injuries. A body injury map is an efficient documentation tool, especially when numerous wounds are present. Be as specific as possible. For example, "multiple contusions and lacerations" will not convey a clear picture to a judge or jury, but "contusions and lacerations at the base of the anterior neck" will back up allegations of attempted strangulation. Record other evidence of abuse, such as torn clothing and jewelry. Do not forget to document the patient's demeanor and behavior objectively.

Whenever possible, obtain color photographs of all injuries. Photographs should be taken with the permission of the victim as a means of supplementing (not replacing) the information written in the medical record. Photograph the same injury from different angles and ranges.

Include full body pictures, midrange views, and close-ups. Each injury should be photographed at least twice. A ruler or a common item, such as a quarter, can be placed near the wound to provide context to injury size. Print the patient's name, photographer's name, and date of treatment on each picture and add descriptive information if the injury location is not obvious (e.g., left flank wound). Photographs should remain with the medical record.

Avoid long descriptions and quotations that deviate from the medical problem (e.g., "He was angry at me because I let the kids go to the movies."). This type of information is inadmissible in court and actually could prove counterproductive if it is inconsistent with court testimony. If the patient states that the injury was caused by abuse, record the information verbatim and write, "patient states" before the quotation. For example, you would record "Patient states she was 'hit in the face by my husband's fist.'"

Patients with suspicious injuries may deny abuse or assault. In such cases write, "The patient's explanation of the injury is inconsistent with physical findings," or "Injuries are suggestive of assault."

References

1. Bureau of Justice Statistics: *Intimate partner violence, 1993-2001,* Washington, DC, 2003, Department of Justice, Office of Justice Programs, Bureau of Justice Statistics.
2. Heise L, Ellsberg M, Gottemoeller N: Ending violence against women, *Population Reports,* series L, No. 11, Baltimore, Johns Hopkins University School of Public Health, Population Information Program, 1999.
3. World Health Organization: World report on violence and health. Retrieved from http://www.who.int/violence_injury_prevention/violence/world_report/en/.
4. Tjaden P, Thoennes N: *Extent, nature, and consequences of intimate partner violence against women: findings from the National Violence Against Women Survey,* Washington, DC, 2000, National Institute of Justice.
5. Family Violence Prevention Fund: Get the facts: domestic violence and health care. Retrieved from http://endabuse.org/programs/display/php3?DocID=25.
6. Coben J: Domestic violence. Retrieved February 4, 2003, from http://www.ahrq.gov/news/ulp/women/ulpwomn5.htm.
7. Black Womens Health: Domestic violence: when love becomes hurtful. Retrieved from http://www.blackwomenshealth.com/domestic_violence.htm.
8. Coker AL et al: Physical health consequences of physical and psychological intimate partner violence, *Arch Fam Med* 9(5):451-457, 2000.
9. Frye V: Examining homicide's contribution to pregnancy-associated deaths, *JAMA* 285(11):1510-1511, 2001 (comment).
10. Nannini A et al: Pregnancy-associated mortality at the end of the twentieth century: Massachusetts, 1990-1999, *J Am Med Womens Assoc* 57(3):140-143, 2002 (see comment).
11. Domestic Violence Safety Assessment, Pittsburgh Mercy Health Care System, May 2001.

51

Sexual Assault

Anita Johnson RN, BSN

Sexual assault is not limited to any particular victim age, race, gender, sexual preference, socioeconomic level, or cultural background.[1,2] Females are the most common victims, and women between the ages of 16 and 19 experience the highest assault rates.[3] Eighty percent to 90% of cases are estimated to go unreported. Legal definitions of sexual assault vary from state to state, but the cornerstone of all definitions is sexual contact imposed against a victim's will. Sodomy, vaginal rape, and molestation are included in this definition. Importantly, sexual assault is not a crime of passion, but one of power, anger, and control. Physical force and psychological coercion are significant elements of sexual assault.[2]

Feelings of guilt, self-blame, shame, embarrassment, fear, vulnerability, and helplessness are typical victim responses. Survivors of sexual assault suffer an overall sense of personal violation. Rape trauma syndrome is described as a cluster of symptoms experienced by survivors of sexual assault that includes somatic, behavioral, and psychological reactions.[1,2,4]

Emergency departments are mandated by federal law to have policies and procedures in place for providing care to victims of sexual assault. The role of emergency department staff members in the management of this patient population is as follows:

- To identify and treat any acute medical conditions and minimize psychological trauma to the victim
- To facilitate the collection and preservation of physical evidence (e.g., blood, semen, saliva, hair, clothing, debris, and objects) for use by the criminal justice system
- To ensure that community resource referrals are made for follow-up physical and psychological care[1-3]

Under many state laws, when the survivor discloses a rape or sexual assault, emergency departments are required to report the alleged crime. However, this practice of reporting without the patient's permission is controversial, given the stigma of rape. Assault victims have the right to refuse a forensic examination and may choose to receive medical care only

following an attack. Ensure that patients who forgo a forensic examination are offered the following:
- Prophylaxis for sexually transmitted diseases and pregnancy[1]
- Comprehensive discharge teaching
- Referrals to community agencies for psychological counseling, support, and follow-up care[1]

Most state laws allow adolescents to request a sexual assault examination without parental knowledge or consent. However, consent laws vary from state to state and should be reviewed for your location.[1] In all states, neither the child victim nor the parents can refuse to participate in the investigation of an alleged child sexual assault.

APPROACH TO THE SEXUAL ASSAULT PATIENT

SART: The Team

Many communities have adopted the sexual assault response/resource team (SART) approach to meeting the needs of the sexual assault survivor. Ideally a SART consists of the following:
- A sexual assault forensic examiner. This is a registered nurse, physician, or forensic odontologist who has successfully completed a course in evidentiary examinations.
- Law enforcement officers
- Patient advocates
- Prosecutors
- Forensic laboratory personnel[5]

SART: The Process

The following is an example of how the SART process works:
- A local law enforcement agency is notified of the assault. Police officers initiate the SART process.
- A sexual assault nurse examiner (SANE) and SART patient advocate are notified.
- Initial disclosure is completed between law enforcement personnel and hospital staff.
- The forensic examination process begins.
- The patient advocate accompanies the victim through the hospital process and provides referrals for community resources, crisis counseling, and patient-witness assistance.
- Evidence is handed over from the hospital to the appropriate agencies.
- The case is referred for investigation.
- Depending on the circumstances, the investigation is handled by the district or city attorney's office.
- Judicial proceedings begin.[5]

Sexual Assault Nurse Examiner

Since the establishment of the first SANE program in 1976, the number of programs has grown steadily. The basic goals of a SANE program are the following:
- To provide forensic sexual assault evidence collection in a consistent and objective manner
- To meet the medical, psychological, and educational needs of the individual requesting care[1]

Triage

Medically nonurgent patients

Most victims of sexual assault do not require emergent medical care in an emergency department. Whenever possible, usher the patient and any family or friends to a private, quiet, and comfortable area away from the routine of the emergency department. A nursing assessment should occur as soon as possible. Expediting the forensic examination (evidence collection process) preserves as much evidence as possible and addresses the physical and emotional needs of the patient. If a victim presents at triage before contacting the police, the nurse can institute the sexual assault procedure of the emergency department and contact local law enforcement. Typically, a patient advocate—such as a rape crisis counselor—is called as well. Departments served by a SANE program also will notify the SANE at this time.

Every attempt should be made to ensure that the patient is not left alone. A designated professional support person (a social worker, a rape crisis counselor, or an advocate) can provide critical psychological intervention to patients, family members, and significant others. The designated support person collaborates with the SANE and emergency department personnel to do the following:
- Explain procedures
- Offer issue-oriented counseling
- Share information regarding the criminal justice process
- Provide community referrals
- Describe victim compensation programs

Medically urgent or emergent patients

When a sexually assaulted patient is medically urgent or emergent, try to consider the effect of every procedure on the forensic evidence collection process. Initiate procedures for reporting and treating sexual assault as soon as possible. After initial stabilization of life-threatening problems, ongoing patient management and treatment can occur concurrently with evidence collection.[1]

NURSING ASSESSMENT

As with any patient presenting to the emergency department for care, a registered nurse has the responsibility to complete an assessment of the sexual assault patient. In some systems, all or part of this evaluation may be delegated to the SANE.

Subjective Data

History of events

- Date, time, and place of the alleged assault
- Description of the assailant
- Information regarding all acts, as reported by the patient
- Injuries associated with the assault
- Postassault activity (e.g., bathing, douching, eating, drinking, and clothing changes)[3]

Medical history

- Date of the last normal menstrual period
- Reproductive history: Age of menarche and menopause, gravity, parity, and current pregnancy status
- Current method of contraception
- Time(s) of any consenting intercourse within the last 72 hours
- History of any sexually transmitted diseases, including pelvic inflammatory disease
- General medical and surgical histories
- Mental health history
- Current medications
- Allergies
- Tetanus and hepatitis B immunization status[3]

Objective Data

Objective data to collect during the assessment include the following:
- Assess for serious trauma, particularly if the history indicates possible neck injuries, blunt blows, choking, or the use of drugs or objects during the assault. Always address major injuries before (or concurrent with) evidence collection.
- Obtain a complete set of vital signs.
- If the patient has only minor injuries, treatment usually can wait until after evidence collection.
- Observe the victim's general emotional state for signs of acute rape trauma syndrome.[2]

SEXUAL ASSAULT EVIDENCE COLLECTION

Basic Principles

The following is a list of basic principles of evidence collection from patients who have been raped or otherwise sexually assaulted:
- To maintain the chain of evidence, all evidence collected from a victim must remain with the collector or be locked in a secure area until released to a law enforcement agency.
- All items collected or released by any emergency department professional involved in the care of a sexual assault victim must be documented in the medical chart.
- Sexual assault evidence collection kits are packaged according to Food and Drug Administration regulations. All evidence collected should be placed and sealed in the containers provided in the approved kit.
- Properly seal and initial all specimens and label them with the following information:
  - The hospital name, patient name, and patient identification number
  - The date and time of collection
  - A description of the specimen and its collection site
  - The name and signature of the person collecting the evidence[5]
- Any objects (e.g., knife, bullets, or clothing) that are removed from the patient must be placed individually in a paper evidence bag, sealed, and labeled as described before.
- Whenever possible, any clothing removed should be unbuttoned or unzipped for removal. If clothes must be cut, do not slice through stains, holes, tears, or buttonholes.
- When moisture is needed to collect biological samples, slightly moisten (vs. saturate) the tip of a cotton swab. Moisture dilutes biological samples, thereby reducing the chance of detecting scant amounts of DNA. Dry the samples and place them in a separate, labeled envelope obtained from the rape kit.

- All physical evidence of the crime collected from the victim should be air dried. Fold clothing without shaking; take care not to cross-contaminate the surfaces. Place individual items in paper collection containers that are sealed and labeled as described before.
- Collect biological samples before any activity or procedure (catheter insertion, voiding, eating, smoking, drinking) that could result in the destruction of evidence. Dry the sample and place it in a separate, labeled envelope obtained from the evidence collection kit.
- After drying, each cotton-tipped applicator is placed bulb end first into a separate, labeled envelope obtained from the evidence collection kit. Ensure that all envelopes are sealed properly.
- Never place moist evidence in plastic or glass containers. Heat and moisture promote growth of mold and other organisms that destroy evidence.

Other Evidence Considerations

Who

A SANE, advanced practice nurse, or registered nurse and physician may collect physical evidence of sexual assault in accordance with emergency department policies and procedures.

Consent

The routine emergency department consent form covers permission for medical treatment of sexual assault victims. Obtain an additional, written, informed consent (or refusal) from adult victims before the evidentiary examination. The consent form should contain a clause allowing the hospital to release physical evidence to law enforcement agencies. Stipulate that physical evidence includes biological specimens, clothing or objects, photographs, and written documentation.[1]

What

In most states, standardized examination kits have been developed for evidence collection. Local law enforcement representatives often provide these kits, which are usually available to hospitals at little or no charge. Included in the kit is information regarding specimen collection, instructions for maintaining the chain of custody, and a list of documentation requirements.[1]

When

Most national, state, and institutional protocols recommend forensic examinations within 72 hours of assault.[1,5] This time limit was established based on the presumption that this was the optimum period for detection of injuries and collection of evidence. However, as laboratory and forensic testing techniques improve, this guideline may be changed. Survivors presenting after 72 hours still should receive a forensic examination if they are symptomatic, exhibit injuries, or have evidence available for collection.[1]

Gather all supplies and have them available in the examination room *before* the start of evidence collection. Open the kit only *after* the examiner is certain that the evidence collection process can be continued without interruption until the kit is resealed. If the examiner leaves the room with the kit opened, the kit is considered abandoned and the chain of evidence breached.

How

Patients who have survived a sexual assault deserve to have professional nursing care and retain the right to have some control over the course of their treatment. Information regarding the process of evidence collection can serve to reassure the patient and decrease anxiety. Staff members who feel uncomfortable caring for the sexual assault patient should delegate this responsibility to another professional.

The Forensic Interview

Verbal history of the incident

"Tell me what happened to you tonight" is an example of an open-ended statement that can be used to begin the forensic interview. Closed questions that require only "yes" or "no" answers are discouraged but can be used to clarify statements made by the patient. "Did Billy rape you tonight?" is an example of a closed question. This type of inquiry should be avoided. Standardized sexual assault documentation tools facilitate consistent and unbiased recording of the patient's recollection of events. Gather the following information:

- Date, time, and location of the alleged assault
- Method of approach used by the assailant
- Whether the assailant is known or unknown to the victim
- Number of assailants
- Race and gender of the assailant(s)
- Weapon use (blunt or sharp objects, gun, rope)
- Type of force used (e.g., physical force, verbal threats, a weapon, or other threats)
- Assault details (e.g., kissing, touching, exposure; or oral, vaginal, or anal penetration)
- Penetrating object(s) used (finger, penis, tongue, other)
- Any oral contact by the assailant and on what body part
- Erection and/or ejaculation by the assailant
- Condom or lubricant use
- Any patient activities after the assault that may affect evidence retrieval (e.g., tooth brushing, bathing, vomiting, changing clothes, douching, defecating, urinating, eating, drinking, or smoking)

During the forensic interview, key answers should be documented as quotations whenever possible. After the forensic interview, explain the evidence collection process *before* each procedure begins and as needed throughout the examination.

Medical photography

Consider the following when photographing forensic evidence:

- Colposcopy with video or photographic capability is considered the best technique for documenting the forensic examination.[1]
- A 35-mm camera can be used for forensic photography when colposcopy is not available.
- Visible injuries or evidence of force should be photographed serially.

Physical Examination

The purpose of clothing collection is to demonstrate the use of force (ripped or torn clothing) and to look for the presence of biological and trace evidence (semen, blood, other stains, debris). Body fluids place the offender with the victim; debris places the victim at the crime scene. Change gloves whenever cross-contamination of evidence might occur. All findings should be documented clearly.

Observe the following procedures:

- Carefully follow the sexual assault evidence collection instructions provided in the kit.
- Before the patient undresses, place a clean hospital sheet on the floor, under the collection paper.
- Allow the patient to remove and place each piece of clothing in a separate paper bag. Handle all clothing with gloved hands to prevent evidence contamination.
- Note all injuries and record their location, size, and a complete description of any trauma. Look for bite wounds, strangulation marks, or areas of tenderness especially around the mouth, breasts, thighs, wrists, upper arms, legs, back, and anogenital region.
- Check the patient for the presence of any biological evidence or foreign debris, but do not disturb it at this time.
- Photograph sites before specimen collection.
- Recover any trace evidence, including sand, soil, leaves, grass, and secretions. Document their location on the body.
- Identify moist secretions and recover them with a dry swab.
- Look for areas of debris and dried secretions stuck to the skin; these can be flaked off onto a piece of paper. Fold the paper well to prevent loss of material. Recover any material remaining on the site using a swab moistened with one drop of water (tap water is acceptable).
- Document the patient's Tanner stage (a scale used to evaluate sexual development) and describe the level of physical maturity.
- Toluidine blue dye may be used to identify minor external injuries to the genitals and anus, but it can cause discomfort in prepubertal children.[6]
- When a vaginal examination is performed, lubricate the speculum with tap water only. Other lubricants may decrease sperm motility and affect test results.
- A vaginal speculum is never used in prepubertal children without general anesthesia.
- When drug or alcohol-facilitated sexual assault is suspected, collect blood and/or urine for toxicologic studies.[5]

Specimen Collection

Evidence collection procedures change as technology evolves. The emergency nurse must keep abreast of the current practices of the state crime laboratory to collect and preserve as much evidence as possible.[5] Core evidence consists of oral, vaginal, and anal samples, as appropriate. Pubic and head hair, fingernail scrapings, and a blood reference sample are also routine components of evidence collection. Staff members who participate in evidence collection should be required to demonstrate competency.

The following are general rules of forensic evidence collection:

- Each patient has only one opportunity for evidence collection. Therefore when in doubt, collect.
- Air dry specimens; never use heat. Heat will degrade biological samples.
- If the specimen was once living (e.g., blood or other body fluids), refrigerate it after collection.
- Collect and store specimens using paper or glass only, never plastic. Plastic does not breathe, and mold will grow.
- Seal, label, and initial everything to maintain the chain of custody. Do not lick envelopes or your DNA will be on the envelope.
- Separate items as they are collected so that there is no transfer of trace evidence between objects.
- Do not touch objects that may contain fingerprints (knife, gun, bullet, cartridge case). Package the evidence to preserve the prints.

- Buccal samples can be used in lieu of blood for DNA testing.
- Optimally, samples will be collected without water. If necessary, place one drop of tap water (not saline) on a swab and rub it against the biomaterial.
- Sterile collection is not essential but it is important to change gloves between sites to avoid cross-contamination.[5]

Penile specimen collection

In the event of an assault involving a male victim's penis, collect biological evidence from the penile area following these steps:
- Inspect the external structures of the penis for injury or disease using colposcopy.
- With a cotton-tip applicator, thoroughly swab the penile shaft and glans area.
- If the assault included oral copulation with the penis, swab along the penile shaft hairline and scrotal sack for saliva.
- Prepare a slide smear as directed by the forensic laboratory.
- Dry all penile swabs and slides and place them in separate, labeled envelopes provided in the kit.

Alternate light source screening

When available, a Wood's lamp or another alternate light source (infrared, ultraviolet) is used in a darkened room to screen the body and clothing for biological stains and injury. Take swabs or scrapings from any sites identified.[1]

DNA

DNA typing now is used extensively in victim and assailant identification.[1] Collection protocols—including preservation and chain of evidence—are developed by regional or state crime laboratories.

Blood standard collection

A blood standard is collected as a reference for the victim's own DNA:
- Collection tubes for the patient's blood standard usually are included in the evidence collection kit.
- Label each tube according to law enforcement and hospital policy.
- Carefully package samples placed in a rape kit to avoid breakage. Kits containing blood must be labeled as biohazardous. Refrigerate blood after collection.
- Until the kit is claimed by a law enforcement agent, the evidence collection kit may be stored in a secured refrigerator.

Blood, urine, and culture collection for medical tests

Perform toxicologic screens per protocol or as indicated, especially if the victim may have been drugged. Date rape drugs (see Chapter 49) are used for their sedative hypnotic effect on the victim. Flunitrazepam (Rohypnol) and gamma hydroxybutyric acid (GHB) are well-publicized date rape drugs, but ethanol and marijuana are by far the most common.[1,7] Other agents include ketamine, scopolamine, chloral hydrate, opiates, and barbiturates.[1] Some experts have found that a patient's elevated ethanol level is helpful in court on the basis that severely impaired victims are unable to consent to sexual relations. Nonetheless, there is also a potential for damaging the case.

Sexually transmitted disease testing

Sexually transmitted disease (STD) testing of sexual assault victims is controversial. In court, positive baseline test results may focus excessive attention on the victim's sexual history or lifestyle.[1] Although no uniform guidelines exist for postassault STD testing, the Centers for Disease Control and Prevention recommend the following baseline studies at the time of the initial examination:

- Obtain cultures for *Neisseria gonorrhoeae* and *Chlamydia trachomatis* from any site of penetration or attempted penetration.
- Collect vaginal swabs for wet mount and culture to check for *Trichomonas vaginalis*. Consider a wet mount for bacterial vaginitis and candidiasis as well if discharge, odor, or itching are present.
- Draw serum samples for human immunodeficiency virus (HIV), hepatitis B, and syphilis studies.[8]

With the patient's consent, collect vaginal cultures and other screening tests *after* evidence samples have been obtained. Any medical test that potentially can injure tissue (e.g., a Pap smear) is discouraged at this time. When collected according to protocol, initial test results are considered baseline, and positive cultures are not presumed to be the result of rape. Repeat STD tests within 1 to 2 weeks of the assault.[8] Although screening is not recommended on asymptomatic minors, positive STD results in children are reportable to the state department of children's services.

Securing and Transferring the Evidence

When securing and transferring the evidence to legal authorities, be aware of the following:

- All packaged evidence should be kept in a separate, secured, temperature-controlled location.
- If whole blood is in the evidence kit, keep the kit refrigerated in a separate and secure location until custody is transferred.
- The investigating law enforcement officer, or any agent authorized in the jurisdiction, can transfer evidence to the forensic laboratory.
- To maintain the chain of evidence, have all parties sign the evidence label, date and time the exchange, and copy the documentation for your records.

MEDICAL TREATMENT

Prophylaxis for pregnancy (females) and STDs (all patients) is recommended if the patient is at potential risk. After screening for treatment contraindications, provide prophylaxis for each of the following conditions.

Sexually Transmitted Diseases

The CDC guidelines recommend treating survivors with an empiric antimicrobial regimen for chlamydia, gonorrhea, trichomonas, and bacterial vaginitis:

- 125 mg ceftriaxone (Rocephin) intramuscularly in a single dose *plus*
- 1g azithromycin (Zithromax) orally in a single dose *plus*
- 2 g metronidazole (Flagyl) orally in a single dose *or*
- 100 mg doxycycline orally twice daily for 7 days[8]

Hepatitis B

Administer the first dose of a hepatitis B vaccine series to sexual assault survivors unimmunized at the time of the initial examination.[8]

Tetanus

Check the tetanus immunization status of patients with wounds; update as needed.

Human Immunodeficiency Virus

The following are the recommendations of the Centers for Disease Control and Prevention for the postexposure HIV assessment of patients who present within 72 hours of sexual assault:

- Review local HIV/acquired immunodeficiency syndrome epidemiology, and assess for HIV infection risks in the assailant.
- Evaluate any circumstances of the assault that may affect the risk for HIV transmission.
- Consult with an HIV treatment specialist if postexposure prophylaxis is considered.
- If the survivor chooses to receive antiviral therapy, prescribe just enough medication to last until the return visit. Reevaluate the patient 3 to 7 days after the incident to assess medication tolerance.
- Perform an HIV antibody test at the time of the original examination. Repeat studies at 6 weeks, 3 months, and 6 months.[8]

Emergency Contraception

For emergency contraception, do the following:

- Test patients for a preexisting pregnancy. Victims who test negative can be offered emergency contraception.
- A "morning after pill" is a postcoitus emergency contraceptive drug. Ovral, a combination estrogen and progesterone birth control pill, traditionally has been prescribed. Patients take two tablets immediately and another two in 12 hours. Given within 72 hours of unprotected vaginal intercourse, this drug (and several similar agents) is capable of preventing pregnancy. An antiemetic (e.g., promethazine) routinely is prescribed as well to combat the side effects of nausea and vomiting.
- See Table 45-4 for further information on emergency contraception.

Follow-up Recommendations

Historically, sexual assault survivors have been difficult to follow up for medical concerns and counseling. Several factors influence ongoing care:

- Some victims who later seek care fail to disclose their sexual assault history, making it difficult for providers to assess their postassault health and well-being fully.
- Emergency nurses and SANEs are in a position to offer comprehensive education and immediate support. This can allay concerns regarding follow-up. For example, patients can be referred to an anonymous HIV testing center or free STD clinic.
- Follow-up information should include *written* instructions.

Patient Education and Discharge Instructions

Include the following in your patient education and discharge information:

- Discuss relative STD and pregnancy risks following sexual assault.
- Teach victims the signs and symptoms of STD infection.

- Describe potential medication reactions.
- Advise patients to use condoms during intercourse until all STD screening test results are negative.
- Teach patients how to care for perineal or other injuries.
- Refer survivors to appropriate health care systems for follow-up.
- Advise medical follow-up in 2 to 4 weeks to repeat STD studies.[9]
- Inform patients about community resources such as rape crisis centers, court advocacy, and victim's compensation.

COMMUNICATION OF SEXUAL ASSAULT INFORMATION

Documentation

Figure 51-1 is an example of a documentation tool for the forensic examination. Sexual assault documentation should include the following elements.

Subjective

The subjective portion of the history summarizes the chief complaint and quotes the patient's statements and answers to the interviewer's questions.

Objective

The objective portion describes observed findings such as the character and location of injury. This portion may include drawings, photographs, and any laboratory tests and results. Note positive pregnancy and STD findings.

Assessment

The assessment portion of your documentation should avoid legal terms, such as *rape, sexual assault,* or *child abuse.* Courts actually may refuse to admit into evidence reports in which foregone legal conclusions are documented on the medical or evidentiary record. In addition, if the legal outcome does not support the medical assessment of rape or child abuse, the provider may be found liable for misdiagnosis or even malpractice. For the same reason, some prosecutors prefer that the word *patient* rather than *victim* be used.

Plan

The plan should include prescribed medical treatments and referrals.

Testimony

When called on to give testimony regarding an alleged sexual assault, the emergency nurse should consider the following points:
- Each person involved in the process of evidence collection after the complaint of a felony (such as rape) is subject to the court of jurisdiction where prosecution is a possibility.
- A fact witness is not the same as an expert witness.
- Fact witnesses may testify to items about which they have "personal knowledge."
- Personal knowledge is obtained by actual observation while participating in, or witnessing, an event.

THE UNIVERSITY HOSPITAL
CENTER FOR EMERGENCY CARE
EVIDENTIARY REPORT FOR REPORTED SEXUAL ASSAULT

SXASLT

Patient Name______________________________

Date__________ Sex _____ Age_______

S. W.

Police __________________ Badge# ________ District/Agency _________

I voluntarily consent to this examination and the gathering of potential evidence including photographs of injured areas. In some cases, this may include the use of a magnifying camera called a colposcope to document internal vaginal injuries.

I authorize the hospital to release this record and all evidence collected to the police.

SIGNATURE ______________________ Date/Time __________

TUH-412, Rev. 8/04, Page 1 of 2

S A N E

Date of Exam:________________Time of Exam:______________Hours Since Assault :___________LNMP: _____________

Bath/Shower: Yes ____ No ____Douche: Yes____ No ____ Urinated: Yes______ No _____ Defecated: yes ______ no ______

Changed Clothes: Yes ______ No ______ Smoked/Ate: Yes ______No________ Mouthwash/Brushed Teeth: Yes _____ No _____

History as stated by patient: (Patient's description of pertinent details of the assault: (oral, rectal vaginal, penetration: digital, penile, foreign objects), (oral contact), (ejaculation location, if known by the patient):

____

____

____

____

____

____

____

____

____

____

____

____

PHYSICAL EVIDENCE OF EXTRA-GENITAL TRAUMA: (Include all details of trauma - tears, lacerations, abrasions, ecchymosis, redness, bitemarks, presence of blood or other secretions.):

____

____

____

____

____

____

____

photos taken ________

Legend: T - tear, E - eechymosis, A - abrasion, R - redness, S - swelling

Signature______________________________ RN Date/Time _______________

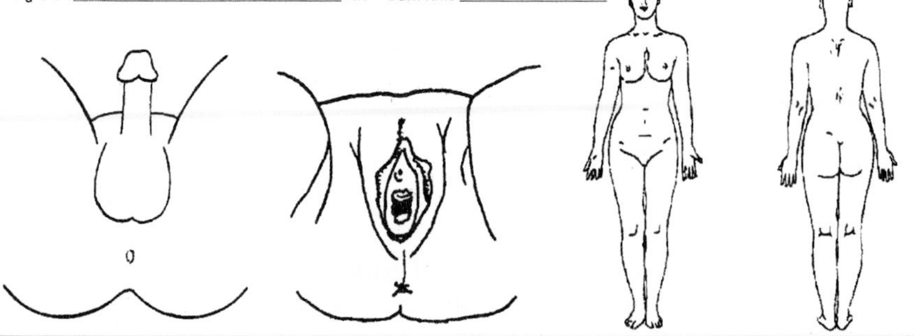

White - Medical Records; Yellow - Billing; Pink -SS; Goldenrod -Police

Figure 51-1. Sexual assault forensic form. (Courtesy University Hospital, Center for Emergency Care, Cincinnati, Ohio.)

Continued

```
*SXASLT*
```

THE UNIVERSITY HOSPITAL
CENTER FOR EMERGENCY CARE
EVIDENTIARY REPORT FOR REPORTED SEXUAL ASSAULT

TUH-412, Rev. 8/04, Page 2 of 2

S

GENITAL EXAM: (Describe any trauma. Use common English terms): Trauma Visible: Yes _____ No _____

Labia Majora: _____

Labia Minora: _____

Posterior Fourchette: _____

Hymen: _____

Vagina _____

Cervix _____

A

Penis _____

Scrotum: _____

Rectal Exam: _____

$\bar{c}$-with $\bar{s}$-without   NTN-no trauma noted   o-none   N/A-not applicable

EVIDENCE COLLECTION: (Collect and initial items below. Use stamped labels to seal envelopes. Use evidence tape to seal paper bags, blood and urine tubes. Collector dates and initials all labeled specimen envelopes; discard unused envelopes.)

N

Initial:

_____ **A. Clothing** Flouresce each item and place any stained clothing in a separate paper bag sealed with label and evidence tape.

_____   Articles submitted: _____

_____ **B. Saline swab of fluorescing body stains** (examine in dark room using Wood's lamp):

_____   Location _____

_____ **C. Loose hair on body**

_____ **D. Foreign Material** (e.g., burrs, grass, twigs)

_____ **E. Bite Mark Swabs**

E

_____ **F. Pulled head hairs** from various areas of head

_____ **G. Clipped Fingernails/Scraped** (only if blood or tissue present or freshly broken)

_____ **H. Oral Swab** (roof of mouth and lower gum line) (four dry and smear)

_____ **I. Combed Pubic Hair**

_____ **J. Clipped pubic hairs** from four different quadrants

_____ **K. Tampons/Pads** (Dry and place in envelope - never in plastic)

_____ **L. Vaginal Swabs** (at least four dry)-smear

_____ **M. Rectal Swab** (four dry)-smear

_____ **N. Penile Swab** (four dry)

_____ **O. Blood filter paper**

_____ **P. Other evidence:** _____

_____ **Q. Photographs of trauma:** (Use ruler in photo to document size) # _____

_____ **R. Colposcopy Exam**

_____ **S. #** _____ **Blood/Urine Tubes**

S A N E / S W

Examiner's Signature: _____ RN Initials: _____ Print Last Name: _____ Date/Time _____

Number of Evidence Parcels Secured: _____ Initials/Signature _____ Date/Time _____

Evidence Released By: _____ Date: _____ Time: _____

Evidence Released To: _____ Badge #: _____ Unit: _____

Figure 51-1. *Continued*

- Fact witnesses can be compelled to testify about matters personally observed.
- An expert witness is a qualified person whose role is to provide an unbiased and neutral opinion.
- The expert's opinion must be scientifically sound regarding the evidence or fact.
- An expert witness cannot be compelled to testify about his or her opinion.
  Other tips to follow when called on to give testimony are these:
- Listen to the complete question before responding.
- Respond to the question by facing the jury.
- Tell the truth.
- Remain calm.
- Be objective.
- Avoid becoming defensive or angry.
- Be prepared to spell and define medical terms.
- Ask for clarification of any question you do not understand.
- Answer only the question you are asked.
- Ask the judge for permission to speak if you feel an explanation is needed.
- Wait to answer until the judge has ruled on an objection.
- Confidently say "I do not know" when you do not know.[2]

References

1. Houmes B et al: Establishing a sexual assault nurse examiner (SANE) program in the emergency department, *J Emerg Med* 25(1):111-118, 2003.
2. Ruiz-Contreras A: Sexual assault. In Newberry L, editor: *Sheehy's emergency nursing: principles and practice,* ed 5, St Louis, 2003, Mosby.
3. Bureau of Justice Statistics, National Crime Victimization Survey: *Criminal victimization 1999: changes 1998-1999 with trend 1993-99,* Washington, DC, 2000, US Department of Justice.
4. Jordan K: Obstetrical and gynecological emergencies. In Jordan K, editor: *Emergency nursing core curriculum,* ed 5, Philadelphia, 2000, WB Saunders.
5. American College of Emergency Physicians: *Evaluation and management of the sexually assaulted or sexually abused patient,* Dallas, 1999, American College of Emergency Physicians.
6. American Academy of Pediatrics: Guidelines for the evaluation of sexual abuse of children: subject review, *Pediatrics* 103(1):188, 1999.
7. Slaughter L: Involvement of drugs in sexual assault, *J Reprod Med* (45):425-430, 2000.
8. Center for Disease Control and Prevention: Sexual assault and STDs, *MMWR* 52:69-74, 2003.
9. Botello S et al: The SANE approach to care of the adult sexual assault survivor, *Top Emerg Med* 25(3): 218-222, 2003.

Index

A

Abandonment, elder, 795
ABCDE mnemonic, 16t
Abciximab, 347t
Abdominal assessment, 84t
Abdominal emergency, 391-403. *See also* Abdominal pain
 bleeding varices as, 398-399
 Boerhaave's syndrome as, 397
 cholecystitis as, 401
 in elderly, 791
 esophageal, 395-407
  esophagitis as, 395-396
  obstruction as, 395-396
 gastritis as, 399-401
 incarcerated hernia as, 403-404
 intestinal obstruction as, 404-405
 irritable bowel syndrome as, 405-406
 Mallory-Weiss syndrome as, 396
 pancreatitis as, 402-403
 peptic ulcer as, 400
 toxic megacolon as, 407
 ulcerative colitis as, 406-407
 upper gastrointestinal bleeding as, 397
Abdominal pain, 389-407. *See also* Abdominal emergency
 assessment of, 390-395, 391t, 392t
 chronic conditions causing, 390b
 diagnostic studies for, 394-395
 endometriosis causing, 821-822
 referred, 390, 390t
 somatic, 390b
 sources of, 390t
 surgery for, 393b
 visceral, 389
Abdominal trauma, 678-689
 assessment of, 680
 to bladder, 682, 683b
 blunt, 678
 in child, 785-786
 diagnosis of, 684-688
  algorithm for, 685f
  computed tomography for, 684

Abdominal trauma *(Continued)*
  focused sonography for, 684, 680f
  peritoneal lavage for, 686-688, 687f
 to diaphragm, 683-684
 gastric, 682
 hypovolemic shock in, 679b
 intestinal, 683, 684b
 to liver, 681, 681b
 to major vessels, 684
 pancreatic, 682
 penetrating, 678-679
 in pregnant patient, 688
 renal, 682, 682b
 signs and symptoms of, 679b
 splenic, 681
 ureteral, 682
 urethral, 683
Abducens nerve
 function of, 94t
 in head injury, 615
Abortion
 care after, 802-803
 complete, 801
 incomplete, 801
 inevitable, 801
 missed, 802
 septic, 802
 spontaneous, 800b
 threatened, 801
Abrasion
 corneal, 754
 wound care for, 201-202
Abruptio placentae, 776, 805-806
Abscess
 dental or periodontal, 593
 perinephric, 512
 peritonsillar, 591-592
 wound care for, 202
Abuse
 child, 857-869
  approach to child, 865-868
  behavioral signs of, 860-861
  categories of, 858-859
  conditions mimicking, 867b
  duty to report, 859-860
  emotional, 859, 859t

The letter b indicates a box, f indicates a figure, and t indicates a table.

Abuse *(Continued)*
  factors contributing to, 860b
  Munchausen syndrome by proxy as, 861,
    856-857, 866t
  prevention of, 868
  signs of, 861, 862t, 863f, 856f
  elder, 795
  sexual, 862t, 907-920. *See also* Sexual assault
  substance, 887-888, 891-900. *See also*
    Substance abuse
Abuse and neglect, 857-869
Accelerated rhythm
  idioventricular, 163t, 163f
  junctional escape, 152, 152f, 153t
Access device, vascular, 128
Accident
  cerebrovascular, 382-385
  vehicular
    elderly and, 794-795
    mechanism of injury in, 600t
Acetabulum fracture, 708-709, 709f
Acetaminophen
  antidote for, 487t
  dose and duration of, 237t
  poisoning with, 467-468
Acetylsalicylic acid, 237t
Achilles tendon rupture, 716
Acid burn of eye, 755
Acoustic nerve
  function of, 94t
  in head injury, 615
Acquired immunodeficiency syndrome
  as blood-borne infection, 529-531
  sexually transmitted, 524t
Across-the-room assessment, 68-69, 69t
Activated charcoal, 460-461, 460b, 461b
Acute condition
  adrenal insufficiency, 438-439
  anxiety attack, 876-877
  cystitis, 515
  delirium, 886
  grief, 877
  laryngotracheobronchitis, 839
  narcosis, 894
  psychotic reaction, 881-883
  subdural hematoma, 630
  transplant rejection, 421
Acute coronary syndrome, 337-347. *See also*
  Coronary syndrome, acute
Acute vs. chronic pain, 229t
Acute respiratory distress syndrome,
  319-321, 320b

Addison's disease, 438-439
Adjunct, airway, 298-301, 300f
Adjuvant for pain, 236, 240t
Adolescent
  growth and development of, 828t-829t
  immunization recommendations for, 535f
Adrenal insufficiency, 438-439
Adrenalin
  in topical anesthetic, 237t
  in wound management, 201
Adult abuse, 868-869
Advance directive, 28, 28t, 245-246,
  246t, 248t
Advanced life support, 279, 288-289, 288b
  for asystole, 285t-286t
  for child, 832
  for pediatric pulseless arrest, 287f
  for pulseless electrical activity,
    283t-284t
  for pulseless ventricular tachycardia,
    280t-282t
Adverse reaction to transfusion, 121t, 122
Advocate
  communication through, 4
  for victim of domestic violence, 904
AEIOU_TIPS, 378b
Affect, assessment of, 873
African American culture, 19t
Afterload
  in cardiogenic shock, 361
  definition of, 178b
Age
  abdominal pain and, 389
  immunization schedule by, 529f-531f
  of suicidal patient, 879
  vital signs related to, 88t
Age-specific assessment, 85t
Agnosia, 877
AIDS, 516t
Air-borne infection, 536, 536-548. *See also*
  Infection, air-borne
Air-borne precautions, 529b
Air embolism, 508
Air transport
  helicopter, 36t, 37-38
  medical record for, 41f-42f
Airway assessment in trauma, 294, 601
  abdominal, 680
  burn injury, 768
  chest, 652
  in child, 783
  facial, 740t

Airway assessment in trauma *(Continued)*
  in head injury, 620
  in pregnant patient, 775
Airway management
  alternate airway devices for, 301
  assessment, 294
  of difficult airway, 302, 304
  history, 294
  nasopharyngeal airway for, 300, 300f
  oropharyngeal airway for, 298-299, 298f
  in pediatric cardiopulmonary arrest, 831t
  in pediatric emergency, 832-833
  tracheal intubation for, 301, 301f
  ventilation for, 299, 301, 305t
Airway obstruction
  allergic reaction causing, 296-297
  angioedema causing, 297-298
  in child, 836-837
  epiglottitis causing, 295, 295f
  foreign body causing, 297
  oxygen therapy for, 298, 298t
Alanine aminotransferase, 134t
Alarm, ventilator, 305t
Albumin, 133t
Albuterol, 563
Alcohol abuse, 892
  CAGE questionnaire related to, 86b
  immunization recommendations in, 534f
  prevention of, 459
Alcohol emergency, 450-455
  acute intoxication as, 450-452
  seizures as, 452
  withdrawal as, 452-453
Alcohol poisoning, 486t-487t, 488
Algorithm
  for abdominal trauma, 685f
  for bradycardia in child, 833f
  for emergency thoracotomy, 674f
  for pediatric pulseless arrest, 287f
  for pulseless arrest in child, 835t
  for tachycardia in child, 826t
Alkali burn of eye, 755
Alkaline phosphatase, 134t
Allen test, 125f
Allergen, 563
Allergy, 563-571
  airway obstruction from, 296-297
  anaphylactic shock in, 358
  to anesthetic, 200
  definition of, 563
  diagnostic tests for, 565
  hypersensitivity reaction in, 561t

Allergy *(Continued)*
  cytotoxic, 561t, 563-564
  delayed, 561t, 564-565
  immediate, 564, 565t, 566-567
  immune complex–mediated,
    561t, 564
  immune response in, 563-564
  immunoglobulins in, 564
  latex, 565-566
  in triage, 71t
Aloe poisoning, 478t
Alpha particle, 222
Alprazolam, overdose of, 469-470
Alteplase, 381b
  for myocardial infarction, 346t
Altered level of consciousness, 378-380,
  378b, 379b
Alternate airway device, 301
Alternate light source screening, 914
Alternative access device
  dialysis, 106
  intraosseous needle, 106-107
Alternative medical system, 262t
Altitude, pulmonary edema and, 323-324
Alveolar osteitis, 594
Alzheimer's disease, 877-878
Amaurosis fugax, 582
Ambulance, paramedic, 35, 36t
American Heart Association
  on advanced life support, 279
  on basic life support, 277-278
  on monophasic defibrillator, 288
American Hospital Association, 8t
American Indian culture, 19t
Americum, 222t
Amitriptyline
  cardiac arrest caused by, 290t
  for pain, 240t
Amniotic fluid, meconium-stained,
  811-812
Amphetamine, 290t
Amputation
  of ear, 757
  traumatic, 732
Amylase
  measurement of, 135
  normal serum values for, 134t
  in pregnancy, 774t
Analgesic, 236, 237t-240t
  bowel obstruction and, 250
  poisoning with, 463-466
  types of, 236

Anaphylactic shock, 358, 368-370, 369f
Anaphylaxis
    definition of, 563
    latex causing, 566
    as transfusion reaction, 121t
Anatomy, chest, 650, 651f, 642
Anemia, 415-416, 415b, 415t
Anesthesia
    spinal, neurogenic shock in, 370-371,
        370f
    topical, 237t
    in wound management, 199-200
Aneurysm, dissecting aortic
    chest pain in, 328t-329t
    symptoms of, 328t
Angina, 330, 339, 340
    chest pain in, 328t-329t
    common sites for, 340f
    Ludwig's, 592
    symptoms of, 330
    types of, 339t
    unstable, 339
    Vincent's, 593t
Angioedema, 297-298
Angiography in head injury, 618-619
Angiotensin-converting enzyme inhibitor,
    244, 347t
Angle-closure glaucoma, 579
Angle of Louis, 652
Aniline, 487t
Anistreplase, 346t
Ankle
    dislocation of, 720t, 728-729, 728f
    fracture of, 714-716, 715f
Antabuse reaction, 454-455
Anterior cord syndrome, 639
Anterior epistaxis, 587-590, 588f, 589f
Anterior fossa fracture, 623
Antianxiety drug, 469-470
Antibiotic
    in asthma, 316
    ophthalmic, 576b
Antibody, 563
    in immune complex–mediated reaction,
        564
Anticholinergic drug
    antidote for, 487t
    for asthma, 844
Anticoagulant
    antidote for, 487t
    for myocardial infarction, 343, 344t

Antidepressant, tricyclic
    antidote for, 487t
    poisoning with, 467-468, 467b
Antidiuretic hormone
    in diabetes insipidus, 433-434
    inappropriate secretion of, 434-435
    in shock, 359t
Antidote, poison, 486t-487t, 486
Antidysrhythmic drug, 290t
Antigen
    common, 564, 566
    definition of, 563
Antipsychotic dystonic reaction, 888-889
Antisepsis in wound management, 197
Antivenin
    scorpion, 495
    for snakebite, 491
    spider, 493
Anuria, 514
Anxiety disorder
    chest pain with, 330t
    as mental health emergency, 875-879
Aorta, abdominal trauma and, 684
Aortic aneurysm, dissecting
    chest pain in, 328t-329t
    symptoms of, 328t
Aortic disruption, 671-672
Aortic dissection, thoracic, 354-356, 355f
Aortic stenosis, 372
Aortic valve injury, 669
Aphasia, 877
Apnea
    in child, 839-840
    Munchausen syndrome by proxy and,
        866t
Apneustic respiration, 89t
Appearance, assessment of, 873
Appendicitis, 853-854
Applanation tonometry, 580b
Apraxia, 877
Arab culture, 19t
Arachnid bite/sting
    black widow spider, 492-493
    brown recluse spider, 493-494
    scorpion, 494-495
Arbus precatorius, 478t
ARDS, 319-321, 320b
Arm, fractured, 700-704
Arrest, cardiopulmonary, 277-293. See also
        Cardiopulmonary arrest
Arsenic, 486t, 487t

Arterial blood gases
  in asthma, 316
  normal values of, 133t
  in pregnancy, 774t
  specimen collection for, 125-127, 125f
Arterial pressure monitoring, 177-180, 178b, 179b, 179f
  pulmonary, 182-192. *See also* Pulmonary artery pressure monitoring
Arterial puncture, 125-127
Arteritis, temporal, 375
Artery
  in abdominal trauma, 684
  retinal, occlusion of, 576
Aspartate aminotransferase, 134t
Aspiration
  of foreign body, 297
  of joint, 131-132
  nasopharyngeal, 132-133
  percutaneous, 131
Aspirin
  dose and duration of, 237t
  for myocardial infarction, 347t
  poisoning with, 465
Asplenia, 534f
Assault, sexual, 907-920. *See also* Sexual assault
Assaultive behavior, 884-885
Assessment, 82-98
  age-specific considerations in, 85t
  of burn, 768
  CAGE questionnaire in, 86b
  for domestic violence, 86b
  of facial trauma, 745, 747, 748
  gender neutral, 86b
  general, 82-83
  history in, 83, 85, 86b, 87b
  mental health, 871, 872t, 873-874
  of musculoskeletal trauma
    inspection in, 692
    neurovascular, 691-692
    palpation in, 693
  objective, 88
  pain, 87t, 228-236. *See also* Pain, assessment of
    in children, 231, 232t-236t
    documentation of, 231
    in elderly, 236
  of pediatric emergency
    primary, 824-825, 826t-830t
    secondary, 829
  physical examination in, 92-93

Assessment *(Continued)*
  primary survey, 83t
  of respiratory emergency, 307
  secondary, 84t
  of sexual assault victim, 909-910
  subjective, 86-87
  of suicidal patient, 878-879
  systems, 93-97
    cardiovascular, 94-95
    endocrine, 97
    gastrointestinal, 95-96
    genitourinary, 96
    of head, ears, eyes, nose, and throat, 94
    hematologic, 96
    immunologic, 97
    integumentary, 96, 97t
    musculoskeletal system, 96
    neurologic, 93, 93t
    respiratory, 95
  of trauma. *See* Trauma, assessment of
  of unconscious patient, 379b
  of victim of domestic violence, 903
  of vital signs, 88-92
    blood pressure, 90
    height, weight, and head circumference, 91-92
    orthostatic, 90, 91b
    oxygen saturation, 89-90
    pulse, 89
    pulse pressure, 90
    respirations, 89, 89t
    shock index, 91
    temperature, 88
  wound, 197
Asthma
  cardiac arrest in, 291t
  in child, 842-844
  emergency treatment of, 318-320
Asymmetry in facial trauma, 741
Asystole, 164-165, 165t, 165f
  life support for, 285t-286t
Ataxic respiration, 889t
Atenolol
  cardiac arrest caused by, 290t
  for myocardial infarction, 344t
Atrial dysrhythmia, 142-148, 143t, 143f
  fibrillation, 145-146, 145t, 145f
  flutter, 144-145, 145t, 145f
  premature complexes, 143-144, 144t, 144f
  wandering pacemaker, 146-147, 146f, 148t

Atrioventricular block, 153-158
    first-degree, 153, 154t, 154f
    second-degree, 153-156, 155t, 155f
    third-degree, 156-158, 157t, 157f
Atrioventricular junction dysrhythmia,
        147-153
    accelerated junctional rhythm, 152-153,
        152f, 153t
    escape rhythm, 151-152, 151f, 152f
    paroxysmal supraventricular tachycardia,
        147-150, 149t, 149f
    premature complexes, 150-151, 150f, 151t
Auricular laceration, 757
Auscultation
    in abdominal pain, 390
    in assessment, 92
Australasia Triage Scale, 65-66, 66t
Authority in mass casualty incident
        management, 53t
Automatic external defibrillation, 278-279
Automatic implantable cardioverter-
        defibrillator, 288-289
Automobile accident
    elderly and, 794-795
    mechanism of injury in, 600t
Autotransfusion of chest blood, 665-666
Avulsion
    of tooth, 760, 760b
    wound management of, 202-203, 203f
Avulsion fracture, 702t
Axillary crutches, 737
Axis, phlebostatic, 190f
Axis of electrocardiogram, 172, 173b
    deviation in, 338f
Axonal injury, diffuse, 626-627
Azalea poisoning, 478t

B

B cell in immune response, 564
B-type natriuretic peptide, 350b
Babinski reflex, 616
Bacillus cereus, 472t-473t
Back, assessment of, 84t
Bacterial infection. *See also* Infection
    in food poisoning, 472-474, 472t, 473t
    pneumonia, in child, 842t
    in septic shock, 366
    vaginosis, 821
Bag-valve mask, 299t
Barrier against radiation exposure, 222
Bartholin cyst, 812t

Basic life support, 277-278, 278f, 278t
    for asystole, 289t
    for pulseless electrical activity, 283-284t
    for pulseless ventricular tachycardia, 280t
Basilar skull fracture, 622, 623
Battle sign, 624f
Bee sting, 495-496
Behavior, homicidal, 884-885
Behavioral response to pain, 229t
Behavioral signs of abuse, 860-861
Belief about diversity, 16, 16t
Bell's palsy, 568-569, 569f
Benign tumor, pheochromocytoma as, 439
Benzodiazepine
    antidote for, 487t
    poisoning with, 473-474
Beta-adrenergic blocking agent
    antidote for, 487t
    cardiac arrest caused by, 290t
    for myocardial infarction, 344, 344t
Beta particle, 222
Bilirubin
    normal blood values of, 133t
    in pregnancy, 774t
Bioimpedance, 175
Biological-based therapy, 262t
Biological weapon
    categories of, 219b
    infection control for, 220t-221t
    mass prophylaxis for, 218
Biot's respiration, 89t
Birth, 806-811, 806b, 806t, 807f, 808f, 810f
Bite, 207-208
    snake, 486-488
    spider, 492-494
Black widow spider
    bite of, 492-493
    venom of, 486t
Bladder
    infection of, 515
    trauma to, 682, 683b
    urinary retention and, 517-518
Blast injury, 216
Bleeding, 408-419. *See also* Hematologic
        disorder
    after tooth extraction, 594
    in dialysis patient, 526
    at end of life, 250-251
    hematuria and, 514
    in hyphema, 751
    intracranial, 627

Bleeding *(Continued)*
 lower gastrointestinal, 405
 Munchausen syndrome by proxy and, 866t
 postpartum, 815-816
 in pregnancy, 804-806
 in trauma patient, 602
 upper gastrointestinal, 397-398
 vaginal, 816
Bleeding time, normal, 133t
Bleeding varices, 398-399
Blepharitis, 577, 576b
Blindness
 corneal ulcer and, 576
 in glaucoma, 579
 keratitis causing, 580
 retinal artery occlusion causing, 576
 transient monocular, 582
 uveitis causing, 581-582
Block
 atrioventricular, 153-158, 154t, 154f, 155t,
  155f, 157t, 157f
 in wound management, 201
Blood
 autotransfusion of, 665-666
 in hemothorax, 664-666, 664f
 hyphema and, 751
 in semen, 516
 toxicologic study of, 135
 in urine, 514
Blood administration set, 102
Blood-borne infection, 526-532, 535-536
 acquired immunodeficiency syndrome,
  530-531
 hepatitis B, 531-532
 hepatitis C, 532, 535
Blood cell count, white, 135-136
Blood disorder, 408-419. *See also* Hematologic
  disorder
Blood gases, arterial
 in asthma, 316
 normal values of, 133t
 in pregnancy, 774t
Blood glucose, 134
Blood loss by site of injury, 362t
Blood pressure
 assessment of, 88t, 90
 of child, 825
 estimating, 603b
 normal, 179b
 in pregnancy, 803-804
Blood product, 359, 364t

Blood sampling from implanted port, 116
Blood specimen
 in abdominal pain, 390-391
 arterial
  aftercare for, 127
  Allen's test for, 125f
  blood gas values and, 127, 127t
  care of specimen of, 126
  equipment for, 126
  general principles of, 125
  procedure for, 126
 for culture, 129-130
 heel stick for, 127-128, 128f
 normal values of, 133, 133t
 point-of-care testing and, 128-129, 129t
 in sexual assault, 914
 from vascular access device, 128
 venous
  finding vein for, 123-124, 123f
  procedure for, 124-125
Blood transfusion, 117-122. *See also*
  Transfusion
Blood urea nitrogen
 measurement of, 134
 in pregnancy, 774t
Blood vessel trauma, 684
Blunt trauma
 abdominal, 678
 cardiac, 668-669
Board, state, 21-22
Body movement, assessment of, 873
Body piercing, 594, 595f, 595t
 facial trauma and, 741
Boerhaave's syndrome, 397
Bone, 690
 fracture of. *See* Fracture
 osteomyelitis of, 733-734
Bony thorax fracture, 654-658
 clavicular, 658
 flail chest and, 655-657, 656f
 rib, 654-655
 sternal, 657
Bordetella pertussis, 545-546
Botulism, 472t-473t, 474
 antidote for, 486t
Bowel
 intussusception of, 854-855
 irrigation of, 461-462
 irritable, 405-406
 obstruction of, at end of life, 250
 volvulus of, 855

Boyle's law, 507
Bradycardia
    in child, 833f
    fetal, 812-813
Bradypnea, 89t
Brain
    bleeding in, 627
    concussion of, 625-626
    contusion of, 627
    diffuse axonal injury to, 626-627
    epidural hematoma and, 628
    herniation of, 634-635
    metastasis to, 249t
    shock affecting, 360b
    subdural hematoma of, 628-631, 629f,
        630f
Brain death, 257, 257b, 259
Breath odor, 457t
Breathing
    absence of, in child, 831-832
    in allergic reaction, 563
    in pediatric assessment, 825
    in pediatric cardiopulmonary arrest, 831t
    in trauma
        abdominal, 680
        assessment of, 602
        burn injury, 768
        chest, 652
        in child, 780, 781f, 782
        facial, 740t
        head, 620
        in pregnant patient, 775
Breech position of fetus, 813-814, 813f, 814f
Broken tooth, 760
Bronchiolitis, 840-841
Bronchitis
    acute, 317-318
    chronic, 318-319
Bronchodilator
    in asthma, 316
    for chronic obstructive pulmonary
        disease, 319
Broselow tape system, 781f
Brown recluse spider bite, 493-494
Brown-Séquard syndrome, 639
Bruise
    from abuse, 862t
    management of, 203-204, 204f, 205f
Bulbocavernous reflex, 634
Bupivacaine, 200
Buprenorphine, 239t

Burn
    from abuse, 862t, 863f
    assessment of, 768-769
    causes off, 762t
    chemical, 770
    classification of, 763-768
        depth and, 763, 764f
    corneal, 754-755
    in elderly, 794
    electrical, 772
    escharotomy sites in, 770, 771f
    extent of, 763, 765f, 766f, 767-768
    friction, 772
    hydrofluoric acid, 486t
    lightning, 506-507
    Parkland resuscitation formula for, 763b
    severity of, 762-763, 762-772
    tar, 770
    wound care of, 769-770
Bursitis, 730-731
Butorphanol, 239t
Butterfly needle, 103
Bypass graft, coronary artery, 331t

C
Cadmium poisoning, 486t
CAGE questionnaire, 86b
Caladium poisoning, 479t
Calcaneus fracture, 711-712, 712f
Calcium
    cardiac arrest and, 289t
    cardiac rhythm changes and, 440t
    hypercalcemia and, 439
    hypocalcemia and, 442-443
    in pregnancy, 768t
Calcium channel blocker
    cardiac arrest caused by, 290t
    poisoning with, 470-471
Calcium chloride, 447
Calculation of intravenous flow rate, 103b
Calculus, renal, 509
Cambodian culture, 19t
Campylobacter jejuni, 472, 472t-473t
Canadian Triage and Acuity Scale, 66, 66t
Candidal infection, genital, 821
Cane, 736
Cannula, nasal, 299t. *See also* Catheter
Cannulation, central vein, 111
Capnometry, sublingual, 176
Capsicum, 479t
Captopril, 347t

Carbamate, 486t
Carbamate poisoning, 480-481, 481t
Carbamazepine, 240t
Carbon dioxide
  end-expiratory, 175-176, 176b
  normal blood values of, 133t
Carbon monoxide poisoning, 322-323, 322t,
    470-471
  antidote for, 487t
  cardiac arrest caused by, 290t
Carboxyhemoglobin, 322t
Carbuncle, renal, 512
Cardiac emergency, 326-356. *See also*
    Cardiopulmonary arrest
  angina as, 337, 339t, 340f
  assessment in
    of chest pain, 327t, 330, 330t-333t
    of rhythm, 326, 334f-336f, 333, 334f
  chest pain in
    assessment of, 326, 327t, 330t-333t
    differential diagnosis of, 328t-329t
  fetal bradycardia as, 812-813
  heart failure as, 347-335, 348t, 349b,
    349b
  malignant hypertension as, 350-341, 350t
  myocardial infarction as, 338-347. *See also*
    Myocardial infarction
  pericarditis as, 351-353, 351t
  risk factors for, 327b
  tamponade as, 353-354, 354f
  therapeutic interventions in, 340
  thoracic aortic dissection as, 354-356, 355f
Cardiac index, 187b
Cardiac injury
  blunt, 668-669
  penetrating, 669-670
  pericardial tamponade in, 670-6671, 671f
Cardiac marker, 135, 342t
Cardiac output
  in cardiogenic shock, 361
  pulmonary artery pressure monitoring for,
    187-188, 187b, 188f
Cardiac rhythm, electrolytes affecting,
    440t-441t
Cardiac tamponade, 353-354, 354f
Cardiogenic pulmonary edema, 313
Cardiogenic shock, 358, 363-366, 369f
Cardiopulmonary arrest, 277-293
  advanced life support for, 279, 288-289, 288b
  asystole, 285t-286t
  automatic external defibrillation for, 278-279

Cardiopulmonary arrest *(Continued)*
  automatic implantable cardioverter-
    defibrillator for, 288-289
  basic life support for, 277-278, 278f, 278t
  cause of
    drug-related, 290t
    metabolic, 289t
    by system, 291t-292t
  in child, 283t, 831-836, 832t, 833f-835f, 836
  pulseless electrical activity in, 283t-284t
  pulseless ventricular tachycardia in, 280t-282t
  special considerations in, 293
  in unusual settings, 293b
  ventricular fibrillation in, 280t-282t
Cardiopulmonary resuscitation guidelines, 278t
Cardiovascular assessment, 94-95
Cardiovascular system
  age-related changes in, 790t
  age-related considerations in, 85t
  in allergic reaction, 566
  cardiac arrest and, 291t
  cocaine affecting, 892b
Cardioverter-defibrillator, automatic
    implantable, 288-289
Caregiver, Munchausen syndrome by proxy
    and, 861, 856-857, 866t
Carotid artery, 578
Carotid artery angiography, 618-619
Carpal bone fracture, 703-704
Carpal tunnel syndrome, 731
Cartilage, 691
Castor bean poisoning, 478t
Cat bite, 208
Cathartic, 461
Catheter
  for central venous pressure monitoring, 180,
    180t
  for dialysis, 106, 525
  Foley, 590b
  intraosseous, 106-107, 113-114
  for intravenous therapy
    central venous, 104-105
    for child, 109-110, 110f
    in elderly, 111
    midline and midclavicular, 105-106
    peripheral, 103-104
    peripherally inserted central, 105
    sizes of, 104, 104t
  for pulmonary artery pressure monitoring,
    182-183, 183f
  Word, 819, 820f

Cauda equina syndrome, 639
Cavernous sinus thrombosis, 571
Cell in immune response, 564-564
Cell-mediated hypersensitivity reaction,
    564-565
Cellulitis
    in Ludwig's angina, 592
    periorbital, 570
Centers for Medicare and Medical Services, 27
Central American culture, 19t
Central brain herniation, 634-635
Central catheter, peripherally inserted,
    105-106
Central cord syndrome, 639
Central nervous system. *See also* Neurologic
        entries
    age-related changes in, 790t
    in allergic reaction, 566
    cocaine affecting, 892b
    depression of, 866t
Central neurogenic hyperventilation, 89t
Central retinal artery occlusion, 576
Central vein cannulation, 111
Central venous access, 104-105
Central venous pressure, 112, 180-182, 180b,
    180t, 181f, 182f
Cerebral angiography, 618-619
Cerebral perfusion pressure, 619
Cerebrospinal fluid
    collection of, 130-131
    in facial trauma, 741
    in head injury, 619b
Cerebrovascular accident, 382-385
    classification of, 384t
    hemorrhagic stroke and, 384
    interventions for, 385
    ischemic stroke and, 384
    scales for, 382t, 383t
    screening for, 383b
    signs and symptoms of, 384-385
Cerumen impaction, 585, 585b
Cervical spinal immobilization, 645-646, 645f
Cervical spine in facial trauma, 740t
Cesarean delivery, perimortem, 778
Cesium, 222t
Chain of custody of evidence, 29
Chalazion, 576-579
Chancroid, 522-523
Charcoal, activated, 460-461, 460b, 461b
Charcoal hemoperfusion, 462
Chemical, inhalant abuse and, 894-895

Chemical burn
    causes of, 762t
    of eye, 754-755
    hydrofluoric acid, 486t
    management of, 770
Chemical weapon, 216-218
Chest
    assessment of, 84t
        in elderly, 791
    flail, 655-657, 656f
Chest pain
    assessment of, 326, 327t, 330t-333t
    differential diagnosis of, 328t-329t
Chest trauma, 650-677
    anatomy related to, 650, 651f, 642
    aortic disruption in, 671-672
    assessment of
        of airway, 652
        of breathing, 652
        of circulation, 653
        of disability, 653
    breathing assessment in, 602
    cardiac injury in
        blunt, 668-669
        penetrating, 669-670
        pericardial tamponade in, 670-671, 671f
    emergent thoracotomy in, 673, 674f, 675b
    fracture in
        clavicular, 658
        flail chest and, 65-657, 656f
        rib, 654-655
        sternal, 657
    hemothorax in, 664-666, 665f
    lung injury in, 666-668
    pneumothorax in
        open, 662, 663b, 664b
        simple, 658-660, 659f
        tension, 660, 661f
    ruptured diaphragm in, 676
    ruptured esophagus caused by, 668-670
Chest tube, 663, 663b, 664b
Chest x-ray in asthma, 316
Cheyne-Stokes respirations, definition of, 89t
Chief complaint, 71t
Chilblains, 499
Child. *See* Pediatric *entries*
Child-resistant container, 462-463
Childbirth, 806-811
Chinese culture, 19t
CHIPE, 457t
Chipped tooth, 760

Chlamydia trachomatis, 520t
  epididymitis and, 517
Chloral hydrate, 243t
Chlordiazepoxide overdose, 469-470
Chlorhexidine, 197
Chloride
  normal blood values of, 133t
  in pregnancy, 768t
Cholecystitis, 401
  chest pain in, 328t-329t
Choline magnesium, 237t
Chronic obstructive pulmonary disease,
    318-319
  immunization recommendations in, 534f
Chronic paroxysmal hemicrania, 376t-377t
Chronic subdural hematoma, 625
Chronic transplant rejection, 421
Chronic vs. acute pain, 229t
CIAMPEDS mnemonic, 70, 71t-72t
Cigarette burn, 863f
Cimetidine, 563
Cimino-Brescia fistula, 525
Circulation
  in allergic reaction, 563
  in pediatric assessment, 825
  in pediatric cardiopulmonary arrest, 831t
  in trauma, 602-603
    abdominal, 680
    burn injury, 768-769
    chest, 653
    in child, 782
    facial, 740t
    head injury, 620
    in pregnant patient, 775
Circumference, head, 91-92
Clavicular fracture, 696, 698, 698f
Cleaning of equipment in bioterrorism, 220t
Cleansing, of wound, 198
Clorazepate, 469-470
Closed pneumothorax, 658-660, 659f
Clostridium botulinum, 470t-473t, 474
Clostridium perfringens, 470, 470t-473t
Clostridium tetanus, 557-558
  wound management and, 198-199
Closure, wound, 208-212, 209-212
  of contaminated wound, 208
  materials for, 208-209
  suture removal and, 209t
  techniques for, 209-211, 211f, 212f
Clotted dialysis access, 525
Clotting factor, 530f

Club drug, 897-900
  ecstasy, 897-900
  flunitrazepam, 899-900
  gamma hydroxybutyrate, 899
  ketamine, 898-899
Cluster headache, 376t-377t
Coagulation, 133t
Coagulation study, 136
Coarctation of aorta, 372
Cobalt, 222t
Cocaine
  abuse of, 892-893, 892b
  antidote for, 486t
  cardiac arrest caused by, 290t
  chest pain caused by, 331t
  in topical anesthetic, 237t
Codeine, 238t
Cognition, assessment of, 874
Colchicine poisoning, 479t
Cold-induced injury, 499-504
  chilblains, 499
  frostbite, 499-502, 500f
  hypothermia, 502-504, 503t
  immersion foot, 499
Cold shock, 367-368
Colitis, ulcerative, 406-407
Collapsed lung. *See* Pneumothorax
Colles' fracture, 704
Collision
  elderly in, 794-795
  mechanism of injury in, 600t
Color, skin, 97t
Color pain rating scale, 235t
Colubridae, 490-491
Coma
  differential diagnosis of, 378b
  hyperosmolar hyperglycemic nonketotic,
    431-433, 431t
  myxedema, 432
Coma scale, 93, 93t
Combitube, 301
Command system for mass casualty incident
    management, 51, 52f, 53t
Comminuted fracture, 696t, 697f
Communication, 3-13
  American Hospital Association guidelines
    for, 8t
  by child, 827t, 829t
  confidential, 7
  in crisis mode, 3-4
  of critical patient reports, 7-8

Communication (*Continued*)
  diversity and, 16t, 17
  with emergency medical services personnel,
    8-9, 12f
  with inpatient units, 9-11
  in interagency transport, 39-40
  JCAHO documentation of, 6
  in mass casualty incident management, 53t
  with mass media representatives, 7
  of patient identification, 5, 7
  standards for, 5
  technology to aid, 11
  through patient representatives, 4
  written, 4-5
Compartment syndrome, 734-735
Complement deficiency, 530f
Complementary and alternative medicine,
    261-270
  classification of, 262t
  drug-herb interactions and, 263, 264t-271t
  overview of, 261-262
  patient history related to, 262-263
Complete abortion, 801
Complete atrioventricular block, 156-158, 157t,
    157f
Complete blood count
  in asthma, 316
  elements of, 134
  normal, 133t
Complete spinal cord lesion, 639
Comprehensive triage, 63, 63b
Compressed fracture, 696t, 697f
Compression, spinal cord, 250
Computed tomography
  for abdominal trauma, 684
  in head injury, 618
Condition, patient, 8t
Condyloma, 820t
Confidentiality
  of communication, 7
  as legal issue, 22-23
Conium maculatum, 478t
Conjunctival laceration, 753-754
Conjunctivitis, 576-577, 579
Conscious sedation, 201
Consciousness
  altered level of, 378-380, 378b, 379b
  in facial trauma, 740t
Consent
  as legal issue, 24-25
  for organ donation, 258f

Consultation in head injury, 620
Contact dermatitis, 564
  latex-induced, 566
Contact lens removal, 574f
Contact precautions, 529b
Contaminated wound, 208
Contamination, radiation, 219-223
  as emergency, 222
  initial interventions for, 222-223
  ionizing vs. nonionizing, 219
  particles vs. waves, 219
  radionuclides produced by, 222t
Contraception after sexual assault, 916
Contraceptive emergency, 822t
Contractility, cardiac, 178b
Contracture, Volkmann's ischemic, 736
Contraindication for peritoneal lavage, 687-688
Contusion
  of brain, 621
  myocardial, 668-669
  pulmonary, 666-667
  wound management of, 203-204, 204f, 205f
Conversion formula for weight, 91b
Cord
  prolapsed umbilical, 814-815, 815f
  spinal
    compression of, 250
    injury to, 638
Core processes, 6b
Cornea
  abrasion of, 754
  burn of, 754-755
  inflammation of, 576-577
  laceration of, 753-754
  ulcer of, 576-577
Corneal reflex, 616
Coronary artery bypass graft, 331t
Coronary artery in myocardial infarction,
    341t, 341f
Coronary syndrome, acute, 337-347
  angina as, 337, 339t, 340f
  myocardial infarction as. *See* Myocardial
    infarction
Corticosteroid for asthma, 843
Corynebacterium diphtheriae, 546-547
Cough
  triage and, 79t
  whooping,
Cramp, heat, 504
Cranial nerve
  assessment of, 94t

Cranial nerve *(Continued)*
    in Bell's palsy, 568-569, 569f
    in head injury, 620-621
    injury to, 759
Crazy Glue in eye, 582-583
Creatine phosphokinase, 134t
Creatinine
    measurement of, 135
    normal blood values of, 133t
    in pregnancy, 768t
Cricothyrotomy, 304, 305f
Crime, evidence collection and, 28-30, 29b, 30b
Crisis, hyperthyroid, 435-436
Crisis communication, 3-13. *See also*
        Communication
Critical care transport, 35, 36t, 37
CroFab, 487
Crotalidae, 490-491
Croup syndrome, 838-839
Crutches, 736-737
Cryoprecipitate transfusion, 119t, 120
Crystalloid infusion, 359, 364t
Cucyta maculata, 478t
Cultural factors
    dilemmas related to, 18
    in end-of-life care, 18, 19t-20t
    practice model of diversity and, 16-18, 16t
    visibility vs. invisibility and, 15-16
Culture
    in asthma, 315
    blood, 129-130
    reporting of, 8, 9f
    in sexual assault, 914
Customer service representative, 4
Cutaneous allergic reaction, 562
Cyanide
    cardiac arrest caused by, 290t
    in inhalation injury, 321
    poisoning with, 471
Cyanoacrylate exposure, 582-583
Cyst
    Bartholin, 820t
    ovarian, 817
Cystitis, 515
Cytotoxic hypersensitivity reaction, 561t,
        563-564

D

Dalteparin, 344t
Data accuracy in pulmonary artery pressure
        monitoring, 190-191, 190f, 191f, 192f

Date rape drug, 897-900
Datura, 479t
Death
    brain, 257, 257b, 259
    cesarean delivery after, 778
    of child, 252
        by abuse, 857
    cultural practices related to, 19t-20t
    fall-related, 793-794
    fetal, 253
    from Munchausen syndrome by proxy, 861
    notification of, 251-252
    organ donation and, 257, 257b, 259
    sudden infant, 832
Decompression sickness, 509-510
Decontamination
    after chemical weapon attack, 216-218
    after radiation attack, 223
    gut, 462-466
    supplies for, 225t
Deep frostbite, 500-503
Deep partial thickness burn, 763, 764f
Deep tendon reflex, 616
Defibrillation, 288-289, 288b
    automatic external, 278-279
Degenerative disease, 328t-329t
Degloving injury, 203, 203f
Degradation of personal protective equipment,
        226
Dehydration
    delirium and, 249t
    severity of, 852t
Delayed hypersensitivity reaction, 561t,
        564-565
    to latex, 566
Delirium
    acute, 894
    at end of life, 249-250, 249t
    in neuroleptic malignant syndrome, 889
Delirium tremens, 453-454
Delivery of infant, 806-811
    Apgar score chart and, 810t
    complications of, 811-816
    placental separation after, 810
    questions to ask patient, 806b
    stages of labor in, 806t
Delivery system, intravenous, 101-103
    drop factors in, 102-103
    intravenous administration sets in, 101-102
    for patient-controlled anesthesia, 102
    saline or heparin lock in, 102

Dementia, 877-878
    pain assessment in, 236
Dental abscess, 593
Dental emergency, 592-594
Dental injury, 760, 760b
Dental malocclusion, 741
Dependent adult abuse, 868-869
Depressed fracture, 696t, 697f
    skull, 622-623
Depression
    as mental health emergency, 878
    of vasomotor center, 370-371, 370f
Dermal infection, 553-554
Dermatome, 642f
Desirudin, 344t
Destination, selection of, 38
Detachment, retinal, 575-576
Development, child, 826t-830t
Dexamethasone, 240t
Dextroamphetamine, 240t
Dextrose-containing intravenous solution,
    99-100
Dezocine, 239t
Diabetes insipidus, 433-434
Diabetes mellitus
    hyperglycemia in, 428-433
        diabetic ketoacidosis and, 428-431
        hyperosmolar hyperglycemic nonketotic
            coma and, 431-433, 431t
    hypoglycemia in, 428-431
    immunization recommendations in, 534f
Diabetic ketoacidosis, 428-431, 431t
Dialysis access device, 106
Dialysis emergency
    bleeding as, 526
    clotted access as, 525-526
    fistula infection as, 526
Diaphragm
    in abdominal trauma, 683-684
    contraceptive, 822t
    function of, 650, 651f, 642
    ruptured, 676
Diarrhea
    in child, 843-845, 852t
    Munchausen syndrome by proxy and, 866t
    traveler's, 550
    triage and, 79t
Diastolic blood pressure, normal, 179b
Diazepam
    overdose of, 469-470
    as procedural sedation, 243t

Diet, 72t
Diffenbachia amoena, 479t
Difficult airway, 301-303
    cricothyrotomy for, 304
    laryngeal mask for, 302, 304, 303f
    percutaneous transtracheal ventilation for,
        304
Diffuse axonal injury, 626-627
Diflunisal, 237t
Digital block, 201
Digitalis
    antidote for, 486t
    cardiac arrest caused by, 290t
Digitalis purpurea, 478t
Digoxin poisoning, 468-469, 468b
Diltiazem
    cardiac arrest caused by, 290t
    poisoning with, 470
Diphenhydramine, 563
Diphtheria, 546-547
Directive, advance, 245-246, 246t, 248t
Disability
    in allergic reaction, 563
    in head injury, 620
    trauma causing, in child, 778
Disaster drill, 46, 50b
Discharge instructions for sexual assault victim,
    916-917
Discharge management after bioterrorism, 221t
Disciplinary action, 22
Disclosure, wrongful, 23
Disinfection after bioterrorism, 220t-221t
Dislocation, joint
    acromioclavicular separation and, 721-722,
        721f
    ankle, 728-729, 728f
    elbow, 723, 723f
    of finger, 724-725, 725f
    foot, 729
    hand, 724-725, 724f
    hip, 725, 726f
    knee, 726-727, 727f
    location of, 720t
    patellar, 727-728, 728f
    shoulder, 722-723
    signs and symptoms of, 719, 721
    wrist, 724, 724f
Dissecting aortic aneurysm
    chest pain in, 328t-329t
    symptoms of, 330t
Dissection, thoracic aortic, 354-356, 355f

Distal radius fracture, 703-704
Distillate, petroleum, 481
Distraction, spinal, 637
Distress, fetal, 775-776
Distributive shock, 358, 366-371
    anaphylactic, 358, 368-370, 369f
    hyperdynamic phase of, 366-367
    hypodynamic phase of, 367-368
Disulfiram reaction, 454-455
Diversity, 14-20
    areas of, 15t
    dilemmas of, 18
    in end-of-life care, 18, 19t-20t
    practice model of, 16-18, 16t
    staff's sensitivity to, 15
    task force on, 15b
    visibility vs. invisibility and, 15-16
Diving emergency, 509-510, 507t, 509t
DNA typing in sexual assault, 914
Do not resuscitate order, 28t, 246-248, 248t
Documentation
    of child abuse, 859-860
    for interagency transport, 39, 40
    of interfacility transport, 33
    of intimate partner violence, 905
    JCAHO requirements for, 6b
    as legal issue, 26-27
    of pain assessment, 231
    of sexual assault, 917
    of triage, 74-75
Dog bite, 208, 209f
Domestic violence, 901-906. See also Intimate
    partner violence
Donation, organ, 254-260. See also Organ
    donation
Doxepin
    cardiac arrest caused by, 290t
    for pain, 240t
Drainage of abscess, 202
Dressing, wound, 211-212
Drop factor, 102-103
Drug
    for allergic reaction, 563
    for asthma, 314
    blood studies of, 135
    for child, 830-831, 830t, 831t
    delirium and, 249t
    heat stroke related to, 507
    for pain, 236, 237t-240t, 243t
    for procedural sedation, 243t
    in sexual assault, 914

Drug abuse, 891-900 See also Substance abuse
Drug-herb interaction, 263, 264t-271t
Drug overdose
    of acetaminophen, 463-464
    of benzodiazepines, 469-470
    of calcium channel blockers, 466-467
    of digoxin, 468-469, 468b
    of nonsteroidal antiinflammatory drugs,
        465-466
    of salicylates, 464-465
    of tricyclic antidepressants, 467-468, 467b
Drug-related disorder
    cardiac arrest as, 290t
    psychiatric, 887-888
Dry socket, 594
dT(TD) immunization, 199
Dual-lumen peripheral catheter, 104
Dumbcane poisoning, 479t
Dumping of patient, 23-24
Durable power of attorney, 28t
Duty to report, Reporting
Dysrhythmia, 137-173
    asystole, 164-165, 165t, 165f
    atrial, 142-148, 143t, 143f
        fibrillation, 145-146, 146t, 145f
        flutter, 144-145, 145t, 145f
        premature complexes, 143-144, 144t, 144f
        wandering pacemaker, 146-147, 146f, 148t
    from atrioventricular junction, 147-153
        accelerated junctional rhythm, 152-153,
            152f, 153t
        escape rhythm, 151-152, 151f, 152f
        paroxysmal supraventricular tachycardia,
            147-150, 149t, 149f
        premature complexes, 150-151, 150f, 151t
    atrioventricular block, 153-158
        first-degree, 153, 154t, 154f
        second-degree, 153-156, 155t, 155f
        third-degree, 156-158, 157t, 157f
    in child, 167
    electrocardiography of, 138f, 166f, 167-173,
        axis of, 172, 173b
        interpretation of, 167, 167t, 168b,
            169f-171f
        steps in reading, 173b
    five-lead electrocardiogram monitor for, 138f
    in myocardial infarction, 345
    overview of, 137
    pacemaker for, 166
    by point of origin, 139t
    pulseless electrical activity, 164, 164b

Dysrhythmia *(Continued)*
    from sinus node, 139-142
        arrhythmia, 142
        bradycardia, 141, 142t, 142f
        normal sinus rhythm and, 139-140, 139f,
            140t
        tachycardia, 140-141, 140f, 141t
    ventricular, 158-163
        accelerated idioventricular rhythm, 163t,
            163f
        fibrillation, 160-162, 161t, 161f
        idioventricular rhythm, 162-163, 162f,
            163t
        premature complexes, 158-159, 158f, 159t
        tachycardia, 159-160, 160t, 160f
Dystonic reaction, antipsychotic, 888-889

E

Ear
    assessment of, 94
        age-related considerations in, 85t
    cerumen impaction in, 585, 585b
    foreign body in, 590
    injury of, 757-758, 862t
    labyrinthitis and, 587
    mastoiditis and, 586
    otitis externa of, 583-584, 584f
    otitis media of, 584-585
Ear wax impaction, 585, 585b
Ecchymosis
    from abuse, 862t
    periorbital, 624f
Eclampsia, 803-804
Economic abuse, 902
Ecstasy, 897-900
    street names of, 896b
Ectopic pregnancy, 799-800
Edema
    penile, 515
    pulmonary, 309-310
        high-altitude, 323-324
Education, diversity and, 18
Educational neglect, 859
Effusion
    pericardial, 95
    pleural, 311-312, 311b
Elapidae, 490-491
Elbow
    dislocation of, 720t, 723, 723f
    fracture of, 701-702
Elder abuse, 795, 868-869

Elderly. *See* Geriatric patient
Electrical activity, pulseless, 283t-284t
Electrical alternans, 354f
Electrical burn, 772
    causes of, 762t
Electrocardiogram
    axis of, 172, 173b
        deviation in, 338f
    in cardiac emergency, 333, 335f-336f
    of dysrhythmia, 166-173, 167f
    interpretation of, 167, 167t, 168b, 169f-171f
    leads for, 167t, 337
    in myocardial infarction, 335f
    procedure for obtaining, 168b, 169f, 170f
    signs of ischemia and injury in, 171f
    steps in reading, 172t
Electrolyte
    cardiac rhythm changes and, 440t-441t
    in diabetic ketoacidosis, 430-431
    normal blood values of, 133t
    in whole-bowel irrigation, 461
Electromechanical dissociation, 164
Embolism
    air, 508
    fat, 733
    pulmonary, 308-309
        cardiac arrest in, 291t
        in dialysis, 522
        obstructive shock in, 371
Emergency contraception, 822t
    after sexual assault, 916
Emergency medical services, 8-9, 9f
Emergency Medical Treatment and Active Labor
        Act, 23-24
    triage and, 75-76
Emergency preparedness, 44-57. *See also* Mass
        casualty incident management
Emergency severity index, 67, 68f
Emergency transfusion, 117
Emergent condition
    psychiatric, 872t
    transport of patient with, 34t
Emergent thoracotomy, 673, 674f, 675b
EMLA cream, 237t
Emotional abuse
    of child, 859, 859t
    of intimate partner, 902
Emotional neglect, of child, 859
Emphysema, 314-315
Enalapril, 347t
ENCARE program, 463

Encephalopathy, lead, antidote for, 486t
End-expiratory carbon dioxide, 175-176, 176b
End of life, 245-253
  advance directives and, 245-246, 246t, 248t
  common emergencies at, 248-251
    bowel obstruction as, 250
    delirium as, 249-250, 249t
    hemorrhage as, 250-251
    pain as, 249
    seizures as, 250
    spinal cord compression as, 250
  cultural aspects of, 18, 19t-20t
  death notification at, 251-253
  do not resuscitate order and, 246-248, 248t
Endocrine system
  assessment of, 97
    age-related considerations in, 85t
  triage assessment of, 74t
Endotoxin, 362
Energy therapy, 262t
Enoxaparin, 344t
Entrapment, nerve, 731
Environmental emergency, 490-510
  cold-induced, 499-504, 500f, 503t
  diving-related, 507-510, 507t, 509t
  heat-induced, 504-506, 505b
  Hymenoptera sting as, 495-496
  lightning injury as, 506-507
  scorpion sting as, 494-495
  snakebite as, 494-496
  spider bite as, 492-494
  tick-borne illness and, 496-499
    Lyme disease, 498-499
    Rocky Mountain spotted fever, 497-498
Environmental poison
  carbon monoxide as, 470-471
  cyanide as, 471
Enzyme, 134t
Epicondylar fracture, 701-702
Epididymitis, 517-518, 518t
Epidural hematoma, 628
Epiglottitis, 295, 295f
  in child, 838-839
Epinephrine
  for allergic reaction, 563
  for anaphylactic shock, 369
  in topical anesthetic, 237t
  in wound management, 200, 201

Epistaxis, 587-590, 588f, 589f, 589b
  anterior, 587-590
  posterior, 590
Eptifibatide, 347t
Equation, modified Fick, 175-176, 176b
Equipment
  for arterial pressure monitoring, 178b
  for blood gas specimen, 126
  for chest tube insertion, 663b
  for compartment pressure, 735b
  for delivery of infant, 799
  disinfection of, after bioterrorism, 220t-221t
  for emergent thoracotomy, 674b
  for interagency transport, 38-39
  for interfacility transport, 32
  personal protective, 224-226
  for pulmonary artery pressure monitoring, 184b
Erection, priapism and, 516-517
Eritrean culture, 19t
Erythrocyte, 133t
Escape rhythm, atrioventricular junction, 151-152, 151f, 152f
Escharotomy, 770, 771f
Escherichia coli, 470, 470t-473t
Esmolol, 344t
Esophageal disorder
  bleeding varices as, 398-399
  Boerhaave's syndrome as, 397
  chest pain in, 331t
  esophagitis as, 395-396
  Mallory-Weiss syndrome as, 396-397
  obstruction as, 395-396
Esophageal ultrasound, 175, 176f
Esophagitis, 395-396
Esophagus
  injury to, 759
  ruptured, 668-670
Ethanol
  abuse of, 892
  antidote for, 487t
  poisoning by, 478t-481t
Ethiopian, 19t
Ethnicity as suicide risk, 879
Ethylene glycol poisoning, 486t-487t
  antidote for, 487t
Etodolac, 237t
Euphorbia pulcherima, 480t
Eupnea, 89t

Evidence collection, 28-30, 29b, 30b
  in sexual assault, 910-915
    basic principles of, 910-911
    consent for, 911
    examination kit for, 911
    interview in, 912
    photography in, 912
    physical examination in, 912-913
    securing and transferring of, 915
    sexually transmitted disease testing and, 915
    of specimens, 912-913
    timing of, 911
Exercise-induced heat stroke, 501-502
Exhaustion, heat, 504-505
Expectant care area, 224
Expiration, diaphragm and, 651f
Exploitation, financial, 868
Explosive weapon, 215-216
Exposure in trauma patient, 604
Express consent, 24-25, 25t
External defibrillation, automatic, 278-279
External genital infection, 819, 820t, 821
Extraction, tooth, 594
Extraocular foreign body, 752
Extravasation, 116
Extremity
  amputation of, 732
  assessment of, 84t
    in elderly, 792
  trauma to, 608
    in child, 779-780
Eye, 571-583
  amaurosis fugax of, 582
  anatomy of, 573f
  assessment of, 94
    age-related considerations in, 85t
    in facial trauma, 741
  blepharitis of, 577, 578b
  central retinal occlusion in, 576
  chalazion of, 578-579
  conjunctivitis of, 576-577, 579
  corneal ulcer in, 576-577
  cyanoacrylate exposure of, 582-583
  glaucoma of, 579-580
  in head injury, 620
  hordeolum of, 578
  injury to, 750-758
    conjunctival and corneal laceration in, 753-754
    corneal abrasion as, 755

Eye (Continued)
    corneal burn as, 754-755
    eyelid laceration in, 750-751
    foreign body causing, 752
    hyphema with, 750-751
    impalement, 753
    to optic nerve, 753
    ruptured globe in, 752-753
    subconjunctival hemorrhage in, 750
  irrigation of, 575b, 575f
  keratitis of, 580-581
  periorbital cellulitis and, 570
  raccoon, 623f
  retinal detachment in, 575-576
  triage assessment of, 74t
  uveitis ini, 581-582
Eye opening in Glasgow Coma Scale, 93t
Eyeglasses as protection, 750
Eyelash, hordeolum and, 578
Eyelid laceration, 750-751

F
Face
  assessment of, 84t
    in trauma patient, 606
  body piercing and, 594, 595f, 595t
Face mask for oxygen therapy, 299t
Facial emergency, 568-571
  Bell's palsy as, 568-569, 569f
  cavernous sinus thrombosis as, 571
  periorbital cellulitis as, 570
  trigeminal neuralgia as, 569-570
Facial nerve, 615
Facial trauma, 739-760
  assessment of, 739, 740t, 741
  dental injury in, 760, 760b
  to ear, 757-758
  to eye, 750-758. See also Eye entries
  fracture caused by, 743-749
    mandibular, 747, 749, 749f
    maxillary, 746-747, 747f, 748t
    nasal, 743-744
    orbital, 745-746, 746f
    zygomatic, 744-745, 744f
  general care of, 735b
  soft tissue, 742-743
Fall, 793-794
Family
  patient transport and, 40, 43
  of trauma patient, 605
Fasciotomy, 770

FAST, 684
Fat embolism syndrome, 733
Faxed report, 9, 11
Febrile nonhemolytic transfusion reaction,
    121t
Febrile seizure, 380
    in child, 846-847
Femoral fracture
    of head, 708-710, 709f
    of knee, 712
    of shaft, 710-711, 710f
Fentanyl
    cardiac arrest caused by, 290t
    dose and duration of, 239t
    as procedural sedation, 243t
Fetal bradycardia, 812-813
Fetal death, 253
Fetal distress, 775-776
Fetus
    abortion of, 800-803
    breech position of, 813-814, 813f, 814f
Fever
    in child, 836
    Munchausen syndrome by proxy and,
        866t
    seizure with, 380, 846-847
    in transfusion reaction, 121t
    triage and, 78t-79t
    typhoid, 551
Fibrillation
    atrial, 145-146, 146t, 145f
    ventricular, 160-162, 161t, 161f
        life support for, 280t-282t
Fibrinogen in pregnancy, 768t
Fibrinolytic therapy
    for myocardial infarction, 345, 346t
    for stroke, 385b
Fick equation, modified, 175-176, 176b
Filipino culture, 19t
Financial abuse, 868
Finger
    dislocation of, 724-725, 725f
    fracture of, 705-706, 705f
Fire ant sting, 495
Fistula infection, 526
Five interventions in trauma, 605
Five-lead electrocardiogram monitor, 138f
Five-level triage, 65, 67
Fixed wing air transport, 36t, 37
FLACC behavioral scale, 236t
Flow rate, intravenous, 103b

Fluid
    cerebrospinal
        collection of, 130-131
        in facial trauma, 741
        in head injury, 619b
    gastric, 129t
    in glaucoma, 579
    meconium-stained, 811-812
    percutaneous aspiration of, 131
    spinal
        collection of, 130-131
Fluid therapy
    in burn injury, 763b
    in diabetic ketoacidosis, 433-434
    in hyperosmolar hyperglycemic nonketotic
        coma, 428-429
Flunitrazepam, 899-900
    street names for, 896b
Flurazepam overdose, 469-470
Flutter, atrial, 144-145, 145t, 145f
Focused abdominal sonography,
    684, 686f
Focused physical assessment, 74t
Foley catheter, 590b
Follicle, eyelash, 578
Food-borne infection, 548-551
    hepatitis A as, 548-549
    hepatitis E as, 549
    traveler's diarrhea as, 550
    typhoid fever as, 551
Food poisoning, 470-474, 472t, 473t
Foot
    dislocation of, 729
    fracture of, 716-717, 717f
    heel stick and, 127, 128f
    immersion, 499
Force of injury, 600, 600b
Forearm crutches, 737
Forearm fracture, 702-703, 703f
Foreign body
    airway obstruction from, 297
    in ear, 586
    in eye, 752
    nasal, 590-591
    wound assessment for, 197
Forensics, 28-30, 29b, 30b
Form
    for organ donation, 258f
    post-recovery assessment, 242f
Formula
    conversion

Formula *(Continued)*
    for central venous pressure, 180b
    for weight, 91b
  Lund and Browder, 766f
  Parkland resuscitation, 763b
Four-lead cardiogram monitor, 334f
Four-level triage, 65
Foxglove poisoning, 478t
  antidote for, 486t
Fracture
  abuse-related, 862t
  ankle, 714-716, 714f
  clavicular, 658, 696, 698
  elbow, 701-702
  facial, 743-749
    blow-out, 745-746, 746f
    mandibular, 747, 749f, 749
    maxillary, 746-747, 749f, 748t
    nasal, 743-744
    orbital, 745-746, 746f
    zygomatic, 744-745, 744f
  femoral shaft, 710-711, 710f
  femoral supracondylar, 706
  finger, 705-706, 705f
  flail chest and, 655-657, 656f
  foot, 716-717, 717f
  forearm, 702-703, 703f
  hand, 705-706, 705f
  heel, 717-718, 718f
  hip, 708-710, 709f
  humeral
    proximal, 700-701, 701f
    of shaft, 700-701, 701f
  knee, 711-712, 712f
  laryngeal, 648, 759
  LeFort, 746-747, 747f, 748t
  patellar, 711-712, 712f
  pelvic, 706-708, 707f
  rib, 654-655
  scapular, 699-700, 699f
  shoulder, 698-699, 699f
  skull, 622-623, 624f, 625
  sternal, 657
  tibia-fibula, 713-714, 714f
  tibial, 712
  toe, 718-719, 719f
  types of, 696t, 697f
  wrist, 703-704
Fresh frozen plasma, 119t, 120
Freshwater drowning, 324
Friction burn, 772

Frostbite, 499-502, 500f
Frozen-deglycerolized packed red blood cells, 118t, 120
Full thickness burn, 763, 764f
Furniture polish, 481

G

Gabapentin, 240t
Gag reflex, 616
Gait training, 737
Gamma hydroxybutyrate, 899
  street names of, 896b
Gas, arterial blood
  in asthma, 316
  normal values of, 133t
  in pregnancy, 768t
  specimen collection for, 125-127, 125f
Gas volume, diving and, 507-508, 507t
Gasoline, 481
Gastric fluid, 129t
Gastric lavage
  collection of material from, 132
  for poisoning, 459-460
Gastric trauma, 676
Gastritis, 399-400, 340f
Gastrointestinal bleeding
  lower, 405
  upper, 397-398
Gastrointestinal disorder
  chest pain in, 328t-329t
  in child, 843-847
    appendicitis as, 853-854
    intussusception as, 854-855
    pyloric stenosis as, 853
    unconscious, 845
    volvulus as, 855
    vomiting and diarrhea as, 851-853, 852t
Gastrointestinal system
  age-related changes in, 85t, 790t
  assessment of, 74t, 95-96
  gut decontamination and, 458-462
Gender neutral interview, 86b
Gender of suicidal patient, 878-879
General assessment, 82-83
Generalized tonic-clonic seizure, 380
Genital herpes, 524t-525t, 532, 820t
Genital infection, 819, 820t, 821
Genitourinary disorder, 515-530
  dialysis emergency and, 525-526
  in male, 515-519
    epididymitis as, 415t, 517-518

Genitourinary disorder *(Continued)*
    hematospermia as, 516
    hydrocele as, 516
    penile or scrotal edema as, 515
    priapism as, 516-517
    prostatitis as, 517
    testicular torsion as, 415t, 518-519
    testicular tumor as, 515
   sexually transmitted, 523, 524t-525t,
      525-530
   of urinary tract, 515-519
    acute cystitis as, 515
    anuria as, 514
    hematuria as, 514
    oliguria as, 514
    perinephric abscess as, 512
    pyelonephritis as, 511-512
    renal calculus as, 513
    renal carbuncle as, 512
    urinary retention as, 509-510
Genitourinary tract
   age-related changes in, 790t
   assessment of, 74t, 96
    in elderly, 791
   sexual abuse and, 862t
Geriatric patient
   abandonment of, 795
   abuse of, 795, 868-869
   intravenous therapy in, 111-112
    catheter insertion for, 111
    central vein cannulation in, 111
    intraosseous, 113-114, 114f
    measuring central venous pressure and,
      112
    subclavian catheter insertion for,
      111-112
    venous cutdown for, 112-113
   musculoskeletal injury in, 686-687
   pain assessment in, 236
   trauma in, 788-796
    assessment of, 609, 789-793, 790t
    burn as, 794
    fall causing, 793-794
    interventions for, 793
    prevention of, 794b
    vehicular collision causing, 794-795
German measles, 543-544
Gestational trophoblastic disease, 817-818
GHB, 899
Gingivitis, 593t
Gland, meibomian, 578-579

Glasgow Coma Scale, 93, 93t, 610t
   in head injury, 615-620
   for trauma patient, 609
Glaucoma, 579-580
Globe, ruptured, 753
Glossopharyngeal nerve
   function of, 94t
   in head injury, 615
Glucose
   cardiac arrest and, 289t
   in hyperkalemia, 444
   hypoglycemia and, 423-431, 428b, 431t
   normal blood values of, 133t
   in pregnancy, 768t
Glue, wound, 211
Glycoprotein IIb/IIIa inhibitor, 345, 347t
Gold poisoning, 486t
Gonorrhea, 521t, 523
Graft, coronary artery bypass, 331t
Graft-versus-host disease, 564
   transfusion-related, 121t
Gram-negative bacteria, 362
Granulocyte transfusion, 118t
Gravida, 800b
Greater trochanter fracture, 708-710, 709f
Greenstick fracture, 696t, 697f
Grief, 877
Ground transport, 35, 36t
Growth and development, child, 826t-830t
Guidelines
   communication, 10t
   for disaster drills, 50b
   for injury triage, 72t
Guillain-Barré syndrome, 386
Gunshot wound, 207
   to heart, 663-664
Gut decontamination, 458-462
   by activated charcoal, 460-461, 460b, 461b
   by cathartics, 461
   by gastric lavage, 459-460
   by hemodialysis, 462, 462b
   by induced emesis, 458, 459t
   by whole-bowel irrigation, 461-462
Gynecologic disorder, 816-818
   abdominal pain with, 391
   contraception and, 822t
   endometriosis as, 821-822
   gestational trophoblastic disease as,
     817-818
   infection as, 818-821
    of external genitalia, 819, 820t, 821

Gynecologic disorder *(Continued)*
     pelvic inflammatory disease, 818, 818t
     toxic shock syndrome as, 818-819
     ruptured ovarian cyst as, 817
     vaginal bleeding as, 816
Gypsy culture, 20t

H

Haemophilus ducreyi, 522-523
Hair, 198
Hallucinogen, nutmeg as, 895-896
Haloperidol, 486t
Hand
     dislocation of, 724-725, 725f
     fracture of, 705-706, 705f
Hard contact lens, 574f
Hazard vulnerability analysis, 46t
     for human event, 49t
     for natural event, 47t
     specific considerations in, 50t
     for technological event, 48t
Head
     assessment of, 84t, 94
          age-related considerations in, 85t
          in elderly, 791
          in trauma patient, 600
     circumference of, 91-92
     delivery of, 809f
Head injury, 613-636
     from abuse, 862t
     assessment of
          angiographic, 618-619
          computed tomography in, 630
          of cranial nerves, 614-615
          Glasgow Coma Scale in, 613-614
          intracranial pressure monitoring in,
               619-620
          pupillary response in, 615
          radiographic, 616-618, 618f
          reflexes in, 616
     to brain
          diffuse, 625-626
          focal, 621-627
     in child, 785
     concussion as, 625-626
     contusion as, 621
     epidural hematoma in, 628
     herniation in, 634-635
     intracerebral hemorrhage in, 26f, 626-627
     intracranial bleeding in, 621
     intracranial pressure in, 633-634

Head injury *(Continued)*
     management of, 614-615
     penetrating, 633
     scalp wounds in, 621-622
     seizures after, 635
     skull fracture, 619, 622-623, 624f
     subarachnoid hemorrhage in, 631-632, 631f
     subdural hematoma in, 629-631, 629f, 630f
Headache
     assessment of, 375-376
     characteristics of, 376t
     chronic paroxysmal hemicrania causing,
          376t-377t
     cluster, 376t-377t
     migraine, 376t-377t
     subarachnoid hemorrhage causing,
          376t-377t
     temporal arteritis causing, 375
     tension, 374-375, 376t-377t
     traumatic, 375, 376t-377t
     triage and, 78t
     vascular, 375
Healing, wound, 195-196
Health Care Financing Administration, 76
Health care precautions, 529b
Heart
     blunt injury to, 668-669
     cardiogenic shock and, 360-362, 369f
     dysrhythmias of, 137-173. *See also*
          Dysrhythmia
     electrolyte disorder and, 440t-441t
     in fetal bradycardia, 812-813
     obstructive shock and, 358
     penetrating injury to, 669-670
     shock affecting, 360b
Heart block, 153-158
     first-degree, 153, 154t, 154f
     second-degree, 153-156, 155t, 155f
     third-degree, 156-158, 157t, 157f
Heart disease, 326-356. *See also* Cardiac
          emergency
     immunization recommendations in, 534f
Heart failure, 347-350, 347t, 349b, 348t, 350b
Heart rate of child, 825
Heart sound, 94
Heat injury, 504-506, 505b
     to airway, 321
Heat stroke, 501-502
Heel fracture, 717-718, 718f
Heel stick, 127, 128f
Height, 91

Helmet removal, 646-647, 647f
Helicopter transport, 36t, 37-38
Hematocrit
    normal, 133t
    in pregnancy, 768t
Hematologic disorder, 408-419
    anemia as, 415-416, 415b, 415t
    malignant, leukemia as, 416-417
    sickle cell disease as, 408-412, 413f, 414f
Hematologic system
    assessment of, 96
        age-related considerations in, 85t
    normal values for, 133t-134t
    in pregnancy, 768t
Hematoma
    epidural, 621-622
    management of, 203-204, 204f, 205f
    of pinna, 757-758
    subdural, 629-631, 629f, 630f
Hematospermia, 516
Hematuria, 514
Hemicrania, chronic paroxysmal, 376t-377t
Hemisection of spinal cord, 639
Hemlock poisoning, 478t
Hemodialysis
    emergency in, 525-526
    immunization recommendations in, 534f
    for poisoning, 462, 462b
Hemodynamic monitoring, 174-194
    calculations and normal values in, 189t
    in donor management, 259t
    invasive, 177-192
        of arterial pressure, 177-180, 178b, 179b,
            179f
        of central venous pressure, 180-182, 180b,
            180t, 181f, 182f
        of pulmonary artery pressure, 182-192.
            See also Pulmonary artery pressure
            monitoring
    noninvasive, 174-177
        bioimpedance as, 175
        end-expiratory carbon dioxide as,
            175-176, 176b
        esophageal ultrasound as, 175, 176f
        near infrared spectrometry as, 176-177
        sublingual capnometry as, 176
        tissue Po_2 as, 177
Hemoglobin
    normal values of, 133t
    in pregnancy, 768t
Hemolysis, transfusion-related, 121t

Hemoperfusion, charcoal, 462
Hemophilia
    coagulation cascade in, 413f
    diagnostic studies for, 414
    factors VIII and IX replacement for, 414t
    interventions for, 414
    patient education about, 414-415
    signs and symptoms of, 408, 414
    types of, 413t
Hemorrhage
    assessment of, 88t
    at end of life, 250-251
    intracerebral, 26f, 632-633
    postpartum, 815-816
    retinal, 863f
    subarachnoid, 631-632, 632f
        headache in, 376t-377t
    subconjunctival, 750
Hemothorax, 658-660, 665f
Hemophilia, 412
Heparin
    antidote for, 487t
    drugs for, 343, 344t
Heparin lock, 102
Hepatic stage of acetaminophen poisoning, 464
Hepatic trauma, 681, 681b
Hepatic vein, 684
Hepatitis A, 537t
    immunization for, 529f
    water- or food-borne, 548-549
Hepatitis B
    as blood-borne infection, 527-528
    characteristics of, 537t-536t
    immunization for, 533f
    prophylaxis for, 916
Hepatitis C
    as blood-borne infection, 532, 533
    characteristics of, 536t
Hepatitis D, 536t
Hepatitis E, 536t, 549
Herb-drug interaction, 263, 264t-271t
Hernia, incarcerated, 403-404
Herniation, brain, 634-635
Heroin, 893-894
Herpes simplex virus
    genital, 820t
    sexually transmitted, 520t-511t, 520
Herpes zoster, 554-555
Hiatal esophagus, 395-396
High-altitude pulmonary edema, 323-324
High-pressure injury, 207

Hip
    dislocation of, 720t, 725, 726f
    fracture of, 708-710, 709f
Hispanic culture, 20t
History, patient
    of abdominal pain, 391
    in assessment, 83, 85, 86b, 87b
    of complementary and alternative medicine,
        262-263
    of respiratory emergency, 308
    of sexual assault, 909-910
    in triage, 71t
HITS mnemonic, 86b
Hmong culture, 20t
Hodgkin's lymphoma, 418
Holly poisoning, 480t
Homicidal behavior, 884-885
Hordeolum, 578
Hormone disorder
    adrenal, 438-439
    antidiuretic
        diabetes insipidus as, 433-434
        inappropriate secretion as, 434-435
    thyroid, 435-438
Hornet sting, 495
Hospital-based do not resuscitate order,
    246-247, 248t
Hospital emergency incident command system,
    52f. See also Mass casualty incident
    management
Hospital use in disaster, 51
Hotline, poison control, 462, 462b
Huber tipped needle, 105f
Human immunodeficiency virus infection, 524t
    sexual assault and, 916
Human-related mass casualty incident, 45b, 49t
Humeral fracture
    proximal, 698-699, 699f
    of shaft, 700-701, 701f
Hydatidiform mole, 817-818
Hydrocele, 516
Hydrocodone, 238t
Hydrofluoric acid burn, 486t
Hydrogen peroxide, 197
Hydrogen sulfide, 486t
Hydromorphone
    cardiac arrest caused by, 290t
    dose and duration of, 239t
Hydrophiidae, 490-491
Hydroxyzine, 240t
Hymenoptera sting, 495-496

Hyperacute transplant rejection, 421
Hypercalcemia
    cardiac arrest caused by, 289t
    cardiac rhythm changes in, 440t
    signs and symptoms of, 443
    treatment of, 443
Hypercarbia, 319
Hyperdynamic shock, 366-367
Hyperextension, spinal, 637, 639
Hyperflexion, spinal, 637
Hyperglycemic nonketotic coma,
    hyperosmolar, 431-433, 431t
Hyperkalemia, 447-448
    cardiac arrest caused by, 289t
    cardiac rhythm changes in, 441t
Hypermagnesemia
    cardiac arrest caused by, 289t
    cardiac rhythm changes in, 440t
    interventions for, 445
    signs and symptoms of, 440-441
Hypernatremia, 448-449
Hyperosmolar hyperglycemic nonketotic coma,
    431-433, 431t
Hyperphosphatemia, 446
    cardiac rhythm changes in, 441t
Hypersensitivity reaction, 561t
    anaphylactic shock in, 368
    cytotoxic, 561t, 563-564
    delayed, 561t, 564-565
    immediate, 564, 561t, 563-563
    immune complex–mediated, 561t, 564
Hypertension
    classification of, 351t
    malignant, 350-351, 351t
    pregnancy-induced, 803-804
Hyperthermia
    in child, 836
    in neuroleptic malignant syndrome, 889
Hyperthyroid crisis, 435-436
Hyperventilation
    central neurogenic, 89t
    chest pain in, 328t-329t
Hyphema, 751
Hypocalcemia
    cardiac arrest caused by, 289t
    cardiac rhythm changes in, 440t
    causes of, 446
    interventions for, 442-445
    signs and symptoms of, 442
Hypodermic needle, 105f
Hypodynamic shock, 367-368

Hypoglossal nerve
  function of, 94t
  in head injury, 615
Hypoglycemia, 428-432
  cardiac arrest caused by, 289t
  causes of, 429
  interventions for, 426-427, 426b, 427t
  reactive, 428
  signs and symptoms of, 429-440
Hypokalemia, 446-447
  cardiac arrest caused by, 289t
  cardiac rhythm changes in, 441t
Hypomagnesemia
  cardiac arrest caused by, 289t
  cardiac rhythm changes in, 440t
  interventions for, 447
  signs and symptoms of, 447
Hypomania, 884
Hyponatremia, 448
Hypophosphatemia, 445-446
  cardiac rhythm changes in, 441t
Hypothermia, 502-504, 503t
  in trauma patient, 604
Hypothyroid coma, 437
Hypovolemia, 288t
Hypovolemic shock, 358, 361-363
  in abdominal trauma, 679b
  complications of fluid replacement for,
    364t
Hypoxemia, 319
Hypoxia, 249t

I

Ibuprofen, 237t
Identification, patient, 5, 7
Idioventricular rhythm, 162-163, 162f, 163t
Ilex, 480t
Imaging
  in abdominal pain, 391
  in pediatric trauma, 786-787
Imipramine, 240t
Immediate hypersensitivity reaction, 564, 561t,
    566-567
  to latex, 566
Immersion foot, 499
Immobilization, cervical spinal, 645-646,
    645f
Immune complex–mediated hypersensitivity
    reaction, 561t, 564
Immune response, 563-564
Immune suppression, 419-422, 420b

Immunization
  schedules for, 533f-535f
  in triage, 71t
Immunodeficiency, 530f
Immunoglobulin, 564
  in immune complex–mediated reaction, 564
Immunologic reaction to transfusion, 121t
Immunologic system, 97
  age-related considerations in, 85t
Immunosuppressive agent, 421b
Impacted fracture, 696t, 697f
Impaction, cerumen, 585, 585b
Impalement eye injury, 753
Implantable cardioverter-defibrillator, 288-289
Implanted port, 105, 106f
  accessing of, 115-116
Implied consent, 24, 25t
Incarcerated hernia, 403-404
Incidence report, 26
Incident, mass casualty. *See* Mass casualty
    incident management
Incision, 204-205
Incomplete abortion, 801
Incomplete spinal cord lesion, 639
Incubation period for infection, 528t
Index, shock, 91
India, culture of, 20t
Indomethacin, 237t
Induced emesis, 458, 459t
Inevitable abortion, 801
Infant
  growth and development of, 826t-830t
  scalp vein access in, 110, 110f
Infection, 527-558
  adult respiratory distress syndrome with, 316b
  air-borne, 536, 536-548
    chickenpox as, 541-542
    diphtheria as, 546-547
    influenza as, 536, 541
    measles as, 541-548
    monkeypox as, 538-41
    mumps as, 541-545
    pertussis as, 545-546
    severe acute respiratory syndrome as,
      547-548
    tuberculosis as, 539-541
  blood-borne, 529-532, 535-536
    acquired immunodeficiency syndrome,
      530-531
    hepatitis B, 531-532
    hepatitis C, 532, 533

Infection *(Continued)*
  bronchiolitis, 840-841
  bronchitis, 317-318
  cavernous sinus thrombosis as, 571
  in conjunctivitis, 568-569, 571
  corneal ulcer with, 576
  cystitis as, 515
  dermal, 553-554
  of dialysis access fistula, 522
  in food poisoning, 472-474, 472t, 473t
  gynecologic, 818-821, 820t
    of external genitalia, 819, 820t, 819
    pelvic inflammatory disease, 818, 818t
    toxic shock syndrome as, 818-819
  herpes zoster, 554-555
  hordeolum caused by, 578
  human immunodeficiency virus, 516t
  immunization schedules for, 533f-535f
  incubation periods for, 528t
  keratitis caused by, 580-581
  Lyme disease, 498-499
  mastoiditis, 586
  meningitis, 555-556
    in child, 848-849, 848b
  meningococcemia as, 849-850
  mononucleosis, 556-557
  Munchausen syndrome by proxy and,
      866t
  osteomyelitis, 733-734
  in periorbital cellulitis, 570
  peritonsillar, 591-592
  precautions for, 523-525, 529b
  Rocky Mountain spotted fever, 497-498
  septic shock in, 358, 366, 363f
  sexually transmitted, 519-525. *See also*
      Sexually transmitted disease
    sexual assault and, 915
  tetanus, 557-558
  transfusion-related, 121t
  vector-borne, 552
  from venous access device, 116
  water-borne, 548-549
    hepatitis A as, 548-549
    hepatitis E, 549
    traveler's diarrhea as, 550
    typhoid fever as, 551
Infection control
  for bioterrorism, 220t-221t
  in triage, 76-77, 78t-79t
Inferior vena cava, 684
Infiltration anesthesia, 200

Inflammation
  of bursa, 730-731
  chalazion caused by, 578-579
  corneal, 576-577
  of ear, 583-585
  of epididymis, 517-518, 518t
  in epiglottitis, 838-839
  of esophagus, 395-396
  gastric, 395-397
  in labyrinthitis, 587
  mastoiditis as, 586
  pelvic, 818, 818t
  in periorbital cellulitis, 570
  pneumonia as, in child, 841-842, 842t
  of prostate, 517
  of tendon, 729-730
  of thyroid, 437-438
  in uveitis, 581-582
Influenza, 536, 539
  immunization for, 533f
Informed consent, 24-25, 25t
Infrared burn of eye, 756
Infusion
  crystalloid, 359
  intraosseous, 113
Infusion pump, 102
Ingestion of cocaine, 893
Inhalant abuse, 894-895
Inhalation injury, 321-322
Inhalation of cocaine, 893
Injury. *See* Mechanism of injury; Trauma
Inpatient unit
  communication with, 9, 11
  transport to, 33-34
Insecticide, 481
Insertion of intravenous catheter, 107-109,
      107t, 108b
Insight, 874
Inspection
  in abdominal pain, 390
  in assessment, 92
  of musculoskeletal injury, 692
Inspiration, diaphragm and, 650, 655f
Institutional-based do not resuscitate order,
      246-247, 248t
Insulin
  in diabetic ketoacidosis, 426
  in hyperkalemia, 448
  in hyperosmolar hyperglycemic nonketotic
      coma, 429
  types and characteristics of, 427t

Integumentary system. *See also* Skin *entries*
  age-related changes in, 790t
  assessment of, 96, 97t
    age-related considerations in, 85t
Interaction, drug-herb, 263, 264t-271t
Intercondylar fracture, 701-702
Intercostal space, 646
Interfacility transfer, 23-24
Interfacility transport
  by air
    patient care record of, 41f-42f
    types of, 37-38
  destination selection for, 38
  by ground, 35, 36t, 37-38
  patient education about, 40, 43
  patient preparation for, 39-40
  planning for, 38
  safety of, 40
Interview
  in child abuse case, 865-868
  in mental health assessment, 873
  triage, 69-70
Intestinal decontamination, 458-459
Intestinal obstruction, 404-405
Intestinal symptoms, 391
Intestinal trauma, 683, 684b
Intimate partner violence, 909-914
  assessment of, 903
  documentation of, 905
  epidemiology of, 909
  identifying victim of, 902-904
  inventions for, 903-904
  reporting of, 905
  signs and symptoms of, 902-903
  support services for victim of, 904
  types of, 902
Intoxication, alcohol, 450-452. *See also* Drug
  overdose
Intraarticular femur fracture, 712
Intracellular fluid, 359t
Intracerebral hemorrhage, 26f, 632-633
Intracranial bleeding, 621
Intracranial pressure
  cardiac arrest and, 288t
  in head injury, 615, 633-634
Intrafacility transport, 31-34
  general considerations in, 31-32
  to inpatient unit, 33-34
  to operating room, 33, 34t
  planning for, 32-33
  for procedures, 34

Intramuscular administration, 830t
Intraocular foreign body, 752
Intraosseous catheter, 113-114
Intraosseous needle, 106-107
Intrauterine device, 822t
Intravenous administration of heroin, 893
Intravenous therapy, 99-122
  accessing venous access devices in, 114-116
  alternative access devices for, 106-107
  for blood transfusion, 117-122. *See also*
    Transfusion
  catheters for, 103-107
    for central venous access, 104-105, 105f,
      106f
    midline and midclavicular, 105-106
    peripheral, 103-104
    peripherally inserted central, 105-106
    sizes of, 104
  in child, 109-110, 110f, 830, 821t
  complications of, 108b
  delivery systems for
    drop factors, 102-103
    intravenous administration sets, 101-102
    patient-controlled anesthesia, 102
    saline or heparin lock, 102
  discontinuation of, 117
  in elderly, 111-114, 114f
  flow rate calculation for, 103b
  insertion procedure for, 107-109
    site preparation in, 108
    site selection in, 107, 107t
    venipuncture techniques in, 109
  solutions for
    dextrose-containing, 99-100
    multiple-electrolyte, 100-101
    sodium-containing, 100
Intubation
  tracheal, 301, 301f
  rapid sequence induction, 301t
Intussusception, 854-855
Invasive hemodynamic monitoring,
  177-192. *See also* Hemodynamic
  monitoring, invasive
Involuntary consent, 25, 25t
Iodine, 222t
Ionizing radiation, 219
Ipecac, 458, 459t
Iron
  poisoning with, 475-476
    antidote for, 486t
  in pregnancy, 768t

Irrigation
    of ear, 585b
    whole bowel, 461-462
    of wound, 198
Irritable bowel syndrome, 405-406
Ischemic chest pain, 330t
Ischemic contracture, Volkmann's, 736
Isolation
    in bioterrorism, 220t
    in triage, 71t
Isolation precautions, 527-533, 529b
isopropanol poisoning, 486t-487t
Isotonic solution, 359

J

Jequirity bean poisoning, 478t
Jewelry, body, 594, 595f, 595t
Jimson weed poisoning, 479t
Job action sheet, 53t, 54f
Joint, 691
    aspiration of, 131-132
    dislocation of, 719-729. See also Dislocation,
        joint
    strain of, 694
Joint Commission on Accreditation of
        Healthcare Organizations
    documentation requirements of, 6b, 26b
    on restraint use, 27-28
    triage and, 76
Judgment, 874
JumpSTART triage system, 51, 55f, 56f, 57f
Junction, atrioventricular
    escape rhythm and, 151, 151f, 152t
        accelerated, 152, 152f, 153t
    paroxysmal supraventricular tachycardia
        and, 148-150, 149f, 149f
    premature complexes and, 150-151, 150f,
        151t
    rhythms originating in, 148-153
Junctional premature complex, 150-151,
        150f, 151t

K

Keratitis, 580-581
Kerosene, 481
Ketamine, 898-899
    as procedural sedation, 243t
    street names of, 896b
Ketoacidosis, diabetic, 428-431, 431t
Ketoprofen, 237t
Ketorolac, 237t

Kidney
    shock affecting, 360b
    trauma to, 682
Kidney stone, 513
Knee injury, 711, 712f
    dislocation, 720t, 726-727, 727f
    fracture, 712-713, 712f
Korean culture, 20t
Kussmaul respiration, 89t

L

Labetalol
    cardiac arrest caused by, 290t
    for myocardial infarction, 344t
Labor
    definition of, 800b
    preterm, 776-777
    stages of, 806t
Laboratory report, 7-8, 9f
Laboratory specimen, 123-136
    blood, 123-130, 133-136. See also Blood
        specimen
    of gastric lavage material, 132
    joint aspiration for, 131-132
    percutaneous aspirations for, 131
    respiratory syncytial virus, 132-133
    spinal fluid, 130-131
    sputum, 132
    stool, 132
    throat swab, 132
    urine, 131
Labyrinthitis, 587
Laceration
    abuse-related, 862t
    auricular, 757
    conjunctival, 753
    corneal, 753
    eyelid, 750-751
    management of, 204-205, 205f
Lactated Ringer's solution, 100-101
Lactic dehydrogenase, 134t
Lantana camera, 479t
Large intestine, injury to, 683
Laryngeal fracture, 648
Laryngeal mask, 302, 304, 303f
Laryngotracheobronchitis, 839
Larynx, fracture of, 759
Lateral bend of spine, 637
Lateral transtentorial herniation, 634
Latex allergy, 565-566
Latino culture, 20t

Latrodectus mactans, 492-493
Lavage
    gastric
        collection of material from, 132
        in poisoning, 459-460
    peritoneal, 686-688, 687f
Lead, electrocardiographic, 167t, 337
Lead poisoning, 476-477
    antidote for, 486t
LeFort fracture, 746-747, 747f, 748t
Left coronary artery, 341f
Left ventricular failure, 360-361
"Left without being seen," 76
Legal issues, 23
    advance directives as, 28, 28t
    confidentiality as, 22-23
    consent as, 24-25, 25t
    documentation as, 26-27, 26b
    evidence collection and preservation as,
        28-30, 29b, 30b
    interfacility transfers as, 23-24
    in intimate partner violence, 905
    nurse practice acts as, 21-22
    reportable conditions as, 23b, 25-26
    restraints as, 27-28
    safety as, 27
Lens
    contact, removal of, 570f
    Morgan, 575b, 575f
Lepirudin, 344t
LET, 237t
    in wound management, 201
Leukemia, 530f
Leukocyte
    in immune response, 563
    normal values of, 133t
Leukocyte poor red blood cells, 118t, 120
Level of consciousness
    altered, 378-380, 378b, 379b
    in facial trauma, 740t
Levorphanol, 239t
Liability, 26, 27b
Licensed professional nurse, 21-22
Lidocaine
    for pain, 240t
    for rapid sequence induction intubation,
        302t
    as topical anesthetic, 237t
    in wound management, 200, 201
Life support
    advanced, 279, 288-289, 288b

Life support *(Continued)*
        for asystole, 285t-286t
        for child, 832
        for pediatric pulseless arrest, 287f
        for pulseless electrical activity,
            283t-284t
        for pulseless ventricular tachycardia,
            280t-282t
    basic, 277-278, 278f, 278t
        for asystole, 289f
        for pulseless electrical activity, 283t-284t
        for pulseless ventricular tachycardia, 280t
    in pediatric cardiopulmonary arrest, 831t,
        832
Life-threatening condition, transport of patient
        with, 34t
Ligament, 690
Lighter fluid, 481
Lightning injury, 506-507
Lisinopril, 347t
Liver
    in acetaminophen poisoning, 464
    shock affecting, 360b
    trauma to, 681, 681b
Liver disease, 530f
Living will, 28t
Local anesthetic, antidote for, 487t
Lock, heparin or saline, 102
Lofstrand crutches, 737
Lorazepam
    overdose of, 469-470
    as procedural sedation, 243t
Lower gastrointestinal bleeding, 405
Loxosceles reclusa, 493-494
Ludwig's angina, 592
Lumbar puncture, 130-131
Lund and Browder formula for burn area,
        766f
Lung
    collapsed. *See* Pneumothorax
    contusion of, 666-667
    injury to, 666-668
    parenchymal laceration of, 667
    shock affecting, 360b
Lung injury, transfusion-related, 121t
Lyme disease, 498-499
Lymphocyte
    in immune response, 564
    in pregnancy, 768t
Lymphoma, 417-419
    immunization recommendations for, 534f

M

Magnesium
  cardiac arrest and, 289t
  cardiac rhythm and, 440t
  hypermagnesemia and, 444-445
  hypomagnesemia and, 443-444
Magnesium citrate, 457
Magnesium sulfate, 457
Magnetic resonance imaging in head injury, 618
Major alcohol withdrawal, 453
Major burn, 765, 767
Male patient, genitourinary disorders in,
    515-519. *See also* Genitourinary disorder
Malignancy
  immunization recommendations for, 534f
  leukemia, 416-417, 416t
  lymphoma, 417-419
Malignant hypertension, 350-351, 351t
Mallory-Weiss syndrome, 396-397
Malocclusion, 741
Maltreatment of child, 857-869. *See also* Abuse,
    child
Manchester Triage Scale, 67, 67t
Mandated reporting. *See* Reporting
Mandibular fracture, 747, 748f, 749
Manic psychosis, 884
Manipulative and body-based therapy, 262t
Manometer, manual, 112
Marital status as suicide risk, 879
Marker, cardiac, 342, 342t
  measurement of, 135
Martini's law, 508
Mask
  laryngeal, 302, 303f
  for oxygen therapy, 302t
Mass and velocity in injury, 600-601, 600b
Mass casualty incident management, 44-57.
    See also Weapon of mass destruction
  mitigation in, 45-46, 45b, 46t-50t
  preparedness for
    planning in, 46
    training drills in, 46, 50b, 51
  recovery in, 55
  response in, 51-55
    command system for, 52f, 53t, 54t
    patterns of hospital use and, 51
    triage in, 51, 53, 55, 55f, 56f, 57f
  training drills in, 46, 50b, 51
Mass media, 7
Mass prophylaxis after biological terrorism,
    218, 219b

Mastoiditis, 586
Maxillary fracture, 746-747, 748t, 749f
MDMA, 897-898
Mean arterial pressure
  in head injury, 619
  normal, 179b
Measles, 541-544
Measles, mumps, rubella immunization, 533f
Mechanical irrigation of wound, 198
Mechanical ventilation, 304, 306, 306t
Mechanism of injury, 598-600, 600b
  in Achilles tendon rupture, 716
  in compartment syndrome, 734
  in dislocation, 720t
    acromioclavicular, 721
    elbow, 717
    foot, 729
    hand or finger, 724
    hip, 725
    knee, 726
    patellar, 727
    shoulder, 722
    wrist, 724
  in fracture
    ankle, 709
    clavicular, 696
    elbow, 701
    femoral shaft, 710
    foot, 716
    forearm, 702
    hand, 705-706
    heel, 717
    hip, 715
    humeral shaft, 700-701
    knee, 711, 712
    pelvic, 706
    scapular, 699
    shoulder, 698
    tibia-fibula, 714
    toe, 718-719
    wrist, 703-704
  in repetitive motion disorder
    bursitis, 730
    carpal tunnel syndrome, 731
    tendinitis, 729
  in spinal trauma, 637-638
  in subdural hematoma, 629f
  in vehicular collision, 600t
Meconium-stained fluid, 811-812
Media, communication with, 7
Mediastinum, widened, 671f

Medical directive, 28t
Medical history, 71t. *See also* History, patient
Medical neglect, 858
Medical psychiatric disorder, 877-879
Medical record
    air transport and, 41f-42f
    interagency transport and, 39
    as legal document, 26-27
Medication, 71t. *See also* Drug *entries*
Medication administration, in child, 830-831,
    830t, 831t
Megacolon, toxic, 407
Meibomian gland, 578-579
Membrane, tympanic, ruptured, 758
Meningitis, 555-556
    in child, 848-849, 848b
Meningococcal immunization, 533f
Meningococcemia, 849-850
Mental health, terrorism and, 226-227, 226b
Mental health emergency, 871-890. *See also*
    Psychiatric emergency
Mental health neglect, 859
Mental status examination, 861, 872b
Meperidine
    cardiac arrest caused by, 290t
    dose and duration of, 238t
    as procedural sedation, 243t
Mercury poisoning, 486t
Mesenteric vein, 684
Metabolic disorder
    acidosis as, 453t
    adrenal, 438-439
    cardiac arrest in, 289t
    coma in, 378b
    delirium and, 249t
    in diabetes, 428-437. *See also* Diabetes mellitus
    electrolyte disorder and, 439-449
    pituitary, 429-431
        diabetes insipidus as, 433-434
        inappropriate secretion of antidiuretic
            hormone as, 434-435
    thyroid, 435-436
        myxedema coma as, 437
        thyroid storm as, 435-436
        thyroiditis as, 437-438
    in unconscious child, 838
Metacarpal fracture, 705-706, 705f
Metastasis, delirium and, 249t
Metatarsal fracture, 716-717, 717f
Metered volume chamber intravenous
    administration set, 101-102

Methadone, 239t
Methamphetamine, 290t
Methanol poisoning, 486t-487t
    antidote for, 487t
3,4-Methylenedioxymethamphetamine,
    897-898
Methylphenidate, 240t
Methylprednisolone, 563
Metoprolol, 344t
Mexican culture, 20t
Mexiletine, 240t
Midazolam
    overdose of, 469-470
    as procedural sedation, 243t
    for rapid sequence induction intubation,
        302t
Midclavicular catheter, 105-106
Middle ear inflammation, 570-585
Middle fossa fracture, 623
Midface fracture, 746-747, 747f
Midline catheter, 105-106
Migraine headache, 376t-377t
Mild hypothermia, 502
Mind-body therapy, 262t
Mineral oil, 481
Mini-Mental Status Examination, 871, 872b
Minnesota tube, 399f
Minor alcohol withdrawal, 452-453
Minor burn, 767
Miscarriage, 800-803
Missed abortion, 802
Mistletoe poisoning, 480t
Mitigation in emergency management, 45-46,
    45b, 46t-50t
Mitral valve
    penetrating injury to, 669
    prolapse of, 331t
Mnemonic
    ABCDE, 16t
    CIAMPEDS, 70, 71t-72t
    HITS, 86b
    MUDPILES, 457t
    PQRST, 86, 87t, 229
    SAMPLE, 86b
    TIDES, 738-739
    for toxic exposures, 457t
Mobitz type I heart block, 153-156, 155t, 155f
Mobitz type II heart block, 155-156, 156t, 156f
Moderate burn, 767
Moderate hypothermia, 499-500, 503t
Moderate sedation, 201

Modified Fick equation, 175-176, 176b
Molar pregnancy, 817-818
Monitoring
    hemodynamic, 174-194. *See also*
        Hemodynamic monitoring
    of trauma patient, 608-609
Monocyte, 564
Mononucleosis, 564-565
Monophasic defibrillator, 288
Monosodium glutamate, 330t
Monteggia's fracture, 702
Mood, assessment of, 763
Morgan lens, 575b, 575f
Morphine
    cardiac arrest caused by, 290t
    dose and duration of, 238t-239t
    for myocardial infarction, 343t
    as procedural sedation, 243t
Mortality
    delirium tremens and, 453
    thyroid storm and, 435
Motor function
    of child, 826t, 828t
    in Glasgow Coma Scale, 93t
    in head injury, 614
Motor nerve, 642f
Motor vehicle accident
    elderly in, 794-795
    mechanism of injury in, 600t
Mouth
    dental emergencies and, 592-594
    in Ludwig's angina, 592
MUDPILES, 457t
Multipara, 800b
Multiple-dose activated charcoal, 461, 461b
Multiple-electrolyte solution for intravenous
        therapy, 100-101
Mumps, 544-545
    immunization for, 533f
Munchausen syndrome by proxy, 861, 856-857,
        866t
Murmur, heart, 95
Muscarinic effects of pesticide poisoning,
        481t
Muscle strain, 694
Musculoskeletal system
    age-related changes in, 790t
    assessment of, 96
        age-related considerations in, 85t
    chest pain and, 326t
    components of, 691-692

Musculoskeletal trauma
    Achilles tendon rupture, 716
    age-related characteristics of, 692-693
    assessment of
        inspection in, 692
        neurovascular, 691-692
        palpation in, 692
    complications of
        compartment syndrome as, 734-735,
            735b
        fat embolism as, 733
        osteomyelitis embolism as, 733-734
        Volkmann's ischemic contracture as, 736
    dislocation as, 719-729. *See also* Dislocation
    fracture. *See* Fracture
    of joints and muscle
        sprains as, 694-695
        strains as, 694
    of knee, 711-712, 712f, 713f
    nerve entrapment in, 731
    patient education about, 736-737
    of peripheral nerves, 695, 696t
    prevention of, 737
    from repetitive motion, 729-731
    splinting in, 693
    subluxation, 719, 720t, 721
    triage assessment of, 74t
Mushroom poisoning, 477
Myasthenia gravis, 386-387
Mycobacterium tuberculosis, 535-537
Mycoplasmal pneumonia, 842t
Myocardial contusion, 668-669
Myocardial infarction
    cardiac arrest in, 291t
    chest pain in, 328t-329t
    clinical findings in, 339-340
    coronary arteries in, 341t
    drugs for
        angiotensin-converting enzyme inhibitor,
            345, 347t
        anticoagulant, 343, 344t
        beta-blockers, 344, 344t
        fibrinolytic, 345, 346t
        glycoprotein IIb/IIIa inhibitors, 345, 347t
        MONA, 342t
    electrocardiography in, 334f
    markers of, 342t
    signs and symptoms of, 340
    symptoms of, 330t
Myocardium, penetrating injury to, 669
Myxedema coma, 432

N

Nabumetone, 237t
Nalbuphine, 239t
Naproxen, 237t
Narcosis
    acute, 894
    nitrogen, 508-509, 509t
Nasal cannula, 299t
Nasal foreign body, 590-591
Nasal fracture, 743-744
Nasopharyngeal airway, 300, 300f
Nasopharyngeal obstruction, 837
Nasopharyngeal wash, 132-133
National Clearinghouse of Child Abuse and
        Neglect, 857
Natriuretic peptide, B-type, 350b
Natural disaster
    examples of, 45b
    hazard vulnerability analysis for, 47t
Navicular bone fracture, 704
Near-drowning, 324-325
Near infrared spectrometry, 176-177
Neck
    assessment of, 84t
        in trauma patient, 600-601
    injury to, 752-754, 752t
        mechanism of, 637-638
    in Ludwig's angina, 592
    soft tissue injury of, 648-649
Necrotizing ulcerative gingivitis, 593t
Needle
    intraosseous, 106-107
    winged, 103
Needle thoracostomy, 660b
Nefazodone, 240t
Negative nonverbal communication, 17
Neglect of child, 858-859
Neisseria gonorrhoeae, 521t, 523
    epididymitis and, 521
Neonate
    Apgar score of, 810t
    care of, 811
    delivery of, 806-811
Nephrogenic diabetes insipidus, 433-434
Nerium oleander, 478t
Nerve
    in Bell's palsy, 568-569, 569f
    optic, injury to, 753
    phrenic, 646
    spinal, 638t, 642f
Nerve block, 201

Nerve entrapment syndrome, 731
Nerve injury, peripheral, 695, 696t
Nerve root, dermatomes and, 642f
Nervous system. *See also* Neurologic *entries*
    age-related changes in, 790t
    in allergic reaction, 562
    cardiac arrest and, 288t
    cocaine affecting, 892b
    depression of, 866t
    in shock, 359t
    triage assessment of, 74t
Neuralgia, trigeminal, 569-570
Neurogenic diabetes insipidus, 433-434
Neurogenic emergency, 374-388
    altered level of consciousness as, 378-380,
        378b, 379b
Neurogenic hyperventilation, central, 89t
Neurogenic pulmonary edema, 313
Neurogenic shock, 358, 370-371, 370f
Neuroleptic drug, antidote for, 486t
Neuroleptic malignant syndrome, 889
Neurologic assessment, 93, 93t
    age-related considerations in, 85t
    in pediatric trauma, 778
    in trauma, 603-604
Neurologic emergency
    in child, 836-843
        febrile seizures as, 846-847
        meningitis as, 848-849, 848b
        meningococcemia as, 849-850
        unconsciousness as, 845-846
        ventriculoperitoneal shunt malfunction
            as, 850-851
    headache as, 374-377, 376t-377t
    meningitis as, 555-556
    Munchausen syndrome by proxy and, 866t
    neuromuscular disorder as, 386-387
    psychiatric, 877-879
    seizure as, 380-382
    shunt problem as, 387
    stroke as, 382-385
        classification of, 384t
        hemorrhagic, 384
        interventions for, 381
        ischemic, 384
        scales for, 378t, 379t
        screening for, 379b
        signs and symptoms of, 384-385
Neuropathic pain, 230t
Neurosurgical consultation, 620
Neurovascular assessment, 691-692

Neutropenia, 416-417
Newborn
    Apgar score of, 810t
    care of, 811
    delivery of, 806-811
Nicotinic effects of pesticide poisoning, 481t
Nightshade poisoning, 479t
Nitrite, 487t
Nitrogen, blood urea, 133t, 134
Nitrogen narcosis, 508-509, 509t
Nitroglycerin, 343t
Nitroglycerin administration set, 102
Non-English-speaking patient, 17
Non-Hodgkin's lymphoma, 418
Nonambulatory victim of chemical
        contamination, 217-218
Noncoring needle, 105f
Nonimmunologic reaction, to transfusion, 121t
Noninvasive hemodynamic monitoring,
        174-177
    bioimpedance as, 175
    end-expiratory carbon dioxide as, 175-176,
        176b
    esophageal ultrasound as, 175, 176f
    near infrared spectrometry as, 176-177
    sublingual capnometry as, 176
    tissue Po$_2$ as, 177
Noninvasive positive pressure ventilation,
        304
Nonionizing radiation, 219
Nonketotic coma, hyperosmolar
        hyperglycemic, 431-433, 431t
Nonnurse triage, 62
Nonopioid analgesic, 236, 237t
Nonpharmacologic intervention for pain,
        240-241, 241t
Nonsteroidal antiinflammatory drug, 465-466
Nonthermal burn, 764, 766
    causes of, 762t
    of eye, 754-755
    hydrofluoric acid, 486t
    management of, 764
Nonurgent mental health condition, 872t
Nonverbal communication, 17
Nose
    assessment of, 85t, 94
    foreign body in, 590-591
    fracture of, 743-744
Nosebleed, 587-590, 588f, 589f, 590b
Nullipara, 800b
Numeric pain rating scale, 231f, 234t

Nurse, forensic, 30b
Nurse practice act, 21-22
Nutmeg abuse, 895-896

O

Objective
    in mass casualty incident management, 53t
    of triage interview, 70
Objective assessment, 88
Objective data in triage, 73
Oblique fracture, 696t, 697f
Obsessive compulsive disorder, 875, 878
Obstetric emergency, 773-778, 799-816. *See also*
        Pregnancy
Obstetrics, cocaine and, 884b
Obstruction
    airway, in child, 836-837
    esophageal, 395-396
    intestinal, 404-405
        at end of life, 250
    nasopharyngeal, in child, 837
    oropharyngeal, 873-830
    of venous access device, 116
    of ventricular shunt, 387
Obstructive pulmonary disease, chronic, 318-319
    immunization recommendations in, 534f
Obstructive shock, 358, 371-373
Occlusion, retinal artery, 576
Occurrence report, 26
Ocular disorder, 571-583, 750-758. *See also* Eye
Oculomotor nerve
    function of, 94t
    in head injury, 609, 615
Odor, breath, 457t
Ointment, ophthalmic, 578b
Oleander poisoning, 478t
    antidote for, 486t
Olfactory nerve
    function of, 94t
    in head injury, 614-615
Oliguria, 514
Onset of illness or injury, 71t-72t
Open-angle glaucoma, 579
Open pelvic fracture, 707f, 708
Open pneumothorax, 662, 663b, 664b
Operating room, transport to, 33, 34t
Ophthalmic ointment, 578b
Opioid, 236, 238t-239t
    antidote for, 487t
    bowel obstruction and, 250
    cardiac arrest caused by, 290t

Optic nerve
  function of, 94t
  in head injury, 615
  injury to, 753
Oral contraceptive, 822t
Orbital fracture, 745-746, 746f
Orbital rim trauma, 745
Organ donation, 254-260
  consent form for, 258f
  criteria for, 256, 256b
  critical pathway for, 257t
  cultural practices related to, 19t-20t
  determination of death for, 257, 257b
  donor management for, 259-260, 259t
  history of, 255b
  organs available, 255b
  procurement process for, 260
  United Network for Organ Sharing for,
    254, 256t
  West Nile virus and, 256-257
    cultural aspects, 256-257
Organophosphate poisoning, 480-481, 481t
Oropharyngeal airway, 298, 300f
Oropharyngeal obstruction, 837-838
Orthopedic injury. *See* Musculoskeletal
  trauma
Orthostatic tilt testing, 91b
Orthostatic vital signs, 90, 91b
Osmolality in pregnancy, 768t
Osteitis, alveolar, 594
Osteomyelitis, 733-734
Otitis externa, 583-584, 584f
Otitis media, 584-585
Ottawa ankle rules, 715b
Oucher pain rating scale, 232t
Out-of-hospital do not resuscitate order,
  247-248, 248t
Ovarian cyst rupture, 817
Over-the-needle catheter, 103-104
Overdose, drug, 463-470
  of acetaminophen, 463-464
  of benzodiazepines, 469-470
  of calcium channel blockers, 466-467
  of digoxin, 468-469, 468b
  of nonsteroidal antiinflammatory drugs,
    465-466
  of salicylates, 464-465
  of tricyclic antidepressants, 467-468, 467b
Overrotation, spinal, 637
Oxycodone, 238t
Oxygen saturation, 88t, 89-90

Oxygen therapy, 298, 298t
  for chronic obstructive pulmonary disease,
    319
  for myocardial infarction, 343t
  in trauma, 602
Oxymorphone, 239t

P
Pacemaker for dysrhythmia, 166
Packaging, for interagency transport, 40
Packed red blood cells, 117, 118t, 120
Pain, 228-244, 229t
  abdominal, 389-407. *See also* Abdominal
    pain
  acute vs. chronic, 229t
  angina, 340f
  assessment of, 86-87, 87t, 228-236
    documentation of, 231
    in elderly, 236
  in child, 231, 232t-236t, 827t, 829t
  dental, 592-593
  drugs for, 236, 237t-240t, 243t
    misconceptions about, 231b
  at end of life, 249
  endometriosis causing, 821-822
  in epididymitis, 518t
  nonpharmacologic interventions for,
    240-241, 241t
  physiological sources of, 230t
  procedural sedation for, 241, 242f, 243t,
    244b
  renal calculi causing, 513
  in testicular torsion, 518t
  in trigeminal neuralgia, 569-570
Pallor, 692
Palpation
  in assessment, 92
  of musculoskeletal injury, 692
Palsy, Bell's, 568-569, 569f
Pancreatic trauma, 676
Pancreatitis, 402-403
Panic disorder, 875
Paralysis
  facial, 568-569, 569f
  in neurovacular assessment, 692
Paramedic ambulance, 35, 36t
Paranoia, 883
Parenchymal laceration of lung, 667
Paresthesia, 692
Parkland burn resuscitation formula, 769
Paroxetine, 240t

Paroxysmal hemicrania, chronic, 376t-377t
Paroxysmal supraventricular tachycardia, 147-150, 149t, 149f
Partial rebreather mask, 299t
Partial seizure, 380
Partial thickness burn, 763, 764f
Partial thromboplastin time, 136
Particle, radiation, 219
Past medical history, 71t. *See also* History, patient
Patellar dislocation, 720t, 727-728, 728f
Patellar fracture, 712-713, 712f, 713f
Patient-controlled anesthesia, 102
Patient identification, 5, 7
Patient representative, 4
Patient Self-Determination Act, 28
Pediatric assessment triangle, 69, 69t
Pediatric emergency
    bradycardia as, 833f
    cardiopulmonary arrest as, 831-832, 831t, 833f-835f, 836
    fever and, 836
    gastrointestinal, 851-855
        appendicitis as, 853-854
        intussusception as, 854-855
        pyloric stenosis as, 853
        volvulus as, 855
        vomiting and diarrhea as, 851-853, 852t
    neurologic, 836-843
        febrile seizures as, 846-847
        meningitis as, 848-849, 848b
        meningococcemia as, 849-850
        unconsciousness as, 845-846
        ventriculoperitoneal shunt malfunction as, 850-851
    primary assessment of, 824-825, 826t-830t
    psychiatric, 879
    pulseless arrest as, 835f
    respiratory, 836-838. *See also* Respiratory emergency, in child
    secondary assessment of, 829
    sudden infant death syndrome as, 832
    tachycardia as, 834f
    triage of, 70, 824
Pediatric patient
    death of, 252
    drug administration for, 830-831, 830t
    dysrhythmia in, 167
    growth and development of, 826t-830t
Pediatric patient (*Continued*)
    immunization recommendations for, 535f
    intravenous therapy for, 109-110, 110f
    musculoskeletal injury in, 692
    neurologic emergency in, 836-843. *See also* Neurologic emergency, in child
    pain assessment in, 231, 232t-236t
    pulseless arrest in, algorithm for, 287f
    respiratory emergency in, 844. *See also* Respiratory emergency, in child
    vital signs of, 825, 828t
Pediatric trauma, 785-787
    abdominal, 785-786
    assessment of, 609
    diagnostic tests for, 786-787
    of extremity, 786
    head injury, 785
    secondary survey of, 784-785
Pelvic inflammatory disease, 818, 818t
Pelvic pain from endometriosis, 821-822
Pelvis
    fracture of, 706-707, 707f
    in trauma patient, 613-614
Penetrating trauma
    abdominal, 678-679
    cardiac, 669-670
    head, 633
    to neck, 648, 649
Penetration of personal protective suit, 226
Penile edema, 515
Penile specimen collection, 914
Penis, priapism of, 516-517
Pentazocine, 238t
Pepper poisoning, 479t
Peptic ulcer, 400
Peptide, B-type natriuretic, 350b
Percussion
    in abdominal pain, 390
    in assessment, 92-93, 92t
Percutaneous aspiration, 131
Percutaneous transtracheal ventilation, 304, 305f
Perfusion
    assessment of, 95
    skin, 603
Perfusion pressure, cerebral, 619
Pericardial effusion, 95
Pericardial tamponade, 670-671, 671f
    cardiac arrest in, 291t
    obstructive shock in, 368

Pericarditis, 351-354
   causes of, 352t
   chest pain in, 328t-329t
   symptoms of, 330t
Pericoronitis, 593t
Perimortem cesarean delivery, 778
Perinephric abscess, 512
Periodontal abscess, 593
Periodontitis, 593t
Periorbital cellulitis, 570
Periorbital ecchymosis, 624f
Peripheral catheter, 103-104
   for intravenous therapy, 103-104
Peripheral intravenous site, 107-109, 107t
Peripheral nerve injury, 695, 696t
Peripheral venipuncture, 109
Peripherally inserted central catheter, 105-106
Peritoneal lavage, 686-688, 687f
Peritonsillar abscess, 591-592
Permeation time, 225
Perphenazine, 290t
Personal protective equipment, 224-226
Pertussis, 545-546
Pesticide poisoning, 480-481, 481t
Phalanx fracture
   of finger, 705-706, 705f
   of toe, 718-719, 719f
Pharyngeal injury, 759
Pharyngotracheal lumen airway, 301
Phencyclidine
   abuse of, 888-889
   cardiac arrest caused by, 290t
   street names of, 896b
Phenothiazine, antidote for, 486t
Phenytoin, 240t
Pheochromocytoma, 439
Phlebostatic axis, 190f
Phoradendron flavescens, 481t
Phosphorus
   cardiac rhythm and, 441t
   hypophosphatemia and, 445-446
   as radionuclide, 222t
Phrenic nerve, 646
Physical abuse, 859
   of intimate partner, 902
Physical examination
   in assessment, 92-93, 92t
   of trauma patient, 605-606
Physical neglect, 858
Physiologic response to pain, 229t
Phytolacca americana, 479t

Piercing, body, 594, 595f, 595t
Pink eye, 568-569, 571
Pinna
   hematoma of, 751
   piercing of, 595t
Piroxicam, 237t
Pit viper bite, 490-491
Placenta, delivery of, 818
Placenta previa, 804-805
Placental abruption, 805-806
Planning
   for mass casualty incident, 46
   for transport
      interfacility, 38
      intrafacility, 32
Plantar puncture wound, 207
Plastic catheter, 104
Platelet
   normal values of, 133t
   transfusion of, 119t, 120
Platelet count
   measurement of, 136
   in pregnancy, 768t
Pleural effusion, 311-312, 311b
Plutonium, 222t
Pneumococcal infection, 533f
Pneumonia, 312-313
   in child, 841-842, 842t
Pneumothorax
   chest pain in, 331t, 328t-329t
   obstructive shock in, 368-369
   open, 662, 663b, 664b
   simple, 658-660, 659f
   spontaneous, 310, 331t
   tension, 660, 661f, 662
Po$_2$, tissue, 177
Pocket mask, 299t
Poinsettia poisoning, 481t
Point-of-care testing, 128-129, 129t
Poison control, 458, 459b
Poison ivy, 481t
Poison Prevention Act, 458-459
Poisoning, 456-489
   alcohol, 478t-481t, 488
   analgesic, 463-466
   antidotes for, 486t-487t, 489
   carbon monoxide, 322-323, 322t
   diagnostic clues to, 457t
   drugs causing
      acetaminophen, 463-464
      benzodiazepines, 469-470

Poisoning *(Continued)*
  calcium channel blockers, 466-467
  digoxin, 468-469, 468b
  nonsteroidal antiinflammatory drugs,
    465-466
  salicylates, 464-465
  tricyclic antidepressants, 467-468, 467b
  environmental
    carbon monoxide, 470-471
    cyanide, 471
  food
    bacterial, 472-474, 472t, 473t
    botulism, 470
  gut decontamination for, 458-462
    by activated charcoal, 460-461, 460b,
      461b
    by cathartics, 461
    by gastric lavage, 459-460
    by hemodialysis, 458, 458b
    by induced emesis, 458, 459t
    by whole-bowel irrigation, 461-462
  intentional, 862t
  metal, 475-477
  Munchausen syndrome by proxy and, 866t
  overview of, 456-458
  pesticide, 480-481, 481t
  petroleum distillates causing, 481
  plants causing, 477, 478t-480t, 480
  poison control centers for, 458
  prevention of, 462-463
  smoke, 321-322
Poker Chip pain rating scale, 233t
Pokeweed poisoning, 479t
Polymorphonuclear leukocyte, 768t
Pontocaine, 201
Port
  for central venous pressure monitoring,
    180, 180t
  implanted, 105, 106f
    accessing of, 115-116
Port-A-Cath, 105
Positioning of child, 782f
Positive pressure ventilation, noninvasive,
  304
Post-recovery assessment form, 242f
Post-traumatic stress disorder, 880-881
Postabortion care, 802-803
Postconcussion syndrome, 626
Posterior cord lesion, 639
Posterior epistaxis, 585f, 590
Posterior fossa fracture, 623

Postmortem care, 252-253
  after bioterrorism, 221t
Postpartum hemorrhage, 815-816
Postural vital signs, 90
Posturing in head injury, 616
Potassium
  cardiac arrest and, 289t
  cardiac rhythm and, 441t
  deficit of, 446-447
  excess of, 447-448
  normal blood values of, 133t
  in pregnancy, 768t
Povidone-iodine, 197
Power of attorney, 28t
PQRST mnemonic, 86, 87t, 229
  for abdominal pain, 391, 391t
Practice act, nurse, 21-22
Precordial lead, 334f
Preeclampsia, 803
Pregnancy
  aborted, 800-903
  bleeding in, 804-806
  delivery complications in
    breech position as, 813-814, 813f, 814f
    fetal bradycardia as, 812-813
    meconium staining as, 811-812
    prolapsed cord as, 814-815, 815f
  ectopic, 799-800
  emergent delivery in, 806-811, 806t,
    807f-812f, 810t
  hypertension in, 803-804
  immunization recommendations in, 534f
  molar, 817-818
  postpartum hemorrhage and, 815-816
  terminology about, 800b
  trauma in, 779-781
    abdominal, 688
    abruptio placentae caused by, 776
    assessment of, 773-776
    perimortem cesarean delivery in, 778
    physiologic changes of pregnancy and, 781t
    preterm labor caused by, 776-777
    uterine rupture caused by, 777
Pregnancy-induced hypertension, 803-804
Preload, definition of, 178b
Premature complex
  atrial, 143-144, 144t, 144f
  of atrioventricular junction, 150-151, 150f,
    151t
  junctional, 150-151, 150f, 151t
  ventricular, 158-159, 158f, 159t

Preparedness, emergency, 44-57. *See also* Mass casualty incident management
Preschool-age child, 826t-830t
Preservation of evidence, 28-30, 29b, 30b
Pressure
    arterial, 177-180, 178b, 179b, 179f
    central venous, 180-182, 180b, 180t, 181f, 182f
    cerebral perfusion, 619
    compartment, 735b
    high-pressure injury and, 207
    intracranial
        cardiac arrest and, 288t
        in head injury, 633-634
    pulmonary artery, monitoring of, 182-192. *See also* Pulmonary artery pressure monitoring
    pulse, 90
    underwater, 507t
Preterm labor, 776-777
Prevention
    of child abuse, 868
    of falls in elderly, 794b
    of infection
        AIDS, 531
        chickenpox, 538
        diphtheria, 543
        hepatitis C, 531
        herpes zoster, 551
        influenza, 535
        measles, 540
        meningitis, 552
        monkeypox, 543
        mononucleosis, 553
        mumps, 541
        pertussis, 545-546
        severe acute respiratory syndrome, 544
        tetanus, 554
        tuberculosis, 536
        typhoid fever, 551
        West Nile virus, 552
    injury, 731
    of latex exposure, 564-565
    of poisoning, 462-463
    of ringworm, 553-554
    of scabies, 553
    of substance abuse, 892
Priapism, 516-517
Prilocaine, 237t
Primary assessment, 83t
Primary intravenous administration set, 101

Primary open-angle glaucoma, 579
Primary survey in trauma
    geriatric, 789-790
    pediatric, 780, 780t, 781t, 782-784
Primigravida, 800b
Primipara, 800b
Prinzmetal angina, 339t
Procedural sedation, 241, 244
    drugs for, 243t
    guidelines for, 244b
    post-recovery assessment form for, 242f
Prolapsed umbilical cord, 814-815, 815f
Prophylaxis
    antibiotic, 199
    for biological terrorism, 218, 219b
    rabies, 208, 209b
    for sexually transmitted disease, 916
Propoxyphene, 238t
Propranolol
    cardiac arrest caused by, 290t
    for myocardial infarction, 344t
Prostatitis, 517
Protective equipment, personal, 224-226
Prothrombin time, 136
Protriptyline, 290t
Proximal humeral injury, 698-699, 699f
Psychiatric assessment, 74t
Psychiatric disorder
    coma in, 378b
    medical or neurologic, 877-879
    Munchausen syndrome by proxy as, 861, 856-857, 866t
    psychotic, 881-884
Psychiatric emergency, 871-890
    antipsychotic drug reaction as, 888-889
    in child or adolescent, 887
    disposition of patient with, 881-882
    drug-related, 887-888
    general management of, 874-875
    homicidal and assaultive behavior as, 884-885
    medical or neurologic, 877-879
        acute delirium as, 886
        dementia as, 877-878
    neuroleptic malignant syndrome as, 889
    nonpsychotic, 875-881
        acute grief as, 877
        anxiety as, 875-879
        depression as, 878
        post-traumatic stress disorder as, 880-881
        suicide as, 878-880

Psychiatric emergency *(Continued)*
  psychotic, 881-884
    acute, 881
    hypomania/manic, 884
    paranoia as, 883
    schizophrenia as, 882-883
    violent patient and, 881-882, 882b
  triage of, 871, 872b, 872t, 873-874
Psychological abuse
  of child, 859, 859t
  of intimate partner, 902
Psychological aspects of terrorism, 226-227, 226b
Psychosis, manic, 884
Psychosocial function of child, 826t, 828t
Psychotic reaction, 881-883
Puerto Rican culture, 20t
Pulmonary artery pressure monitoring, 182-192
  cardiac output determination and, 187-188, 187b
  catheter for, 182-183, 183f
  complications of, 186
  data accuracy of, 190
  equipment for, 184b
  normal values in, 186b
  occlusive pressure waveform analysis in, 186, 187f
  patient preparation for, 183-184
  phlebostatic axis and, 190f
  square wave test and, 191f, 192f
  systemic vascular resistance and, 188, 189b
  therapeutic interventions for, 187
  waveform analysis of, 184, 185f, 186, 186f
Pulmonary contusion, 666-667
Pulmonary disease, chronic obstructive, 318-319
  immunization recommendations in, 534f
Pulmonary edema, 313-314
  high-altitude, 319-320
Pulmonary embolism, 308-309
  cardiac arrest in, 291t
  in dialysis, 525
  obstructive shock in, 371
Pulmonary system
  age-related changes in, 790t
  cardiac arrest and, 291t
  cocaine affecting, 892b
Pulse
  assessment of, 88t, 89
  in neurovascular assessment, 692
  in trauma patient, 602-603

Pulse pressure, 90
Pulseless arrest in child, 835t
  algorithm for, 287f
Pulseless electrical activity, 164, 164b
  life support for, 283t-284t
Pulseless ventricular tachycardia, 280t-282t
Pump, infusion, 102
Puncture wound, 206-207, 206f
Pupillary response in head injury, 615
Pyelonephritis, 507-508
Pyloric stenosis, 853
Pyorrhea, 593t

Q
Q wave, 171f
Qualifications of triage nurse, 77, 80
Questions in triage, 70, 72t

R
Rabies prophylaxis, 208, 209b
Raccoon eyes, 623f
Race as suicide risk, 879
Radiation, 223b
Radiation burn
  causes of, 762t
  of eye, 762
Radiation contamination, 219-223
  as emergency, 222
  initial interventions for, 222-223
  ionizing vs. nonionizing, 219
  particles vs. waves, 219
  radionuclides produced, 222t
Radiographic evaluation of head injury, 616-617, 623f
Radiology report, 8, 9f
Radius
  dislocation of, 720t
  fracture of, 702-703, 703f
Radius fracture, distal, 703-704
Ramipril, 347t
Ranitidine, 563
Rapid sequence induction intubation, 301t
Rapid sequence induction medication, 302t
Rash
  Munchausen syndrome by proxy and, 866t
  triage and, 78t
Rating, triage severity, 73
Rattle snake venom, 486t
Reactive hypoglycemia, 428
Recognition of terrorist attack, 214-215

Record, medical
    interagency transport and, 39
    as legal document, 26-27
Recovery from mass casualty incident, 55
Red blood cell transfusion, 118t, 119, 120
Referral
    for dental emergency, 593t
    transport and, 38
Referred abdominal pain, 390, 390t
Reflex
    bulbocavernous, 634
    in child, 827t, 829t
    in head injury, 616
Rejection, transplant, 421-422, 421b
Renal calculus, 513
Renal carbuncle, 512
Renal failure, 534f
Renal function in shock, 360b
Renal trauma, 682
Renin-angiotensin-aldosterone system, 359t
Repetitive motion disorder
    bursitis as, 730-731
    tendinitis as, 729-730
Report
    faxed, 9, 11
    laboratory, 7-8, 9f
    written, 11, 12f
Reporting
    of child abuse, 856-860
    of elder/dependent adult abuse, 869
    of intimate partner violence, 905
    mandatory, 25-26
Respiration, 89, 89t
Respiratory disorder, allergic, 562
Respiratory emergency, 307-325
    acute respiratory distress syndrome as,
        319-321, 316b
    assessment of, 307
    asthma as, 314-316
    bronchitis as, 317-318
    carbon monoxide poisoning as, 322-323,
        322t
    in child
        airway obstruction as, 836-837
        apnea as, 839-840
        asthma as, 842-844
        bronchiolitis as, 832-833
        croup syndromes as, 838-839
        nasopharyngeal obstruction as, 837
        oropharyngeal obstruction as, 837-838
        pneumonia as, 841-842, 842t

Respiratory emergency (Continued)
        status asthmaticus as, 844
        unconscious, 845
    chronic obstructive pulmonary disease as,
        318-319
    high-altitude pulmonary edema as,
        319-320
    history of, 308
    inhalation injury as, 321-322
    pleural effusion as, 311-312
    pneumonia as, 312-313
    pulmonary edema as, 313-314
    pulmonary embolus as, 308-309
    spontaneous pneumothorax as, 310
    status asthmaticus as, 316-317
    submersion injury as, 324-325
Respiratory infection
    influenza, 536, 539
    tuberculosis, 535-537
Respiratory protection from radiation exposure,
    222
Respiratory rate of child, 825
Respiratory syncytial virus, 132-133
Respiratory system
    age-related changes in, 790t
    assessment of, 95
    cardiac arrest and, 291t
    cocaine affecting, 892b
    triage assessment of, 74t
Restraint
    documentation of, 6b
    as legal issue, 27
Resuscitation
    fluid, Parkland formula for, 769
    in pediatric cardiopulmonary arrest, 831t,
        832
Retention, urinary, 509-510
Reteplase, 346t
Retinal artery occlusion, 576
Retinal detachment, 575-576
Retinal hemorrhage, 863f
Revised trauma score, 610t
Rhododendron, 478t
Rhythm, cardiac, electrolytes affecting,
    440t-441t
Rib fracture, 654-655
Ricinus communis, 478t
Rickettsia rickettsii, 497-498
Right coronary artery, 341f
Right ventricular failure, 360-361
Rim, orbital, 745

Ringer's solution, 100-101
Ringworm, 553-554
Risk, legal, 27b
Risk factor
    for cardiac emergency, 327b
    for lymphoma, 418
    for pulmonary embolus, 308
    for suicide, 879
    for violence, 881-882, 882b
Rocky Mountain spotted fever, 497-498
Rohypnol, 899-900
    street names for, 896b
Role of triage nurse, 80
Roma culture, 20t
Root injury, spinal, 639
Rosenbaum vision screener, 568b
Rubella, 541-544
Rubella immunization, 533f
Rubeola, 541-545
Rule of nines, 763, 765f
Rules, Ottawa ankle, 715b
Rupture
    of Achilles tendon, 716
    of diaphragm, 676
    esophageal, 668-670
    of globe, 753
    of ovarian cyst, 817
    of tympanic membrane, 758
    uterine, 777
Russian culture, 20t

S
Safety
    of interagency transport, 40
    of interfacility transport, 33
    as legal issue, 27
    in triage, 73-74
Salicylate poisoning, 464-465
Saline lock, 102
Saline-washed red blood cells,
        118t, 120
Saliva, testing of, 129t
Salmonella food poisoning, 472,
        472t-473t
SAMPLE mnemonic, 86b
SANE program, 908-909
Saphenous vein, 112-113
Sarcoptes scabiei, 553
SART team, 908
Scabies, 524t, 553
    genital, 820t

Scale
    Glasgow coma, 609, 610t
    mental health triage, 872t
    pain, 231f, 232t-236t
Scalp vein access, 110, 110f
Scalp vein needle, 103
Scalp wound, 621-622
Scaphoid bone fracture, 698
Scapular fracture, 699-700, 700f
Schiøtz tonometry, 580b
Schizophrenia, 882-883
School-age child, 828t-829t
Scorpion sting, 494-495
Scrotal edema, 515
Seawater drowning, 324
Secondary assessment, 84t
Secondary glaucoma, 579
Secondary intravenous administration
        set, 101
Security, 73-74
Sedation
    in asthma, 316
    procedural, 241, 242f, 243t, 244b
    in wound management, 201
Sedimentation rate
    normal values of, 133t
    in pregnancy, 768t
Seizure
    at end of life, 250
    febrile, 838-839
    in head injury, 629
    management of, 381-382
    Munchausen syndrome by proxy and, 866t
    types of, 380
Semen, blood in, 512
Semicircular canal, inflamed, 587
Semiurgent mental health condition, 872t
Sensory nerve, 642f
Sepsis, delirium in, 249t
Septic abortion, 802
Septic shock, 358, 366, 367f
Serum electrolyte
    measurement of, 135
    normal values for, 134t
Serum iron in pregnancy, 768t
Serum marker, cardiac, 342
Serum sickness, 564
Severe acute respiratory syndrome, 79t,
        547-548
Severe hypothermia, 499-500, 503t
Severity rating, triage, 73

Sexual assault, 859, 862t, 907-920
  approach to victim of, 908-909
  documentation of, 917, 918f-919f
  evidence collection after, 910-915
  of intimate partner, 910
  medical treatment after, 915-917
  nursing assessment of, 909-910
  overview of, 907-920
  testimony about, 917, 920
Sexual assault nurse examiner, 908-909
Sexual assault response/resource team, 908
Sexually transmitted disease, 519-525
  acquired immunodeficiency syndrome as, 520t
  chancroid as, 521-523
  Chlamydia trachomatis as, 521-524
  epididymitis and, 517-518, 518t
  genital herpes as, 524t-525t, 524
  genital warts as, 521t
  gonorrhea as, 521t, 523
  hepatitis B as, 521t
  scabies as, 520t
  syphilis as, 522t, 522-523
  testing for, 915
  treatment of, 915-916
  urethritis as, 519, 522
Shaft fracture
  femoral, 710-711, 710f
  humeral, 700-701, 701f
Shaken baby syndrome, 863f
Shigella, 472t-473t
Shingles, 554-555
Shock, 361-373
  acute respiratory distress syndrome with, 316b
  cardiogenic, 358, 363-366, 369f
  classification of, 357-358
  compensatory mechanisms in, 359t
  distributive, 358, 366-371
    anaphylactic, 358, 368-370, 369f
    hyperdynamic phase of, 366-367
    hypodynamic phase of, 367-368
    neurogenic, 358, 370-371, 370f
    septic, 358, 366, 367f
  hypovolemic, 358, 361-363
    in abdominal trauma, 679b
    blood loss in, 358t, 359t
    complications of fluid replacement for, 364t
    development of, 369f
  obstructive, 358, 371-373
  pathophysiology of, 359-360, 359t, 360b
Shock index, 91

Shoulder
  dislocation of, 720t, 722-723
  fracture of, 692-693
Shunt malfunction
  ventricular, 387
  ventriculoperitoneal, 850-851
Sickle cell disease, 408-410, 409f, 410f, 411b
Sign, Battle, 624f
Silver fork deformity, 704
Simple pneumothorax, 658-660, 659f
Simple triage and rapid treatment system, 51, 55f, 57f
Sinus arrhythmia, 142
Sinus bradycardia, 141, 142t, 142f
Sinus rhythm, 139-142, 139f, 140t
Sinus tachycardia, 140-141, 140f, 141t
Sinus thrombosis, cavernous, 571
Skin
  age-related changes in, 85t, 790t
  in allergic reaction, 562
  assessment of, 96, 97t
  in elderly, 792
  radiation exposure and, 222
  triage assessment of, 74t
Skin antisepsis, 197-198
Skin infection, 553-554
Skin perfusion, 603
Skull fracture, 619, 622-623, 624f
Skull in head injury, 617-618
Small intestine, injury to, 682
Smoke inhalation, 321
Snakebite, 490-492
Snellen eye chart, 568b
Socket, dry, 594
Sodium
  cardiac rhythm and, 441t
  hyponatremia and, 448
  in intravenous fluid, 100
  normal blood values of, 133t
  in pregnancy, 768t
Sodium bicarbonate in hyperkalemia, 448
Sodium citrate, 457
Sodium polystyrene sulfonate, 448
Soft tissue injury
  facial, 742-743
  of neck, 648-649
Solanum, 479t
Solution for intravenous therapy
  dextrose-containing, 99-100
  multiple-electrolyte, 100-101
  sodium-containing, 100

Somatic pain, 230t
  abdominal, 389
Sorbitol, 457
Sound, heart, 94
South Asian culture, 20t
Space, intercostal, 646
Specimen, 123-136. *See also* Laboratory
      specimen
  in sexual assault, 912-913
Spectrometry, near infrared, 176-177
Speech, assessment of, 873
Spider bite, 492-494
Spider venom, 486t
Spinal accessory nerve
  function of, 94t
  in head injury, 609
Spinal anesthesia, neurogenic shock in,
      379-371, 370f
Spinal cord
  compression of, 250
  in elderly, 791
Spinal fluid, 130-131. *See also* Cerebrospinal
      fluid
Spinal injury, 638-639
  anatomy in, 641f
  assessment of, 640
  cervical stabilization in, 645-646, 645f
  complete cord, 639
  dermatomes and, 642f
  diagnosis of, 643
  helmet removal in, 646-647, 647f
  incomplete cord, 639
  interventions for, 643-650,
      651f, 651t
  mechanism of, 637-638
  neurogenic shock in, 370-371, 370f
  prevention of, 643
  signs and symptoms of, 640, 637
  vertebrae in, 640
Spinal nerve, 638t
Spinal root injury, 639
Spinal stabilization in child, 780
Spine
  assessment of
    in elderly, 791
    in trauma patient, 602-603
  in facial trauma, 740t
  in head injury, 617
Spiral fracture, 696t, 697f
Spleen, 681
Splenectomy, 534f

Splint
  instructions about, 736
  for orthopedic injury, 693
Spontaneous abortion, 800b
Spontaneous pneumothorax, 310
  chest pain in, 331t
Spot check triage, 63
Sprain, 694-695
  knee, 711-712
Sputum
  in asthma, 315
  collection of, 132
Square wave test, 191f, 192f
Stab wound
  abdominal, 678-679
  to heart, 669-670
  management of, 206-207, 206f
Stable angina, 339t
Stable pelvic fracture, 707f, 708
Staff, diversity sensitivity of, 15b
Staffing, transport of patient
      impacting, 34
Standard catheter, 105
Standard precautions, 527-529
Standards, communication, 5
Staphylococcus aureus
  in cavernous sinus thrombosis, 571
  food poisoning with, 472, 472t-473t
  hordeolum caused by, 578
  in osteomyelitis, 733-734
  in toxic shock syndrome, 818-819
Stapling of wound, 210-211, 212f
START triage system, 51, 55f, 57f
State law on reportable conditions,
      25-26
State nurse practice act, 21-22
Status asthmaticus, 316-317
  in child, 844
Status epilepticus, 381-382
Stenosis
  aortic, 372
  pyloric, 853
Sternal fracture, 657
Steroid for asthma, 843
Stiff neck, 78t
Stimulant, cardiac arrest caused by, 290t
Sting
  bee or wasp, 495-496
  scorpion, 494-495
Stomach, trauma to, 676
Stone, renal, 513

Stool
  in abdominal pain, 391
  abnormal, 388b
  collection of, 132
  point-of-care testing of, 129t
  in triage, 72t
Storm, thyroid, 435-436
Strain, knee, 711
Street names of drugs, 896b
Streptococcus
  in cavernous sinus thrombosis, 571
  food poisoning with, 472t-473t
Streptokinase, 346t
Stress, post-traumatic, 880-881
Strip and rinse decontamination, 217-218
Stroke, 382-385
  classification of, 384t
  heat, 501-502
  hemorrhagic, 384
  interventions for, 385
  ischemic, 380
  scales for, 382t, 383t
  screening for, 379b
  signs and symptoms of, 384-385
Strontium, 222t
Stump, amputation, 732
Sty, 578
Subacute subdural hematoma, 630-631,
    632
Subarachnoid hemorrhage, 631-632, 631f
  headache in, 376t-377t
Subclavian catheter, 111-112
Subconjunctival hemorrhage, 750
Subdural hematoma, 629-631, 629f, 630f
Subjective assessment, 86-87, 87t
Sublingual capnometry, 176
Subluxation, 719, 720t, 721
Submersion injury, 324-325
Substance abuse, 883-892
  alcohol, 892
  of club drugs, 897-900
    ectasy, 897-900
    flunitrazepam, 899-900
    gamma hydroxybutyrate, 899
    ketamine, 898-899
  cocaine, 892-893, 892b
  epidemiology of, 883
  heroin, 893-894
  inhalants, 894-895
  nutmeg, 895-896
  phencyclidine, 896-897

Substance abuse *(Continued)*
  prevention of, 459, 900
  street names of drugs in, 896b
Subungual hematoma, 204, 204f, 205f
Suctioning, airway, 301
Sudden infant death syndrome, 832
Suicidal patient, 878-880
Sulfonylurea, antidote for, 487t
Sulindac, 237t
Sumatriptan, 240t
Super Glue in eye, 582-573
Superficial frostbite, 500
Superficial partial thickness burn, 763
Supplies for interfacility transport, 32
Support services for domestic violence
    victim, 904
Supportive care area, 224
Supracondylar fracture, 701-702, 712
Supraventricular tachycardia, paroxysmal,
    147-150, 149t, 149f
Surgery
  transport to, 33, 34t
Survival time of severed limb, 732
Suture
  removal of, 209t
  types of, 210-211
Swab, throat, 129t, 132
Swimmer's view, 617, 618f
Sympathetic nervous system, 359t
Sympathomimetic agent, 888-889
Syndrome of inappropriate secretion of
    antidiuretic hormone, 434-435
Syphilis, 521t, 524
Systemic vascular resistance, 188, 189b
Systolic blood pressure, normal, 179b

T
T cell, 564
T wave, 171f
Tabletop exercises in mass casualty incident
    management, 51
TAC, 237t
  in wound management, 201
Tachycardia
  chest pain with, 326t
  in child, 826t
  paroxysmal supraventricular, 147-150,
    149f, 149t
  ventricular, 159-160, 160t, 160f
    pulseless, 280t-282t
Tachypnea, 89t

Tamponade
    cardiac, 353-354, 354f
        signs of, 95
    pericardial, 670-671, 671f
        obstructive shock in, 368
Tape for wound closure, 210, 211f
Tape system, Broselow, 781f
Tar burn, 770
Taxus, 478t
Team, SART, 908
Tear
    aortic, 671-672
    from body jewelry, 741
    esophageal, 393-394
    retinal, 575-576
Technologic event, hazard vulnerability
        analysis for, 48t
Technology, communication, 11
Teeth
    avulsed, 760, 760b
    dental emergencies of, 592-594
Telephone reporting of laboratory
        results, 8
Telephone triage, 77
Temazapam, 469-470
Temperature
    assessment of, 88
    in child, 825
    frostbite and, 500f
    heat injury and, 504-506
    metabolism and, 505b
Temporal arteritis, 375
Tendinitis, 729-730
Tendon, 690
Tendon rupture, Achilles, 716
Tenecteplase, 346t
Tension headache, 374-375, 376t-377t
Tension pneumothorax, 660, 661f, 662
    cardiac arrest in, 288t
    obstructive shock in, 368-369
Terrorism, 214-227. *See also* Mass casualty
        incident management; Weapon of mass
        destruction
Testicular torsion, 521, 521t
Testimony about sexual assault, 917, 918f-919f,
        920
Tetanus, 557-558
Tetanus immunization, 198-199, 533f
Tetracaine, 201, 237t
Thermal injury to airway, 321

Thermal burn
    causes of, 762t
    of eye, 750-758
Thioxanthene, 486t
Thoracic aortic dissection, 354-356, 355f
Thoracic cavity, 650, 651f, 642
Thoracic trauma, 650-677. *See also* Chest trauma
Thoracostomy, needle, 660b
Thoracostomy, tube, 657, 657b, 658b
Thoracotomy, emergent, 673, 674f, 675b
Thought control, 875
Threat of violence, 881-882, 882b
Threatened abortion, 801
Three-lead electrocardiogram monitor, 138f,
        333f
Three-level triage, 65
Throat
    age-related considerations in, 85t
    assessment of, 94
    Ludwig's angina and, 592
    peritonsillar abscess of, 591-592
Throat swab, 132
    point-of-care testing of, 129t
Thrombosis, cavernous sinus, 571
Through-the-needle catheter, 104
Thyroid disorder
    hyperthyroid storm as, 435-436
    myxedema coma as, 432
    thyroiditis as, 437-438
Thyroiditis, 437-438
Tibia-fibula fracture, 713-714, 714f
Tibial fracture, 712
Tic douloureux, 569-570
Tick-borne illness, 496-499
    Lyme disease as, 498-499
    Rocky Mountain spotted fever as, 497-498
TIDES mnemonic, 738-739
Tilt testing, orthostatic, 91b
Time limits on use of restraints, 28
Tinea corporis, 553-554
Tirofiban, 347t
Tissue donation, 254-260
    criteria for, 256, 256b
    critical pathway for, 257t
    history of, 255b
    procurement process for, 260
    West Nile virus and, 256-257
        cultural aspects, 256-257
Tissue Po$_2$, 177
Toddler, 826t-827t

Toe fracture, 718-719, 719f
Tong placement, 644f
Tongue piercing, 594, 595f, 595t
Tonometry, 580b
Tooth
  avulsed, 760, 760b
  dental emergency and, 592-594
  extraction of, 594
Topical anesthesia, 237t
  in wound management, 201
Torsion, testicular, 518, 518t
Toxic megacolon, 407
Toxic shock syndrome, 818-819
Toxic substance as weapon, 216-218
Toxicity
  coma in, 378b
  of complementary and alternative therapy,
    263, 264t-271t
Toxicologic blood study, 135
Toxicologic emergency, 456-489. *See also*
    Poisoning
Toxin in cardiac arrest, 290t
Tracheal intubation, 301
Tracheobronchial tree injury, 667-668
Traffic director triage, 62
Tramadol, 238t
Transfer, interfacility, 23-24
Transferring of evidence, 915
Transfusion, 117-122
  adverse reactions to, 121t, 122
  of blood products, 117, 118t-119t, 120
  of cryoprecipitate, 120
  emergency, 117
  of fresh frozen plasma, 120
  process of, 122
Transient monocular blindness, 582
Translation, consent and, 25
Transmission-based precautions, 529b
Transplant
  immunosuppression and, 420
  rejection of, 421-422, 421b
Transport
  in bioterrorism, 220t
  interfacility, 35-43. *See also* Interfacility
    transport
  intrafacility, 31-34, 34t
Transtentorial herniation, uncal, 634
Transtracheal ventilation, percutaneous,
    304, 305f
Transverse fracture, 696t, 697f

Trauma
  abdominal, 678-689. *See also* Abdominal
    trauma
  Achilles tendon rupture and, 716
  adult respiratory distress syndrome with, 316b
  amputation caused by, 732
  assessment of, 611t
    of airway, 601
    of breathing, 602
    of circulation, 602-603
    of disability, 603-604, 603b
    documentation of, 609
    environmental control and, 604
    Glasgow Coma Scale for, 609
    laboratory tests in, 605b
    musculoskeletal, 691-692
    of pediatric or geriatric patient, 609
    of posterior surfaces, 608
    systematic approach to, 600-601
    of vital signs, 604-605
  blast injury and, 216
  chest, 650-677. *See also* Chest trauma
  comfort measures in, 605
  in compartment syndrome, 734
  dislocation from. *See* Dislocation
  epidemiology of, 605
  to eye, 750-758. *See also* Eye, injury to
  fracture and. *See* Fracture
  in geriatric patient, 788-796. *See also*
    Geriatric patient
  hypovolemic shock in, 358, 361-363, 360t
  inhalation injury and, 321-322
  from intimate partner violence, 909-914.
    See also Intimate partner violence
  mechanism of injury in, 605-604, 605b, 605t
  neck, 648-649
  obstetric, 773-778
    abruptio placentae caused by, 776
    assessment of, 773-776
    perimortem cesarean delivery in, 777
    physiologic changes of pregnancy and, 775t
    preterm labor caused by, 776-777
    uterine rupture caused by, 777
  ocular. *See* Eye, injury to
  patient history of, 605-606
  physical examination in
    of abdomen, 607
    of chest, 607
    of neck, 606-607
    of pelvis, 607-608

Trauma *(Continued)*
  in repetitive motion disorder
    bursitis, 730
    carpal tunnel syndrome, 731
    tendinitis, 729
  spinal, 637-638
  subdural hematoma in, 629f
  submersion, 324-325
  triage of, 72t
  vehicular collision causing, 500t
Traumatic headache, 375, 376t-377t
Traveler's diarrhea, 550
Trazodone, 240t
Trench mouth, 593t
Treponema pallidum, 521t, 524
Triage, 61-81, 69t
  across-the-room assessment in, 68-69
  CIAMPEDS, 71t-72t
  documentation of, 74-75, 75b
  Emergency Medical Treatment and Active
    Labor Act and, 75-76
  focused physical assessment in, 74t
  infection control in, 76-77, 78t-79t
  of injury, 72t
  interfacility transfers and, 24
  interview in, 69-70
  Joint Commission on Accreditation of
    Healthcare Organizations and, 76
  of mass casualties, 51, 53, 55, 55f, 55t, 56f,
    57f, 223-224
  of mental health emergency, 871, 872b,
    873t, 873-874
  objective data in, 73
  overview of, 61-62
  patient leaving without being seen and, 76
  pediatric, 70, 824
  qualifications for, 77, 80
  questions to ask in, 72t
  radiologic, 223
  role of, 80
  safety and security of, 73-74
  severity rating systems of, 73
    Australasian, 65-66, 66t
    Canadian, 66, 66t
    emergency severity index, 67, 68f
    five-level, 65
    four-level, 65
    Manchester, 67, 67t
    three-level, 65
    two-level, 64
  of sexual assault victim, 917

Triage *(Continued)*
  by telephone, 77
  two-tiered, 63-64
  type I, 62, 62t
  type II, 63
  type III, 63
  vital signs at, 70, 73
Triazolam, 469-470
Trichomonas vaginalis, 821
Tricyclic antidepressant
  antidote for, 487t
  cardiac arrest caused by, 290t
  poisoning with, 467-468, 467b
Trigeminal nerve
  function of, 94t
  in head injury, 609
Trigeminal neuralgia, 569-570
Trigger
  for asthma, 314-315
  for migraine, 372t
Trochanter fracture, 708-710, 709f
Trochlear nerve
  function of, 94t
  in head injury, 609
Trophoblastic disease, 817-818
Troponin I, 134t
Tube
  chest, 663, 663b, 664b
  Minnesota, 399f
Tube thoracostomy, 663, 663b, 664b
Tuberculosis, 535-537
Tumor, pheochromocytoma, 439
Tunneled catheter, 105
  for venous access, 114-115
Turpentine, 481
Twelve-lead electrocardiogram, 333
Two-tiered triage system, 63-64
Tympanic membrane, ruptured, 758
Typhoid fever, 551

U
Ulcer
  corneal, 576-577
  peptic, 400
Ulcerative colitis, 406-407
Ulcerative gingivitis, necrotizing, 593t
Ulnar dislocation, 720t
Ulnar fracture, 702-703, 703f
  distal, 703-704
Ultrasound, esophageal, 175, 176f
Ultraviolet burn of eye, 756

Umbilical cord, prolapsed, 814-815, 815f
Uncal transtentorial herniation, 634
Unconscious patient, 378-380, 379b
   child, 845-846
   hypoglycemia in, 426-427
Underwater pressure, 507t
Uniform Anatomical Gift Act, 259
United Network for Organ Sharing, 254, 256t
Unstable angina, 339t
Unstable pelvic fracture, 707f, 708
Upper arm fracture, 700-701, 701f
Upper gastrointestinal bleeding, 397-398
Urea nitrogen
   measurement of, 134
   normal blood values of, 133t
Ureteral trauma, 676
Urethral trauma, 683
Urethritis, sexually transmitted, 523, 524
Urgent condition
   mental health, 872t
   transport of patient with, 34t
Urinary retention, 513-514
Urinary tract disorder, 515-519
   abdominal pain with, 391, 392t
   acute cystitis as, 515
   anuria as, 514
   hematuria as, 514
   oliguria as, 514
   perinephric abscess as, 512
   pyelonephritis as, 515-516
   renal calculus as, 513
   renal carbuncle as, 512
   urinary retention as, 513-514
Urine
   blood in, 514
   as clue to toxic exposure, 457t
   collection of, 131
   normal serum values for, 134t
   oliguria or anuria, 514
   point-of-care testing of, 129t
   in triage, 72t
Urine specimen, in sexual assault, 914
Urologic injury, 682-683, 683b
Urticaria, transfusion-related, 121t
Uterine bleeding, abnormal, 816
Uterine rupture, 777
Uveitis, 581-582
Uvula, piercing of, 595t

V

Vaginal bleeding, 816
Vaginosis, bacterial, 821
Vagus nerve
   function of, 94t
   in head injury, 609
Valve, cardiac, penetrating injury to, 669
Variance report, 26
Varicella immunization, 533f
Varices, bleeding, 398-399
Vascular access device, 128
Vascular headache, 375
Vascular resistance, systemic, 188, 189b
Vascular trauma, abdominal, 678
Vasogenic shock, 358, 362-367
   anaphylactic, 358, 368-370, 369f
   hyperdynamic phase of, 366-371
   hypodynamic phase of, 367-368
   neurogenic, 358, 370-371, 370f
   septic, 358, 366, 367f
Vasomotor center depression, 370-371, 370f
Vector-borne infection, 552
   rabies, 208, 209b
   Rocky Mountain spotted fever as, 497-498
   West Nile virus as, 552
Vehicular accident
   elderly in, 794-795
   mechanism of injury in, 600t
Vein
   in abdominal trauma, 678
   for blood collection, 123-124, 124f, 125f
   scalp, for intravenous access, 110, 110f
Velocity in injury, 600-601, 600b
Vena cava, 678
Venipuncture, 109
Venom
   snake, 490-481
   spider, 486t, 492-494
Venous access device
   accessing of, 114-116
      blood sampling via, 116
      catheters for, 114-115
      implanted port for, 115-116
   complications of, 116
Venous blood sample, 123-124, 124f, 125f
Venous cannulation, central, 111
Venous cutdown, 112-113
Venous pressure, central, 180-182, 180b, 180t, 181f, 182f

Ventilation
  mechanical, 306, 306t
  noninvasive positive pressure, 304
  percutaneous transtracheal, 304, 305f
  in trauma, 602
Ventricular dysrhythmia, 158-163
  accelerated idioventricular rhythm, 163t,
    163f
  fibrillation, 160-162, 161t, 161f
  idioventricular rhythm, 162-163, 162f, 163t
  premature complexes, 158-159, 158f, 159t
  tachycardia, 159-160, 160t, 160f
Ventricular failure, 360-361
Ventricular fibrillation, 280t-282t
Ventricular shunt malfunction, 387
Ventricular tachycardia, pulseless, 280t-282t
Ventriculoperitoneal shunt malfunction,
    850-851
Venturi mask, 299t
Verapamil
  cardiac arrest caused by, 290t
  poisoning with, 466
Verbal assessment
  in Glasgow Coma Scale, 93t
  in head injury, 614
Vertebra
  anatomy of, 641f
  in trauma patient, 602-603
  spinal cord injury and, 638
Vessel in abdominal trauma, 678
Vibrio cholerae, 472t-473t
Victim of intimate partner violence, 902-903
Vincent's angina, 589t
Violation
  of Emergency Medical Treatment and Active
    Labor Act, 24
  of Health Insurance Portability and
    Accountability Act, 23
Violence, intimate partner, 909-914
Violent patient, 881-882
Viperidae, 490-491
Viral infection
  bronchiolitis, 840-841
  chickenpox, 541-542
  hepatitis A as, 548-549
  hepatitis B, 527-532
  hepatitis C, 532, 533
  hepatitis E, 549
  herpes zoster, 554-555
  HIV, 530-531, 534f
  immunization schedules for, 533f-535f

Viral infection (Continued)
  influenza, 536, 539
  measles, 541-544
  monkeypox, 542-543
  mononucleosis, 556-557
  mumps, 541-545
  pneumonia, 842t
  severe acute respiratory, 547-548
Visceral pain, 230t
  abdominal, 389
Visual acuity testing, 571-582, 568b, 568t
Visual analogue pain rating scale, 234t
Vital signs
  in abdominal pain, 389
  age-related considerations in, 85t
  assessment of, 88-92, 88t
    blood pressure, 90
    height, weight, and head circumference,
      91-92
    orthostatic, 90, 91b
    oxygen saturation, 89-90
    pulse, 89
    pulse pressure, 90
    respirations, 89, 89t
    shock index, 91
    temperature, 88
  in newborn, 811b
  pediatric, 825, 829t
  in trauma patient, 604-605
  at triage, 70-71, 73
Volkmann's ischemic contracture, 736
Volvulus, 855
Vomiting
  abdominal pain with, 391
  in child, 851-853, 842t
  induced, 458, 459t
  Mallory-Weiss syndrome and, 396-397
  Munchausen syndrome by proxy and,
    866t
Von Willebrand disease, 412, 409f, 409t,
    414, 414t
Vulvovaginitis, 819, 820t, 821

W
Wandering pacemaker, atrial, 146-147,
    146f, 148t
Warfarin, 487t
Warm shock, 366-367
Wash, nasopharyngeal, 132-133
Washed red blood cells, 118t, 120
Wasp sting, 495-496

Water-borne infection, 548-549
  hepatitis A as, 548-549
  hepatitis E as, 549
  traveler's diarrhea as, 550
  typhoid fever as, 551
Water hemlock poisoning, 478t
Wave, radiation, 219
Waveform analysis
  arterial pressure, 179, 179f
  central venous pressure, 181-182, 181f, 182f0
  pulmonary artery pressure, 184, 185f, 186b, 186f, 187f
Weapon of mass destruction, 214-227. *See also* Mass casualty incident management
  biological, 218, 219b
    infection control for, 220t-221t
  chemical, 216-218
  decontamination and, 215
  explosive, 215-216
  interacting with victims of, 226-227, 226b
  Internet resources about, 227
  mental health aspects of, 226
  personal protective equipment for, 224-226
  radiation as, 219-223
    as emergency, 222
    initial interventions for, 222-223
    ionizing vs. nonionizing, 219
    particles vs. waves, 219
    radionuclides produced, 222t
  recognition and identification of, 214-215
  triage for, 223-224
Weight, 91
Wenckebach heart block, 153-154, 155t, 155f
West Indian culture, 20t
West Nile virus, 552
  organ donation and, 256-257
Wheezing in asthma, 314
White blood cell count
  measurement of, 135-136
  in pregnancy, 768t
White blood cell differential, 135-136
Whole blood transfusion, 117, 118t
Whole-bowel irrigation, 461-462
Whooping cough, 542
Widened mediastinum, 671f
Winged needle, 103
Withdrawal, alcohol, 452-453
Wong-Baker FACES pain rating scale, 231, 232t

Wood's lamp, 914
Word catheter, 819, 820f
Word-Graphic pain rating scale, 233t-234t
Wound
  burn, 769-770
  percutaneous aspiration of, 131
  scalp, 621-622
Wound management, 195-213
  for abrasion, 201-202
  for abscess, 202
  aftercare in, 211-212
  anesthesia in, 199-201
  assessment in, 197
  of avulsion, 202-203, 203f
  basic considerations in, 195
  of bite, 207-208, 209b
  closure in, 208-212
    of contaminated wound, 208
    materials for, 208-209
    suture removal and, 209t
    techniques for, 209-211, 211f, 212f
  of contusion, 203-204, 204f, 205f
  dressing in, 211-212
  general principles of, 196-197
  healing and, 195-196
  of incision and lacerations, 204-205, 205f
  prophylactic antibiotics in, 199
  for puncture, 206-207, 206f
  tetanus immunization in, 198-199
  wound preparation in, 197-198
Wrist dislocation, 724, 724f
Wrist fracture, 703-704
Written communication, 4-5
Written report, 11, 12f

X
XAP, 201
Xylocaine, 201

Y
Yeast infection, 821
Yellow sage poisoning, 479t
Yellowjacket sting, 495-496
Yew poisoning, 478t

Z
Zone of chemical contamination, 216
Zygomatic fracture, 744-745, 744f

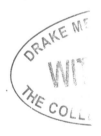